Chemoinformatics

METHODS IN MOLECULAR BIOLOGY™

John M. Walker, SERIES EDITOR

METHODS IN MOLECULAR BIOLOGY™

Chemoinformatics

Concepts, Methods, and Tools for Drug Discovery

Edited by

Jürgen Bajorath

Albany Molecular Research Inc.
Bothell Research Center, Bothell, WA
and University of Washington, Seattle, WA

Humana Press ✳ Totowa, New Jersey

© 2004 Humana Press Inc.
999 Riverview Drive, Suite 208
Totowa, New Jersey 07512

www.humanapress.com

This publication is printed on acid-free paper. ∞
ANSI Z39.48-1984 (American Standards Institute)

Permanence of Paper for Printed Library Materials.

Cover illustration: *Background*: Figure 3 from Chapter 7. *Foreground*: Illustration supplied by Jürgen Bajorath.

Cover design by Patricia F. Cleary.

For additional copies, pricing for bulk purchases, and/or information about other Humana titles, contact Humana at the above address or at any of the following numbers: Tel.: 973-256-1699; Fax: 973-256-8341; E-mail: humana@humanapr.com; or visit our Website: www.humanapress.com

Photocopy Authorization Policy:

Authorization to photocopy items for internal or personal use, or the internal or personal use of specific clients, is granted by Humana Press Inc., provided that the base fee of US $25.00 per copy is paid directly to the Copyright Clearance Center at 222 Rosewood Drive, Danvers, MA 01923. For those organizations that have been granted a photocopy license from the CCC, a separate system of payment has been arranged and is acceptable to Humana Press Inc. The fee code for users of the Transactional Reporting Service is: [1-58829-261-4/04 $25.00].

Printed in the United States of America. 10 9 8 7 6 5 4 3 2 1
Library of Congress Cataloging in Publication Data
Chemoinformatics : concepts, methods, and tools for drug discovery / edited by Jürgen Bajorath.
     p. cm. — (Methods in molecular biology ; v. 275)
     Includes bibliographical references and index.
     ISBN 1-58829-261-4 (alk. paper) eISBN 1-59259-802-1
     1. Chemoinformatics. I. Bajorath, Jürgen. II. Series: Methods in
     molecular biology (Clifton, N.J.) ; v. 275.
     RS418.C48 2004
     615'.19—dc22   2004047477

Preface

In the literature, several terms are used synonymously to name the topic of this book: chem-, chemi-, or chemo-informatics. A widely recognized definition of this discipline is the one by Frank Brown from 1998 (*1*) who defined chemoinformatics as the combination of "all the information resources that a scientist needs to optimize the properties of a ligand to become a drug." In Brown's definition, two aspects play a fundamentally important role: decision support by computational means and drug discovery, which distinguishes it from the term "chemical informatics" that was introduced at least ten years earlier and described as the application of information technology to chemistry (not with a specific focus on drug discovery). In addition, there is of course "chemometrics," which is generally understood as the application of statistical methods to chemical data and the derivation of relevant statistical models and descriptors (*2*). The pharmaceutical focus of many developments and efforts in this area—and the current popularity of gene-to-drug or similar paradigms—is further reflected by the recent introduction of such terms as "discovery informatics" (*3*), which takes into account that gaining knowledge from chemical data alone is not sufficient to be ultimately successful in drug discovery. Such insights are well in accord with other views that the boundaries between bio- and chemoinformatics are fluid and that these disciplines should be closely combined or merged to significantly impact biotechnology or pharmaceutical research (*4*). Clearly, from an algorithmic or methodological point of view, bio- and chemoinformatics are much more similar to each other than many of their applications would suggest, at least on a first glance. It is fair to assume that the application of information science and technology to chemical or biological problems will further develop and mature, as well as continue to define, and redefine, itself.

If we wish to focus on chemoinformatics in a more narrow sense, what should we really consider? First, methods that support decision making in the context of pharmaceutical research (*2*) (such as compound design and selection) or methods that help interfacing computational and experimental programs (*4*) [such as virtual and biological screening (*5*)] are without doubt essential components. Second, equally important to developing methods and research tools is building and maintaining computational infrastructures to collect, organize, manage, and analyze chemical data. Third, I would propose that it has also become increasingly difficult to distinguish between chemoinformatics and chemometrics, since statistical methods, models, and descriptors play a crucial role in, for example, similarity and diversity analysis or virtual screening. Fourth, approaches to explore (and exploit) structure–activity or structure–property relationships can hardly be excluded from chemoinformatics research, much of which aims at helping to identify or make better molecules. This means that approaches that are long disciplines in their own right such as QSAR or structure-based design can—and perhaps should—also be considered to contribute and belong to chemoinformatics. Lastly, evaluation of drug-likeness and prediction of downstream ADME characteristics of compounds have become highly relevant topics for chemoinformatics and drug discovery research and are approached using rather different concepts and algorithms.

Being confronted with the task of putting *Chemoinformatics: Concepts, Methods, and Tools for Drug Discovery* together, I decided to focus on authors and their individual contributions, rather than trying to address everything possible that could be covered under the chemoinformatics umbrella, as discussed above. It was my sincere hope that this approach would do justice to this still evolving and rather diverse field. Therefore, a variety of researchers (including well-recognized pioneers, senior scientists, and junior-level investigators) from diverse professional environments (academia, large pharmaceutical industry, and biotech companies) were asked to contribute. Chemoinformatics-relevant subject areas were initially outlined to provide some guidance, but authors were given as much freedom as possible in choosing their topics and designing their chapters. The result we are looking at is the rather diverse array of chapters I had initially hoped for. Certainly, many chapters go well beyond the introduction of single methods and protocols that is a major theme of the *Methods in Molecular Biology* series, at least as far as experimental science is concerned. Our contributions range from the description of specific methods or applications to the discussion of fundamentally important concepts and extensive review articles. On the other hand, some of the topics I initially envisioned to cover are missing, for example, neural network simulations or chemical genetics, to name just two. By contrast, some contributions present and discuss similar methods, for example, compound selection or library design, in rather different ways, which I find particularly interesting and stimulating.

Chemoinformatics: Concepts, Methods, and Tools for Discovery begins with an elaborate theoretical discussion of the concept of molecular similarity by Maggiora & Shanmugasundaram that is one of the origins and cornerstones of chemoinformatics as we understand it today. Chapter 2 by Willett follows up on this theme and extends the discussion to molecular diversity, a related

—yet distinct—and equally fundamental concept. Following these method-ological considerations, Bembenek & colleagues describe a computational infra-structure to enable pharmaceutical researchers to efficiently access basic chemoinformatics tools and help in decision-making. Chapters 4 and 5 by Parker & Schreyer and Lajiness & Shanmugasundaram describe efforts to interface chemoinformatics approaches with high-throughput screening and with screening and medicinal chemistry, respectively. As discussed above, the formation of such interfaces is one of the major challenges—and opportunities—for chemoinfor-matics in pharmaceutical research.

Esposito & colleagues provide an extensive discussion of QSAR approaches in Chapter 6. The authors review basic principles and methods and then focus on the latest developments in multidimensional QSAR analysis. In the following chap-ter, Gomar & colleagues describe the development of a lipophilicity descriptor that alleviates the molecular alignment problem in QSAR and discuss exemplary appli-cations. In general, the majority of chemoinformatics applications critically depend on the use of descriptors of molecular structure and properties, and Chapter 8 by Labute presents a good example of descriptor design. The author describes the gen-eration of a novel class of molecular surface property descriptors that can be readily calculated from 2D representations of molecular structures.

The next four chapters focus on partitioning algorithms and classification methods that have become very popular for the analysis of large compound databases, screening sets, and virtual screening for active molecules. Xue & colleagues describe cell-based partitioning based on principal component analysis and, to contrast with chemical space dimension reduction methods, Godden & Bajorath introduce a statistically based partitioning algorithm that directly oper-ates in higher-dimensional, albeit simplified, chemical descriptor spaces. In the following back-to-back chapters, Lam & Welch first apply clustering and cell-based partitioning methods for the selection of active compounds from the HIV data set of the National Cancer Institute. Based on their computational scheme and results, Young & Hawkins apply recursive partitioning (another statistical approach) to the same data set, thus enabling direct comparisons.

Following these compound classification and selection methods, Chap-ters 13–15 describe different approaches to compound library design. Gillet discusses a genetic algorithm-based method to simultaneously optimize mul-tiple objectives or properties when designing libraries. Schnur & colleagues describe various approaches to focus compound libraries on families of thera-peutic targets, which represents a major trend in drug discovery, and Zheng introduces simulated annealing as a stochastic approach to library design.

In Chapter 16, Lavine & colleagues return to a compound classification prob-lem by using a combination of principal component analysis and a genetic algorithm that is here applied to an optimization problem different from the one discussed by Gillet. In the next chapters, Crippen introduces novel ways of describing molecular chirality and conformational parameters with relevance for the analysis of structure–activity relationships, and Pick provides a brief review of scoring functions for structure-based virtual screening. The book ends with an extensive and detailed description by Jalaie & colleagues of different types of methods, including structure-based approaches, to predict drug-like character of compounds and basic ADME properties based on modeling their putative interactions with cytochrome P450 isoforms, which are important drug metabolizing enzymes. This discussion complements other major themes represented herein including molecular similarity, structure-activity relationships, and compound classification and design.

First and foremost, I would like to thank our authors whose diverse contributions have made this project a (hopefully, interesting!) reality.

Jürgen Bajorath

References

1. Brown, F. K. (1998) Chemoinformatics: What is it and how does it impact drug discovery. *Ann. Rep. Med. Chem.* **33**, 375–384.
2. Goodman, J. M. (2003) Chemical informatics. *Chem. Inf. Lett.* **6** (2); http://www.ch.cam.ac.uk/MMRG/CIL/cil_v6n2.html#14
3. Claus, B. L. and Underwood, D. J. (2002) Discovery informatics: Its evolving role in drug discovery. *Drug Discov. Today* **7**, 957–966.
4. Bajorath, J. (2001) Rational drug discovery revisited: Interfacing experimental programs with bio- and chemo-informatics. *Drug Discov. Today* **6**, 989–995.
5. Bajorath, J. (2002) Integration of virtual and high-throughput screening. *Nature Rev. Drug Discov.* **1**, 882–894.

Contents

Contributors

RIEKO ARIMOTO • *Discovery Technologies, Pfizer Global Research and Development, Ann Arbor, Michigan, USA*

JÜRGEN BAJORATH • *Computer Aided Drug Discovery, Albany Molecular Research Inc., Bothell Research Center, Bothell, Washington, and Department of Biological Structure, University of Washington, Seattle, Washington, USA*

SCOTT D. BEMBENEK • *Computer Aided Drug Discovery and Cheminformatics, Johnson & Johnson, Pharmaceutical Research & Development, L.L.C., San Diego, California, USA*

BRETT R. BENO • *Computer Aided Drug Design, Pharmaceutical Research Institute, Bristol-Myers Squibb Company, Princeton, New Jersey, USA*

CURT BRENEMAN • *Department of Chemistry, Rensselaer Polytechnic Institute, Troy, New York, USA*

PIERRE ALAIN CARRUPT • *Institute of Medicinal Chemistry, School of Pharmacy, University of Lausanne, Lausanne, Switzerland*

STEVEN J. COATS • *High-Throughout Chemistry, Johnson & Johnson Pharmaceutical Research & Development, L.L.C., Spring House, Pennsylvania, USA*

GORDON M. CRIPPEN • *College of Pharmacy, University of Michigan, Ann Arbor, Michigan, USA*

CHARLES E. DAVIDSON • *Department of Chemistry, Clarkson University, Potsdam, New York, USA*

EMILIO XAVIER ESPOSITO • *Department of Chemistry and Biochemistry, Duquesne University, Pittsburgh, Pennsylvania, USA*

ERIC GIFFORD • *Discovery Technologies, Pfizer Global Research and Development, Ann Arbor, Michigan, USA*

VALERIE J. GILLET • *Department of Information Studies, University of Sheffield, Sheffield, United Kingdom*

ELIE GIRAUD • *Aventis Pharmaceuticals, Bridgewater, New Jersey, USA*

JEFFREY W. GODDEN • *Computer Aided Drug Discovery, Albany Molecular Research Inc., Bothell Research Center, Bothell, WA, USA*

JÉRÔME GOMAR • *Synt:em, Nimes, France*

ANDREW GOOD • *Computer Aided Drug Design, Pharmaceutical Research Institute, Bristol-Myers Squibb Company, Princeton, New Jersey, USA*

DOUGLAS M. HAWKINS • *School of Statistics, University of Minnesota, Minneapolis, Minnesota, USA*

ANTON J. HOPFINGER • *Department of Medicinal Chemistry and Pharmacognosy, College of Pharmacy, University of Illinois at Chicago, Chicago, Illinois, USA*

MEHRAN JALAIE • *Discovery Technologies, Pfizer Global Research and Development, Ann Arbor, Michigan, USA*

WILLIAM KAAT • *Department of Chemistry, Rensselaer Polytechnic Institute, Troy, New York, USA*

PAUL LABUTE • *Chemical Computing Group Inc., Montreal, Quebec, Canada*

ROGER LAHANA • *Synt:em, Nimes, France*

MICHAEL S. LAJINESS • *Structural and Computational Sciences, Lilly Corporate Center, Eli Lilly and Company, Indianapolis, Indiana, USA*

RAYMOND L.H. LAM • *Department of Data Exploration Sciences, GlaxoSmithKline, King of Prussia, Pennsylvania, USA*

BARRY K. LAVINE • *Department of Chemistry, Clarkson University, Potsdam, New York, USA*

JEFFRY D. MADURA • *Department of Chemistry and Biochemistry, Duquesne University, Pittsburgh, Pennsylvania, USA*

GERALD M. MAGGIORA • *Division of Medicinal Chemistry, College of Pharmacy, University of Arizona, Tucson, Arizona, USA*

CHRISTIAN N. PARKER • *Novartis Institute for BioMedical Research, Cambridge, Massachusetts, USA*

DANIEL PICK • *Computational Science Research Center, San Diego State University, San Diego, California, USA*

CHARLES H. REYNOLDS • *Computer Aided Drug Discovery, Johnson & Johnson Pharmaceutical Research & Development, L.L.C., Spring House, Pennsylvania, USA*

SABINE SCHEFZICK • *Discovery Technologies, Pfizer Global Research and Development, Ann Arbor, Michigan, USA*

DORA SCHNUR • *Computer Aided Drug Design, Pharmaceutical Research Institute, Bristol-Myers Squibb Company, Princeton, New Jersey, USA*

SUZANNE K. SCHREYER • *Chemical Computing Group Inc., Montreal, Quebec, Canada*

VEERABAHU SHANMUGASUNDARAM • *Computer Assisted Drug Design, Pfizer Global Research and Development Ann Arbor, Michigan, USA*

FLORENCE L. STAHURA • *Computer Aided Drug Discovery, Albany Molecular Research Inc., Bothell Research Center, Bothell, Washington, USA*

ANDREW TEBBEN • *Computer Aided Drug Design, Pharmaceutical Research Institute, Bristol-Myers Squibb Company, Princeton, New Jersey, USA*

BRETT A. TOUNGE • *Computer Aided Drug Discovery, Johnson & Johnson Pharmaceutical Research & Development, L.L.C., Spring House, Pennsylvania, USA*

DAVID TURNER • *Synt:em, Nimes, France*

CHRIS L. WALLER • *Discovery Technologies, Pfizer Global Research and Development Ann Arbor, Michigan, USA*

WILLIAM J. WELCH • *Department of Statistics, University of British Columbia, Vancouver, British Columbia, and Department of Statistics and Actuarial Science, University of Waterloo, Waterloo, Ontario, Canada*

PETER WILLETT • *Krebs Institute for Biomolecular Research and Department of Information Studies, University of Sheffield, Sheffield, United Kingdom*

LING XUE • *Computer Aided Drug Discovery, Albany Molecular Research, Inc., Bothell Research Center, Bothell, Washington, USA*

S. STANLEY YOUNG • *National Institute of Statistical Sciences, Research Triangle Park, North Carolina, USA*

WEIFAN ZHENG • *Lead Generation Chemistry, Eli Lilly and Company, Research Triangle Park, North Carolina, USA*

1

Molecular Similarity Measures

Gerald M. Maggiora and Veerabahu Shanmugasundaram

Abstract

Molecular similarity is a pervasive concept in chemistry. It is essential to many aspects of chemical reasoning and analysis and is perhaps the fundamental assumption underlying medicinal chemistry. Dissimilarity, the complement of similarity, also plays a major role in a growing number of applications of molecular diversity in combinatorial chemistry, high-throughput screening, and related fields. How molecular information is represented, called the representation problem, is important to the type of molecular similarity analysis (MSA) that can be carried out in any given situation. In this work, four types of mathematical structure are used to represent molecular information: sets, graphs, vectors, and functions. Molecular similarity is a pairwise relationship that induces structure into sets of molecules, giving rise to the concept of a chemistry space. Although all three concepts—molecular similarity, molecular representation, and chemistry space—are treated in this chapter, the emphasis is on molecular similarity measures. Similarity measures, also called similarity coefficients or indices, are functions that map pairs of compatible molecular representations, that is, representations of the same mathematical form, into real numbers usually, but not always, lying on the unit interval. This chapter presents a somewhat pedagogical discussion of many types of molecular similarity measures, their strengths and limitations, and their relationship to one another.

Key Words: Molecular similarity; molecular similarity analyses (MSA); dissimilarity.

1. Introduction

Similarity is a fundamental concept that has been used since before the time of Aristotle. Even in the sciences, it has been used for more than two centuries *(1)*. Similarity is subjective and relies upon comparative judgments—there is no absolute standard of similarity, rather "like beauty, it is in the eye of the beholder." Because of this subjectivity it is difficult to develop methods for unambiguously computing the similarities of large sets of molecules *(2)*. Moreover, there is no absolute standard to compare to so that assessing the validity of any similarity-based method remains subjective; basically, one must rely upon the

From: *Methods in Molecular Biology, vol. 275:*
Chemoinformatics: Concepts, Methods, and Tools for Drug Discovery
Edited by: J. Bajorath © Humana Press Inc., Totowa, NJ

judgment of experienced scientists. Nevertheless, numerous approaches have been developed over the years to address this difficult but important problem *(3–5)*.

The notion of similarity is fundamental to many aspects of chemical reasoning and analysis; indeed, it is perhaps the fundamental assumption underlying medicinal chemistry, and falls under the general rubric of *molecular similarity analysis* (MSA). Determining the similarity of one "molecular object" to another is basically an exercise in pattern matching—generally called the *matching problem*. The outcome of the exercise is a value, the *similarity measure*, that characterizes the degree of matching, association, proximity, resemblance, alignment, or similarity of pairs of molecules as manifested by their "molecular patterns," which are made up of sets of features. The terminology "proximity" is sometimes used in a more general sense to refer to the similarity, dissimilarity, or distance between pairs of molecules. Similarity is generally considered to be a symmetric property, that is, "A" is as similar to "B" as "B" is to "A," and most studies are based upon this property. Tversky *(6)*, however, has argued persuasively that certain similarity comparisons are inherently asymmetric. Although his work was directed toward psychology, it nonetheless has applicability in studies of molecular similarity. An example will be presented that illustrates the nature of asymmetric similarity and how it can be used to augment the usefulness of the usual symmetric version of similarity. Recently, Willett et al. *(7)* presented a comprehensive overview of many of the similarity measures in use today. Their review included a table that summarized the form of the various measures with respect to the type of representation used and should be consulted for further details.

Choosing an appropriate feature set and an associated mathematical structure (e.g., set, vector, function, or graph) for handling them is called the *representation problem* and underlies all aspects of MSA. Because similarity is subjective, choosing a feature set depends upon the background of the scientist doing the choosing and to some extent on the problem being addressed. For example, a synthetic organic chemist may focus on the nature of a molecular scaffold and its substituent groups while a physical chemist may be more interested in three-dimensional (3-D) shape and electrostatic properties.

Closely allied with the notion of molecular similarity is that of a *chemistry space*. Chemistry spaces provide a means for conceptualizing and visualizing molecular similarity. A chemistry space consists of a set of molecules and a set of associated relations (e.g., similarities, dissimilarities, distances, and so on) among the molecules, which give the space a "structure" *(8)*. In most chemistry spaces, which are coordinate-based, molecules are generally depicted as points. This, however, need not always be the case—sometimes only similarities or "distances" among molecules in the population are known. Nevertheless, this type of pairwise information can be used to construct an appropriate coordinate system that optimally preserves the information using methods such as multi-dimensional scaling (MDS) *(9)*, principal-component analysis (PCA) *(10)*, or nonlinear mapping (NLM) *(11)*. Coordinate-based chemistry spaces can also be partitioned into cells and are usually referred to as cell-based chemistry spaces *(12)*. Each particular type of representation of chemistry space has its strengths and weaknesses so that it may be necessary to use multiple types of representations to satisfactorily treat specific problems.

Identifying the appropriate molecular features is crucial in MSA, as the number of potential features is quite large and many contain redundant information. Typical types of molecular features include molecular size, shape, charge distribution, conformation states, and conformational flexibility. In general, only those features deemed relevant or necessary to the matching task at hand are considered. Features are mimicked by any number of descriptors that, ideally, capture the essential characteristics of the features. For example, numerous descriptors of molecular shape exist, such as the Jurs shape indices *(13)* or the Sterimol parameters *(14)*, as well as descriptors of charge distributions, such as the venerable Mulliken population analysis *(15)* or charged partial surface areas, which conveniently incorporate both charge and shape information *(16)* and descriptors of conformational flexibility, such as the Kier molecular flexibility index Φ *(17)*. Sometimes the term "feature" is used interchangeably with "descriptor." As is seen in the above discussion, features are more general than descriptors, but this distinction is generally not strictly adhered to in most research papers including this one. Other chapters in this work should be consulted for detailed discussion of the many types and flavors of descriptors in use in chemoinformatics and chemometrics today.

Similarity measures for assessing the degree of matching between two molecules given a particular representation constitutes the main subject matter of this chapter. These measures, also called similarity coefficients or indices, are functions that map pairs of compatible molecular representations, that is, representations of the same mathematical form, into real numbers usually, but not always, lying on the unit interval. Set, graph, vector, and function-based representations use a variety of distance and "overlap" measures. Graph-based representations use chemical distance or related graph metrics *(18,19)*, although numerous graph invariants have been used as descriptors in vector-based representations *(20–22)*. All of the similarity and related measures have at least some idiosyncratic behavior, which can give rise to misleading assessments of similarity or dissimilarity *(2)*. Similarity measures are sometimes referred to as similarity coefficients or similarity indices and these terminologies will be used somewhat interchangeably in this work.

From the above discussion it is clear that similarity measures provide assessments that are inherently subjective in nature. Thus, the inconsistencies of various measures are not entirely surprising and sometimes can be quite daunting. An interesting approach was recently developed by Willett's group using a technique called "data fusion"*(23)*. They showed that values obtained from multiple similarity methods combined using data fusion led to an improvement over values obtained utilizing a single similarity measure. Alternatively, less sophisticated approaches, such as taking the mean of multiple similarity values, can also be used.

A brief introduction to the types of molecular representations typically encountered in MSA is presented at the beginning of **Subheading 2.** followed in **Subheading 2.1.** by a discussion of similarity measures based on chemical-graph representations. Although graph-based representations are the most familiar to chemists, their use has been somewhat limited in similarity studies due to the difficulty of evaluating the appropriate similarity measures. This section is followed by a discussion of similarity measures based on finite vector representations, the most ubiquitous types of representations. In these cases, the vector components can be of four types:

$$
\begin{array}{ll}
\text{B} & \text{Boolean Variables } \{0,1\} \\
\text{K} & \text{Categorical Variables } \{\text{finite, ordered set}\} \\
\text{N}_o & \text{Non-Negative Integer Variables } \{0,1,2,3,...\} \\
\text{R} & \text{Real Variables } \{\text{uncountably infinite set}\}
\end{array}
\qquad (1.1)
$$

the first of which, called "binary vectors," "bit vectors," or "molecular fingerprints," is by far the most prevalent in applications and is discussed in detail in **Subheading 2.2.1.** Although the terminology "vector" is used, these objects mathematically are classical sets. Thus, the associated similarity measures are set-based rather than vector-based measures. In addition to the more traditional symmetric similarity measures, a discussion of asymmetric similarity measures associated with binary vectors is also presented.

Vectors whose components are based upon categorical or integer variables are described in **Subheading 2.2.3.** As was the case for binary vectors, these vectors are also classical sets, and, as was the case in the previous subsection, the associated similarity measures are set-based rather than vector-based. Here it will also be seen that the form of the set measures are, in some cases, modified from those associated with traditional classical sets.

Subheading 2.3. describes the last class of finite feature vectors, namely, those with continuous-valued components, where the components (i.e., features) are usually obtained from computed or experimentally measured properties. An often-overlooked aspect of continuous feature vectors is the inherent non-orthogonality of the basis of the "feature space." The consequences of this are discussed in **Subheading 2.3.2.** Similarity measures derived from continuous vectors are generally related to Euclidean distances or to cosine or correlation coefficients, all of which are "true" vector-based measures, and are discussed in **Subheading 2.3.3.** Finally, a new "molecule-based" approach to continuous feature vectors that automatically accounts for the inherent non-orthogonality of the feature basis is presented in **Subheading 2.3.4.**

Essentially none of the previously discussed approaches deals with the three-dimensionality of molecules. This is dealt with in **Subheading 2.4.**, which describes the application of field-based functions to 3-D molecular similarity. The fields referred to here are related to the steric, electrostatic, and lipophilic properties of molecules and are represented by functions (i.e., "infinite-dimensional vectors"), which are usually taken to be linear combinations of atomic-centered Gaussians. Similarity measures totally analogous to those defined for finite-dimensional, continuous-valued feature vectors (*see* **Subheading 2.3.3.**) also apply here and are treated in **Subheading 2.4.2.** An added difficulty encountered in 3-D MSA arises from the conformational flexibility of most molecules of interest in chemoinformatic applications. Two general approaches to this problem are described here. One approach involves the identification of a set of conformational prototypes and the other approach involves the simultaneous maximization of the similarity measure and minimization of the conformational energy of the molecules being aligned. The former approach is more computationally demanding because it involves $M \times N$ pairwise comparisons, where M and N are the respective numbers of prototype conformations for each pair of molecules.

The role of chemistry spaces in chemoinformatics is treated briefly in **Subheading 3.** The treatment includes a discussion of coordinate-based and coordinate-free chemistry spaces, how they can be transformed into one another, and how the usually high dimension of typical chemistry spaces can be reduced in order to facilitate visualization and analysis.

This work is not intended as a comprehensive review of the similarity literature. Rather, it is intended to provide an integrated and somewhat pedagogical discussion of many of the simple, complex, and confounding issues confronting scientists using the concept of molecular similarity in their work.

2. Molecular Representations and their Similarity Measures

How the structural information in molecules is represented is crucial to the types of "chemical questions" that can be asked and answered. This is certainly true in MSA where different representations and their corresponding similarity measures can lead to dramatically different results *(2)*. Four types of mathematical objects are typically used to represent molecules—sets, graphs, vectors, and functions. Sets are the most general objects and basically underlie the other three and are useful in their own right as will be seen below. Because of their importance a brief introduction to sets, employing a more powerful but less familiar notation than that typically used, is provided in the Appendix.

Typically chemists represent molecules as "chemical graphs" *(24)*, which are closely related to the types of graphs dealt with by mathematicians in the field of graph theory *(25)*. Most chemical graphs describe the nature of the atoms and how they are bonded. Thus, chemical graphs are sometimes said to provide a 2-D representation of molecules. They do not typically contain information on the essential 3-D features of molecules, although chemical graphs have been defined that do capture some of this information *(26)*. Three-dimensional structures are also used extensively, especially now that numerous computer programs have been developed for their computation and display.

While chemical graphs provide a powerful and intuitive metaphor for understanding many aspects of chemistry, they nevertheless have their limitations especially when dealing with questions of interest in chemometrics and chemoinformatics (*vide infra*). In these fields molecular information is typically represented by *feature vectors*, where each component corresponds to a "local" or "global" feature or property of a molecule usually represented by one of a number of possible descriptors associated with the chosen feature. Local features include molecular fragments ("substructures"), potential pharmacophores *(27)*, various topological indices *(28)*, and partial atomic charges, to name a few. Global features include properties such as molecular weight, log*P*, polar surface area, various BCUTs *(29)*, and volume.

More recently, with the significant increases in computer power even on desktop PCs, methods for *directly matching* 3-D features of molecules have become more prevalent. Features here generally refer to various types of molecular fields, some such as electron density ("steric") and electrostatic-potential fields are derived from fundamental physics *(30,31)* while others such as lipophilic potential fields *(32)* are constructed in an *ad hoc* manner. Molecular fields are typically represented as continuous functions. Discrete fields have also been used *(33)* albeit somewhat less frequently except in the case of the many CoMFA-based studies *(34)*.

2.1. Chemical Graphs

Chemical graphs are ubiquitous in chemistry. A chemical graph, G_k, can be defined as an ordered triple of sets

$$G_k = (V_k, E_k, L_k) \ ,$$
(2.1)

where V_k is a set (see the Appendix for notation) of *n* vertices ("atoms")

$$\begin{aligned} V_k &= \{V_k(x_1), V_k(x_2), ..., V_k(x_n)\} \\ &= \{v_{k,1}, v_{k,2}, ..., v_{k,n}\} \end{aligned} ,$$
(2.2)

where the lower expression for the vertex set in **Eq. 2.2** is used to designate all vertices in the set for which $V(x_i) = 1$. E_k is the corresponding set of m edges ("bonds")

$$E_k = \{e_{k,1}, e_{k,2}, ..., e_{k,m}\} \, , \tag{2.3}$$

where each edge corresponds to an unordered pair of vertices, that is $e_{k,i} = \{v_{k,p}, v_{k,q}\}$, and L_k is a set of r symbols

$$L_k = \{\ell_{k,1}, \ell_{k,2}, ..., \ell_{k,r}\} \tag{2.4}$$

that label each vertex ("atom") and/or edge ("bond"). Typical atom labels include hydrogen ("H"), carbon ("C"), nitrogen ("N"), and oxygen ("O"); typical bond labels include single ("s"), double ("d"), triple ("t"), and aromatic ("ar"), but other possibilities exist. Whatever symbol set is chosen will depend to some degree on the nature of the problem being addressed. In most chemoinformatics applications *hydrogen-suppressed* chemical graphs, which are obtained by deleting all of the hydrogen atoms, are used. **Figure 1** depicts an example of two hydrogen-suppressed chemical graphs, G_1 and G_2, which are clearly related to a chemist's 2-D representation of a molecule. Chemical graphs of 3-D molecular structures are described by Raymond and Willett *(26)*, but their use has been much more limited.

The notion of a subgraph is also important. If G_k' is a subgraph of G_k, written $G_k' \subseteq G_k$, then

$$G_k' \subseteq G_k \Rightarrow V_k' \subseteq V_k \text{ and } E_k' \subseteq E_k \, , \tag{2.5}$$

that is, the vertex and edge sets V_k' and E_k' associated with the subgraph, G_k', are subsets of the corresponding vertex and edge sets V_k and E_k of the graph, G_k. Many operations defined on sets can also be defined on graphs. One such operation is the norm or cardinality of a graph,

$$|G_k| = |V_k| + |E_k| \tag{2.6}$$

which is a measure of the "size" of the graph. Another measure the *edge norm*, which is of interest in this work, is given by

$$|G_k|_E = |E_k| \, , \tag{2.7}$$

where the subscript E explicitly denotes that the cardinality refers only to the edges ("bonds") of the graph. For the two chemical graphs depicted in **Fig. 1**, $|G_1|_E = 22$ and $|G_2|_E = 20$. Note that only the number of bonds and not their multiplicities (e.g., single, double) are considered here. However, many other possibilities exist, and their use will depend on the problem being addressed *(18)*.

A key concept in the assessment of molecular similarity based on chemical graphs is that of a *maximum common substructure*, $MCS(G_i, G_j)$, of two chem-

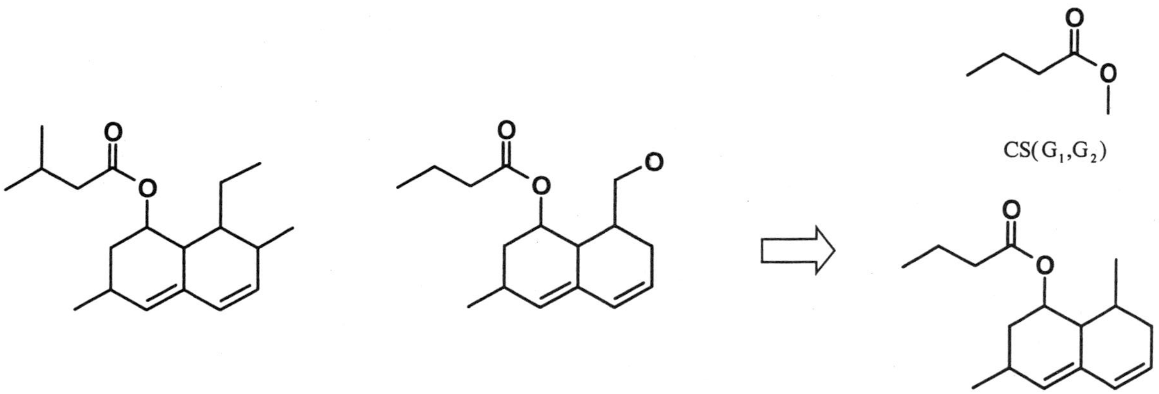

G_1 G_2 $CS(G_1,G_2)$ $MCS(G_1,G_2)$

$|G_1|_E = 22$

$|G_2|_E = 20$

$|MCS(G_1,G_2)|_E = 19$

$$S_{Tan}(G_i,G_j) = \frac{|G_i \cap G_j|_E}{|G_i \cup G_j|_E} = \frac{|MCS(G_i,G_j)|_E}{|G_i|_E + |G_j|_E - |MCS(G_i,G_j)|_E} = \frac{19}{22 + 20 - 19} = 0.83$$

$$d(G_i,G_j) = |G_i|_E + |G_j|_E - 2|MCS(G_i,G_j)|_E = 22 + 20 - 2(19) = 4$$

Fig. 1. An example of two hydrogen-suppressed graphs G_1, G_2, and a common substructure CS(G_1,G_2) and the maximum common substructure MCS(G_1,G_2) are shown above. The Tanimoto similarity index and the distance between the two chemical graphs are computed below.

ical graphs, which derives from the concept of maximum common subgraph employed in mathematical graph theory. There are several possible forms of MCS *(19,26)*. Here we will focus on what is usually called the maximum common edge substructure, which is closest to what chemists perceive as "chemically meaningful" substructures *(35)*, but we will retain the simpler and more common nomenclature MCS. A common (edge) substructure (CS) of two chemical graphs is given by

$$CS(G_i, G_j)_{k,\ell} = E_i^k \cap E_j^\ell = E_i^k = E_j^\ell \; , \tag{2.8}$$

where E_i^k and E_j^l are subsets of their respective edge sets, $E_i^k \subseteq E_i$ and $E_j^l \subseteq E_j$, and are equivalent. Thus, the intersection (or union) of these two equivalent subsets is equal to the sets themselves. As there are numerous such common substructures, $CS(G_i, G_j)_{k,l}$, $k,l = 1,2,3, \ldots$, determining the MCS between two chemical graphs is equivalent to determining the edge intersection-set of maximum cardinality, that is

$$MCS(G_i, G_j) = CS(G_i, G_j)_{p,q} \text{ such that } \left| CS(G_i, G_j)_{p,q} \right|_E = \max_{k,\ell} \left| CS(G_i, G_j)_{k,\ell} \right|_E \tag{2.9}$$

Thus,

$$G_i \cap G_j \equiv MCS(G_i, G_j) \; , \tag{2.10}$$

that is, the MCS is equivalent to "graph intersection," which is equivalent to the maximum number of edges in common between the two molecules. Note that multiple solutions may exist and that some of the solutions could involve disconnected graphs. However, to obtain "chemically meaningful" results only *connected* MCS's are usually considered.

The edge cardinality of the intersection and union of two chemical graphs is given, respectively, by

$$\left| G_i \cap G_j \right|_E = \left| MCS(G_i, G_j) \right| \tag{2.11}$$

and

$$\left| G_i \cup G_j \right|_E = \left| G_i \right|_E + \left| G_j \right|_E - \left| MCS(G_i, G_j) \right| \; . \tag{2.12}$$

These two expressions form the basis for several measures such as Tanimoto similarity (see **Subheading 2.2.** for an extensive discussion)

$$S_{\mathrm{Tan}}(G_i, G_j) = \frac{\left| G_i \cap G_j \right|_E}{\left| G_i \cup G_j \right|_E} = \frac{\left| MCS(G_i, G_j) \right|_E}{\left| G_i \right|_E + \left| G_j \right|_E - \left| MCS(G_i, G_j) \right|_E} \tag{2.13}$$

and the distance between two chemical graphs

$$d(G_i, G_j) = \left| G_i \right|_E + \left| G_j \right|_E - 2\left| MCS(G_i, G_j) \right|_E \; . \tag{2.14}$$

The edge cardinality is explicitly designated in **Eqs. 2.9** and **2.11–2.14** in order to emphasize that a particular norm has been chosen. **Equation 2.13** is the graph-theoretical analog of the well-known Tanimoto similarity index (*see* **Eq. 2.19**), which is symmetric and bounded by zero and unity. **Equation 2.14** corresponds to the distance between two graphs *(36)*, which is the number of bonds that are not in common in the two molecules depicted by G_i and G_j. Another distance measure called "chemical distance" is similar to that given in **Eq. 2.14** except that lone-pair electrons are explicitly accounted for *(19)*. The Tanimoto similarity index of the two chemical graphs in **Fig. 1** and the distance between them are given by $S_{Tan}(G_i, G_j) = 0.83$ and $d(G_i, G_j) = 4$, respectively.

A similarity index called "subsimilarity," which is short for substructure similarity, has been developed by developed by Hagadone *(37)*. In form it is identical to one of the family of asymmetric similarity indices developed by Tversky *(6)* that is discussed in **Subheading 2.2.2.**,

$$S_{Tve}(G_Q, G_T) = \frac{\left|G_Q \cap G_T\right|_E}{\left|G_Q\right|_E} = \frac{\left|MCS(G_Q, G_T)\right|_E}{\left|G_Q\right|_E} , \qquad (2.15)$$

where G_Q is the substructure query and G_T is a target molecule. In contrast to $S_{Tan}(G_i, G_j)$, $S_{Tve}(G_i, G_j)$ is not symmetric, although zero and unity also bound it.

Although chemical graphs are intuitive to those trained in the chemical sciences, they have not been widely used in MSA primarily because of the computational demands brought on by the need to compute $MCS(G_i, G_j)$, which for large complex systems can be quite daunting. Approximate algorithms do exist, however *(26,37)*, and with the ever-increasing power of computers, the use of graph-based similarity may become more prevalent in the future. Interestingly, there is a close analogy between determination of the MCS and alignment of the 3-D molecular fields of molecules (*see* **Subheading 2.4.**) except that in the former the optimization is discrete while in the latter it is continuous.

2.2. Discrete-Valued Feature Vectors

The components of discrete feature vectors may indicate the presence or absence of a feature, the number of occurrences of a feature, or a finite set of binned values such as would be found in an ordered, categorical variable.

2.2.1. Binary-Valued Feature Vectors

Each component of an *n*-component binary feature vector, also called *bit vectors* or *molecular fingerprints*,

$$\mathbf{v}_A = \left(v_A(x_1), v_A(x_2), ..., v_A(x_k), ..., v_A(x_n)\right) \qquad (2.16)$$

indicates the presence or absence of a given feature, x_k, that is

$$v_A(x_k) = \begin{cases} 1 & \text{Feature present} \\ 0 & \text{Feature absent} \end{cases} . \tag{2.17}$$

A wide variety of features have been used in bit vectors, including molecular fragments, 3-D "potential pharmacophores," atom pairs, 2-D pharmacophores, topological torsions, and variety of topological indices.

Binary feature vectors are completely equivalent to sets (see the Appendix for further discussion). Care must be exercised when using them to ensure that appropriate mathematical operations are carried out. The number of components in a bit vector is usually quite large, normally $n \gg 100$. In some cases n can be orders of magnitude larger, sometimes exceeding a million components *(27,38)*. Bit vectors of this size are not handled directly because many of the components are zero, and methods such as hashing *(39)* are used to reduce the size of the stored information.

Bit vectors live in an n-dimensional, discrete hypercubic space, where each vertex of the hypercube corresponds to a set. **Figure 2** provides an example of sets with three elements. Distances between two bit vectors, $\mathbf{v}_A$ and $\mathbf{v}_B$, measured in this space correspond to Hamming distances, which are based on the city-block l_1 metric

$$d_{Ham}(\mathbf{v}_A, \mathbf{v}_B) = |\mathbf{v}_A - \mathbf{v}_B| = \sum_{k=1}^{n} |v_A(x_k) - v_B(x_k)| . \tag{2.18}$$

Because these vectors live in an n-dimensional hypercubic space, the use of non-integer distance measures is inappropriate, although in this special case the square of the Euclidean distance is equal to the Hamming distance.

The most widely used similarity measure by far is the Tanimoto similarity coefficient S_{Tan}, which is given in set-theoretic language as (cf. **Eq. 2.13** for the graph-theoretical case)

$$S_{Tan}(A,B) = \frac{|A \cap B|}{|A \cup B|} . \tag{2.19}$$

Using the explicit expressions for set cardinality, intersection, and union given in **Eqs. 5.10, 5.5,** and **5.6,** respectively, **Eq. 2.19** becomes

$$S_{Tan}(A,B) = \frac{\sum_k \min[A(x_k), B(x_k)]}{\sum_k \max[A(x_k), B(x_k)]} . \tag{2.20}$$

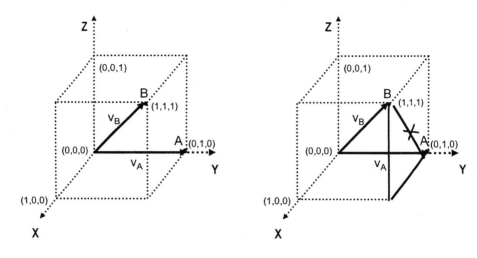

$$d_{\text{Ham}}(\mathbf{v}_A, \mathbf{v}_B) = |\mathbf{v}_A - \mathbf{v}_B| = \sum_{k=1}^{n} |v_A(x_k) - v_B(x_k)| = [1-0] + [1-1] + [1-0] = 2$$

Fig. 2. Distance between two binary-valued feature vectors $\mathbf{v}_A$ and $\mathbf{v}_B$ is not given by the Euclidean distance but the Hamming distance between the two.

By changing the form of the denominator (*see* **Eq. 5.15**), S_{Tan} is also given by

$$S_{\text{Tan}}(A,B) = \frac{|A \cap B|}{|A-B| + |B-A| + |A \cap B|}$$

$$= \frac{a}{a+b+c} \qquad (2.21)$$

where

$$a = |A \cap B| \qquad \text{Number of features common to A and B}$$
$$b = |A-B| \qquad \text{Number of features common to A but not to B} \qquad (2.22)$$
$$c = |B-A| \qquad \text{Number of features common to B but not to A}$$

The Tanimoto similarity coefficient is symmetric,

$$S_{\text{Tan}}(A,B) = S_{\text{Tan}}(B,A) \; , \qquad (2.23)$$

as are most of the similarity coefficients in use today, and is bounded by zero and unity,

$$0 \leq S_{\text{Tan}}(A,B) \leq 1 \; . \qquad (2.24)$$

From the form of these equations it can be seen that the method is biased when there is a great disparity in the size of the two molecules being compared. Consider, for example, the case when $|Q| << |T|$, where Q is a query molecule and T is a target molecule that could be obtained in a similarity search. If Q is much smaller than T, $|Q \cup T| \approx |T|$, and because $|Q| \leq |Q \cap T|$, it follows that $S_{Tan}(Q,T) \approx |Q| / |T|$. A consequence of this relationship is that in similarity-based searching Q will tend to recover other small molecules, T, because as T gets larger S_{Tan} becomes smaller in value, which works against the selection of larger molecules in the search. This is not generally a problem except in cases where a substructure of a large target molecule is quite similar to the smaller query molecule. If the query were biologically active, the larger target molecule containing a similar substructure to the query, which is bioactive, would be missed. The same holds true for a large molecule query, that is, it will tend to recover larger molecules. Thus, molecules with a strong *substructural relationship* to the query molecule will likely be missed, but this could be important in drug design as the substructure may contain the key atoms of the pharmacophore. As will be seen in the next section, the use of an asymmetric similarity measure can compensate for this to some degree. The above argument carries through completely to the case of chemical-graph-based similarity indices (see **Subheading 2.1.**).

A number of other similarity indices are in use today. The recent work by Willett et al. *(7)* should be consulted for examples of many of them, including a comprehensive discussion of their properties.

2.2.2. Asymmetric Similarity Indices

Most similarity measures for binary-valued feature vectors in use today are symmetric; Tversky *(6)*, however, has defined an infinite family of *asymmetric* measures

$$S_{Tve}(A,B) = \frac{|A \cap B|}{\alpha |A - B| + \beta |B - A| + |A \cap B|} , \qquad (2.25)$$

where $\alpha, \beta \geq 0$. This generalizes the typical symmetric Tanimoto similarity measure given in **Eq. 2.21**, which obtains when $\alpha = \beta = 1$. For all other values of α and β $S_{Tve}(A,B)$ is asymmetric, that is, $S_{Tve}(A,B) \neq S_{Tve}(B,A)$. Only the two extreme forms will, however, be considered here, namely, those when $\alpha = 1$ and $\beta = 0$ and $\alpha = 0$ and $\beta = 1$. Their set-theoretic forms are given by

$$S_{Tve}^{*}(A,B) = \frac{|A \cap B|}{|A - B| + |A \cap B|}$$

Fraction of A similar to B   (2.26)

$$= \frac{|A \cap B|}{|A|}$$

$$S^*_{Tve}(B,A) = \frac{|A \cap B|}{|B - A| + |A \cap B|}$$

Fraction of B similar A   (2.27)

$$= \frac{|A \cap B|}{|B|}$$

Using **Eqs. 5.5** and **5.10** both of the above equations can be written in a form similar to that for S_{Tan} given in **Eq. 2.20**. For example, **Eq. 2.26** becomes

$$S^*_{Tve}(A,B) = \frac{\sum_k \min[A(x_k), B(x_k)]}{\sum_k A(x_k)} \quad .$$

(2.28)

In analogy to **Eq. 2.21** the asymmetric similarity indices are given, respectively, by

$$S^*_{Tve}(A,B) = \frac{a}{a+b} \quad \text{and} \quad S^*_{Tve}(B,A) = \frac{a}{a+c} \quad .$$

(2.29)

As was the case for the symmetric similarity coefficient

$$0 \le S^*_{Tve}(A,B), S^*_{Tve}(B,A) \le 1 \quad ,$$

(2.30)

although generally $S^*_{Tve}(A,B) \ne S^*_{Tve}(B,A)$.

Asymmetric similarity can provide some benefits in similarity searches not afforded by its symmetric competitors. For example, consider as in **Subheading 2.2.1.**, the query and target molecules, Q and T, respectively, and the asymmetric similarity coefficients given in **Eqs. 2.26** and **2.27**. If Q is relatively "small" (N.B. "small" and "large" are used here refer to the size of the set and not to the size of the corresponding molecule), that is, if $|Q| << |T|$, then target molecules for which Q is an approximate subset will be selected using **Eq. 2.26**, that is,

$$S^*_{Tve}(Q,T) = \frac{|Q \cap T|}{|Q|} \Rightarrow 1 \quad \text{as} \quad Q \cap T \Rightarrow Q \quad .$$

(2.31)

This result is approximately independent of the size of T given that Q is an approximate subset of T. A comparable selection of molecules would not be obtained using the symmetric similarity coefficient in **Eq. 2.19** or the asymmetric similarity coefficient given by **Eq. 2.27** because as the target molecule increased in size the denominator would reduce the overall similarity values making selection less likely. If, on the other hand, Q is a relatively "large," that is, if $|Q| >> |T|$, then using the lower expression for asymmetric similarity in **Eq. 2.27** will produce similar results

$$S^*_{Tve}(T,Q) = \frac{|Q \cap T|}{|T|} \Rightarrow 1 \quad \text{as} \quad Q \cap T \Rightarrow T$$

(2.32)

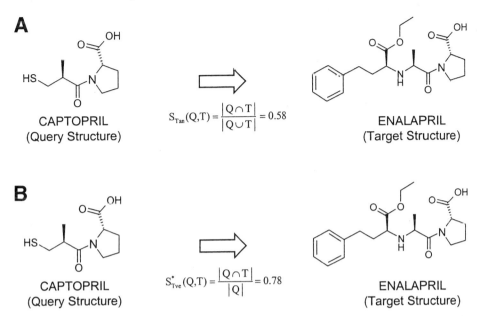

Fig. 3. Asymmetric similarity searching might provide some benefits not afforded by symmetric similarity searching. **(A)** Database searching using ISIS keys and symmetric similarity searching, S_{Tan}, will not yield enalapril as a "database hit" because the similarity value is too low, 0.58. **(B)** Whereas database searching using asymmetric similarity searching, S_{Tve}^*, could yield enalapril as a "database hit" because the asymmetric similarity value is 0.78.

except that the target molecules retrieved will be smaller than Q and will also be approximate subsets of Q. An example of this is shown in **Figs. 3** and **4**. Interestingly, choosing $S_{Pet_{min}}$ (A,B) given below in **Eq. 2.34**, where A = Q and B = T, will always yield the maximum similarity value for a given (Q,T) pair regardless of the "size" of the query molecule Q. Thus, $S_{Pet_{min}}$ (Q,T) may be the preferred similarity index in certain types of similarity searches (cf. the example given in **Figs. 3** and **4**).

The "extreme" forms, but not the intermediate forms, of asymmetric similarity defined by Tversky (6) given in **Eqs. 2.26** and **2.27** can be transformed into two symmetric measures by taking the maximum and minimum of the set cardinalities in the denominators of the two equations. The forms of these equations are obtained in analogy to those developed by Petke (33) for vectors and field-based functions (see **Subheadings 2.3.** and **2.4.** for further details):

$$S_{Pet_{max}}(A,B) = \frac{|A \cap B|}{max(|A|,|B|)} \tag{2.33}$$

A

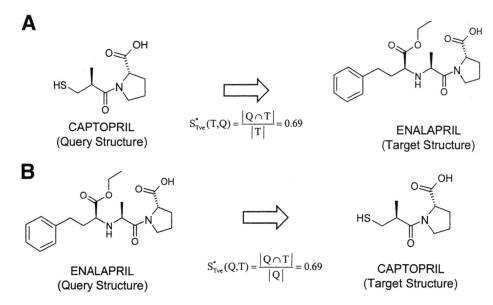

CAPTOPRIL
(Query Structure)

$$S^{*}_{Tve}(T,Q) = \frac{|Q \cap T|}{|T|} = 0.69$$

ENALAPRIL
(Target Structure)

B

ENALAPRIL
(Query Structure)

$$S^{*}_{Tve}(Q,T) = \frac{|Q \cap T|}{|Q|} = 0.69$$

CAPTOPRIL
(Target Structure)

Fig. 4. **(A)** The other asymmetric Tversky similarity index, S^{*}_{Tve}, has a value of 0.69. Exchanging the roles of the query and target molecules (Q⇔T) gives **(B)**, which shows that smaller target molecules are more likely to be retrieved from a large query structure using the asymmetric Tversky similarity index than the Tanimoto similarity index.

and

$$S_{Pet_{min}}(A,B) = \frac{|A \cap B|}{min(|A|,|B|)} .$$ (2.34)

As is the case for asymmetric similarity indices, both $S_{Pet_{max}}(A,B)$ and $S_{Pet_{min}}(A,B)$ are bounded by zero and unity, but are ordered with respect to each other and with respect to Tanimoto similarity, that is,

$$0 \le S_{Pet_{max}}(A,B) \le S_{Tan}(A,B) \le S_{Pet_{min}}(A,B) \le 1.$$ (2.35)

2.2.3. Integer- and Categorical-Valued Feature Vectors

Feature vectors with integer- or categorical-valued components are identical in form to binary-valued vectors (*see* **Eq. 2.16**). In contrast, however, each component takes on a finite number of values

$$v(x_k) = \begin{cases} \text{Finite, Ordered Set of Non-Negative Integers} \\ \text{Finite, Ordered Set of Values} \end{cases}$$ (2.36)

In the integer case, these values usually refer to the frequency of occurrence of a given feature such as, for example, a molecular fragment. In the categorical case the values may refer to a binned variable. In both cases the vectors live in discrete, lattice-like "hyperrectangular" spaces, which are generalizations of the hypercubic spaces inhabited by bit vectors. Such spaces can also be described by multisets *(40)*, but this formalism will not be used in this work.

Distances in these spaces should be based upon an l_1 or city-block metric (*see* **Eq. 2.18**) and not the l_2 or Euclidean metric typically used in many applications. The reasons for this are the same as those discussed in **Subheading 2.2.1.** for binary vectors. Set-based similarity measures can be adapted from those based on bit vectors using an *ansatz* borrowed from fuzzy set theory *(41,42)*. For example, the Tanimoto similarity coefficient becomes

$$S_{\text{Tan}}(\mathbf{v}_A, \mathbf{v}_B) = \frac{\sum_k \min[v_A(x_k), v_B(x_k)]}{\sum_k \max[v_A(x_k), v_B(x_k)]} \quad (2.37)$$

As noted in Klir and Yuan *(41)* there are many possible denominators that can be used in place of $|A \cup B|$, each of which gives rise to a different similarity measure.

The asymmetric similarity coefficients become, in an analogous fashion (*see* **Eq. 2.28**)

$$S_{\text{Tve}}^*(\mathbf{v}_A, \mathbf{v}_B) = \frac{\sum_k \min[v_A(x_k), v_B(x_k)]}{\sum_k v_A(x_k)}$$

$$S_{\text{Tve}}^*(\mathbf{v}_B, \mathbf{v}_A) = \frac{\sum_k \min[v_A(x_k), v_B(x_k)]}{\sum_k v_B(x_k)} \quad (2.38)$$

As was the case in the previous section for bit vectors, it can be shown that the similarity coefficients defined here are also bounded

$$0 \le S_{\text{Tan}}(\mathbf{v}_A, \mathbf{v}_B) \le S_{\text{Tve}}(\mathbf{v}_A, \mathbf{v}_B), S_{\text{Tve}}(\mathbf{v}_B, \mathbf{v}_A) \le 1 \quad (2.39)$$

It should be noted here that these expressions only apply to the case of non-negative integer-valued vector components. Other modifications are needed to accommodate non-integer values. Maggiora et al., *(43)* have discussed this issue in general for the case of field-based continuous functions, but their work also applies to vectors.

In a methodology they developed called holographic QSAR *(44)*, Hurst and Patterson have used integer-valued vectors to characterize the frequency of occurrence of molecular fragments. However, they do not use the vectors in their "native" form but rather fold them into a smaller vector by hashing.

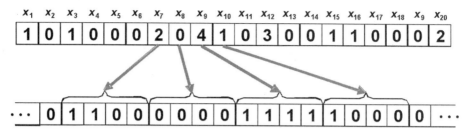

Fig. 5. In the scheme shown above, a 20-bit integer-valued vector (maximum integer value for each bit is 4) is converted into a 80-bit binary vector by converting each integer bit into a binary bit of four-bit length {0=0000; 1 = 1000; 2 = 1100; 3=1110; 4=1111}.

Schneider et al. *(45)* have also used integer-valued vectors to characterize what they call 2-D pharmacophores.

Integer- and categorical-valued vectors can be converted into equivalent binary vectors by augmenting the components of a typical bit vector as shown in **Fig. 5**. The process is straightforward for integer-valued variables, and Bajorath *(46)* has developed a novel binning approach for variables with continuous values, basically converting them into categorical variables. Once the mapping to the augmented bit vector has been completed all of the usual bit-vector-based similarity measures (see **Subheading 2.2.2.** for further discussion) can be applied.

There are many other expressions for similarity that can be used for integer- and categorical-valued vectors. Again, the comprehensive discussion provided by Willett et al. should be consulted for additional details *(7)*. Many of the features of discrete vector-based representations do not capture all of the relevant 3-D information in any substantive way, although they do capture some 3-D information indirectly, and this is why some feature vector procedures are referred to as "2.5-D" methods.

2.3. Continuous-Valued Feature Vectors

Vectors whose components have continuous values correspond to the more "traditional" types of vectors found in the physical sciences. They are of identical form to the discrete-valued vectors (*see* **Eq. 2.16**) except that the components, $v_A(x_k)$, are continuous valued. In chemoinformatics, however, the nature of the components is considerably different from those typically found in physics. For example, physiochemical properties, such as log*P*, solubility, melting point, molecular volume, Hammett $\sigma\rho$ parameters, and surface charge, as well as other descriptors derived explicitly for the purpose, such as BCUTs *(29)*, have routinely been used. The use of continuous-valued vectors is usually confined to relatively low-dimensional chemistry spaces, generally less than

10 dimensions (*see* **Subheading 3.** for further discussion). This is in sharp contrast to those discussed in the previous sections, where the dimensions are generally manifold larger.

Although it is ubiquitous in chemoinformatics applications, the term vector should be used with caution as vectors are properly the objects of vector spaces and must satisfy the axioms of vector spaces. For example, vectors in BCUT chemistry spaces do not form a vector space because the sum of two BCUT vectors may not lie in the space *(29)*. However, as long as this rather fine distinction is borne in mind, significant problems should not arise, and the term vector, taken in its broadest sense, will be used here.

2.3.1. Property-Based Continuous-Valued Feature Vectors

The components of most continuous-valued feature vectors are based on a variety of molecular properties such as solubilities, log$P$s, melting points, polar surface areas, molecular volumes, various shape indices (*vide supra*), and BCUTs, which are related to the charge, polarizability, and hydrogen-bonding properties of molecules. Because these properties have a wide range of values, they are typically scaled using the usual "z-transform" $z_i = (x_i - \bar{x})/\sigma_x$ favored by statisticians, where $\bar{x}$ is the average property value and σ_x^2 is its variance. Other transforms have also been used; one of the most popular is $x_i' = (x_i - x_{min})/(x_{max} - x_{min})$, where the values of the property, x_i, are mapped into the unit interval [0,1]. Simple scaling can be used to expand or contract the unit interval if desired.

An advantage of the z-transform is that it establishes a well-defined point of reference for the property-based vectors (the mean) as well as scaling the values of all of the variables to unit variance. BCUTs have a more complicated scaling, and relevant papers should be consulted for further details *(29)*. Because distances between vectors are invariant to the origin of the coordinate system, mean centering does not affect the result. However, the transformations used in all of the above procedures involve some form of scaling, and thus distances are not preserved between the original and scaled coordinate systems. Care must be exercised in the case of cosine similarity indices between vectors because they are both origin and scale dependent.

2.3.2. Inherent Non-Orthogonality of Descriptor Coordinate Systems

An often-overlooked issue is the *inherent non-orthogonality* of coordinate systems used to portray data points. Almost universally a Euclidean coordinate system is used. This assumes that the original *variables* are orthogonal, that is, are uncorrelated, when it is well known that this is generally not the case. Typically, principal component analysis (PCA) is performed to generate a putative orthogonal coordinate system each of whose axes correspond to directions of maximum variance in the transformed space. This, however, is not quite correct. Because an orthogonal similarity transformation is used to carry out the PCA, and because such transformations rigidly rotate the original coordinate system, the angles among the coordinate vectors are unchanged. By exactly reversing the rigid rotation of the orthogonal principal-component coordinate system, one regenerates the original coordinate system, which is thus seen to be orthogonal. This clearly contradicts the general observation that most variables used in practice tend to be statistically correlated, that is, are non-orthogonal. Importantly, even when the variables are properly uncorrelated, this does not mean that they are necessarily *statistically independent (47)*. To correctly handle such correlated variables one must first orthogonalize the original variables, and then perform PCA to orient the orthogonal coordinate system along directions of maximum variance of the data points. This is rarely done in current practice, but what are the consequences of not doing this? As is well known from the theory of tensors *(48)* both distances and angles between data vectors are affected by the angles between the coordinate axes. Conclusions drawn using, for example, either cosine similarity indices or distances will be affected *quantitatively* but not *qualitatively*. This is a manifestation of the fact that the topology (i.e., neighborhood relationships) of the space is preserved but its geometry (i.e., distances and angles) is not. The consequences of this are the following. The order of nearest neighbors from a given reference molecule in a chemistry space (*see* **Subheading 3.** for further details) will remain unchanged but the magnitude of their distances from the reference molecule will change. Thus, if one is only interested in, say, obtaining the 50 most similar molecules to a given reference molecule, nothing will change by modifying the angles of the coordinate axes. If, one the other hand, one is interested in finding all molecules with similarities greater than or equal to, say, 0.85 with respect to that reference molecule, the results obtained will change because they depend on the angles of the coordinate vectors.

In many cases, however, problems brought about by skewed coordinate axes due to significant correlations among the variables are somewhat ameliorated by procedures, such as genetic algorithms, used for variable selection. Although such procedures tend to remove highly correlated variables, this may not always be the case so that coordinate system skew may still be a problem. However, if the variables are not too correlated, the skew of a coordinate system will not significantly influence the overall results. A methodology is described in **Subheading 2.3.4.** that includes, in a natural way, the non-orthogonality of the coordinate system.

2.3.3. Proximity Measures for Continuous-Valued Vectors

Because of the continuous nature of the vector components described in this section, other types of distance and similarity measures have been used.

Although the Hamming distance (*see* **Eq. 2.18**) also applies for continuous vectors, Euclidean distances are typically used

$$
\begin{aligned}
d_{\text{Euc}}(\mathbf{v}_A, \mathbf{v}_B) &= \| \mathbf{v}_A - \mathbf{v}_B \| \\
&= \sqrt{\langle (\mathbf{v}_A - \mathbf{v}_B), (\mathbf{v}_A - \mathbf{v}_B) \rangle} \\
&= \sqrt{\sum_{k=1}^{n} (v_A(x_k) - v_B(x_k))^2}
\end{aligned}
\tag{2.40}
$$

In some instances, however, Minkowski distances are employed

$$
d_{\text{Minkow}}(\mathbf{v}_A, \mathbf{v}_B) = \| \mathbf{v}_A - \mathbf{v}_B \|_{\ell_r} = \left[\sum_{k=1}^{n} |v_A(x_k) - v_B(x_k)|^r \right]^{\frac{1}{r}},
\tag{2.41}
$$

where $r \geq 0$. Minkowski distances include both Hamming ($r = 1$) and Euclidean ($r = 2$) distances as special cases. Continuous distances can be converted into similarities using an appropriate monotonically decreasing function of distance, d, such as $\exp(-\eta \cdot d)$ or $1/(1 + \eta \cdot d)$, which both map to the unit interval, $[0,1]$ for finite, non-negative values of η.

The most prevalent among the similarity coefficients is the so-called *cosine similarity index* or *correlation coefficient*. For the field functions discussed in **Subheading 2.4.** it is usually called the *Carbó similarity index*, and this nomenclature will be used here as well,

$$
\begin{aligned}
S_{\text{Car}}(\mathbf{v}_A, \mathbf{v}_B) &= \frac{\langle \mathbf{v}_A, \mathbf{v}_B \rangle}{\sqrt{\| \mathbf{v}_A \|^2 \cdot \| \mathbf{v}_B \|^2}} \\
&= \frac{\langle \mathbf{v}_A, \mathbf{v}_B \rangle}{\| \mathbf{v}_A \| \cdot \| \mathbf{v}_B \|}
\end{aligned}
\tag{2.42}
$$

where the term in brackets in the numerator is the *inner product* of the two vectors

$$
\langle \mathbf{v}_A, \mathbf{v}_B \rangle = \sum_{k=1}^{n} v_A(x_k) \cdot v_B(x_k) = \| \mathbf{v}_A \| \cdot \| \mathbf{v}_B \| \cos(\mathbf{v}_A, \mathbf{v}_B)
\tag{2.43}
$$

and their magnitudes are given by the Euclidean norm

$$
\| \mathbf{v}_X \| = \sqrt{\langle \mathbf{v}_X, \mathbf{v}_X \rangle} = \sqrt{\sum_{k=1}^{n} v_X(x_k)^2} , \quad X = A, B .
\tag{2.44}
$$

It is important to note that the expressions in the latter two equations implicitly assume, as we shall see in **Subheading 2.4.**, that the basis of the vectors is orthonormal.

As this similarity index is origin-dependent, there generally is a difference between the values computed for the cosine similarity index and correlation coefficients, because the latter is always computed at the mean of the data. Moreover, if the components of the vectors are all non-negative, then $S_{Car}(\mathbf{v}_A,\mathbf{v}_B)$ is also non-negative. When this is not the case, however, $S_{Car}(\mathbf{v}_A,\mathbf{v}_B)$ may become negative, a situation that also obtains for the other similarity indices discussed in the remainder of this section. Maggiora et al. *(43)* have treated this case in great detail for continuous field functions, but the arguments can be carried through for finite vectors as well.

As has been pointed out numerous times, if $\mathbf{v}_A = \kappa\mathbf{v}_B \Rightarrow S_{Car}(\mathbf{v}_A,\mathbf{v}_B) = 1$, for all κ. This prompted Hodgkin and Richards *(49)* to define a slightly modified form of the similarity, usually called the Hodgkin similarity index, that does not suffer from this problem, namely,

$$S_{Hod}(\mathbf{v}_A,\mathbf{v}_B) = \frac{\langle \mathbf{v}_A, \mathbf{v}_B \rangle}{\frac{1}{2}\left(\left\| \mathbf{v}_A \right\|^2 + \left\| \mathbf{v}_B \right\|^2\right)} \quad . \tag{2.45}$$

Petke *(33)* has developed two additional indices that bound both the Carbó and Hodgkin similarity indices, namely,

$$S_{Pet_{min}}(\mathbf{v}_A,\mathbf{v}_B) = \frac{\langle \mathbf{v}_A, \mathbf{v}_B \rangle}{\min\left(\left\| \mathbf{v}_A \right\|^2, \left\| \mathbf{v}_B \right\|^2\right)} \tag{2.46}$$

and

$$S_{Pet_{max}}(\mathbf{v}_A,\mathbf{v}_B) = \frac{\langle \mathbf{v}_A, \mathbf{v}_B \rangle}{\max\left(\left\| \mathbf{v}_A \right\|^2, \left\| \mathbf{v}_B \right\|^2\right)} \quad , \tag{2.47}$$

that are analogous to those given, respectively, in **Eqs. 2.26** and **2.27** for the case of sets or binary vectors. Recently, a comprehensive analysis has been given for continuous, field-based functions of all of the similarity coefficients of this general form, which characterizes their linear ordering and their upper and lower bounds *(43)* (*see* **Eq. 2.85**). Because field-based functions also satisfy the postulates of linear vectors spaces, their approach can be taken over in its entirety to the case of finite-dimensional vectors covered in this section. Thus, the bounds of the similarity indices in **Eqs. 2.42, 2.45, 2.46,** and **2.47,** are given by

$$0 \le S_{Pet_{max}}(\mathbf{v}_A,\mathbf{v}_B) \le S_{Hod}(\mathbf{v}_A,\mathbf{v}_B) \le S_{Car}(\mathbf{v}_A,\mathbf{v}_B) \le 1 \le S_{Pet_{min}}(\mathbf{v}_A,\mathbf{v}_B) \le \infty. \tag{2.48}$$

All of the indices except $S_{Pet_{min}}(\mathbf{v}_A,\mathbf{v}_B)$ have upper bound of unity.

2.3.4. Molecule-Based Approach to Continuous-Valued Feature Vectors

In the "traditional" molecular-fragment approach the coefficients of the vector components are usually binary- or positive integer-valued. A continuous vector representation can be constructed in the following way. Choose a set of f molecular fragments, or whole molecules, as a "molecular basis" for representing chemistry space

$$\Phi = \{\phi_1, \phi_2, ..., \phi_k, ..., \phi_f\} . \tag{2.49}$$

which can be written as the row vector

$$\Phi = (\phi_1, \phi_2, ..., \phi_k, ..., \phi_f) . \tag{2.50}$$

Consider the similarities of all of the elements of the molecular basis with respect to each other. This generates a similarity matrix

$$
\mathbf{S} = \langle \Phi, \Phi \rangle
$$
$$
= \begin{pmatrix}
\langle \phi_1, \phi_1 \rangle & \langle \phi_1, \phi_2 \rangle & \cdots & \langle \phi_1, \phi_f \rangle \\
\langle \phi_2, \phi_1 \rangle & \langle \phi_2, \phi_2 \rangle & \cdots & \langle \phi_2, \phi_f \rangle \\
\vdots & \vdots & \ddots & \vdots \\
\langle \phi_f, \phi_1 \rangle & \langle \phi_f, \phi_2 \rangle & \cdots & \langle \phi_f, \phi_f \rangle
\end{pmatrix}, \tag{2.51}
$$

$$
\mathbf{S} = \begin{pmatrix}
S_{1,1} & S_{1,2} & \cdots & S_{1,f} \\
S_{2,1} & S_{2,2} & \cdots & S_{2,f} \\
\vdots & \vdots & \ddots & \vdots \\
S_{f,1} & S_{f,1} & \cdots & S_{f,f}
\end{pmatrix} . \tag{2.52}
$$

whose diagonal elements are unity and where the matrix elements can, depending on the nature of the molecular basis, be evaluated in a number of different ways. For example, suppose the $\phi_i \Uparrow G_i$, that is, the ith element of the molecular basis, is a *labeled chemical graph* of a molecular fragment or complete molecule. Then $S_{i,j} = \langle \phi_i, \phi_j \rangle = S_{Tan}(Gi, Gj)$, where the Tanimoto similarity, S_{Tan}, is evaluated as in **Eq. 2.13**. The set of labeled graphs $G = \{G_1, G_2, ..., G_f\}$ will be referred to as a "fragment graph basis" or a "chemical graph basis" depending on whether molecular fragments or complete molecules are used, respectively. Note that similarities could also be computed using a bit-vector representation, especially in cases where complete molecules are used. The molecular basis could be related to the 3-D structures of molecules or their fragments or, alternatively, to their 3-D fields. In such cases, evaluation of the similarities can be accomplished as described in **Subheading 2.4.**

Because $0 \leq S_{i,j} \leq 1$, the elements of **S** are completely analogous to the basis-set overlap integrals familiar in quantum chemistry *(50)*. As the off-diagonal elements of the matrix are non-zero, that is, $S_{i,j} \neq 0$ for all $i \neq j$, the basis is non-orthogonal. In some applications **S** is equivalent to what is typically called the metric matrix; *in statistics* **S** *is equivalent to the correlation matrix.*

Consider a given molecule, A, within a set of n molecules that can, in matrix notation, be represented in the Φ-basis as

$$\mathbf{v}_A = \mathbf{\Phi}\mathbf{v}_A \ , \tag{2.53}$$

where the column vector of coefficients is given by

$$\mathbf{v}_A = \begin{pmatrix} v_A(x_1) \\ v_A(x_2) \\ \vdots \\ v_A(x_k) \\ \vdots \\ v_A(x_n) \end{pmatrix} . \tag{2.54}$$

To compute the various cosine-like similarity indices it is necessary to evaluate, respectively, the inner product $\langle \mathbf{v}_A, \mathbf{v}_B \rangle$ and Euclidean norms $||\mathbf{v}_X|| = \sqrt{\langle \mathbf{v}_X, \mathbf{v}_X \rangle}$ (*see* also **Eqs. 2.43** and **2.44**):

$$\langle \mathbf{v}_A, \mathbf{v}_B \rangle = \langle \mathbf{\Phi}\mathbf{v}_A, \mathbf{\Phi}\mathbf{v}_B \rangle$$
$$= \mathbf{v}_A^T \langle \mathbf{\Phi}, \mathbf{\Phi} \rangle \mathbf{v}_B \ , \tag{2.55}$$

which in expanded form is

$$\langle \mathbf{v}_A, \mathbf{v}_B \rangle = \left(v_A(x_1), v_A(x_2), ..., v_A(x_n) \right) \begin{pmatrix} S_{1,1} & S_{1,2} & \cdots & S_{1,f} \\ S_{2,1} & S_{2,2} & \cdots & S_{2,f} \\ \vdots & \vdots & \ddots & \vdots \\ S_{f,1} & S_{f,1} & \cdots & S_{f,f} \end{pmatrix} \begin{pmatrix} v_B(x_1) \\ v_B(x_2) \\ \vdots \\ v_B(x_n) \end{pmatrix} . \tag{2.56}$$

In "summation form" **Eq. 2.56** becomes

$$\langle \mathbf{v}_A, \mathbf{v}_B \rangle = \sum_i \sum_j v_A(x_i) \cdot v_B(x_j) \cdot S_{i,j} \ , \tag{2.57}$$

where $S_{i,j} = 1$ for $i = 1, 2, \ldots, f$. Comparing **Eq. 2.57** with **Eq. 2.43** shows that the elements of the **S**-matrix modulate the product of the vector components and the cross-terms, $v(x_i) \cdot v(x_j)$, remain. When the basis is orthonormal, and $\mathbf{S} = \mathbf{I}$ and **Eq. 2.57** reduces to **Eq. 2.43**. Similarly, the Euclidean norm is given by

$$\| \mathbf{v}_X \| = \sqrt{\sum_i \sum_j v_X(x_i) \cdot v_X(x_j) \cdot S_{i,j}} \quad , \tag{2.58}$$

which reduces to **Eq. 2.44** when $\mathbf{S} = \mathbf{I}$. These relationships clearly show the important role play by the metric matrix $\mathbf{S}$. Importantly, because the various cosine-like similarity indices all depend on the quantities given in **Eqs. 2.57** and **2.58**, it follows these indices also depend upon $\mathbf{S}$, but this dependence is routinely neglected in most calculations. Euclidean (*see* **Eq. 2.40**) and other distances are likewise affected by the metric matrix:

$$
\begin{aligned}
d_{\text{Euc}}(\mathbf{v}_A, \mathbf{v}_B) &= \| \mathbf{v}_A - \mathbf{v}_B \| \\
&= \sqrt{\langle (\mathbf{v}_A - \mathbf{v}_B), (\mathbf{v}_A - \mathbf{v}_B) \rangle} \\
&= \sqrt{\sum_i \sum_j \left(v_A(x_i) - v_B(x_i) \right) \cdot \left(v_A(x_j) - v_B(x_j) \right) \cdot S_{i,j}}
\end{aligned}
\tag{2.59}
$$

As was the case in the two cases above, **Eq. 2.59** reduces to **Eq. 2.40** in an orthonormal basis.

There are numerous ways in which to orthonormalize a basis. Here we choose to employ the *symmetric orthonormalization* procedure described by Löwdin *(51)*, which has the benefit over other orthogonality procedures that the new basis is as close as possible, in a least squares sense, to the original basis *(52)*

$$\mathbf{\Lambda} = \mathbf{\Phi S}^{-\frac{1}{2}} \quad , \tag{2.60}$$

where

$$\mathbf{\Lambda} = (\lambda_1, \lambda_2, ..., \lambda_k, ... \lambda_f) . \tag{2.61}$$

Computing the inner product, $\langle \mathbf{\Lambda}, \mathbf{\Lambda} \rangle = \left\langle \mathbf{\Phi S}^{-\frac{1}{2}}, \mathbf{\Phi S}^{-\frac{1}{2}} \right\rangle = \mathbf{S}^{-\frac{1}{2}} \langle \mathbf{\Phi}, \mathbf{\Phi} \rangle \mathbf{S}^{-\frac{1}{2}} = \mathbf{S}^{-\frac{1}{2}} \mathbf{S} \, \mathbf{S}^{-\frac{1}{2}} = \mathbf{I}$, shows that the basis is indeed orthonormal.

Right multiplying the terms in **Eq. 2.60** by $\mathbf{S}^{\frac{1}{2}}$ gives $\mathbf{\Phi} = \mathbf{\Lambda S}^{\frac{1}{2}}$, which upon substitution into **Eq. 2.53** yields

$$
\begin{aligned}
\mathbf{v}_A &= \mathbf{\Phi} \mathbf{v}_A \\
&= (\mathbf{\Lambda S}^{\frac{1}{2}}) \mathbf{v}_A = \mathbf{\Lambda} (\mathbf{S}^{\frac{1}{2}} \mathbf{v}_A) , \\
&= \mathbf{\Lambda} \, \mathbf{v}_A^{\lambda}
\end{aligned}
\tag{2.62}
$$

where the "expansion coefficients" (i.e., components) in the new, *orthonormal basis* are given by

$$\mathbf{v}_A^{\lambda} = \mathbf{S}^{\frac{1}{2}} \mathbf{v}_A \quad . \tag{2.63}$$

As was the case for the basis above, **Eq. 2.60** can be rearranged to give the expansion coefficients in the original, non-orthogonal basis, that is,

$$\mathbf{v}_A = \mathbf{S}^{-\frac{1}{2}}\, \mathbf{v}_A^\lambda \ . \tag{2.64}$$

Thus, this equation provides the means for determining the components of $\mathbf{v}_A$ in the original basis given the components in the orthonormal basis, which as we will see are easily determined. This can be accomplished by first taking the inner product of, say, the kth orthonormal basis element with $\mathbf{v}_A$ using **Eq. 2.57**

$$\begin{aligned}
\langle \lambda_k, \mathbf{v}_A \rangle &= \langle \lambda_k, \Lambda \rangle \mathbf{v}_A^\lambda \\
&= \sum_{\ell=1}^{f} \langle \lambda_k, \lambda_\ell \rangle v_A^\lambda(x_\ell)
\end{aligned} \tag{2.65}$$

Because $\langle \lambda_k, \lambda_\ell \rangle = \delta_{k,\ell}$, where the Kronecker delta, $\delta_{k,k} = 1$ and $\delta_{k,\ell} = 0$ for $k \neq \ell$, the kth component of $\mathbf{v}_A^\lambda$ is given by

$$v_A^\lambda(x_k) = \langle \lambda_k, \mathbf{v}_A \rangle \text{ for } k = 1, 2, ..., f \ . \tag{2.66}$$

Because $\mathbf{v}_A^\lambda$ is normalized with respect to the Euclidean norm

$$\sum_{k=1}^{f} v_A^\lambda(x_k)^2 = 1 \tag{2.67}$$

the square of each component value, $v_A^\lambda(x_k)$, gives the fraction of the "molecule" represented by its corresponding basis element λ_k.

To evaluate the inner product $\langle \lambda_k, \mathbf{v}_A \rangle$, λ_k must be expanded in terms of the non-orthogonal ϕ-basis (*see* **Eq. 2.60**), that is

$$\lambda_k = \sum_{\ell=1}^{f} \phi_\ell\, S_{k,\ell}^{-\frac{1}{2}} \ . \tag{2.68}$$

Substituting **Eq. 2.68** into **Eq. 2.66** yields

$$v_A^\lambda(x_k) = \sum_{\ell=1}^{f} S_{k,\ell}^{-\frac{1}{2}} \langle \phi_\ell, \mathbf{v}_A \rangle \ . \tag{2.69}$$

The inner-product terms $\langle \phi_\ell, \mathbf{v}_A \rangle$ can now be evaluated in exactly the same manner as was described earlier. For example, $\langle \phi_\ell, \mathbf{v}_A \rangle = S_{\text{Tan}}(G_l, G_A)$, where ϕ_ℓ is the labeled graph corresponding to lth "basis fragment," $\mathbf{v}_A$ is the labeled graph corresponding to molecule A, and $S_{\text{Tan}}(G_l, G_A)$ is the chemical graph-theoretical Tanimoto similarity coefficient.

This approach can, in many instances, be extended even to cases where the basis is comprised of physicochemical, topological, or other such parameters. The similarity matrix is replaced in these cases by the correlation matrix computed with respect to the "basis set" of parameters (*vide supra*).

Agrafiotis et al. *(53)* developed a similar approach to generate vectors for input into neural nets. Although these authors did not account for the inherent non-orthogonality of the "basis," in their work the issue of the orthogonality of the basis may be less critical than it is here, and the mappings they generated seem to be sufficiently stable. Another related approach comes from Villar and co-workers *(54)*. In this case, however, the basis consisted of a set of proteins. The interaction of each molecule in the training set to each of the proteins in the "basis" was measured experimentally, and the expansion coefficients were determined using a least squares procedure. Again, non-orthogonality of the basis was not explicitly addressed, although the choice of the basis proteins did involve an assessment of correlations among them.

Randic *(55–57)* has investigated the role of orthogonalized descriptors in multivariate regressions. In his work he points out that, although the predictions obtained with orthogonal or non-orthogonal descriptors are the same, the stability of the regression coefficients is much greater in the former case. Also, adding a new, orthogonal descriptor to set of orthogonal descriptors does not affect the values of the previously determined regression coefficients. This is definitely *not* the case for non-orthogonal descriptors where addition of a new descriptor can cause all of the coefficients to fluctuate significantly depending on the degree of collinearity of the new descriptor with those in the original set.

2.4. Field-Based Functions

Many methods exist for assessing 3-D molecular similarity. Lemmen and Lengauer *(58)* provide a comprehensive review of most of the methods in use today, a large class of which utilizes some form vector-based representation of 3-D molecular features such as 3-D pharmacophores *(59)* and various types of 3-D shape descriptors *(60)*. The components of these vectors can be binary, integer, categorical, or continuous as discussed in the last three sections, respectively. Most 3-D methods, however, involve some type of direct alignment of the molecules being considered. Early on RMS deviations between specific atoms in the molecules being compared were employed, but this required identifying the key atoms, a non-trivial computational task. A variety of other 3-D methods exist *(58)*, but the bulk of the 3-D methods utilize some form of field-based function to represent the fields or *pseudo*-fields, which can be either continuous or discrete, surrounding molecules. Examples include "steric," electrostatic potential, and lipophilic fields *(32)*. Several workers have also developed a field-based methodology for directly aligning molecules based on their electric fields *(33,49)*, which differs from the usual scalar potential fields that are typically matched, but these approaches have only been implemented as discrete procedures. Use of continuous electric fields has not been carried out at this time.

Interestingly, there is a close analogy between the alignment of 3-D molecular fields and the determination of maximum common substructures of two chemical graphs (see **Subheading 2.1.**). Both cases involve the search for optimal overlays or alignments: The former requires continuous optimizations of non-linear similarity indices that give rise to large numbers of solutions and to great difficulties in clearly identifying the global maximum solution. The latter requires discrete optimizations, but the problem is NP complete and thus does not scale well computationally.

A major factor differentiating 3-D from 2-D similarity methods, regardless of the type of 3-D method employed, is the need to account in some manner for conformational flexibility. There are two ways this is generally accomplished. One way involves carrying out a conformational analysis and selecting a subset of "appropriate" conformations. All pairwise alignments are then considered. The other way involves some form of conformational search carried out simultaneously with the alignment process *(61,62)*. Because of its importance in similarity-based alignments of molecules, the remainder of the discussion in this section will focus on field-based methods.

2.4.1. Representation of Molecular Fields

Field-based methods generally utilize linear combinations of appropriate functions that are associated in some way with the atoms of the molecule under study:

$$F_A^\alpha(\mathbf{r}) = \sum_{i \in \text{atoms}} a_i^\alpha f_i(\mathbf{r}) \ , \qquad (2.70)$$

where "α" designates the specific type of field or property being considered. The coefficients a_i^α weight the atom-based functions and in many cases are used to characterize specific properties attributed to the individual atoms (*vide infra*). Unnormalized, spherically symmetric Gaussian functions, "Gaussians" for short, are by far the most ubiquitous functions used in field-based applications:

$$f_i(\mathbf{r}) = \exp\left(-\kappa_i |\mathbf{r} - \mathbf{R}_i|^2\right) \ , \qquad (2/71)$$

where R_i is the location of the Gaussian, generally at an atomic center, and κ_i is its "width," which is the reciprocal of the variance, that is $\kappa_i = 1/\sigma_i^2$. The variance is sometimes referred to as the orbital radius, $\rho_i = \sigma_i^2$, of a Gaussian *(63)*. As $\kappa_i \to 0$, $f_i(\mathbf{r})$ becomes more spread out and conversely as $\kappa_i \to \infty$, $f_i(\mathbf{r})$ becomes sharper until, in the limit, it approaches an infinitely sharp delta function. In the latter case atoms are essentially represented as points, while in the former case they are represented as "soft spheres," which is illustrated in **Fig. 6**.

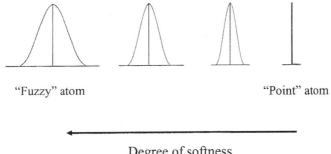

"Fuzzy" atom   "Point" atom

← Degree of softness

Fig. 6. Gaussian curves as a function of increasing width. As the degree of softness increases, the curves represent "fuzzy" atoms, and as the degree of softness deceases, the Gaussian converges to a "point" atom model.

A useful property of Gaussians is that the integral of the product of two Gaussians *(50)* is given by another Gaussian that is a function of their distance of separation, that is,

$$\int f_i(\mathbf{r}) \cdot f_j(\mathbf{r}) d^3\mathbf{r} = \left(\frac{\pi}{\kappa_i + \kappa_j}\right)^{3/2} \exp\left(-\frac{\kappa_i \kappa_j}{\kappa_i + \kappa_j} |\mathbf{R}_i - \mathbf{R}_j|^2\right). \quad (2.72)$$

Thus, the "overlap" of two molecules, A and B, with respect to the field of property α, $\Omega(F_A^\alpha, F_B^\alpha)$, is given by

$$\begin{aligned} \Omega(F_A^\alpha, F_B^\alpha) &= \int F_A^\alpha(\mathbf{r}) \cdot F_B^\alpha(\mathbf{r}) d^3\mathbf{r} \\ &= \sum_{i \in A} \sum_{j \in B} a_i^\alpha \cdot b_j^\alpha \int f_i(\mathbf{r}) f_j(\mathbf{r}) d^3\mathbf{r} \\ &= \sum_{i \in A} \sum_{j \in B} a_i^\alpha \cdot b_j^\alpha \left(\frac{\pi}{\kappa_i + \kappa_j}\right)^{3/2} \exp\left(-\frac{\kappa_i \kappa_j}{\kappa_i + \kappa_j} |\mathbf{R}_i - \mathbf{R}_j|^2\right) \end{aligned} \quad , \quad (2.73)$$

$$\Omega(F_A^\alpha, F_B^\alpha) = \sum_{i \in A} \sum_{j \in B} \tilde{a}_i^\alpha \cdot \tilde{b}_j^\alpha \exp\left(-\frac{\kappa_i \kappa_j}{\kappa_i + \kappa_j} |\mathbf{R}_i - \mathbf{R}_j|^2\right), \quad (2.74)$$

where the modified coefficients, $\tilde{a}_i^\alpha$ and $\tilde{b}_j^\alpha$, are obtained by including the square root term equally into the two field (property) coefficients a_i^α and b_j^α given in **Eq. 2.73**. In most cases the width parameters, κ_i and κ_j, are chosen to be the same for all atoms.

Equation 2.74 is a general form that is used in a number of field-based approaches to 3-D molecular alignment and similarity. For example, in the program Seal *(64)* the coefficients given either in **Eq. 2.73** or **Eq. 2.74** are subsumed into a single "property coefficient," $\tilde{a}_i^{\alpha} \cdot \tilde{b}_j^{\alpha} \Rightarrow w_{i,j}$, which may account for the effect of multiple types of properties,

$$\Omega_{\text{``Seal''}}(A, B) = \sum_{i \in A} \sum_{j \in B} w_{i,j} \exp\left(-\kappa \left| \mathbf{R}_i - \mathbf{R}_j \right|^2\right) . \tag{2.75}$$

The exponential coefficient, κ, determines the spread of the Gaussian and is taken be identical for all atom pairs. Some methods assign property values directly to the coefficients $\tilde{a}_i^{\alpha}$ and $\tilde{b}_j^{\alpha}$ *(62,65)*.

An alternative approach *(30)* treats the steric and electrostatic potential fields directly. The steric field is generally given by an expression similar to that in **Eq. 2.70**,

$$F_A^{\text{st}}(\mathbf{r}) = \sum_{i \in \text{atoms}} a_i^{\text{st}} f_i(\mathbf{r}) , \tag{2.76}$$

where the coefficients are usually to be unity, that is, $a_i^{\text{st}} = 1$, the field functions, $f_i(\mathbf{r})$, are usually taken to be Gaussians (*see* **Eq. 2.71**), and the width parameters, κ_i, are either held constant for all atoms or are adjusted for each specific "atomic environment" *(30)*. In the case of the molecular electrostatic potential (el) field

$$F_A^{\text{el}}(\mathbf{r}) = \sum_{i \in \text{atoms}} \frac{q_i}{\left| \mathbf{r} - \mathbf{R}_i \right|} \tag{2.77}$$

the "$1/r$" term, which becomes singular at each atomic nucleus, presents a computational problem that was solved by Good et al., *(66)* who developed a Gaussian expansion of the "$1/r$" term,

$$\frac{1}{\left| \mathbf{r} - \mathbf{R}_i \right|} \approx \sum_{k \in A_i} c_k f_{i,k}(\mathbf{r}) , \tag{2.78}$$

that significantly expedites computations. In this expression $f_{i,k}(\mathbf{r})$ is the kth Gaussian in the expansion of $1/r$ about the ith atom, A_i, of molecule A. The expansion usually consists of two or three terms, and the expansion coefficients, c_k, are obtained by least-squares minimization. Note that the width parameters, κ_k, are independent of the atom center and differ significantly from each other in order to fit the $1/r$ term with sufficient accuracy *(66)*. Substituting **Eq. 2.78** into **Eq. 2.77** converts it into a sum of Gaussians, and thus most field-based similarity measures (*vide infra*) only require calculation of Gaussian overlap integrals (*see*, for example, **Eqs. 2.72** and **2.73**) when dealing with steric or electrostatic potential fields. Thus, many of the issues that plague similarity calculations carried out within a discrete lattice framework are no longer a problem in the case of continuous field-based functions.

2.4.2 Field-Based Similarity Indices

Field-based similarities are usually evaluated by the cosine or correlation function similarity measure employed initially by Carbó and co-workers (67) to compute molecular similarities based upon quantum mechanical wavefunctions. Such a measure, which is usually called a Carbó similarity index, is given by

$$
S_{Car}\left(F_A^\alpha, F_B^\alpha\right) = \frac{\left\langle F_A^\alpha, F_B^\alpha \right\rangle}{\left\| F_A^\alpha \right\| \cdot \left\| F_B^\alpha \right\|}
$$

$$
= \frac{\left\langle F_A^\alpha, F_B^\alpha \right\rangle}{\sqrt{\left\| F_A^\alpha \right\|^2 \cdot \left\| F_B^\alpha \right\|^2}} ,
$$

(2.79)

where the inner product in the numerator is now given by an integral rather than a summation because the objects considered here are field functions, F_A^α and F_B^α, not vectors, that is,

$$
\left\langle F_A^\alpha, F_B^\alpha \right\rangle = \int F_A^\alpha(\mathbf{r}) \cdot F_B^\alpha(\mathbf{r}) d^3\mathbf{r} ,
$$

(2.80)

and the Euclidean norm of the functions is given by

$$
\left\| F_X^\alpha \right\| = \sqrt{\int F_X^\alpha(\mathbf{r})^2 d^3\mathbf{r}} , \quad X=A,B .
$$

(2.81)

Note the similarity of **Eqs. 2.43** and **2.44** with **Eqs. 2.80** and **2.81** because both the vectors in the former equations and the functions of the latter are all elements of linear vector spaces. The main difference arises in the way in which the inner products are evaluated. Also, as was the case for vectors, if the field functions are non-negative functions, $S_{Car}(F_A^\alpha, F_B^\alpha)$ will be non-negative. When this is not the case, however, $S_{Car}(F_A^\alpha, F_B^\alpha)$ may become negative, a situation that also obtains for the other similarity indices discussed in the remainder of this section. Maggiora et al. (43) have treated this case in great detail for continuous field functions, but the arguments can be carried through for finite vectors as well (*vide supra*).

As discussed in the previous section for vectors, if F_A^α and F_B^α differ only by a constant, that is, if $F_A^\alpha = K \cdot F_B^\alpha$, then $S_{Car}(F_A^\alpha, F_B^\alpha) = 1$ regardless of the specific form of the functions. While this is not a likely occurrence in practical applications, Hodgkin and Richards (49) nonetheless defined a slightly altered similarity measure, usually referred to as the Hodgkin similarity index, which is not affected by this problem and is given by

$$
\left\| F_X^\alpha \right\| = \sqrt{\int F_X^\alpha(\mathbf{r})^2 d^3\mathbf{r}} , \quad X=A,B .
$$

(2.82)

where the terms in the denominator of **Eqs. 2.79** and **2.82** are, respectively, the geometric and arithmetic means of the squared norms of F_A^α and F_B^α. As has been shown by Maggiora et al. *(43)*, a family of similarity indices can be defined in terms of the means of the squared norms in their denominators.

The Petke indices, defined earlier for vectors (*see* **Eqs. 2.46** and **2.47**), are given by

$$S_{\text{Pet}_{\min}}\left(F_A^\alpha, F_B^\alpha\right) = \frac{\left\langle F_A^\alpha, F_B^\alpha \right\rangle}{\min\left(\left\| F_A^\alpha \right\|^2, \left\| F_B^\alpha \right\|^2\right)} \tag{2.83}$$

and

$$S_{\text{Pet}_{\max}}\left(F_A^\alpha, F_B^\alpha\right) = \frac{\left\langle F_A^\alpha, F_B^\alpha \right\rangle}{\max\left(\left\| F_A^\alpha \right\|^2, \left\| F_B^\alpha \right\|^2\right)}. \tag{2.84}$$

All of the same bounding properties described in the previous section for vectors (*see* **Eq. 2.48**) obtain here as well, including the fact that all of the indices except $S_{\text{Pet}_{\min}}$ are bounded from above by unity:

$$0 \le S_{\text{Pet}_{\max}}\left(F_A^\alpha, F_B^\alpha\right) \le S_{\text{Hod}}\left(F_A^\alpha, F_B^\alpha\right) \le S_{\text{Car}}\left(F_A^\alpha, F_B^\alpha\right) \le 1 \le S_{\text{Pet}_{\min}}\left(F_A^\alpha, F_B^\alpha\right) \le \infty. \tag{2.85}$$

None of the cosine/correlation-like similarity indices or their complements (*see* **Subheading 2.5.**) are true metrics, that is, they do not obey the distance axioms. Petitjean *(68,69)*, however, has developed a distance-based methodology, but it has not been applied in many cases.

Similarity indices corresponding to different fields can be combined into an overall similarity index, for example,

$$S_X(F_A, F_B) = \lambda \cdot S_X(F_A^{\text{st}}, F_B^{\text{st}}) + (1 - \lambda) \cdot S_X(F_A^{\text{el}}, F_B^{\text{el}}), \tag{2.86}$$

where X = Carbó, Hodgkin, Petke, or other appropriate index *(43)* and λ is the weighting coefficient. Mestres et al. *(30)* have used a value ($\lambda \approx 0.66$), arrived at pragmatically, that weights steric to electrostatic-potential similarity in a $2:1$ ratio.

2.4.3. Addressing Conformational Flexibility

As noted in the introduction of this section, computing 3-D molecular similarities of a set of molecules requires physically aligning the appropriate fields of the molecules, while accounting for their conformational flexibility, which can be accomplished in two ways, either by rigid body superpositions of selected conformations of each of the molecules being aligned or by simultaneous conformational sampling during the alignment process. In the rigid-body case, one molecule is generally chosen as the *reference molecule*, which remains fixed, while the other *adapting molecule* is translated and rotated until a maximum of the similarity index is obtained. Because the similarity index is a non-linear function, it generally has multiple solutions,

$$S_X(F_A, F_B)^1 \geq S_X(F_A, F_B)^2 \geq \cdots \geq S_X(F_A, F_B)^k \geq \cdots \qquad (2.87)$$

although it is difficult to know if the global maximum has been attained. To increase the chances that all of the best solutions are obtained, multiple starting geometries are usually sampled.

An added difficulty in rigid-body alignment is that all "relevant" conformations, say N, of the reference molecule must be aligned with all "relevant" conformations, say M, of the adapting molecule—$N \times M$ alignments must be carried out where, as discussed above, each alignment involves multiple starting geometries. This is a significant computational burden for the alignment of a single pair of molecules, and thus carrying out alignments for a large set of molecules is not computationally feasible at this time.

There are some approaches that hold promise for speeding up the computations. A novel procedure based on Fourier transforms was developed by Nissink et al. *(70)* and used by Lemmen et al. *(65)* The method separates the translational and rotational motions needed to align pairs of molecules and thus allows the separate optimization of each, thereby facilitating the overall alignment process. While this certainly speeds up the computations, it does not significantly alter the significant time requirements of rigid body alignments.

An alternative approach that combines conformational searching with similarity-based structure alignment perhaps holds more promise in terms of speeding up the process of aligning conformationally flexible molecules. In contrast to the rigid alignment process where one molecule is held fixed (reference molecule) and one is allowed to move rigidly (adapting molecule), here both molecules are treated on an equal footing and are allowed to move and conformationally flex. In the approach of Blinn et al. *(61)*, which is similar to that developed by Labute *(62)*, the energy of the combined system of the two molecules being aligned, $E_{A,B}^{total}$, is given by

$$E_{A,B}^{total} = E_A^{conf} + E_B^{conf} + E_{A,B}^{sim}, \qquad (2.88)$$

where E_A^{conf} is the conformational energy of molecule A, E_B^{conf} is the conformational energy of molecule B, and $E_{A,B}^{sim}$ is a pseudo-energy penalty term, which is given by

$$\begin{aligned} E_{A,B}^{sim} &= K_{sim} \cdot [1 - S_X(F_A, F_B)] \\ &= K_{sim} \cdot D_X(F_A, F_B) \end{aligned} \qquad (2.89)$$

where K_{sim} is an adjustable proportionality constant, which lies in the range of 5–20 kcal/mol. The dissimilarity (see **Subheading 2.5.**) $D_X(F_A,F_B)$ is used rather than similarity because the penalty term should vanish when the fields of the two molecules are in perfect alignment, that is, when $S_X(F_A,F_B) = 1 \rightarrow D_X(F_A,F_B) = 0 \rightarrow E_{A,B}^{sim} = 0$, and, alternatively, the maximum penalty should be assessed when

$$S_X(F_A,F_B) = 0 \rightarrow D_X(F_A,F_B) = 1 \rightarrow E_{A,B}^{sim} = K_{sim}. \qquad (2.90)$$

Other forms for the pseudo-energy penalty term have also been investigated *(61,62)*. In any case, pseudo-energy penalty term acts as a constraint on the overall energy of the system, which is a balance between favorable conformational energies and overall molecular alignment as measured by field-based similarity (dissimilarity).

2.4.4. Deriving Consistent Multimolecule Alignments

As has been shown by Mestres et al. *(71)* the optimal solution, $S_X(F_A,F_B)^1$, may not correspond to the correct "experimentally derived" molecular alignment. To address this problem, Mestres et al. *(71)* developed the concept of *pairwise consistency*, which is depicted in **Fig. 7**. Consider the similarities of three molecules A, B, and C. Suppose molecule A is the reference molecule, which is held fixed, and molecules B and C are the adapting molecules. Now determine the optimal similarity solutions for $S_X(F_A,F_B)^1$ and $S_X(F_A,F_C)^1$ using an appropriate similarity index. Both molecules B and C are now aligned to molecule A. Keeping their positions relative to molecule A fixed, compute $S_X(F_B,F_C)^*$, which is not necessarily equal to the optimized solution, that is, $S_X(F_B,F_C)^* \neq S_X(F_B,F_C)^1$. Pairwise consistency holds only in the case when equality obtains, otherwise the solutions are said to be pairwise inconsistent. Sometimes pairwise consistency is obtained when one of the lower similarity solutions is considered, say, for example, $S_X(F_A,F_C)^2$. In such cases, the alignments given by $S_X(F_A,F_B)^1$, $S_X(F_A,F_B)^2$, and $S_X(F_B,F_C)^* = S_X(F_B,F_C)^1$ are assumed to be the correct alignments. In many cases, it is not possible to identify pairwise consistent sets of solutions. In such cases, the fields of three molecules are *simultaneously aligned* using the average of the pairwise similarities

$$S_X(F_A,F_B,F_C) = \tfrac{1}{3}\big[S_X(F_A,F_B) + S_X(F_A,F_C) + S_X(F_B,F_C)\big]. \qquad (2.91)$$

This procedure automatically generates pairwise consistent solutions, and it can be continued to higher orders until consistent solutions are obtained to all orders, a computationally very demanding task that has not been pursued in most cases because the ternary similarities are generally sufficient for molecular design purposes.

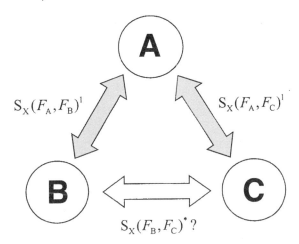

Fig. 7. Depiction of *pairwise consistency* among three molecules, A, B, and C.

2.5 Dissimilarity Measures

Dissimilarity is generally taken to be the complement of similarity, that is,

$$D(A,B) = 1 - S(A,B) .\tag{2.92}$$

Although this is mathematically reasonable, and is thus used extensively, psychologically the two concepts are not so simply related. This stems from the fact that assessing the similarity of two objects is easier than assessing their dissimilarity. As two objects become less and less similar, a point is reached, say, for a similarity value of 0.35, below which it is very difficult to assign a value to their similarity. Because dissimilarity is just the complement of similarity, it follows that humans can only properly assess the dissimilarity of two objects if they are not too dissimilar. Thus, even though we can assign dissimilarities ~1.0 using **Eq. 2.33**, its "meaning" is not easily grasped. This is why we have focused our discussion on similarity rather than dissimilarity, even though the concept of dissimilarity has important practical applications in studies of molecular diversity. Martin *(72)* has edited an interesting account of the development and implementation of the concepts of molecular dissimilarity and diversity in chemoinformatics and combinatorial chemistry.

3. Chemistry Spaces

This section on chemistry spaces, while important, is not presented with the same level of mathematical detail as given in earlier sections. The object here is to provide a general overview of some of the important characteristics of chemistry spaces. Cited references should be consulted for additional information.

The concept of a chemistry space derives from the notion of a space used in mathematics and is taken here to be a set of molecules along with one or more relationships defined on the set. The nature of a given chemistry space depends, directly or indirectly, on how the molecular information is represented (**Subheading 2.**); the representation used strongly influences what can be known about the set of molecules under study. *Unlike the case in physics, however, the underlying relationships in chemistry spaces are not invariant to representation.* For example, neighborhood relationships that obtain in one chemistry space may not also obtain in another chemistry space *(2,73)*. Thus, there is loss of topological invariance, which is much more severe than the loss of the purely geometric features such as the distances between molecules or the angles between vectors representing the locations of molecules in chemistry spaces, which may also occur. Loss of topological invariance can have dire consequences in subset selection procedures *(2)* because it can change the rank ordering of nearest neighbors.

3.1. Dimensionality of Chemistry Spaces

Chemistry spaces can be grouped into two broad classes, namely, *coordinate-based* and *coordinated-free*. In coordinate-based chemistry spaces molecules are represented as points distributed throughout the space as illustrated in **Fig. 8**. Points in close proximity are considered to represent similar molecules, while distant points represent dissimilar molecules. An important feature of coordinate-based chemistry spaces is that the *absolute position* of a molecule within the space is known, not just its position relative to the other molecules in the space. This is not the case with coordinate-free chemistry spaces. In such spaces the relationship of a given molecule to its near and far neighbors is known but not its location within the space. Thus, finding "compound voids" in a coordinate-free chemistry space is a much more difficult task than it is in a coordinate-based chemistry space (*vide infra*). An additional useful feature of coordinate-based chemistry spaces is their ability to portray the distribution of compounds in ways that, in many cases, can enhance our understanding of the space. However, as is seen in the following paragraph, the high dimensionality of these spaces can frustrate attempts to visualize them.

The dimension of a coordinate-based chemistry space is simply the number of independent variables used to define the space. As seen in earlier discussions, the dimension of such spaces can be quite large, and there are a significant number of examples where the dimension can exceed one million *(27,38)*. Even for spaces of much lower dimension, say around 10 or greater, the effects of the *curse of dimensionality (74,75)* can be felt. Bishop *(76)* provides an excellent example, which shows that the ratio of the volume of a hypersphere inscribed in a unit hypercube of the same dimension goes to zero as the dimen-

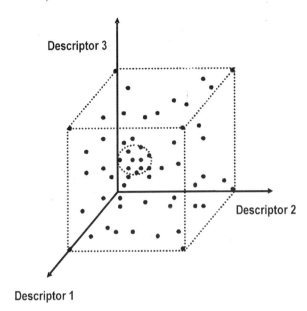

Fig. 8. In coordinate-based chemistry space points in close proximity are considered to be similar. For instance, the compounds within the sphere shown here are quite similar to each other compared to compounds in the extremities of this 3-D chemistry space.

sionality goes to infinity. Actually, even for the 10-dimensional case, the volume of the hypersphere is less than 10% of that of the corresponding hypercube. In addition, most of the spaces of extremely high dimension are discrete, a feature that can present additional problems (*vide infra*). This is not the case in coordinate-free chemistry spaces. Moreover, it is possible in such spaces to rigorously construct coordinates within a Euclidean space (the embedding problem) for any set of molecules in the space. The caveat is that faithfully representing the intermolecular proximities may require that the space may be of quite high dimension, possibly equal to one less than the number of molecules in the set, although this would be a very extreme case. As will be discussed in the following section, a number of methods exist for constructing low-dimensional Euclidean spaces for both high dimensional coordinate-based and coordinate-free representations of molecules.

3.1.1. Constructing Reduced-Dimension Chemistry Spaces

This section provides a brief discussion on the construction of reduced-dimension chemistry spaces for sets of molecules described by coordinate-free or by high-dimensional coordinate-based representations. Inherently low-dimensional

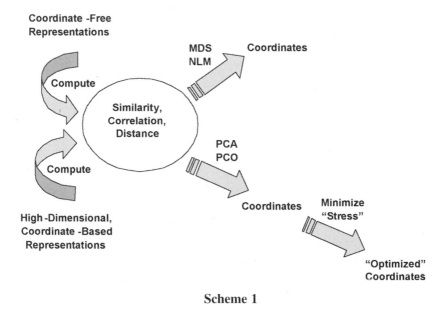

Scheme 1

chemistry spaces such as those generated, for example, by BCUT descriptors are not considered. It is important to note that all of the issues surrounding the inherent non-orthogonality of coordinate systems described in **Subheading 2.3.2.** are applicable here as well, and that section should be consulted for further details.

Scheme 1 illustrates the various routes for the "construction" of reduced-dimension coordinate systems. As is seen in the scheme, similarity, correlation, or distance play a central role in the process. The first step in reducing the dimension of either coordinate-free or high-dimensional coordinate-based representations is computation of some proximity measure of the similarity, correlation, or distance between all the pairs of molecules in the set of interest. This can be accomplished using the methods described earlier in this work. For example, in the coordinate-free case (N.B. that this is a bit of a misnomer in some cases because, for example, the functions used in 3-D field-based similarity matching are essentially infinite-dimensional vectors) similarity can be computed using the graph-theoretical approach described in **Subheading 2.1.**, the field-based approach described in **Subheading 2.4.**, or other less well-known approaches such as shape-group *(77)* and feature-tree *(78)* methods. In high-dimensional coordinate-based cases all of the vector-based approaches described in **Subheadings 2.2.** and **2.3.** are applicable.

Once a proximity measure has been computed for all of the molecules, basically two paths exist for determining a lower-dimensional coordinate-based representation. In the upper path in **Scheme 1** coordinates are determined using either multidimensional scaling (MDS) *(79)* or non-linear mapping (NLM) *(80)* procedures, both of which require minimization of some sort of error function. In the past, both procedures were somewhat limited and could only deal effectively with datasets of less than approx 2000 molecules. In addition, they encountered difficulty in treating new sets of compounds that were not included in the original set without redoing the calculations for the entire augmented set. These limitations have been removed by the work of Agrafiotis and his colleagues *(81,82)*, who developed a clever neural-net approach that learned the non-linear mapping based on the use of training sets of relatively small sample size (approx 1000 compounds). Once the mapping function was learned, new compounds can be mapped with relative ease.

The lower path is somewhat more complicated. The first step in the path involves either PCA *(83)* or principal-coordinate analysis (PCO) *(83)*. This step can be followed by optimization of a function that minimizes the error between the proximity measure computed in the reduced-dimension and full coordinate systems if desired. Xie et al. *(84)* recently published an interesting paper along these lines. Kruscal stress *(79)* is a widely used function in this regard

$$K_{stress} = \sqrt{\frac{\sum_i \sum_{j>i} (\hat{d}_{i,j} - d_{i,j})^2}{\sum_i \sum_{j>i} \hat{d}_{i,j}^2}} \quad , \tag{3.1}$$

where $\hat{d}_{i,j}$ is the distance computed in the reduced-dimension space and $d_{i,j}$ is the distance computed in the full space.

PCA is designed to deal directly with correlation matrices, but not directly with similarity or distance matrices. However, as pointed out by Kruscal *(85)*, the similarity matrix (or other proximity matrix) can be treated as a normal data matrix upon which principal component analysis is performed, that is,

$$\mathbf{S} \underset{\substack{\text{mean}\\\text{center}\\\text{columns}}}{\Rightarrow\Rightarrow} \mathbf{\bar{S}} \underset{\substack{\text{form}\\\text{matrix}\\\text{product}}}{\Rightarrow\Rightarrow} \mathbf{\bar{S}^T\bar{S}} \underset{\substack{\text{diagonalize}\\\text{matrix}}}{\Rightarrow\Rightarrow} \mathbf{V^T \left(\bar{S}^T\bar{S}\right) V = \Lambda} \; , \tag{3.2}$$

where the columns of the eigenvector matrix $\mathbf{V}$ are the principal components and the elements of the diagonal matrix Λ are the corresponding eigenvalues. The coordinates in the transformed, PC coordinate system, usually called the "scores," are given by the matrix $\mathbf{T}$, where

$$\mathbf{T} = \mathbf{\bar{S}V} \; . \tag{3.3}$$

PCO *(83)* works in an analogous fashion except that the similarity matrix is used directly without the additional multiplications given in **Eq. 3.2**. Gower has described the relationship between PCA and PCO *(86)*. Because both approaches utilize matrix diagonalization procedures, the size systems that they can practically treat are limited to approx 2000 molecules. This computational obstacle can be overcome for PCA using one of the neural-net methods for determining principal components *(87)*. Benigni and Giuliani *(88)* described an analogous method based on a matrix of Euclidean distances computed from high-dimensional vectors representing a set of molecules. Analogous dissimilarity-based methods have also been developed.

An important question is whether the proximity measures are compatible with those of these references addresses the important issue of whether the proximity measure is compatible with embedding in a Euclidean space. For example, satisfying the distance axioms does not in itself guarantee that any distance matrix associated with a given set of molecules be compatible as the distance axioms are still satisfied in a non-Euclidean space. Gower has written extensively on this important issue, and his work should be consulted for details *(89–91)*. Benigni *(92)*, and Carbó *(67)* have also contributed interesting approaches in this area.

4. Summary and Conclusions

This chapter provides an overview of the mathematics that underlies many of the similarity measures used in chemoinformatics. Each similarity measure is made up of two key elements: (1) A mathematical representation of the relevant molecular information and (2) some form of similarity index or coefficient that is compatible with the representation. The mathematical forms typically used are sets, graphs, vectors, and functions, and each is discussed at length in this chapter.

As was described in **Subheading 2.1.**, chemical graphs are a subclass of mathematical graphs, and thus many of the features of the latter can be taken over to the former. A number of graph metrics, such as the size of a graph and the distance between two graphs, have been applied to chemical graphs. In addition, similarity measures, such as the Tanimoto similarity index, also have their corresponding graph-theoretical analogs and have been used in a number of cases, albeit on relatively small sets of molecules. Although chemical graphs are the most familiar and intuitive representation of molecular information to chemists, they have been used relatively rarely in MSA, primarily due to computational difficulties brought on by the need to evaluate the MCS, an NP-complete computational problem that is required by most graph-based distance and similarity measures.

Subheading 2.2. describes the properties of discrete-valued feature vectors, with components given by finite, ordered sets of values. The most prevalent class is that of vectors with binary-valued components, which are mathematically equivalent to classical sets. Here features are either in the set (component value of "1") or not in the set (component value of "0"). Because we are essentially dealing with sets, the distance and similarity measures used are typically related to set measures (i.e., cardinalities) and not to the types of inner (scalar) products defined on linear vector spaces. A hypercubic mathematical space can be associated with classical sets, where the dimension of the space is equal to the number of elements in the universal set and each vertex of the hypercube corresponds to a subset, including the null and universal sets. Distances in these spaces are appropriately Hamming distances that satisfy an l_1 metric. Although Euclidean distances are sometimes used, they are inappropriate in such hypercubic spaces. Most similarity indices are taken to be symmetric ("A is as similar to B as B is similar to A"), but Tversky defined an infinite family of asymmetric indices related to the Tanimoto similarity index, some of which may be useful for similarity-related tasks such as similarity searching.

Another class of discrete-valued feature vectors useful in MSA is integer- and categorical-valued feature vectors. Here the vectors are mathematically equivalent to multisets and not directly to classical sets, although multisets can be reformulated as classical sets. The components of the vectors now indicate the number of times a given feature occurs or the ordered set of categorical values corresponding to the given feature or property. Although care must be taken, distance and similarity measures analogous to those used for binary-valued vector components can be used here as well.

In **Subheading 2.3.** the important class of vectors with continuous-valued components is described. A number of issues arise in this case. Importantly, since the objects of concern here are vectors, the mathematical operations employed are those applied to vectors such as addition, multiplication by a scalar, and formation of inner products. While distances between vectors are used in similarity studies, inner products are the most prevalent type of terms found in MSA. Such similarities, usually associated with the names Carbó and Hodgkin, are computed as ratios, where the inner product term in the numerator is normalized by a term in the denominator that is some form of mean (e.g., geometric or arithmetic) of the norms of the two vectors.

The notion of an orthogonal set of "basis vectors" is also of significance here and is particularly important because, as discussed in **Subheading 2.3.2.**, it is in many instances ignored. In a non-orthogonal basis the associated similarity matrix defines the metric of the space in which the vectors "live." Thus, "measurements" such as the distance or the angle between two vectors in the space are dependent on the metric of that space. **Subheading 2.3.4.** describes a general approach for dealing with non-orthogonal bases and explores some of the consequences of ignoring non-orthogonality. While most of the discussion deals with substructural descriptors, the method can also deal with physico-chemical, topological, or other such descriptors. However, in these cases the correlation matrix replaces the similarity matrix.

Subheading 2.4. addresses the use of field-based functions in MSA. Field-based functions, which can be thought of as infinite-dimensional vectors, are used primarily in 3-D MSA. Here, molecular fields (e.g., steric or electrostatic) or pseudo-fields (e.g., lipophilic) of the molecules being compared are matched, using various similarity measures, the most popular being those of Carbó or Hodgkin. Conformational flexibility adds a new degree of difficulty to studies of 3-D molecular similarity, and this has been dealt with in a number of ways. The most widespread approach is by standard conformational analysis. Because such an analysis leads to many conformations, clustering is usually used to group the conformations as a basis for identifying a smaller set of prototypical conformations. Molecular similarity is then carried out by pairwise matching the fields generated by each conformational prototype in one molecule with each conformational prototype in the other molecule being compared. This represents a rather substantial computational problem that has been ameliorated somewhat using Fourier transforms to separate translational from rotational motions in the optimization process. Alternatively, several procedures have been developed that combine conformational analysis with 3-D similarity matching simultaneously in the optimization process. Both approaches are, however, computationally demanding although the latter is somewhat better in this regard. In either case, the need to assess the consistency of the 3-D alignment solutions is paramount, and this is dealt with in **Subheading 2.4.4.**

Subheading 2.5. provides a very brief discussion of molecular dissimilarity measures that are basically the complement of their corresponding molecular similarity measures. This section also presents reasons as to why similarity is preferred over dissimilarity, except in studies of diversity, as a measure of molecular resemblance.

The concept of chemistry space pervades, either explicitly or implicitly, much of the literature in chemoinformatics. As is discussed in **Subheading 3.**, chemistry spaces are induced by various similarity measures. The different similarity measures do not, however, give rise to topologically equivalent chemistry spaces—nearest-neighbor relations are generally not preserved among chemistry spaces induced by different similarity measures. The consequences of this are manifold. An especially egregious consequence is that the results of similarity searches based on different similarity measures can differ substantially. And there is no easy solution to this problem.

Chemistry spaces fall into two broad categories, coordinate-based and coordinate-free. Coordinate-based chemistry spaces tend to be of high dimension and thus cannot be visualized directly. Coordinate-free chemistry spaces cannot be visualized directly since coordinates do not exist. In both cases it is possible to develop reduced-dimension representations that are easier to work with theoretically and also afford possibilities for visualization. Dimensionality reduction is a difficult problem that pervades many fields, and methods developed in these fields have proved useful in chemoinformatics, albeit to varying degrees.

Molecular similarity analysis has developed substantially over the years, especially as digital computers became faster, more compact, and widely available to scientists. Handling large sets of molecules is generally not a problem. The main problem confronting MSA is the problem of the lack of topological invariance of the chemistry spaces induced by the various similarity measures. Unfortunately, this problem may be fundamentally related to the inherent subjectivity of similarity and thus cannot be addressed in any simple manner.

5. Appendix—A New Notation for Classical Sets

Sets are very general mathematical objects that are used in many branches of mathematics. Here the focus is on *finite* sets, that is, sets with a finite set of elements. A key concept in set theory is that of the *universal set*, U, sometimes called the *universe of discourse*, which is an unordered collection of n elements $x_1, x_2, \ldots, x_k, \ldots, x_n$ and is given by

$$U = \{x_1, x_2, \ldots, x_k, \ldots, x_n\}. \tag{5.1}$$

All sets in this "universe," including U and the null or empty set $\varnothing$, are subsets of U. A subset A is typically written as, for example,

$$A = \{x_1, x_3, x_9, x_{12}, x_{17}, x_{18}, \ldots\}, \tag{5.2}$$

but this notation can become awkward and cumbersome for large, complex sets. A more general and powerful notation, which utilizes the concept of a *characteristic function*, $A(x_k)$, is illustrate in **Eq. 5.3**:

$$A = \{A(x_1), A(x_2), \ldots, A(x_k), \ldots, A(x_n)\}, \tag{5.3}$$

where $A(x_k)$ characterizes the membership of each element in the set and is given by

$$A(x_k) = \begin{cases} 1 \text{ if } x_k \in A \\ 0 \text{ if } x_k \notin A \end{cases}. \tag{5.4}$$

Thus, in the universal set $A(x_k) = 1$ for $k = 1, 2, \ldots, n$, that is, all elements of the universal set have a membership-function value of unity.

Note that this representation differs from that usually used (*see* **Eq. 5.2**) where only those elements actually in the set, that is, those elements for which $A(x_k) = 1$, are included explicitly. All possible sets A, including the empty and universal sets ∅ and U, are subsets of U, i.e., A ⊆ U. Although this notation may be unfamiliar, it is completely equivalent to that used for binary vectors or "bit vectors." Fuzzy sets, although not treated in this chapter, can also be represented in this notation with the modification that elements of the set are no longer confined to the binary values {0,1}; fuzzy sets can take on all values between and including zero and unity *(41)*.

A number of useful operations between two sets, A and B, are given in the notation introduced above:

$$A \cap B = \min_k [A(x_k), B(x_k)] \qquad \text{Set Intersection} \qquad (5.5)$$

$$A \cup B = \max_k [A(x_k), B(x_k)] \qquad \text{Set Union} \qquad (5.6)$$

$$A^c = \{1 - A(x_1), 1 - A(x_2), ..., 1 - A(x_n)\}$$
$$= \{A^c(x_1), A^c(x_2), ..., A^c(x_n)\} \qquad \text{Set Complementation} \quad (5.7)$$

$$A - B = A \cap B^c = \min_k [A(x_k), 1 - B(x_k)]$$
$$= \min_k [A(x_k), B^c(x_k)] \qquad \text{Set Difference} \qquad (5.8)$$

$$A \subseteq B = A(x_k) \le B(x_k) \text{ for all } k \qquad \text{Subsethood} \qquad (5.9)$$

$$|A| = \sum_k A(x_k) \qquad \text{Cardinality} - \text{Set} \qquad (5.10)$$

$$|A \cap B| = \sum_k \min[A(x_k), B(x_k)] \qquad \text{Cardinality} - \text{Set Intersection} (5.11)$$

$$|A \cup B| = \sum_k \max[A(x_k), B(x_k)] \qquad \text{Cardinality} - \text{Set Union} \quad (5.12)$$

$$|A| = |A - B| + |A \cap B| \qquad \text{Cardinality} - \text{Set} \qquad (5.13)$$

$$|A \cup B| = |A| + |B| - |A \cap B| \qquad \text{Cardinality} - \text{Set Union} \quad (5.14)$$

$$|A \cup B| = |A - B| + |B - A| + |A \cap B| \qquad \text{Cardinality} - \text{Set Union} \quad (5.15)$$

Relations, which are also sets, play an important role in set theory and in the similarity theory, but due to space limitations are not formally considered in this work.

Acknowledgment

The authors would like to thank Dr. Tom Doman for his constructive comments on this manuscript.

References

1. Rouvray, D. (1990) The evolution of the concept of molecular similarity. In *Concepts and applications of molecular similarity*, Johnson, M. A. and Maggiora, G. M. (eds.), John Wiley & Sons, New York, Chapter 2.
2. Sheridan, R. P. and Kearsley, S. K. (2002) Why do we need so many chemical similarity search methods? *Drug Discovery Today* **7**, 903–911.
3. Willett, P. (1987) *Similarity and clustering in chemical information systems.* Research Studies Press, Letchworth.
4. Johnson, M. A. and Maggiora, G. M. (eds.) (1990) *Concepts and applications of molecular similarity.* John Wiley & Sons, New York.
5. Dean, P. M. (ed.) (1994) *Molecular similarity in drug design.* Chapman & Hall, Glasgow.
6. Tversky, A. (1977) Features of similarity. *Pyschol. Rev.* **84**, 327–352.
7. Willett, P., Barnard, J. P., and Downs, G. M. (1998) Chemical similarity searching. *J. Chem. Inf. Comput. Sci.* **38**, 983–996.
8. Johnson, M. A. (1989) A review and examination of mathematical spaces underlying molecular similarity analysis. *J. Math. Chem.* **3**, 117–145.
9. Borg, I. and Groenen, P. (1997) *Modern multidimensional scaling.* Springer, New York.
10. Jolliffe, I. T. (2002) *Principal component analysis*, 2nd ed. Springer, New York.
11. Domine, D., Devillers, J., Chastrette, M., and Karcher, W. (1993). Non-linear mapping for structure-activity and structure-property modeling. *J. Chemometrics* **7**, 227–242.
12. Rush, J. A. (1999) Cell-based methods for sampling high-dimensional spaces. In *Rational drug design*, Truhlar, D. G., Howe, W. J., et al. (eds.), Springer, New York, pp. 73–79.
13. Rohrbaugh, R. H. and Jurs, P. C. (1987) Descriptions of molecular shape applied in studies of structure/activity and structure/property relationships. *Anal. Chim. Acta* **199**, 99–109.
14. Verloop, A. (1987) *The STERIMOL approach to drug design.* Marcel Dekker, New York.
15. Mulliken, R. S. (1955) Electronic population analysis on LCAO-MO molecular wave functions. I. *J. Chem. Phys.* **23**, 1833–1840.
16. Stanton, D. T. and Jurs, P. C. (1990) Development and use of charged partial surface area structural descriptors in computer-assisted quantitative structure-property relationship studies. *Anal. Chem.* **62**, 2323–2329.
17. Kier, L. B. (1989) An index of molecular flexibility from kappa shape attributes. *Quant. Struct.-Act. Relat.* **8**, 221–224
18. Kvasnička, V. and Pospíchal, J. (1989) Two metrics for a graph-theoretical model of organic chemistry. *J. Math. Chem.* **3**, 161–191.
19. Kvasnička, V. and Pospíchal, J. (1991) Chemical and reaction metrics for graph-theoretical model of organic chemistry. *J. Mol. Struct. (Theochem.)* **227**, 17–42.
20. Randić, M. (1992) Representation of molecular graphs by basic graphs. *J. Chem. Inf. Comput. Sci.* **32**, 57–69.

21. Baskin, I. I., Skvortsova, M. I., Stankevich, I. V., and Zefirov, N. S. (1995) On the basis of invariants of labeled molecular graphs. *J. Chem. Inf. Comput. Sci.* **35,** 527–531.
22. Skvortsova, M. I., Baskin, I. I., Stankevich, I. V., Palyulin, V. A., and Zefirov, N. S. (1998) Molecular similarity. I. Analytical description of the set of graph similarity measures. *J. Chem. Inf. Comput. Sci.* **38,** 785–790.
23. Ginn, C. M. R., Willett, P., and Bradshaw, J. (2000) Combination of molecular similarity measures using data fusion. *Perspec. Drug Disc. Design* **20,** 1–16.
24. Trinajstić, N. (1992) *Chemical graph theory.* CRC Press, Boca Raton, FL.
25. Harary, F. (1969) *Graph theory.* Addison-Wesley Publishing Company, Reading, MA.
26. Raymond, J. W. and Willett, P. (2002) Maximum common subgraph isomorphism algorithms for the matching of chemical structures. *J. Comput.-Aided Mol. Design* **16,** 521–533.
27. Mason, J. S., Morize, I., Menard, P. R., Cheney, D. L., Hulme, C., and Labaudiniere, R. F. (1999) New 4-point pharmacophore method for molecular similarity and diversity applications: overview of the method and applications, including a novel approach to the design of combinatorial libraries containing privileged substructures. *J. Med. Chem.* **42,** 3251–3264.
28. Devillers, J. and Balaban, A. T. (eds.) (1999) *Topological indices and related descriptors in QSAR and QSPR.* Gordon and Breach Science Publishers, Amsterdam, The Netherlands.
29. Pearlman, R. S. and Smith, K. M. (1998) Novel software tools for chemical diversity. *Perspec. Drug Disc. Design* **9/10/11,** 339–353.
30. Mestres, J., Rohrer, D. C., and Maggiora, G. M. (1997) MIMIC: A molecular-field matching program. Exploiting applicability of molecular similarity approaches. *J. Comput. Chem.* **18,** 934–954.
31. Thorner, D. A., Willett, P., Wright, P. M., and Taylor, R. (1997) Similarity searching in files of three-dimensional chemical structures: Representation and searching of molecular electrostatic potentials using field-graphs. *J. Comput.-Aided Mol. Design* **11,** 163–174.
32. Du, Q., Arteca, G. A., and Mezey, P. G. (1997) Heuristic lipophilicity potential for computer-aided rational drug design. *J. Comput.-Aided Mol. Design* **11,** 503–515.
33. Petke, J. D. (1993) Cumulative and discrete similarity analysis of electrostatic potentials and fields. *J. Comput. Chem.* **14,** 928–933.
34. Cramer, R. D., Patterson, D. E., and Bunce, J. D. (1988) Comparative molecular field analysis (CoMFA). 1. Effect of shape on binding of steroids to carrier proteins. *J. Amer. Chem. Soc.* **110,** 5959–5967.
35. McGregor, J. and Willett, P. (1981) Use of a maximal common subgraph algorithm in the automatic identification of the ostensible bond changes occurring in chemical reactions. *J. Chem. Inf. Comput. Sci.* **21,** 137–140.
36. Johnson, M. (1985) Relating metrics, lines, and variables defined on graphs to problems in medicinal chemistry. In *Graph theory and its applications to algorithms and computer science,* Alavi, Y., et al. (eds.), John Wiley & Sons, New York, pp. 457–470.

37. Hagadone, T. R. (1992) Molecular substructure similarity searching: Efficient retrieval in two-dimensional structure databases. *J. Chem. Inf. Comput. Sci.* **32,** 515–521.
38. Rusinko, A., Farmen, M. W., Lambert, C. G., and Young, S. S. (1997) SCAM: Statistical classification of activities of molecules using recursive partitioning. 213th ACS Natl. Meeting, San Francisco, CA, CINF 068.
39. James, C. A., Weininger, D., and Delany, J. (2002) *Daylight theory manual.* Daylight Chemical Information Systems, Inc.
40. Kanerva, P. (1990) *Sparse distributed memory.* MIT Press, Cambridge, MA, pp. 26–27.
41. Klir, G. J. and Yuan, B. (1995) *Fuzzy sets and fuzzy logic: theory and applications.* Prentice Hall PTR, Upper Saddle River, NJ.
42. Miyamoto, S. (1990) *Fuzzy sets in information retrieval and cluster analysis.* Kluwer Academic Publishers, Dordrecht, The Netherlands.
43. Maggiora, G. M., Petke, J. D., and Mestres, J. (2002) A general analysis of field-based molecular similarity indices. *J. Math. Chem.* **31,** 251–270.
44. Hurst, T. and Heritage, T. (1997) HQSAR—A highly predictive QSAR technique based on molecular holograms. 213th ACS Natl. Meeting, San Francisco, CA, CINF 019.
45. Schneider, G., Neidhart, W., Giller, T., and Schmid, G. (1999) "Scaffold-hopping" by topological pharmacophore search: A contribution to virtual screening. *Angew. Chem. Int. Ed.* **38,** 2894–2896.
46. Xue, L., Godden, J. W., and Bajorath, J. (1999) Database searching for compounds with similar biological activity using short binary bit string representations of molecules. *J. Chem. Inf. Comput. Sci.* **39,** 881–886.
47. Hyvarinen, A., Karhunen, J., and Oja, E. (2001) *Independent component analysis.* John Wiley & Sons, New York.
48. Kay, D. C. (1988) *Theory and problems of tensor calculus, Schaum's Outline Series.* McGraw-Hill, New York.
49. Hodgkin, E. E. and Richards, W. G. (1987) Molecular similarity based on electrostatic potential and electric fields. *Int. J. Quantum Chem.: Quantum Biol. Symp.* **14,** 105–110.
50. Szabo, A. and Ostlund, N. S. (1982) *Modern quantum chemistry—introduction to advanced electronic structure theory.* Macmillan Publishing Company, New York.
51. Löwdin, P. O. (1992) On linear algebra, the least square method, and the search for linear relations by regression analysis in quantum chemistry and other sciences. *Adv. Quantum Chem.* **23,** 83–126.
52. Carlson, B. C. and Keller, J. M. (1957) Orthogonalization procedures and the localization of Wannier functions. *Phys. Rev.* **105,** 102–103.
53. Agrafiotis, D. K., Rassokhin, D. N., and Lobanov, V. S. (2001) Multi-dimensional scaling and visualization of large molecular similarity tables. *J. Comput. Chem.* **22,** 1–13.
54. Kauvar, L. M., Higgins, D. L., Villar, H. O., et al. (1995) Predicting ligand binding to proteins by affinity fingerprinting. *Chemistry & Biology* **2,** 107–118.

55. Randic, M. (1991) Resolution of ambiguities in structure-property studies by use of orthogonalized descriptors. *J. Chem. Inf. Comput. Sci.* **31,** 311–320.

56. Randic, M. (1991) Correlation of enthalpy of octanes with orthogonal connectivity indices. *J. Mol. Struct. (Theochem.)* **233,** 45–59.

57. Randic, M. (1993) Fitting non-linear regressions by orthogonalized power series. *J. Comput. Chem.* **14,** 363–370.

58. Lemmen, C. and Lengauer, T. (2000) Computational methods for the structural alignment of molecules. *J. Comput.-Aided Mol. Design* **14,** 215–232.

59. Güner, O. F. (ed.) (2000) *Pharmacophore perception, development and use in drug design.* International University Line, La Jolla, CA.

60. Mansfield, M. L., Covell, D. G., and Jernigan, R. L. (2002) A new class of molecular shape descriptors. Theory and properties. *J. Chem. Inf. Comput. Sci.* **42,** 259–273.

61. Blinn, J. R., Rohrer, D. C., and Maggiora, G. M. (1998) Field-based similarity forcing in energy minimization and molecular matching. In *Pacific symposium on biocomputing '99*, Altman, R. B., et al. (eds.), World Scientific, Singapore, pp. 415–424.

62. Labute, P. (1999) Flexible alignment of small molecules. *J. Chem. Comput. Group,* Spring 1999 Edition [http://www.chemcomp.com/feature/malign.htm].

63. Christoffersen, R. E. and Maggiora, G. M. (1969) *Ab initio* calculations on large molecules using molecular fragments. Preliminary investigations. *Chem. Phys. Letts.* **3,** 419–423.

64. Kearsley, S. K. and Smith, G. M. (1990) An alternative method for the alignment of molecular structures: Maximizing electrostatic and steric overlap. *Tetrahedron Comput. Meth.* **3,** 615–633.

65. Lemmen, C., Hiller, C., and Lengauer, T. (1998) RigFit: A new approach to superimposing ligand molecules. *J. Comput.-Aided Mol. Design* **12,** 491–502.

66. Good, A. C., Hodgkin, E. E., and Richards, W. G. (1992) Utilization of Gaussian functions for the rapid evaluation of molecular similarity. *J. Chem. Inf. Comput. Sci.* **32,** 188–191.

67. Carbó, R. and Calabuig, B. (1990) Molecular similarity and quantum chemistry. In *Concepts and applications of molecular similarity*, Johnson, M. A. and Maggiora, G. M. (eds.),Wiley-Interscience, New York, pp. 147–171.

68. Petitjean, M. (1995) Geometric molecular similarity from volume based distance minimization: Application to Saxitoxin and Tetrodotoxin. *J. Comput. Chem.* **16,** 80–90.

69. Petitjean, M. (1996) Three-dimensional pattern recognition from molecular distance minimization. *J. Chem. Inf. Comput. Sci.* **36,** 1038–1049.

70. Nissink, J. W. M., Verdonk, M. L., Kroon, J., Mietzner, T., and Klebe, G. (1997) Superposition of molecules: Electron density fitting by application of Fourier transforms. *J. Comput. Chem.* **18,** 638–645.

71. Mestres, J., Rohrer, D. C., and Maggiora, G. M. (1999) A molecular-field-based similarity study of non-nucleoside HIV-1 reverse transcriptase inhibitors. *J. Comput.-Aided Mol. Design* **13,** 79–93.

72. Martin, Y. C. (2001) Diverse viewpoints on computational aspects of molecular diversity. *J. Comb. Chem.* **3,** 231–250.
73. Patterson, D. E., Cramer, R. D., Ferguson, A. M., Clark, R. D., and Weinberger, L. E. (1996) Neighborhood behavior: A useful concept for validation of molecular diversity. *J. Med. Chem.* **39,** 3049–3059.
74. Bellman, R. E. (1961) *Adaptive control processes.* Princeton University Press, Princeton, NJ.
75. Hastie, T., Tibshirani, R., and Friedman, J. (2001) *The elements of statistical learning.* Springer, New York.
76. Bishop, C. (1995) *Neural networks for pattern recognition.* Clarendon Press, Oxford.
77. Walker, P. D., Maggiora, G. M., Johnson, M. A., Petke, J. D., and Mezey, P. G. (1995) Shape group-analysis of molecular similarity—Shape similarity of 6-membered aromatic ring-systems. *J. Chem. Inf. Comput. Sci.* **35,** 568–578.
78. Rarey, M. and Dixon, J. S. (1998) Feature trees: A new molecular similarity measure based on tree matching. *J. Comput.-Aided Mol. Design* **12,** 471–490.
79. Borg, I. and Groenen, P. (1997) *Modern multidimensional scaling—theory and applications.* Springer, New York.
80. Domine, D., Devillers, J., Chastrette, M., and Karcher, W. (1993) Non-linear mapping for structure-activity and structure-property modelling. *J. Chemometrics* **7,** 227–242.
81. Agrafiotis, D. K. and Lobanov, V. S. (2000) Nonlinear mapping networks. *J. Chem. Inf. Comput. Sci.* **40,** 1356–1362.
82. Rassokhin, D., Lobanov, V. S., and Agrafiotis, D. K. (2000) Nonlinear mapping of massive data sets by fuzzy clustering and neural networks. *J. Comput. Chem.* **21,** 1–14.
83. Jolliffe, I. T. (2002) *Principal Component Analysis*, Second Edition. Springer, New York.
84. Xie, D., Tropsha, A., and Schlick, T. (2000) An efficient projection protocol for chemical databases: Singular value decomposition combined with truncated-Newton minimization. *J. Chem. Inf. Comput. Sci.* **40,** 167–177.
85. Kruskal, J. (1977) The relationship between multidimensional scaling and clustering. In *Classification and Clustering*, Van Ryzin, J. (ed.), Academic Press, New York.
86. Gower, J. C. (1966) Some distance properties of latent root and vector methods used in multivariate analysis. *Biometrika* **53,** 325–338.
87. Diamantaras, K. I. and Kung, S. Y. (1996) *Principal component neural networks—theory and applications.* John Wiley & Sons, New York.
88. Benigni, R. and Giuliani, A. Analysis of distance matrices for studying data structures and separating classes. *Struct.-Act. Relat.* **12,** 397–401.
89. Gower, J. C. (1971) A general coefficient of similarity and some of its properties. *Biometrics* **27,** 857–874.

90. Gower, J. C. (1984) Distance matrices and their Euclidean approximation. In *Data analysis and informatics, III*, Diday, E., et al. (eds.), Elsevier Science Publishers B.V. (North-Holland), The Netherlands.
91. Gower, J. C. and Legendre, P. (1986) Metric and Euclidean properties of dissimilarity coefficients. *J. Classific.* **3,** 5–48.
92. Benigni, R. (1994) EVE, a distance-based approach for discriminating non-linearly separable groups. *Quant. Struct.-Act. Relat.* **13,** 406–411.

2

Evaluation of Molecular Similarity and Molecular Diversity Methods Using Biological Activity Data

Peter Willett

Abstract

This chapter reviews the techniques available for quantifying the effectiveness of methods for molecular similarity and molecular diversity, focusing in particular on similarity searching and on compound selection procedures. The evaluation criteria considered are based on biological activity data, both qualitative and quantitative, with rather different criteria needing to be used depending on the type of data available.

Key Words: Chemical database; compound selection; library design; molecular diversity; molecular similarity; neighborhood behavior; similar property principle; similarity searching.

1. Introduction

The concepts of molecular similarity *(1–3)* and molecular diversity *(4,5)* play important roles in modern approaches to computer-aided molecular design. Molecular similarity provides the simplest, and most widely used, method for virtual screening and underlies the use of clustering methods on chemical databases. Molecular diversity analysis provides a range of tools for exploring the extent to which a set of molecules spans structural space, and underlies many approaches to compound selection and to the design of combinatorial libraries. Many different similarity and diversity methods have been described in the literature, and new methods continue to appear. This raises the question of how one can compare different methods, so as to identify the most appropriate method(s) for some particular application: this chapter provides an overview of the ways in which this can be carried out, illustrating such comparisons by,

From: *Methods in Molecular Biology, vol. 275:*
Chemoinformatics: Concepts, Methods, and Tools for Drug Discovery
Edited by: J. Bajorath © Humana Press Inc., Totowa, NJ

principally, our experience of similarity and diversity studies that have been carried out in the Chemoinformatics Research Group at the University of Sheffield.

There are two bases for the comparison of similarity and diversity methods. It is possible to compare the *efficiency* of methods, i.e., the resources, typically computer time and computer memory, necessary for the completion of processing. Considerations of efficiency, in particular, theoretical analyses of computational complexity, are important in that they can serve to identify methods that are unlikely to be applicable given the rapidly increasing sizes of current and planned chemical datasets. Here, however, we restrict ourselves to comparing the *effectiveness* of similarity and diversity methods, i.e., the extent to which a method is able to satisfy the user's requirements in terms of identifying similar or diverse sets of compounds. More specifically, we focus on evaluation criteria based on the availability of bioactivity data for the molecules that are being processed, where the data can either be *qualitative*, i.e., a categorical (usually binary) variable, or *quantitative*, i.e., a real-valued variable. The discussion here considers only the criteria that can be used for comparative studies: the reader is referred elsewhere for the results of such studies.

2. Methods

2.1. Molecular Similarity Methods

2.1.1. Introduction

The basic concept of molecular similarity has many applications *(1,2)*, but we focus here on its use for similarity-based virtual screening, which is often referred to as *similarity searching (3)*. Here, a user specifies a *target structure* that is characterized by one or more structural descriptors, and this set is compared with the corresponding sets of descriptors for each of the molecules in the database. These comparisons enable the calculation of a measure of similarity, i.e., the degree of structural relatedness, between the target structure and each of the database structures, and the latter are then sorted into order of decreasing similarity with the target. The output from the search is a ranked list in which the structures that are calculated to be most similar to the target structure, the *nearest neighbors*, are located at the top of the list. These neighbors form the initial output of the search and will be those that have the greatest probability of being of interest to the user, given an appropriate measure of intermolecular structural similarity.

Many different types of similarity measure have been discussed in the literature, but they generally involve three principal components: the *representation* that is used to characterize the molecules that are being compared; the *weighting scheme* that is used to assign differing degrees of importance to the various components of these representations; and the *similarity coefficient* that is used to provide a quantitative measure of the degree of structural relatedness between a pair of structural representations. These three components are closely related and, hence, it is most important that a comparative study should seek to ensure that only one of these components is varied at any one time. For example, only a limited amount of information might be gained from a comparison of the effectiveness of similarity searching using binary fingerprints (e.g., those produced by the UNITY or Daylight software) and the Tanimoto coefficient, with the effectiveness of similarity searching using a set of computed physicochemical parameters (e.g., those produced by the MOLCONN-Z or DiverseSolutions software), some particular standardization method and the Euclidean distance. Given an appropriate evaluation criterion (as discussed below), one might be able to decide that one of these approaches gave better results than the other, but one would not be able to identify the relative contributions of the various components of the overall similarity measures that were being studied.

The basis for all of the evaluation techniques to be discussed here is what is commonly referred to as the *similar-property principle*, which was first stated explicitly by Johnson and Maggiora in their seminal 1990 book *(1)*. The principle states that structurally similar molecules are expected to exhibit similar properties. It is clear that there are many exceptions to the principle as stated *(6,7)*, because even a small change in the structure of a molecule can bring about a radical change in some property; for example, replacement of a small alkyl group by a larger one, e.g., methyl replaced by *t*-butyl, can mean that a molecule is now too large to fit a binding site. The principle does, however, provide a general rule of thumb that is very widely applicable; indeed, if this were not the case, then it would prove difficult indeed to develop meaningful structure-activity relationships of any sort. If the principle does hold for a particular dataset, then the top-ranked molecules in a similarity search are expected to have properties that are related to those of the target structure. We can hence evaluate the effectiveness of a structurally based similarity procedure by the extent to which the similarities resulting from its use mirror similarities in some external property, which in the context of this chapter we take to be biological activity (but could be any type of chemical, biological, or physical property). The next two sections detail the ways in which the principle is applied to the analysis of qualitative and quantitative datasets.

2.1.2. Use of Qualitative Data

In what follows, we shall adopt ideas and terminology from that part of computer science that is normally referred to as *information retrieval (8–10)*. The measurement of search effectiveness has played a large part in the development of information retrieval (or IR) systems, whose principal aim is to identify as many documents as possible that are relevant to a user's query while simulta-

Table 1
**Contingency Table Describing the Output of a Search
in Terms of Active Molecules and Molecules Retrieved
in a Similarity Search Retrieving *n* Molecules**

		Active		
		Yes	No	
Retrieved	Yes	a	$n-a$	n
	No	$A-a$	$N-n-A+a$	$N-n$
		A	$N-A$	N

neously minimizing the number of non-relevant documents that are retrieved. It is possible to apply many of these measures to the evaluation of chemical retrieval systems, where one wishes to identify as many molecules as possible that have the same activity as the target structure while simultaneously minimizing the number of inactive molecules that are retrieved.

The relationship between IR and chemical similarity searching is discussed in detail by Edgar et al. *(11)* who summarize the various effectiveness measures in terms of the 2 × 2 contingency table shown in **Table 1**. In this table, it is assumed that a search has been carried out resulting in the retrieval of the *n* nearest neighbors at the top of the ranked output. Assume that these *n* nearest neighbors include *a* of the *A* active molecules in the complete database, which contains a total of *N* molecules. Then the *recall*, *R*, is defined to be the fraction of the active molecules that are retrieved, i.e.,

$$R = \frac{a}{A},$$

and the *precision*, *P*, is defined to be the fraction of the retrieved molecules that are active, i.e.,

$$P = \frac{a}{n}.$$

A retrieval mechanism should seek to maximize both the recall and the precision of a search so that, in the ideal case, a user would be presented with all of the actives in the database without any additional inactives: needless to say, this ideal is very rarely achieved in practice.

It is inconvenient to have to specify two measures, i.e., recall and precision, to quantify the effectiveness of a search. The Merck group have made extensive use of the *enrichment factor*, i.e., the number of actives retrieved relative to the number that would have been retrieved if compounds had been picked from the database at random *(12)*. Thus, using the notation of **Table 1**, the enrichment factor at some point, n, in the ranking resulting from a similarity search is given by

$$\frac{a/n}{A/N}.$$

Note that because A/N is a constant, the enrichment is monotonic with precision. Rather than specifying the enrichment at some specific point in the ranking, e.g., the top-1000 positions, it can alternatively be specified at that point where some specific fraction, e.g., 50%, of the actives have been retrieved. Examples of the use of enrichment factors are provided by Sheridan and colleagues *(12)* and Gillet et al. *(13)*.

Alternatively, Güner and Henry *(14)* have introduced the G-H score, which is a weighted average of recall and precision. The score was originally developed for evaluating the effectiveness of three-dimensional (3D) database searches but can be applied to the evaluation of any sort of search for which qualitative bioactivity data are available. Using the previous notation, the G-H score is defined to be

$$\frac{\alpha P + \beta R}{2},$$

where α and β are weights describing the relative importance of recall and precision. The lower bound for the G-H score is zero; if both weights are set to unity, then the score is simply the arithmetic mean of recall and precision, i.e.,

$$\frac{P + R}{2}.$$

Examples of the use of the G-H score are provided by Güner and Henry *(15)* and by Raymond and Willett *(16)*, while Edgar et al. discuss other combined measures that can be used for chemical similarity searching *(11)*.

At least three alternative approaches have been used widely. First, the Sheffield group has generally quoted the mean numbers of active compounds identified in some fixed number of the top-ranked nearest neighbors, when averaged over a set of searches for bioactive target structures. An early example of the use of this approach is a comparison of 3D similarity measures based on

Table 2
**Contingency Table Describing the Output of a Search
in Terms of Correctly and Incorrectly Predicted Molecules
in a Classification Experiment Classifying *n* Molecules**

		Classification		
		Active	Inactive	
Truth	Active	*i*	*j*	*i+j*
	Inactive	*k*	*l*	*k+l*
		i+k	*j+l*	*n*

interatomic distances *(17)*, with Briem and Lessel providing a more recent application in their extended comparison of virtual screening methods *(18)*. The use of a fixed cut-off means that this measure is basically a reformulation of precision, which is entirely acceptable in the early stages of a discovery program, when the immediate need is to identify additional active molecules; however, the measure takes no account of recall, which may be an important factor in a detailed comparative study of the behavior of different similarity measures. A second, and alternative, "leave-one-out" classification approach assumes that the activity of one of the molecules in the database, X, is unknown. A similarity search is carried out using X as the target structure and the top-x (where x is odd) nearest neighbors identified. The activity or inactivity of X is then predicted on the basis of a majority vote (hence the requirement for an odd number) of the known activities of the selected nearest neighbors. This process is repeated for each of the N molecules in turn (or just the A active molecules in many cases), yielding a contingency table of the sort shown in **Table 2**. Various statistics can be produced from the elements of this table: perhaps the most common is Cohen's kappa statistic *(19)*. This is defined to be

$$\frac{O-E}{1-E},$$

where O and E are the observed and expected accuracies of classification. These accuracies can be defined in terms of the elements of **Table 2** as follows:

$$O = \frac{i+l}{n}, \text{ and}$$

$$E = \frac{(i+k)(i+j)+(j+l)(k+l)}{n^2}.$$

There are many variants on this basic idea, such as the weighted kappa described by Cohen himself *(20)* and the Rand statistic *(21)*, which is perhaps the most widely used of the measures available for comparing different clusterings of the same set of objects.

Finally, it may be of interest to study the performance of a measure across the entire ranking resulting from a similarity search, rather than the performance for some fixed number of nearest neighbors. In this case, the most popular approach is the use of a *cumulative recall* graph, which plots the recall against the number of compounds retrieved (i.e., a/A against n using the notation of **Table 1**). The best-possible such graph would hence be one in which the A relevant documents are at the top of the ranking, i.e., at rank-positions 1, 2, 3, . . ., A (or at rank-positions, $N - A + 1$, $N - A + 2$, $N - A + 3$, . . ., N in the case of the worst-possible ranking). The use of such diagrams is exemplified by studies of similarity searching using physicochemical descriptors *(12)* and of a range of virtual screening methods for searching agrochemical datasets *(22)*. The cumulative recall plot is closely related to the *receiver operating characteristic* (ROC) curves that are widely used in signal detection and classification problems *(23)*. An ROC curve plots the true positives against the false positives for different classifications of the same set of objects; this corresponds to plotting a against $n - a$ using the notation of **Table 1**, and thus the shape of an ROC curve tends to the shape of a cumulative recall plot when $n \gg a$. An example of the use of ROC plots in chemoinformatics is provided by the work of Cuissart et al. on similarity-based methods for the prediction of biodegradability *(24)*.

2.1.3. Use of Quantitative Data

The similar property principle can also be applied to the analysis of datasets for which quantitative bioactivity data are available, most commonly using a simple modification of the "leave-one-out" classification approach described above. Here, the predicted property value for the target structure X, $P(X)$, is taken to be the arithmetic mean of the observed property values of the selected nearest neighbors. This procedure results in the calculation of a $P(X)$ value for each of the N structures in a dataset, and an overall figure of merit is then obtained by calculating the product moment correlation coefficient between the sets of N observed and N predicted values. This approach can equally well be applied to the evaluation of clustering methods, with the predicted values here being the mean of the other compounds in the cluster containing the chosen molecule, X.

This application of the similar property principle was pioneered by Adamson and Bush *(25,26)* and has since been very extensively applied. For example, Willett and Winterman used it in one of the first detailed comparisons of measures for similarity searching *(27)*, and it also formed the basis for Brown and

Martin's much-cited comparison of clustering methods and structural descriptors for compound selection *(28)*.

2.2. Molecular Diversity Methods

2.2.1. Introduction

The principal aim of molecular diversity analysis is to identify structurally diverse (synonyms are dissimilar, disparate, and heterogeneous) sets of compounds that can then be tested for bioactivity, the assumption being that a structurally diverse set will generate more structure-activity information than will a set of compounds identified at random. The sets of compounds can be selected from an existing corporate or public database, or can be the result of a systematic combinatorial library design process *(4,5)*.

Many of the comments that were made in **Subheading 2.1.1.** regarding similarity measures are equally applicable to diversity methods, in that the latter involve knowledge of the degree of dissimilarity or distance between pairs, or larger groups, of molecules. Here, however, there is also the need to specify a *selection algorithm*, which uses the computed dissimilarities to identify the final structurally diverse set of compounds, and there may also be a *diversity index*, which quantifies the degree of diversity in this set. It is thus important, as with similarity measures, to isolate the effect of the various components of the diversity methods that are being analyzed in a comparative study. There have been many such comparisons, e.g., **refs.** *28–33*. Here, we focus on diversity indices because it is these that measure the overall effectiveness of a method. (In fact, while an index is computed once a selection algorithm has completed its task, there are some types of algorithm that seek explicitly to optimize the chosen index, so that the current value of the index drives the operation of the selection algorithm.)

Many of the early evaluations of the effectiveness of diversity methods used structure-based diversity indices, such as functions of intermolecular dissimilarities in the context of distance-based selection methods or of the numbers of occupied cells in partition-based selection methods *(4)*. A wide range of such indices has been reported, as discussed in the excellent review by Waldman et al. *(34)*. They do, however, have the limitation that they quantify diversity in *chemical space*, whereas the principal rationale for molecular diversity methods is to maximize diversity in *biological space (35)*, and we hence focus here on indices that take account of biological activity.

2.2.2. General Screening Programs

We have noted the importance of the similar property principle, which would imply that a set of compounds exhibiting some degree of structural redundancy, i.e., containing molecules that are near neighbors of each other, will also exhibit some degree of biological redundancy; a structurally diverse subset, conversely, should maximize the number of types of activity exhibited by its constituent molecules. It should thus be possible to compare the effectiveness of different structure-based selection methods by the extent to which they result in subsets that exhibit as many as possible of the types of activity present in the parent dataset. Maximizing biological diversity in this way is the principal aim of general screening programs, which aim to select molecules from a database (or design combinatorial libraries for synthesis) that exhibit the widest possible range of different types of activity. An obvious measure of the diversity of the resulting compounds is hence the number of types of activity exhibited by them. This can be easily tested using one of the public databases that contain both chemical structures and pharmacological activities, such as the *MACCS Drug Data Report* (MDDR, at URL http://www.mdli.com/products/mddr.html) or the *World Drugs Index* (WDI, at URL http://www.derwent.com/worlddrug-index/index.html) databases. Thus, in one of the earliest studies of methods for comparing diverse database subsets, Snarey et al. compared a range of maximum dissimilarity and sphere exclusion methods for dissimilarity-based compound selection by means of the number of different types of activity present in subsets chosen from molecules in the WDI database *(31)*; this approach has been adopted in several subsequent studies.

2.2.3. Focused Screening Programs

In a focused screening program, the aim is to select molecules from a database (or design combinatorial libraries for synthesis) that provide the maximum amount of information about the relationships that exist between structural features and some specific type of biological activity. If these data are qualitative in nature, then a simple count of the active molecules present will suffice to quantify the degree of biological diversity. However, at least some account must additionally be taken of the chemical diversity that is present, to avoid a high level of diversity being ascribed to a cluster of highly similar molecules (such as "me too" or "fast follower" compounds in a drug database). An example of this approach is a comparison of binning schemes for cell-based compound selection by Bayley and Willett *(36)* that selected one molecule from each cell in a grid (thus ensuring that the selected molecules were structurally diverse) and then noted how many of these selected molecules were bioactive (thus quantifying the biological diversity).

Once interest has been focused on some small volume of structural space, large numbers of molecules are synthesized and tested (and often re-tested in the case of HTS data), and the results of these experiments used to develop a quantitative structure-activity relationship (QSAR). It has for long been claimed that the use of diverse sets of compounds will enable more robust QSARs to be developed than can be developed using randomly chosen training sets. That this is in fact the case has been demonstrated recently by Golbraikh and Tropsha *(37)*, and one can hence quantify the effectiveness of a compound selection method by the predictive power of the QSARs that can be derived from the compounds selected by that method. Quantitative bioactivity data also lie at the heart of the neighborhood behavior approach of Patterson et al. *(33)*, which is analogous to the similar property principle but emphasizes the absolute differences in descriptor values and in bioactivity values, rather than the values themselves. Specifically the authors state that a meaningful descriptor for diversity analysis is one for which "small differences in structure do not (often) produce large differences in biology," and then use this idea to compare a wide range of descriptor types by means of a χ^2 analysis; an improved version of this analysis is described by Dixon and Merz *(38)*.

3. Notes

1. The group in Sheffield has over two decades experience of carrying out comparative studies of similarity (and, more recently, diversity) methods. Perhaps the most important single piece of advice we can give to those wishing to carry out comparable studies is the need to use a range of types of data, ideally including both homogeneous and heterogeneous datasets. Only by so doing can one ensure the robustness and general applicability of the methods that are being compared. In particular, one would not wish to encourage the situation that pertained for some time in the QSAR literature, where a new method was normally developed and tested on just a single dataset, most commonly the set of steroids *(39)* first popularized by Cramer et al. *(40)*.

2. In like vein, we would recommend the use of more than just one evaluation measure. That said, it is our experience that different measures usually agree as to the relative merits of different approaches (unless there are only very minor differences in effectiveness): even so, it is always worth carrying out additional analyses to ensure that one's results are, indeed, independent of the evaluation criterion that has been adopted.

3. Having criticized the exclusive use of the steroid dataset, it does have the great advantage that it provides a simple basis for comparison with previous work, and it would be highly desirable if comparable test-sets were available for similarity and diversity analyses. To some extent, this is already happening with increasing use being made of the qualitative bioactivity data in the MDDR and WDI datasets mentioned previously; two other datasets that can be used for this purpose, and which have the advantage that they are available for public download, are the cancer and AIDS files produced by the National Cancer Institute (at URL http://dtp.nci.nih.gov/).

References

1. Johnson, M. A. and Maggiora, G. M. (eds.) (1990) *Concepts and applications of molecular similarity.* Wiley, New York.

2. Dean, P. M. (ed.) (1994) *Molecular similarity in drug design.* Chapman and Hall, Glasgow.
3. Willett, P., Barnard, J. M., and Downs, G. M. (1998) Chemical similarity searching. *J. Chem. Inf Comput. Sci.* **38,** 983–996.
4. Dean, P. M. and Lewis, R. A. (eds.) (1999) *Molecular diversity in drug design.* Kluwer, Amsterdam.
5. Ghose, A. K. and Viswanadhan, V. N. (eds.) (2001) *Combinatorial library design and evaluation: principles, software tools and applications in drug discovery.* Marcel Dekker, New York.
6. Kubinyi, H. (1998) Similarity and dissimilarity—a medicinal chemist's view. *Perspect. Drug. Discov. Design* **11,** 225–252.
7. Martin, Y. C., Kofron, J. L., and Traphagen, L. M. (2002) Do structurally similar molecules have similar biological activities? *J. Med. Chem.* **45,** 4350–4358.
8. Salton, G. and McGill, M. J. (1983) *Introduction to modern information retrieval.* McGraw-Hill, New York.
9. Frakes, W. B. and Baeza-Yates, R. (eds.) (1992) *Information retrieval: data structures and algorithms.* Prentice Hall, Englewood Cliffs, NJ.
10. Sparck Jones, K. and Willett, P. (eds.) (1997) *Readings in information retrieval.* Morgan Kaufmann, San Francisco, CA.
11. Edgar, S. J., Holliday, J. D., and Willett, P. (2000) Effectiveness of retrieval in similarity searches of chemical databases: a review of performance measures. *J. Mol. Graph. Model.* **18,** 343–357.
12. Kearsley, S. K., Sallamack, S., Fluder, E. M., Andose, J. D., Mosley, R. T. and Sheridan, R. P. (1996) Chemical similarity using physiochemical property descriptors. *J. Chem. Inf. Comput. Sci.* **36,** 118–127.
13. Gillet, V. J., Willett, P., and Bradshaw, J. (1998) Identification of biological activity profiles using substructural analysis and genetic algorithms. *J. Chem. Inf. Comput. Sci.* **38,** 165–179.
14. Güner, O. F. and Henry, D. R. Formula for determining the "goodness of hit lists" in 3D database searches. At URL http://www.netsci.org/Science/Cheminform/feature09.html.
15. Güner, O. F. and Henry, D. R. (2000) Metric for analyzing hit lists and pharmacophores. In *Pharmacophore perception, development and use in drug design,* Güner, O. (ed.), International University Line, La Jolla, CA, pp. 193–212
16. Raymond, J. W. and Willett, P. (2002) Effectiveness of graph-based and fingerprint-based similarity measures for virtual screening of 2D chemical structure databases. *J. Comput.-Aid. Mol. Design* **16,** 59–71.
17. Pepperrell, C. A. and Willett, P. (1991) Techniques for the calculation of three-dimensional structural similarity using inter-atomic distances. *J. Comput.-Aided Mol. Design* **5,** 455–474.
18. Briem, H. and Lessel, U. F. (2000) *In vitro* and *in silico* affinity fingerprints: finding similarities beyond structural classes. *Perspect. Drug Discov. Design* **20,** 231–244.

19. Cohen, J. A. (1960) A coefficient of agreement for nominal scales. *Educ. Psychol. Measure.* **20,** 37–46.

20. Cohen, J. A. (1968) Weighted kappa: nominal scale agreement with provision for scale disagreement or partial credit. *Psychol. Bull.* **70,** 213–220.

21. Rand, W. M. (1971) Objective criteria for the evaluation of clustering methods. *J. Amer. Stat. Assoc.* **66,** 846–850.

22. Wilton, D., Willett, P., Mullier, G., and Lawson, K. (2003) Comparison of ranking methods for virtual screening in lead-discovery programmes. *J. Chem. Inf. Comput. Sci.* **43,** 469–474.

23. Egan, J. P. (1975) *Signal detection theory and ROC analysis*, Academic Press, New York.

24. Cuissart, B., Touffet, F., Crémilleux, B., Bureau, R., and Rault, S. (2002) The maximum common substructure as a molecular depiction in a supervised classification context: experiments in quantitative structure/biodegradability relationships. *J. Chem. Inf. Comput. Sci.* **42,** 1043–1052.

25. Adamson, G. W. and Bush, J. A. (1973) A method for the automatic classification of chemical structures. *Inf. Stor. Retriev.* **9,** 561–568.

26. Adamson, G. W. and Bush, J. A. (1975) A comparison of the performance of some similarity and dissimilarity measures in the automatic classification of chemical structures. *J. Chem. Inf. Comput. Sci.* **15,** 55–58.

27. Willett, P. and Winterman, V. (1986) A comparison of some measures for the determination of inter-molecular structural similarity. *Quant. Struct.-Activ. Relat.* **5,** 18–25.

28. Brown, R. D. and Martin, Y. C. (1996) Use of structure-activity data to compare structure-based clustering methods and descriptors for use in compound selection. *J. Chem. Inf. Comput. Sci.* **36,** 572–584.

29. Brown, R. D. (1997) Descriptors for diversity analysis. *Perspect. Drug Disc. Design* **7/8,** 31–49.

30. Bayada, D. M., Hamersma, H., and van Geerestein, V. J. (1999) Molecular diversity and representativity in chemical databases. *J. Chem. Inf. Comput. Sci.* **39,** 1–10.

31. Snarey, M., Terret, N. K., Willett, P., and Wilton, D. J. (1997) Comparison of algorithms for dissimilarity-based compound selection. *J. Mol. Graph. Model.* **15,** 372–385.

32. Matter, H. and Potter, T. (1999) Comparing 3D pharmacophore triplets and 2D fingerprints for selecting diverse compound subsets. *J. Chem. Inf. Comput. Sci.* **39,** 1211–1225.

33. Patterson, D. E., Cramer, R. D., Ferguson, A. M., Clark, R. D., and Weinberger, L. E. (1996) Neighbourhood behaviour: a useful concept for validation of "molecular diversity" descriptors. *J. Med. Chem.* **39,** 3049–3059.

34. Waldman, M., Li, H., and Hassan, M. (2000) Novel algorithms for the optimisation of molecular diversity of combinatorial libraries. *J. Mol. Graph. Model.* **18,** 412–426.

35. Ferguson, A. M., Patterson, D. E., Garr, C. D., and Underiner, T. L. (1996) Designing chemical libraries for lead discovery. *J. Biomol. Screen.* **1,** 65–73.
36. Bayley, M. J. and Willett, P. (1999) Binning schemes for partition-based compound selection *J. Mol. Graph. Model.* **17,** 10–18.
37. Golbraikh, A. and Tropsha, A. (2002) Predictive QSAR modeling based on diversity sampling of experimental datasets for the training and test set selection. *J. Comput.-Aid. Mol. Design* **16,** 357–369.
38. Dixon, S. L. and Merz, K. M. (2001) One-dimensional molecular representations and similarity calculations: methodology and validation. *J. Med. Chem.* **44,** 3795–3809.
39. Coats, E. A. (1998) The CoMFA steroids as a benchmark dataset for development of 3D QSAR methods. *Perspect. Drug Discov. Design* **12/14,** 199–213.
40. Cramer, R. D., Patterson, D. E., and Bunce, J. D. (1988) Comparative molecular field analysis (CoMFA). Effect of shape on binding of steroids to carrier proteins. *J. Am. Chem. Soc.* **110,** 5959–5967.

3

A Web-Based Chemoinformatics System for Drug Discovery

Scott D. Bembenek, Brett A. Tounge, Steven J. Coats, and Charles H. Reynolds

Abstract

One of the key questions that must be addressed when implementing a chemoinformatics system is whether the tools will be designed for use by the expert user or by the "bench scientist." This decision can impact not only the style of tools that are rolled out, but is also a factor in terms of how these tools are delivered to the end users. The system that we outline here was designed for use by the non-expert user. As such, the tools that we discuss are in many cases simplified versions of some common algorithms used in chemoinformatics. In addition, the focus is on how to distribute these tools using a web-services interface, which greatly simplifies delivering new protocols to the end user.

Key Words: Chemoinformatics; databases; information systems; web-based tools; computational tools; combinatorial chemistry.

1. Introduction

Chemoinformatics refers to the systems and scientific methods used to store, retrieve, and analyze the immense amount of molecular data that are generated in modern drug-discovery efforts. In general, these data fall into one of four categories: structural, numerical, annotation/text, and graphical. However, it is fair to say that the molecular structure data are the most unique aspect that differentiate chemoinformatics from other database applications *(1)*. Molecular structure refers to the 1-, 2-, or 3-D representations of molecules. Examples of numerical data include biological activity, pK_a, $logP$, or analytical results, to name a few. Annotation includes information such as experimental notes that are associated with a structure or data point. Finally, any structure

From: *Methods in Molecular Biology, vol. 275:*
Chemoinformatics: Concepts, Methods, and Tools for Drug Discovery
Edited by: J. Bajorath © Humana Press Inc., Totowa, NJ

or data point may have associated graphical information such as spectra or plots. In all cases the data may be experimental or computed and the molecules may be real or "virtual."

Considering the vast number of molecules in most corporate databases (not to mention external sources) and the large quantity of data associated with these molecules, the need for sophisticated information systems is clear. Modern drug discovery requires systems that have the ability to access and manipulate large quantities of data quickly and easily. However, information archival and retrieval is not enough. It is also necessary to have tools that can effectively analyze and organize these data in order to make it useful for effective decision-making. Consequently, chemoinformatics has become an integral part of the drug-discovery process, from lead identification through development.

Companies face a number of important challenges and philosophical decisions when developing and deploying a chemoinformatics system. One issue is whether to target tools primarily to the expert user or the "bench scientist." Expert tools can be more powerful and flexible, but are generally too complex to be used by the general scientist community. General-purpose tools must be simpler in order to make them accessible to the more casual user, but this usually comes at the cost of reduced functionality. Another issue is the system architecture. One option is to implement a large, integrated, and usually home-grown solution. This offers the opportunity to provide a seamless and comprehensive system, but it is expensive to develop and support. Another option is to assemble a collection of commercial off-the-shelf tools that will cover most applications. This results in a more heterogeneous environment, but does not require the development of custom software. Other technical issues include whether the applications run locally, on a server, or using a client–server combination. None of these decisions are easy or clear-cut.

At J&J PRD we have used the following principles to guide the development of our chemoinformatics platform:

1. Deliver the most generally useful chemoinformatics tools directly to the "bench scientist" so that he/she can use them without requiring the intervention of a specialist.
2. Accommodate access to heterogeneous data sources and analysis tools.
3. Make use of commercial visualization and analysis packages where possible.
4. Avoid putting applications directly on the desktop, relying instead on web deployment.
5. Implement a system that allows rapid application development and deployment with a minimum of support overhead.

These principles are embodied in the chemoinformatics system outlined below. This system uses a backend (for database access and computations) that is accessible via a simple web-services interface. The underlying platform is the Pipeline Pilot software package from Scitegic, Inc. *(2)*. We rely on existing desktop tools for data visualization (e.g., DIVA or Accord for Excel from Accelrys) *(3,4)*. This architecture is consistent with the design goals laid out previously. For example, the web interface makes it possible to deliver new protocols quickly and easily. Once a method has been written and tested on the server, it is simply posted as a new web service. This eliminates the need to push new software out to the desktop. In addition, the use of existing desktop tools not only reduces development time and support costs, it also provides the user with an already familiar interface. Finally, this platform is very flexible and allows us to retrieve and manipulate data from multiple and disparate sources.

We will highlight this system by first giving a brief overview of the architecture, followed by some practical examples that cover several common tasks in the drug discovery process. The goal is not to give a detailed account of the methods employed, but rather to illustrate how the system functions in practice. We will present as examples some of the most widely used chemoinformatics applications: customized database access, similarity and substructure searching, reactant selection, and library design.

2. Methods

2.1. Overview of the Architecture

The main page for accessing the web-based tools is shown in **Fig. 1**. This is the chemoinformatics homepage and it serves as the entry point for several different classes of tools (left-hand column of **Fig. 1**). The protocols are categorized by the type of task: for example, substructure/similarity searches, database access, and property calculators. The underlying system driving many of these protocols is outlined in **Fig. 2**. The Pipeline Pilot software serves as the main interface for accessing several different corporate databases and calling third party programs [via command line, Simple Object Access Protocol (SOAP), or remote shell calls]. In addition, we make extensive use of methods within Pipeline Pilot for developing protocols. This functionality is then delivered to the users' desktop using the web-services interface. For example, a protocol can be written that will access the structural and biological data for all compounds for a given project. These data can then be manipulated within the programming environment of Pipeline Pilot (e.g., modify units or add descriptors) to enhance its utility. Once the protocols are finalized, they are placed in a public area where they become accessible from the interface shown in **Fig. 3**.

2.2. Database Access

Whether one is interested in data-mining techniques or simply collecting all the data for a given compound or project, the ability to retrieve data easily and

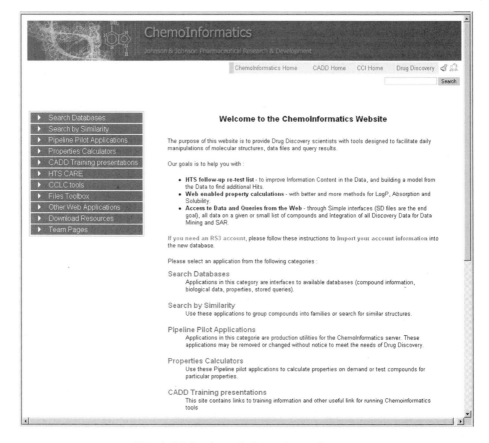

Fig. 1. Main chemoinformatics web page.

accurately from a database is of primary importance. From a bench scientist's perspective much of the retrieval of information is focused around the latter of these two tasks. The types of tools we currently provide to address this need fall into two categories: *ad hoc* queries and custom database access protocols focused around therapeutic team projects. Both are provided using the backend Pipeline Pilot tools in conjunction with existing desktop visualization tools. One of the strengths of this approach is the ability to extract data from multiple databases and join them "on-the-fly" in a way that is transparent to the end user.

2.2.1. Ad Hoc Queries

Before Pipeline Pilot, retrieval of assay data (for us) was done mainly via RS³ for Excel *(5)*. RS³ allows one to obtain information on a given assay or a set of assays with queries that are set up by clicking on the folders containing

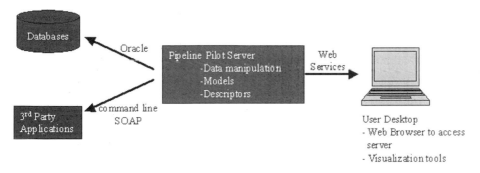

Fig. 2. Schematic drawing of the system architecture.

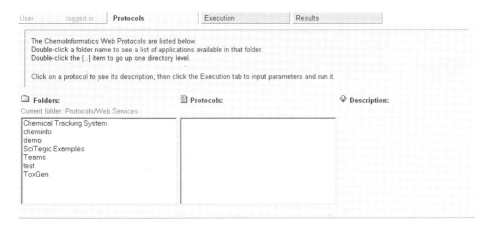

Fig. 3. Main level of the web services interface.

the desired data. This query style is appealing, because it is visual, interactive, and intuitive. The interactive feature makes it easy to expand or focus the search as needed. However, queries involving several assays can be cumbersome to set up. An example would be the queries needed to retrieve data for two or more assays where one wants data if they exist for any of the assays. The natural construct of RS^3 is to impose a constraint upon the existence of data in a single assay and, therefore, multiple assay queries of this "any" type, while possible, are not smoothly implemented. Furthermore, RS^3 does not allow for sophisticated manipulation of the data during the retrieval process such as filtering data based on certain descriptors.

As an alternative, we have made extensive use of the data retrieval and manipulation functions within Pipeline Pilot to provide more powerful querying capabilities without sacrificing ease of use. **Figure 4** shows the user interface for the standard *ad hoc* assay protocol used by most chemists and

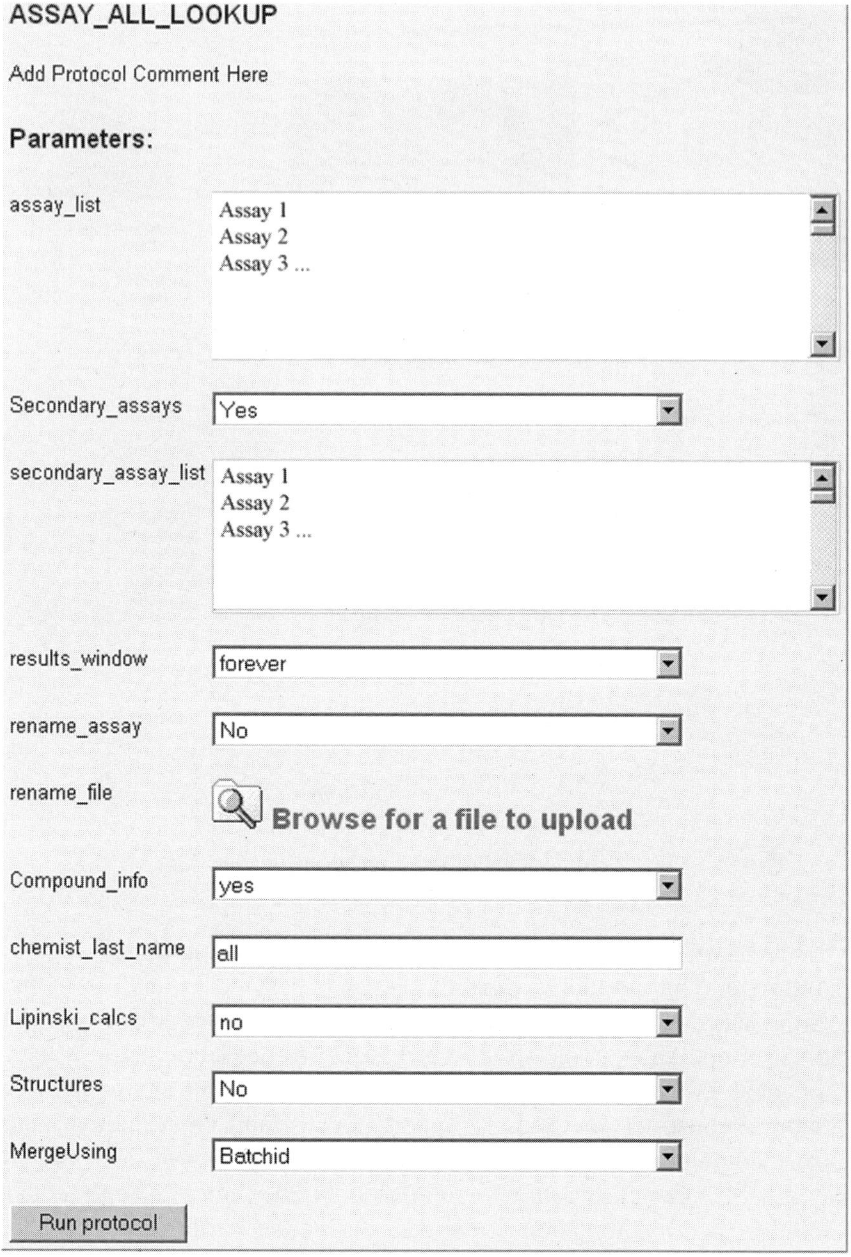

ASSAY_ALL_LOOKUP

Add Protocol Comment Here

Parameters:

assay_list

> Assay 1
> Assay 2
> Assay 3 ...

Secondary_assays   Yes

secondary_assay_list   Assay 1
> Assay 2
> Assay 3 ...

results_window   forever

rename_assay   No

rename_file   **Browse for a file to upload**

Compound_info   yes

chemist_last_name   all

Lipinski_calcs   no

Structures   No

MergeUsing   Batchid

Run protocol

Fig. 4. Interface for the *ad hoc* query tool.

biologists. The two large boxes each contain a list of all the registered assays in our database. The top box specifies the primary assays. This means that for a compound to be returned it must contain an entry for at least one of the assays that are highlighted. The second box provides the option to return additional assay data on the first set of compounds. These secondary assay results are added (if they exist) to the primary assay data for each compound. These two options allow the user to easily define a complex query. The ability to manipulate the data as they are retrieved is exemplified by the additional options shown in **Fig. 4**. The user has the option of filtering on chemist name, obtaining notebook information, filtering on assay date, and calculating Lipinski's rule descriptors *(6)*.

2.2.2. Custom Database Access Protocols

While the protocol described above has proven very useful in its own right, it often serves as the first step in designing custom protocols for a team. Once a user is satisfied with the results returned by the *ad hoc* query, the next step is often to hardwire these queries into a protocol that provides "one-button" access to all the pertinent data for a project. **Figure 5** shows such a protocol used to retrieve data for several assays in a Neuroscience project. This protocol highlights an additional filtering option that we make use of in many of our protocols. The text box ("selected_cmpds_from_list") *(7)* supports the input of a list of identification numbers (in our case either "jnjnumber" or "batchid"). This allows data to be retrieved on select compounds as opposed to all those tested in the assays. This feature is very popular and involves the use of Perl within the Pipeline Pilot protocol. All this work is done on the server and the results are written to a SD file that can be downloaded to the desktop. At this stage either DIVA or Accord for Excel is typically used to view the files.

2.2.3. Data Mining

We have illustrated the capability of Pipeline Pilot to query all the data on a set of compounds from the internal database and perform simple filtering on them. Additionally, the ability of Pipeline Pilot to easily access other (several) databases (or files) besides the internal database provides us with a very powerful tool for data mining. The utility of accessing multiple databases simultaneously is discussed in the following sections. Here we give an example of how being able to access different databases, other than the in-house one, and perform sophisticated filtering on an the data is in itself a tremendous asset.

Figure 6 shows a Pipeline Protocol where the Available Chemicals Directory (ACD) *(8)* was mined for reactants useful in alkylation. This protocol high-

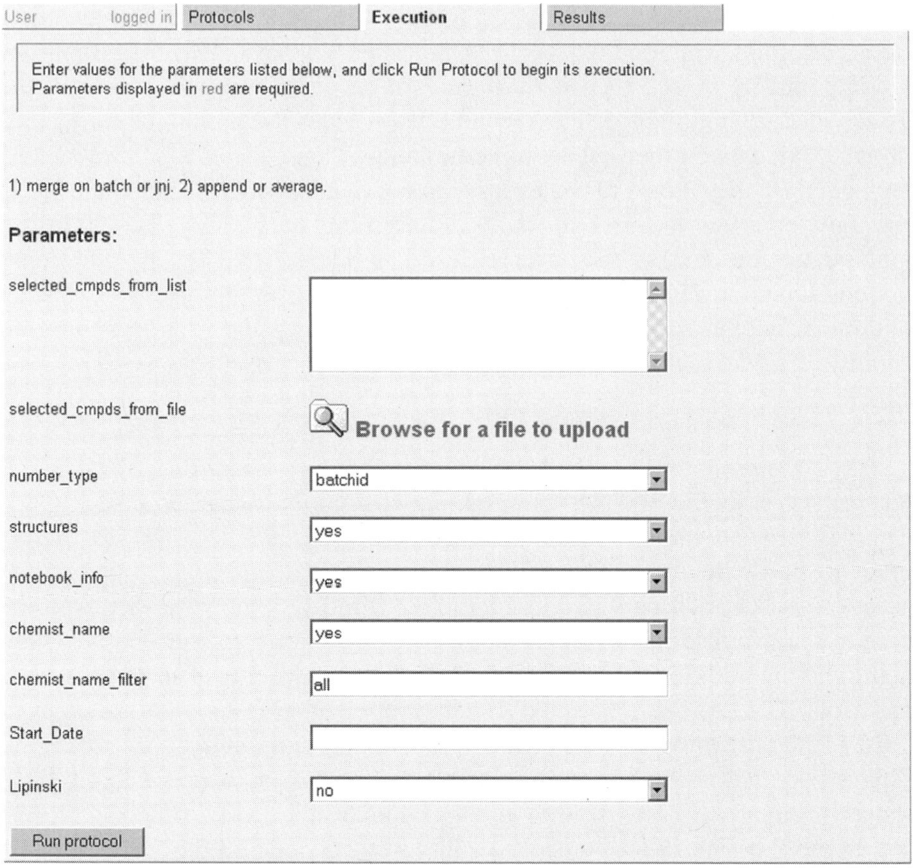

User	logged in	Protocols	Execution	Results

Enter values for the parameters listed below, and click Run Protocol to begin its execution. Parameters displayed in red are required.

1) merge on batch or jnj. 2) append or average.

Parameters:

selected_cmpds_from_list

selected_cmpds_from_file   **Browse for a file to upload**

number_type   `batchid`

structures   `yes`

notebook_info   `yes`

chemist_name   `yes`

chemist_name_filter   `all`

Start_Date

Lipinski   `no`

Run protocol

Fig. 5. User interface for a custom made protocol for a neuroscience project.

lights many of the filtering methods available within the Pipeline Pilot interface. In this case compounds were removed that had high acceptor or donor counts, did not contain a Br or Cl, and contained a Br or Cl attached to a phenyl ring (the latter two cases make alkylation impossible). The resulting subset of ACD compounds was useful [to the computer-aided drug discovery (CADD) group] in modeling possible substitutents to be added to an existing template being used in lead refinement in immunology.

2.3. Similarity and Substructure Searches

2D similarity and substructure searching are among the most widely used methods for mining structural data *(9)*. The basic principle of these methods is that compounds with structural features in common will have similar properties,

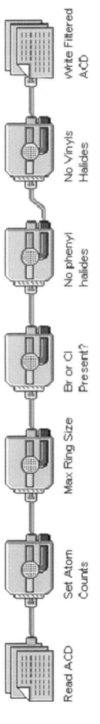

Fig. 6. Pipeline Pilot protocol used to filter reactants useful in alkylation.

Read ACD

Set Atom Counts

Max Ring Size

Br or Cl Present?

No phenyl halides

No Vinyls Halides

Write Filtered ACD

73

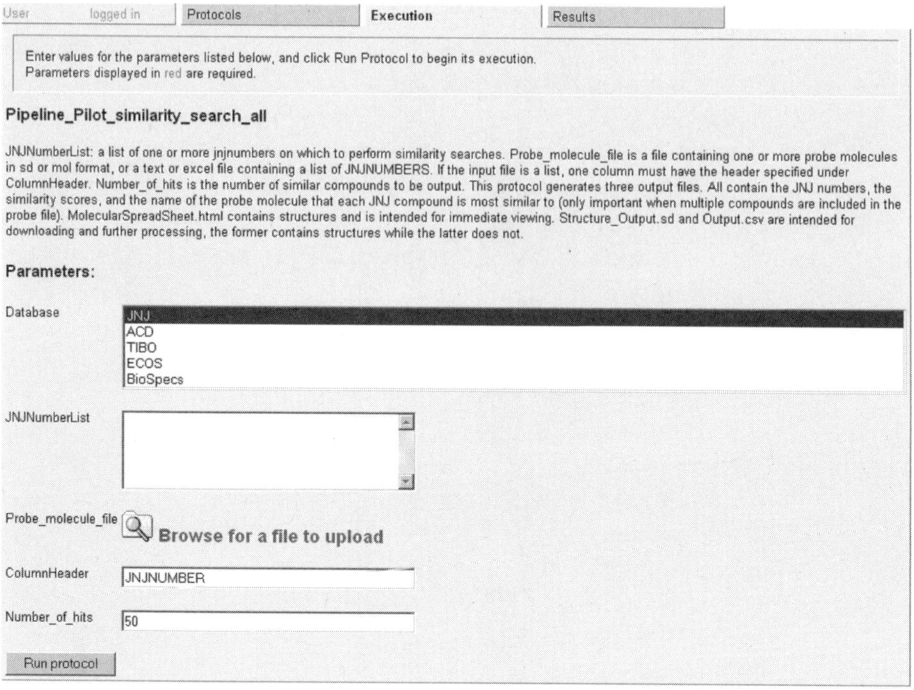

Fig. 7. User interface of the Pipeline Pilot similarity search protocol.

often including biological activity *(10)*. The intuitive nature of this concept undoubtedly has contributed to the popularity of these methods, which makes them perfect candidates for generally available applications. At J&J PRD, similarity and substructure searching have proven to be powerful tools that are widely used to probe internal and external databases for compounds similar to known "actives" or other structures of interest (e.g., literature structures). One of the most systematic applications is following up on high-throughput screening (HTS) hits. In addition, these methods can be used to search for structurally relevant reactants or when "brainstorming" for new chemotypes.

2.3.1. Similarity Searches

Figure 7 shows the web interface for our Pipeline Pilot–based similarity search engine. For similarity searching a connectivity fingerprint (available within the Pipeline Pilot software) is used and the Tanimoto coefficient is calculated. In the text box (labeled "JNJNumberList" under "Parameters") one can type or paste (e.g., from an Excel sheet) a list of identification numbers ("jnjnumber," "batchid") to be used as probes for the search. Alternatively, an

SD structure file or a file containing a list of identification numbers [Excel or Comma Separated Value (CSV) format] can be uploaded. In the Excel or CSV cases the protocol will automatically look up the structure that corresponds to the identification number, as it does for the text box input. A useful feature (see "Databases" under "Parameters" in **Fig. 7**) is the ability to search multiple databases in a single search. This is made possible by the use of Perl in the Pipeline Pilot protocol. The Perl code is very general and easily allows for the addition of new databases as they become available, thereby further increasing the versatility of this protocol.

2.3.2. Substructure Searches

Both DIVA and RS[3] provide some functionality in terms of substructure searches (SSS), although it is somewhat limited. For example, DIVA searches can only be performed on data that have already been queried from the database(s). This pre-queried data need to be readily available to DIVA either via RS[3] or as an SD file. In the case of RS[3], the inclusion of multiple data sources (e.g., searching the corporate database and an external vendor library) is not trivial. As a result, while DIVA and RS[3] are very useful for SSS under certain conditions, they are not as robust when compared to the Pipeline Pilot protocol.

Like the similarity protocol, the user interface for the Pipeline Pilot SSS protocol supports multiple databases and multiple probes in a single query. The input of the probe molecule(s) is accomplished using a SD file, which can be generated in most standard chemical drawing programs. This file is supplied as one of the inputs in the SSS interface. The use of identification numbers is not as applicable here as it is in the case of the similarity protocol since we are most likely not using existing molecules as substructures. Consequently, textbox input is not an option nor is the upload of a list of numbers in CSV or Excel format.

2.4. Library Design

The protocols developed for library design highlight the trade-off between providing a user friendly interface versus providing a more versatile tool for the expert user. For example, in the enumeration interface that will be outlined below we have sacrificed the ability to look at complex multistep reactions for the sake of providing an interface with a few intuitive options. One of the keys to the implementation of this system was the integration of existing desktop tools. In the example outlined below, ISIS/Draw and ISIS/Base *(11)* are used for defining the reaction scheme and queries, Pipeline Pilot provides the enumeration engine and selection and filtering routines, and the visualization is accomplished with DIVA or Accord for Excel. The integration of these tools is best illustrated by stepping through a library design example.

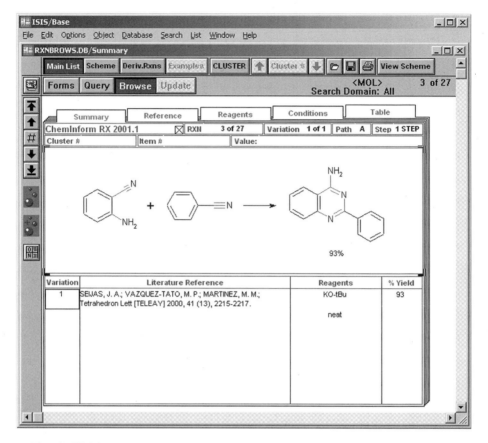

Fig. 8. ISIS/Base reaction browser. This interface can be used to directly export RXN files.

2.4.1. Defining the Reaction

The enumeration engine within Pipeline Pilot uses REACCS RXN files to define the chemistry *(12,13)*. These files can be easily generated using ISIS/Draw or they can be exported directly from the reaction browser of ISIS/Base. For the example here, we start with the reaction browser **(Fig. 8)**. Once the desired reaction is found [in this case a ring formation starting with aminonitriles and nitriles *(14)*] it is exported from ISIS/Base as a RXN file. This file can be used directly for the enumeration, or it can be modified using ISIS/Draw. In this case the nitrile is modified to define a more generic transformation **(Fig. 9)**. The key element to specifying the reaction is the atom-to-atom mapping that can also be seen in **Fig. 9**. This defines which atoms are kept (all reactant atoms that are not mapped to products are deleted) and

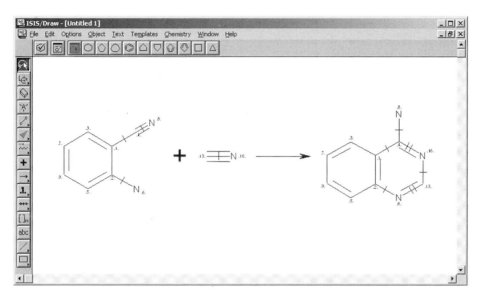

Fig. 9. ISIS/Draw interface used for defining or modify RXN files. The "atom-to-atom" mapping function in ISIS/Draw is used to define the reaction. In this case the reaction taken out of ISIS/Base **(Fig. 8)** has been modified to make it more generic.

defines the placement of the reactant atoms in the final product (which can include stereochemistry information).

2.4.2. Reactant Selection and Filtering

The selection of reactants can be accomplished through two different interfaces that use substructure and similarity searches, respectively. The interface for the substructure searching protocol is shown in **Fig. 10** *(15)*. At the top of the page is a box that lists the databases that can be searched. In addition there is an option to upload a SD file as the search database. Below this box is a list of functional groups with a set of radio buttons that allow users to define their query. For each group they can specify whether they want it to exist at least once ("Must Exist"), only once ("Exist Only Once"), or not at all ("May Not Exist"). The default for each group is to not include it in the query ("No Preference"). The underlying methodology is a predefined set of individual queries (in this case substructures drawn with ISIS/Draw and saved as "mol" files) that are combined at run time into the appropriate Boolean expression *(16)*. For the example here we have chosen to find all compounds with one nitrile group and none of the other functional groups. We also provide the user with the option of searching a custom substructure query. This method was used to find the R1 reactant set (aminonitriles).

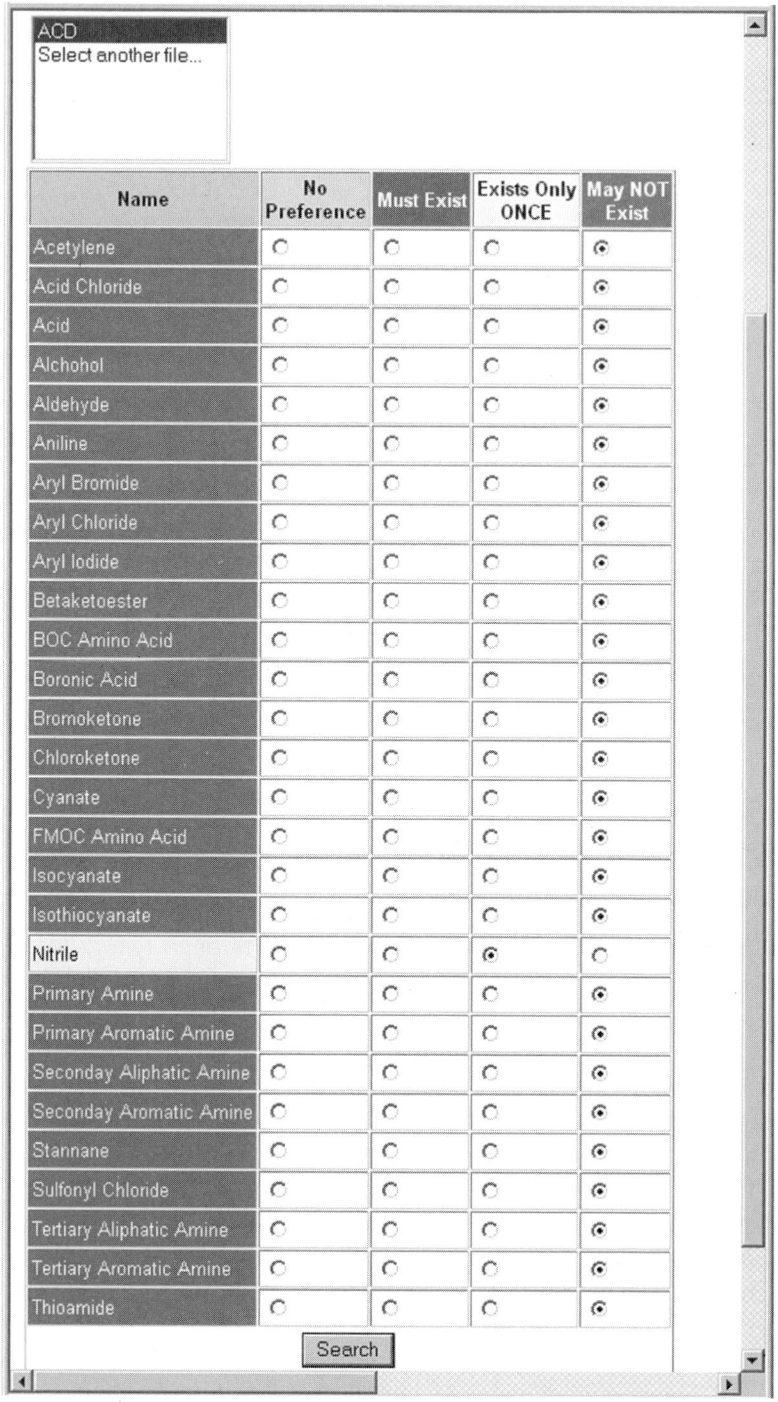

ACD
Select another file...

Name	No Preference	Must Exist	Exists Only ONCE	May NOT Exist
Acetylene	○	○	○	◉
Acid Chloride	○	○	○	◉
Acid	○	○	○	◉
Alchohol	○	○	○	◉
Aldehyde	○	○	○	◉
Aniline	○	○	○	◉
Aryl Bromide	○	○	○	◉
Aryl Chloride	○	○	○	◉
Aryl Iodide	○	○	○	◉
Betaketoester	○	○	○	◉
BOC Amino Acid	○	○	○	◉
Boronic Acid	○	○	○	◉
Bromoketone	○	○	○	◉
Chloroketone	○	○	○	◉
Cyanate	○	○	○	◉
FMOC Amino Acid	○	○	○	◉
Isocyanate	○	○	○	◉
Isothiocyanate	○	○	○	◉
Nitrile	○	○	◉	○
Primary Amine	○	○	○	◉
Primary Aromatic Amine	○	○	○	◉
Seconday Aliphatic Amine	○	○	○	◉
Seconday Aromatic Amine	○	○	○	◉
Stannane	○	○	○	◉
Sulfonyl Chloride	○	○	○	◉
Tertiary Aliphatic Amine	○	○	○	◉
Tertiary Aromatic Amine	○	○	○	◉
Thioamide	○	○	○	◉

Search

Fig. 10. Reagent selector tool. Here we have chosen to look for all compounds that contain only one nitrile and none of the other functional groups.

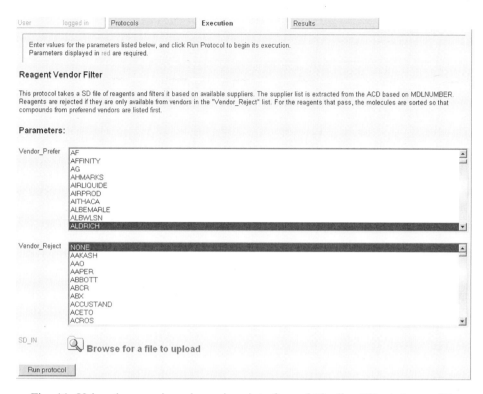

Fig. 11. Using the generic web services interface of Pipeline Pilot it is possible to generate complex input forms. In this case we use different variable types to provide a "Vendor Filter" protocol for selecting reactants.

At this stage several different algorithms could be applied to filter the reactant list *(17,18)*. The simple example we use here allows one to filter reactants based on preferences for vendors. This filter is easy to implement using the Pipeline Pilot web interface (**Fig. 11**). Using this filter, compounds only available from vendors in the "vendor_reject" list are removed. The remaining compounds are then sorted so that reactants from preferred vendors are listed first.

2.4.3. Enumeration

Once the final reactant lists are prepared, they are supplied along with the RXN file defining the reaction to the enumeration engine using the web interface shown in **Fig. 12A**. This interface provides a general framework for specifying up to three reagent files (R1, R2, and R3 inputs). The interface also provides the user with two options for the enumeration. First they can choose whether or not they would like a subset of the library returned or not (simple random percent filter). This smaller subset can be visualized in a web page to

A Library Enumeration

INPUT: Up to 3 reagent Files (SD format)
REACCS RXN File which defines the reaction/transformation
OUTPUT: Enumerated Library in SMILES format
Library Subset (percent_return) as Web page and SD File

Parameters:

R1   **Browse for a file to upload**

R2   **Browse for a file to upload**

R3   **Browse for a file to upload**

Return_subset   no   ▼

percent_return   1

Reaction.rxn   **Browse for a file to upload**

IfMultipleMappings   RejectStartingMaterial   ▼
                       RejectStartingMaterial
                       UseFirstMapping
                       UseAllMappings

[Run protocol]

B

Molecule	R1_MDLNUMBER	R2_MDLNUMBER	Molecular_Weight
	MFCD00179901	MFCD00045606	443.087
	MFCD00007362	MFCD00079701	372.387

check the enumeration before downloading the full library set. The second option determines how reactants that map multiple times are handled. For example, if a compound in the R2 list had two nitrile groups, the user can specify whether that compound should not be used, used once (at the first mapped site), or reacted on each mapped site.

Although we have made use of SD files up to this point, at this stage we switch to SMILES files *(19)*. This becomes necessary because even for small libraries the file size for a fully enumerated set can be quite large. For example, a sample library of just 2500 compounds resulted in 4.85 MB SD file while the SMILES file was only 384 KB. The one caveat with the SMILES format is that there is no standard for handling data fields. Our solution was to reformat the SD file type data field tags into the SMILES file,

SMILES_STRING ;<Data_1>val_1,val_2;<Data_2>val_1,val_2 . . .

where "Data_N" is the property name and "val" . . . "val_N" are all the values associated with that property. Subsequent processing of the library can then be done on this smaller file. Using this format we are able to easily track the MFCD numbers (or some other tracking number) for the reactants that go into each enumerated compound (**Fig. 12B**). These are used later to extract final reactant lists.

2.4.4. Final Library Selection

Just as was the case for the reactant filtering, many methodologies exist for selecting library subsets for synthesis *(18,20–29)*. For this example library we used a simple "Rule of 5" type filter to select a subset of compounds *(6)*. After filtering, the final step in the process is to extract the reactant lists from the selected library subset. Because in each step of the procedure outlined above we have maintained the MFCD numbers for all the reactants (tagged by reactant number), this is simply a matter of extracting these numbers from the final library. For each of the compounds we provide the molecule name, list of vendors, MFCD and CAS (if available) numbers, molecular weight, and information about whether the reactant is available in-house (**Fig. 13**).

Fig. 12. *(see opposite page)* The library enumeration interface (**A**) allows for up to three reactant files to be uploaded. This is also where the preference for how to handled reactants that map multiple times to the substructure as defined in the RXN file is set. These compounds can be rejected, reacted once, or they can be reacted at each matching site. The output of the library subset (**B**) can be visualized in a web page before downloading the entire library.

Molecule	MOLNAME	MDLNUMBER	Vendor	CAS_NUMBER	cts_check	Molecular_Weight
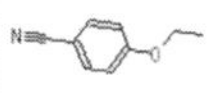	4-ETHOXYBENZONITRILE	MFCD00001819	2 7 ABCR 9 14 ALDRICH 16 23 ALFA-ORG 25 34 APIN 36 41 AVOCADO 43 46 ICN-RF 48 57 LANCASTER 59 65 SYNTEC 67 74 TRANSWLD	25117-74-2	Not in CTS	147.178
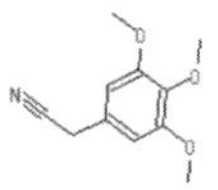	3,4,5-TRIMETHOXYPHENYLACETONITRILE	MFCD00001912	2 7 ACROS 9 14 ADVAN-SYNTH 16 22 ALDRICH 24 29 APIN 31 37 FLUKA 39 42 KNOLL 44 54 LANCASTER 56 61 NARCHEM 63 77 PFALTZ-BAUER	13338-63-1	Not in CTS	207.231

Fig. 13. Final list of R2 reactants extracted from the library. For each compound we check the in-house inventory.

3. Discussion

The ability effectively to access and manipulate chemical and biological data is crucial to the drug-discovery process. Given the number of compounds (internal and external) and corresponding data generated by pharmaceutical research, this ability is a necessity for good information-driven decision-making. The system we have outlined here accomplishes this task by successfully tying together several commercially available packages and making extensive use of web services for the rollout of tools to the end user. Specifically, we have demonstrated that Pipeline Pilot along with commercially available desktop tools such as DIVA and Accord can be integrated to provide a comprehensive chemoinformatics system. There are many advantages to this approach. For example, because the server (Pipeline Pilot) can access multiple data sources and has extensive facilities for data manipulation, we can deliver customized data management tools rapidly that draw from disparate data sources. This approach has the advantage of being relatively independent of any one particular data structure, and provides a great deal of flexibility. New databases can be easily incorporated via Pipeline Pilot obviating the need to clean, filter, and export a new data source to a common data repository. From an implementation perspective, this architecture is appealing because it involves little modification of the standard desktop system supplied to users. As a result, there is no client that needs to be validated, updated, or propagated across the discovery organization. This greatly simplifies the task of maintaining the system.

Of course, there are limitations to this approach that must be kept in mind. First, because we use commercially available components for the data visualization, we are tied to the standard file formats. For the most part these formats are sufficient, but in certain cases they can be limiting. For example, there is no standard for handling multiple entries for a single data field. This becomes an issue when retrieving assay results, because in many cases more than one experiment has been run. Second, this system requires a robust and fast network since many file uploads and downloads to the server are involved. However, in practice we have found these issues to be manageable.

Acknowledgments

The authors would like to thank Frank K. Brown who heads the development of chemoinformatics at J&J PRD. We would also like to recognize Laurent Alquier, Mario Dolbec, Gordon Madise, Greg Rusin, and Andre Volkov for their work in setting up and maintaining the system. Additionally, we acknowledge the contributions of Mike Hack, Mark Seierstad, and Frank Axe in developing protocols for the web services.

References

1. Brown, F. K. (1998) *Chemoinformatics: what is it and how does it impact drug discovery. Annu. Rep. Med. Chem.* **33,** 375–384.
2. Pipeline Pilot (2003) 2.5, SciTegic, Inc.: San Diego, CA.
3. DIVA (2002) 2.1, Accelrys, Inc.: San Diego, CA.
4. Accord for Excel2000 (2000) 3.1, Accelyrs, Inc.: San Diego, CA.
5. RS^3 Discovery for Excel (2000) 2.0, Accelyrs, Inc., San Diego, CA.
6. Lipinski, C. A. (2001) Drug-like properties and the causes of poor solubility and poor permeability. *J. Pharmacol. Toxicol. Methods* **44,** 235–249.
7. The textbox feature discussed in the similarity and substructure protocols and appearing in many other protocols not mention herein is due to an interfacing of Perl code with Pipeline Pilot written by Mike Hack in the J&J PRD La Jolla CADD group.
8. ACD (2000) 2000.2, MDL Information Systems, Inc., San Leandro, CA.
9. Willett, P., Barnard, J. M., and Downs, G. M. (1998) Chemical similarity searching. *J. Chem. Inf. Comput. Sci.* **38,** 983–997.
10. Randic, M. (1990) Design of molecules with desired properties: a molecular similarity approach to property optimization. In *Concepts and applications of molecular similarity*, Johnson, M. A. and Maggiora, G. M. (eds.), John Wiley & Sons, New York, pp. 77–146.
11. ISIS (2000) 2.3; MDL Information Systems, Inc., San Leandro, CA.
12. Chen, L., Nourse, J. G., Christie, B. D., Leland, B. A., and Grier, D. L. (2002) Over 20 years of reaction access systems from MDL: a novel reaction substructure search algorithm. *J. Chem. Inf. Comput. Sci.* **42,** 1296–1310.

13. MDL File Formats, MDL Information Systems, Inc., San Leandro, CA.

14. Seijas, J. A., Vazquez-Tato, M. P., and Martinez, M. M. (2000) Microwave-enhanced synthesis of 4-aminoquinazolines. *Tetrahedron Lett.* **41**, 2215–2217.

15. The pipeline pilot protocol as a well as the initial version of the web interface for the protocol was written by Chris Farmer at Scitegic. The web interface was refined by Andre Volkov from J&J PRD.

16. Leach, A. R., Bradshaw, J., Green, D. V. S., Hann, M. M., and Delany, J. J. I. (1999) Implementation of a system for reagent selection and library enumeration, profiling, and design. *J. Chem. Inf. Comput. Sci.* **39**, 1161–1172.

17. Walters, W. P. and Murcko, M. A. (2000) Library filtering systems and prediction of drug-like properties. *Methods Princ. Med. Chem.* **10**, 15–32.

18. Matter, H., Baringhaus, K., Naumann, T., Klabunde, T., and Pirard, B. (2001) Computational approaches towards the rational design of drug-like compound libraries. *Comb. Chem. High Throughput Screen.* **4**, 453–475.

19. SMILES Format, Daylight Chemical Information Systems, Inc., Mission Viejo, CA.

20. Walters, W. P., Ajay, and Murcko, M. A. (1999) Recognizing molecules with drug-like properties. *Curr. Opin. Chem. Biol.* **3**, 384–7.

21. Sadowski, J. and Kubinyi, H. (1998) A scoring scheme for discriminating between drugs and nondrugs. *J. Med. Chem.* **41**, 3325–3329.

22. Muegge, I., Heald, S. L., and Brittelli, D. (2001) Simple selection criteria for drug-like chemical matter. *J. Med. Chem.* **44**, 1841–1846.

23. Mitchell, T. and Showell, G. A. (2001) Design strategies for building drug-like chemical libraries. *Curr. Opin. Drug Discovery Dev.* **4**, 314–318.

24. Lewis, R. A., Pickett, S. D., and Clark, D. E. (2000) *Computer-aided molecular diversity analysis and combinatorial library design.* Rev. Comput. Chem. Lipkowitz, K. B. and Boyd, D. B. (eds.), VCH Publishers, Inc., NY, vol. 16.

25. Frimurer, T. M., Bywater, R., Nrum, L., Lauritsen, L. N., and Brunak, S. (2000) Improving the odds in discriminating "drug-like" from "non drug-like" compounds. *J. Chem. Inf. Comput. Sci.* **40**, 1315–1324.

26. Ajay, Walters, W. P., and Murcko, M. A. (1998) Can we learn to distinguish between "drug-like" and "nondrug-like" molecules? *J. Med. Chem.* **41**, 3314–3324.

27. Anzali, S., Barnickel, G., Cezanne, B., Krug, M., Filimonov, D., and Poroikov, V. (2001) Discriminating between drugs and nondrugs by prediction of activity spectra for substances (PASS). *J. Med. Chem.* **44**, 2432–2437.

28. Blake, J. F. (2000) Chemoinformatics—predicting the physicochemical properties of "drug-like" molecules. *Curr. Opin. Biotechnol.* **11**, 104–107.

29. Böhm, H.-J. and Stahl, M. (2000) Structure-based library design: molecular modeling merges with combinatorial chemistry. *Curr. Opin. Chem. Biol.* **4**, 283–286.

4

Application of Chemoinformatics to High-Throughput Screening

Practical Considerations

Christian N. Parker and Suzanne K. Schreyer

Abstract

The objective of this chapter is to summarize and evaluate some of the most common chemoinformatic methods that are applied to the analysis of high-throughput-screening data. The chapter will briefly describe current high-throughput-screening practices and will stress how the major constraint on the application of chemoinformatics is often the quality of high-throughput-screening data. Discussion of the NCI dataset and how it differs from most high-throughput-screening datasets will be made to highlight this point.

Key Words: High-throughput screening; chemoinformatics; NCI dataset.

1. Introduction

Screening (and now high throughput screening [HTS]) has always been the method of choice for identifying novel ligands to biological targets (*1*). Even with new methods for detecting ligand binding such as NMR and crystallography (*2,3*), or the application of virtual screening methods using protein structures (*4,5*), there still comes a point at which the compounds of interest must be tested (screened) for activity. As the numbers of compounds available for screening increases (at present there are approx 2 million compounds commercially available through ChemNavigator), advances in assay miniaturization and screening throughput continue to allow more compounds to be tested. However, as more sophisticated assay endpoints are becoming available to monitor increasingly complex biological processes, and so monitor more

From: *Methods in Molecular Biology, vol. 275:*
Chemoinformatics: Concepts, Methods, and Tools for Drug Discovery
Edited by: J. Bajorath © Humana Press Inc., Totowa, NJ

drug targets, the costs associated with screening become larger. These costs increase further now that screening is being used to identify ligands even for proteins of unknown function (so as to identify function) in an effort to validate newly discovered genes as potential drug targets *(6,7)*. As the number of compounds screened becomes larger and larger and the complexity of the analysis increases, the need for methods to help visualize, organize, and exploit these data becomes of increasing importance. Hence, the need for chemoinformatic methods of data analysis. The challenge of being able to organize and understand screening data is made even more difficult due to the intrinsic errors present in screening data. This uncertainty is magnified when one considers that often different assay formats for the same target can give differing results *(8,9)*.

This chapter will provide a critical review of examples where chemoinformatics has been applied to screening data and to highlight the difficulties in routinely applying such methods. Chemoinformatics can be applied before a screening campaign has begun or applied to data that have been collected; in either case the role of chemoinformatics is to help organize, visualize, and thus suggest explanations for the data. Organization and modeling of the data allow hypotheses to be generated that can identify possible false positives or false negatives by identifying differing classes or groups of compounds that may be working by a similar mechanism *(10)*. Therefore, screening can be thought of as one of the "omic" sciences *(11)*, where the aim of the experiment is to obtain, in an unbiased manner, large amounts of data describing how a system responds to different stimuli (in the case of screening structure activity information). These data are then used to develop hypotheses from a variety of different analyses that can be experimentally tested using standard hypothesis-driven science. Many different chemoinformatic methods are proprietary, making their comparison and evaluation difficult. Additionally, even though many of the methods are applied to the NCI cancer or AIDS datasets, such comparisons are of limited value for assessing their utility for data-mining HTS datasets as these datasets do not reflect the data quality or library design usually generated from HTS. Finally, the chapter will suggest possible improvements to the application of chemoinformatics to screening and how these should be assessed.

2. Practical Aspects of High Throughput Screening

HTS has become accepted as a separate area of expertise within the drug-discovery process, requiring scientists able to work at the interface of chemistry, biology, robotics, statistics, database management, and chemoinformatics. Any high throughput screen begins with a series of compounds, usually available as a library of pre-plated DMSO stock solutions. These compound mother plates are then used to transfer compounds to an assay plate where the biological test is conducted, following addition of reagents and incubation, and the assay signal is measured. The results are usually converted to a percentage inhibition or fold stimulation (depending on the assay format) and finally the data are stored in a relational database that links the compound structure to the biological data.

The important points to note are that often the vast majority of compounds are tested just once, at a single concentration, and the results are converted to a percentage inhibition. The result of this is that the error associated with any data point may be quite large and the dynamic range of the data is limited to essentially a range of 1–100. As will be discussed below, this places important constraints on the significant information that can be successfully extracted from HTS data.

3. Application of Chemoinformatics to Screening

As will be briefly discussed in this section, chemoinformatics has been used to aid screening in a number of different ways, including (1) library design, (2) similarity searching and clustering, (3) data modeling, and (4) experimental design of screening strategies.

3.1. Library Design

As HTS became available, there was much debate as to the value of library design with a well-articulated argument that with the development of HTS technologies it should be possible to screen every available compound and not to miss any potential leads *(12)*. However, this may not be feasible as the numbers of compounds that could be synthesized are astronomically large with estimates ranging from 10^{18} to 10^{200} *(13,14)*. One estimate of the number of possibly pharmaceutically relevant small molecules was made by Villar and Koehler *(15)* with the commonly used ISIS-MDL molecular descriptors, this gave a credible estimate of 10^{49} possible molecules. Even if this is a fivefold overestimate of the number of suitable drug-like compounds, this still leaves a possible chemistry space of approx 100 million. So for practical reasons a number of different pharmaceutical companies have chosen to make selections of compounds for screening from either their internal or vendor compound collections and compounds that could be synthesized around combinatorial scaffolds, in order to maximize the efficiency of their screening efforts.

The selections of compounds are made using a variety of methods, such as dissimilarity selection *(16)*, "optiverse" library selection *(17)*, Jarvis–Park clustering *(18)*, and cell-based methods *(19)*. All these methods attempt to choose a set of compounds that represent the molecular diversity of the available compounds as efficiently as possible. A consequence of this is that only a few compounds around any given molecular scaffold may be present in a HTS screening dataset. Consistent with this statement is the observation by Nilakantan et al. (using historical screening data and ring-scaffold descriptors of the molecules tested) that it may be necessary to test as many as 100 compounds from a particular group of related compounds in order to be confident that actives in this group of compounds would have been identified *(20)*. We have conducted a similar empirical analysis of our own historical screening data using molecular equivalence numbers (structural browsing indices) *(21)* to organize the compounds similarly to Nilakantan et al. This analysis showed that more than 30 compounds from any group of compounds needed to be tested to determine if a particular compound scaffold might contain actives. This estimate was determined after analysis of screening data where the compounds were first grouped according to their ring scaffold, then second by the identifying the ring scaffolds that contained no actives. Thus, it was possible to show that scaffolds containing more than 30 compounds, all of which were inactive, would not contain actives even if additional such compounds were tested. Clearly, the density with which chemistry space needs to be explored may be greater than was initially thought and may explain the earlier assertions that all compounds need to be tested in order not to miss a potential lead (**Fig. 1**).

As mentioned above, it is now common for pharmaceutical companies to select a diverse set of compounds for screening that represent the available compounds (either internal or commercially available). Yet, this is not so for compound collections that have grown as sets of compounds, have been synthesized, or have been acquired for particular projects. This is an important reason why many examples of data-mining techniques when applied to the NCI dataset work so well and may help explain why such methods often do not perform as well against different HTS datasets *(22)*.

One approach to screening subsets of available compounds is to screen sets of compounds that, although not representative of the molecular diversity of the available compound collection, do contain as much structure activity relationship information as possible. An example of this was the "Informer Library" strategy proposed by CombiChem (which was eventually purchased by DuPont Pharmaceuticals in 1999) *(23)*. Unfortunately, there have been no published applications of this screening strategy that assess its success or failure.

3.2. Clustering and Similarity or Nearest-Neighbor Searching

A consequence of screening dissimilar libraries is that by their very nature they should contain only a small representation of any particular scaffold. As a result, there are usually few actives of similar structure; this prevents the formulation of hypotheses as to the possible substructure responsible for activity. Thus, similarity searching around initial hits is very important to permit sufficient information to be acquired to allow such hypotheses to be made and

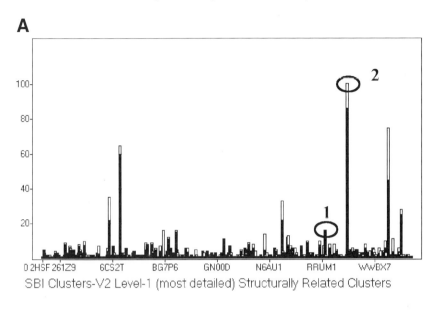

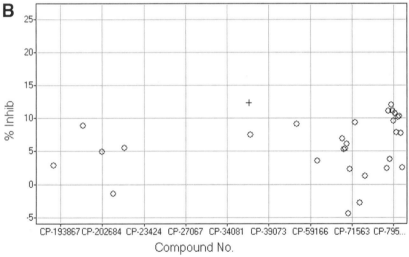

Fig. 1. Empiric observation that more than approx 20 compounds from any scaffold need to be tested in order to be sure that an active will be found. **(A)** This shows the results from a whole cell assay in which the compounds have been classified using the Level 1 Ring System of the Structural Browsing Index (SBI) also known as molecular equivalence numbers or meqnums, which is the most-detailed level. The most-populated SBI containing only inactives is labeled 1, it contains 16 compounds. The most-populated SBI containing actives is labeled 2. **(B)** Looking at only the compounds present in the most-populated SBI (2 above) and arranging the compounds in this SBI randomly, the smallest set of compounds in which an active (indicated by +) can be found is approx 30 compounds.

tested. Another application of similarity searching has been the discovery of compounds with similar biological activity but different chemical structure (or at least different enough to allow patenting of the new structure); this has been termed "leapfrogging" or "scaffold hopping" (24,25).

Recently there has been debate over the validity of the assumption that similar compounds behave similarly, with the observation that compounds similar to a probe molecule may not have the desired activity (26). This observation should not really come as a surprise when one considers that often the molecular descriptors used for similarity searching of large databases do not take into account the stereochemistry or salt forms (which can have vastly different aqueous solubilities) of the compounds. In addition, generation of most QSAR models requires a range of activities spanning 1000-fold, and yet most HTS is conducted at a single concentration. So it should be obvious that primary screening data can not detect the subtle structure activity relationships present in a class of active compounds. It is for this reason that when following up on confirmed hits from a high throughput screen we routinely assay similar compounds (even if they tested inactive in the primary screen) and will conduct dose responses starting at concentrations greater than the original screening concentration, if possible.

It should be noted that comparison between different similarity methods applied to different assays is further compromised by differences in the compound collections and differences in the molecular descriptors used. For example, Martin and Brown (27,28) have recommended using Wards Clustering with MACCS keys and a similarity cutoff of 85% for clustering compounds with similar biological activity. Yet this estimate was derived from only a limited number of screens using only the Abbott compound collection. Another example where published results may be difficult to extrapolate is that of Stanton et al. (24), which presented a logistic regression model relating the biological activity of the compound to its similarity to an initial search compound. While this example was derived from the results of 11 different similarity searches, it used only one biological assay and the BCUT molecular descriptors used to calculate similarity were normalized to the collection of available compounds. Therefore, these results should not be extrapolated to other biological screens or different chemistry spaces, making it impossible to apply conclusions drawn from this data set to other compound libraries.

Two recent papers further highlight the difficulty of choosing which similarity searching method to use (29,30). Given the vast array of different molecular descriptors available and the vast number of different similarity measures, this field has been the subject of many publications espousing different methods. As similarity searching and clustering are the easiest, yet very useful, chemoinformatic techniques available to screeners, they continue to be the subject of continued improvements and alterations.

3.3. Methods for Modeling Data

As with measures of similarity, this subject is under constant development with different data-mining packages using various data-mining algorithms being described. These include recursive partitioning, rule-based organization of screening data, binary QSAR, pharmacophore modeling, and design of experiment methods.

3.3.1. Recursive Partitioning

Recursive partitioning was originally called the decision tree method *(31)*; the goal of this method is to divide the dataset up using a series of simple rules, i.e., divide the dataset between compounds with or without a certain group or physical characteristics. Using such a series of rules, each generating an additional branch in the decision tree, it is possible to classify compounds into groups with similar structural and biological features. The advantage of this methodology is that it can work with very large datasets with large numbers of descriptors. Recursive partitioning is possibly the most commonly used data-mining method applied to HTS data *(32)*. This may be partially due to the groundbreaking efforts of S. Young and co-workers at GlaxoSmithKline. Initially, this technique was used to retrospectively model data to help in the identification of suitable lead compound classes for further follow-up and evaluation *(33)*. However, this was expanded to data modeling and used prospectively to guide subsequent sequential rounds of directed screening *(34)*. In these earlier studies the screened compounds were described using atom-pair descriptors owing to the computational ease with which these descriptors could be generated and presented as binary descriptors. However, additional fragment-based descriptors *(35)* as well as whole molecule descriptors *(36,37)* have also been applied to recursive partitioning. The value of this method is apparent by the fact that it has been accepted and exploited by other groups *(38)* and other recursive methodologies have been developed *(39)*. Not only have novel descriptors been used to improve the performance of recursive partitioning but also strategies to generate multiple decision trees and using the average prediction of these trees to better model the data, i.e., Decision Forests *(40)*, and combining recursive partitioning with K nearest neighbors *(41)*.

3.3.2. Rule Based Evaluation

Methods in which compounds are described using predefined molecular substructures have been applied to HTS data usually because of the ease with which such molecular descriptors can be generated *(42,43)*. However, such descriptors may have the disadvantage that relationships between compounds in different categories can be lost. This has been addressed with the LeadScope software package, which arranges the groupings hierarchically so as to maintain the relationship between compounds. Other means of categorizing compounds by the structural features they contain include ring-based heuristic systems *(44)* and extended to structural browsing indices *(43)*, which categorize compounds dependent on a dictionary of structural features. The compounds are readily partitioned in these molecular equivalence classes based on the structural features present in the compounds, and these molecular equivalence classes can then be ordered so as to maintain the relationship between the particular classes. As initially developed, these methods function mainly as tools for the visualization and organization of HTS data.

This approach to organizing HTS data has evolved, with novel methods being developed to identify larger associations of substructures with activity, using recursive partitioning and simulated annealing to further optimize the possible associations *(34)*.

3.3.3. Binary QSAR

Another approach that has been described for modeling HTS data is Binary Quantitative Structure Activity Relationships (Binary QSAR) *(45)*. This methodology uses a Bayesian approach to correlate structural features present in a compound with activity. A very similar strategy has been described for identifying substructures that are associated with activity, called CASE *(46)*, and this has been extended to include further structural and physicochemical modulators to allow more accurate modeling of the observed activity *(47)*. These methods have not only been used to model existing data describing inhibition of tubulin polymerization, but have successfully been used to guide subsequent rounds of screening to identify a novel lead compound (discodermolide) that has been taken on for further evaluation and drug development *(48)*.

As with recursive partitioning, binary QSAR has been the focus of continued development with novel molecular descriptors being evaluated *(49)*. As the number of potential descriptors has grown, methods to select the most appropriate descriptors, such as binary or whole molecule descriptors, have been described *(50)*. The methodology has been expanded to include kernel discrimination of activity data *(51)*. It might be expected that such a methodology might have a better chance of dealing with HTS data where the uncertainty, or error, associated with the activity data is usually greatest around the active/inactive cutoff. This method therefore tries to include within the model this uncertainty by inclusion of a kernel function to describe the error associated with the original activity estimate. One of the strongest points of this approach is that it utilizes nonparametric statistics and thus makes no assumption about the distribution of error in the data making the method robust to noise in the dataset. Another strength of this method is the acceptance by the authors that no one method for predicting activity is sufficient, especially as the goal of HTS is to identify as many different classes of active molecules as possible.

The application of binary QSAR presented by Gao and Bajorath *(52)* highlights one of the common weaknesses present in data-mining literature, where the reported activity of a set of known compounds is taken as defining activity, and this limited set of compounds are then added to a much larger set of compounds (say the MDDR), which are arbitrarily designated as inactive. Although this assumption can generally be accepted, it fails to take into account that in reality the assay may well pick up a number of false negatives, false positives, or even true positives not present in the artificial training set. For example, a training set of quinolone compounds used to develop a model for inhibition of topoisomerases, while possibly able to identify other classes of similar compounds such as doxorubicin or 9-aminoacridine, would fail to identify topoisomerase inhibitors such as cyclothalidine, novobiocin, or microcin B17, all of which inhibit topoisomerases but which act by very different mechanisms at different sites on the target *(53)*. It also overlooks the possibility that true positives may be identified that can be used for different therapeutic indications. In fact exploitation of such side activities has been used as the starting point for novel drug discovery *(54)*.

3.3.4. Pharmacophore Modeling

Pharmacophore modeling has been used in library design once common pharmacophores from known actives have been identified. Initially designed for smaller datasets, pharmacophore modeling is being increasingly applied to HTS data *(55,56)*. The advantage this methodology offers to the researcher is that it suggests common structural themes even from a diverse set of active compounds. This can then help rationalize the observed activity and much more quickly suggest directions in which the actives can be modified to optimize activity (i.e., helping in the hit to lead optimization stage of discovery).

Although the programs for this type of application were initially developed for relatively small numbers of compounds, they have also been applied to sets of screening data. Software to identify common structural features associated with active compounds, yet not present in the inactive compounds, using 2D descriptions of the compounds has been developed *(57,58)*.

The one caveat common to all these methods is that the model is only able to perceive compounds that fit into the pharmacophore known for the target. This means that even for targets of known function, new hits will only be identified that are perceived to be similar by the program to those already identified.

3.3.5. Design of Experiments (DOE)

While not exactly the same as the methods described above in that DOE cannot be applied retrospectively to diverse datasets, it has been used very successfully to guide the selection and evaluation of compounds from combinatorial libraries *(59,60)*. However, DOE has been successfully applied only in cases where limited libraries of related compounds (e.g., peptides) were being evaluated. The reason for this is intuitively obvious, as one of the assumptions of DOE is that variability in the descriptors is continuous and related to activity over a smooth response surface, so that trends and patterns can be readily identified. With HTS data both of these assumptions are generally not true, as molecules can display discontinuous responses to changing features, and the SAR of even related compounds does not map to a smooth continuous response surface (for example, **Fig. 2**).

A successful application of DOE to a high throughput screening campaign remains to be reported in the literature.

3.3.6. Data Shaving

All the previously described methods use information from active compounds to choose new compounds for further testing. However, this makes the assumption that the chemistry space has been tested evenly and that false positives or negatives are not a significant source of error. Analysis of a series of Pharmacia datasets derived from different screens using three sets of diverse compounds reveals that, even though these libraries sample the same chemistry space (**Fig. 3**), they do not overlap. This can be seen most clearly by comparing the molecular equivalence number or structural browsing indices (SBI) in which actives were identified from the three libraries (**Fig. 4**). This figure shows that in a number of cases actives from a particular SBI are present only in one of the three libraries.

To address this issue the concept of "data shaving" has been introduced *(61)*, in which screening data are used to identify structural features that are commonly associated with inactive compounds. Then, in subsequent rounds of screening, compounds containing such features can be deprioritized. In effect this presents a logical strategy to generate rules for when to stop screening certain types of compounds that may be inactive and to thus focus on either classes of compounds containing actives or on classes of compounds that have not yet been explored sufficiently to generate a "stopping rule."

In concept this is very similar to the molecular fingerprint scaling suggested by Xue et al. *(62)* or activity-weighted chemical hyperstructures *(63)* in which a consensus fingerprint or pattern (hypergraph) is computed for a series of compounds acting on a common target. This method gives additional weight to the structural features found associated with active compounds. Data shaving in

A

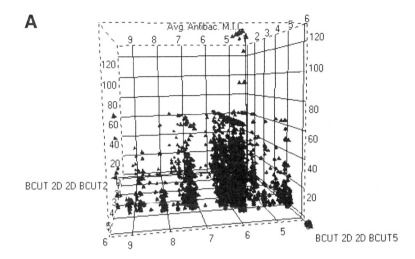

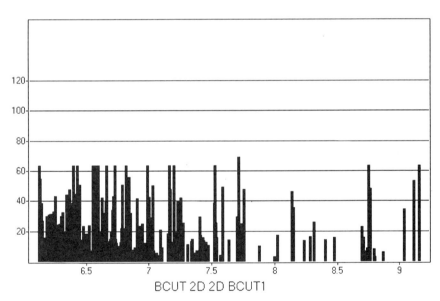

Fig. 2. Example of rough activity landscape. This figure shows the activity landscape for a series of related antibacterial compounds plotted in using the 2D BCUT descriptors to arrange the compounds. (**A**) Shows how the compounds are arrayed in a 2D representation of the chemistry space with the height of the marker being proportional to the minimum inhibitor concentration of the compounds [the smaller the minimum inhibitory concentration (MIC) the more potent the compound]. (**B**) This second panel presents the upper figure as a 2D figure to enhance the sharp cutoff between active and inactive compounds, emphasizing the point that activity landscapes are rarely smooth continuous functions.

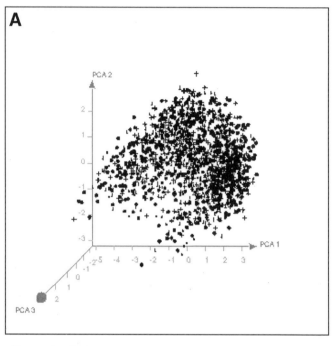

Shape by Set
■ BRO ● CAC ✚ DTC

Fig. 3. Coverage of chemistry space by four overlapping sublibraries. **(A)** Different diversity libraries cover similar chemistry space but show little overlap. This shows three libraries chosen using different dissimilarity measures to act as different representations of the available chemistry space. The compounds from these libraries are presented in this representation by first calculating the intermolecular similarity of each of the compounds to all of the other compounds using fingerprint descriptors and the Tanimoto similarity index. Principal component analysis was then conducted on the similarity matrix to reduce it to a series of principal components that allow the chemistry space to be presented in three dimensions.

contrast identifies features common to inactive compounds. This has the following advantages: (1) the majority of screening data identify inactive compounds, so rules are generated on greater amounts of data, and (2) the error associated with inactivity may have less impact on the validity of the model generated. Then regions of chemistry space occupied predominantly by inactive compounds are removed from subsequent analysis, generating a dataset much more evenly distributed around active compounds to be used to model features conferring activity.

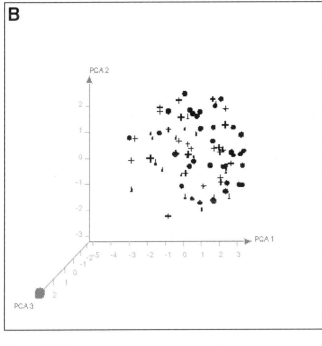

Shape by Set

▲ BRO ● CAC ✚ DTC

Fig. 3. *(continued)* **(B)** The non-overlapping nature of these different libraries is emphasized if one only considers the active compounds identified in a given screen from these libraries. As shown below almost none of the active compounds overlap and many appear in regions of space where no similar and active compounds from the other libraries were found.

3.3.7. Different Methods Applied to One Project

Given the large number of different molecular descriptors and data-mining methods available, it is increasingly difficult to identify the appropriate ones to use for the analysis of data from any given screen. One approach that has been suggested to circumvent this is to use the strategy of consensus scoring developed for improving virtual docking of ligands to protein structures *(64)*. In this approach a series of different methods are used to score the affinity of a compound for a given protein target; the results from the different methods are then rank ordered and combined in order to arrive at a consensus score for a given set of compounds.

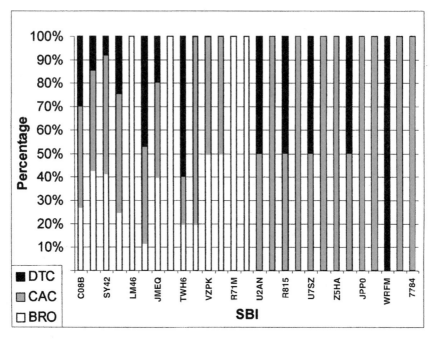

Fig. 4. Comparision of molecular equivalence numbers or structural browsing indices (SBI) containing active molecules from four different sublibraries. This figure shows how, even though the libraries described in **Fig. 3** occupy similar chemistry spaces, they still undersample certain areas so that some active classes are only found when screening one particular sublibrary and not the others. This figure takes the active compounds represented in **Fig. 3B** using structural Browsing Indices and shows which library the actives came from. This serves to emphasize how active compounds with particular structural features may be identified in only one of the three sublibraries, e.g., compounds containing the SBI 7704 are only found in the CAC sublibrary.

We have applied a similar strategy to the expansion and evaluation of hits identified from one screen using a total of five different methods to identify additional compounds similar to the original hit. **Table 1** lists the different methods used and the relative success rates of the different methods in identifying additional actives. Although it is not possible to give details concerning this experiment, one feature that should be highlighted is how the different methods each identified not only compounds with similar scaffolds to the initial hit, but also new actives with slightly different scaffolds, enlarging the choice of compounds for subsequent expansion. The fact that each method generated similar but not totally overlapping compounds for subsequent testing

Table 1
**Results of Multiple Methods to Model HTS Screening Data
and to Then Identify Novel Hits**

Method	Hits Rate
Random Screening	0.45%
Identification of additional compounds for testing similar to an initial hit using the following methods:	
Similarity Searching Methods	
SBI[a]	18%
Cousin Descriptors[b]	26%
BCUT Descriptors[c]	2%
Data Modeling Methods	
Binary QSAR[d]	5%
Recursive Partitioning[e]	2.2%
Data Mining with Enterprise Miner[f]	16%

[a]Similar compounds were chosen by selecting untested compounds with common cyclic ring systems using the SBI descriptors *(43)*.

[b]Compounds were chosen for further testing using Cousin fingerprint descriptors *(73)* and the Tanimoto similarity coefficient with a 67% similarity cutoff.

[c]Similar compounds were selected for further testing using BCUT descriptors and Euclidean distance to identify the untested compounds closest to the initial hit *(24)*.

[d]A Binary QSAR model was created using the initial screening results and then used to select additional compounds for testing as described previously *(50)*

[e]Recursive partitioning, using the ChemTree software package (available from Golden Helix, http://www.goldenhelix.com/recursivepartitioningbenefits.html), was used to model the initial screening data. Then the bin containing the target compound was used to select compounds for further testing.

[f]The Enterprise Miner software package was used to model the initial screening data and select additional compounds for testing as described previously *(74)*

and follow-up reiterates the point made by Harper et al. *(51)* that no one method will be able to fully describe the structure activity relationships present in HTS data.

4. Critical Review of Chemoinformatic Applications

Although there have been a great number of publications describing potential chemoinformatic methods for screening strategies, most describe methods applied retrospectively to screening data. These methods have great value in helping to model, explore, and ultimately understand the screening data; to improve the choice of actives for follow up; and to direct subsequent lead optimization. However, such strategies are rarely applied prospectively to screening campaigns. This is not due to a reluctance of the screeners to apply such strategies, but rather the constraints of reality. Sets of compounds for screening are often chosen using some diversity function and then are made up as a master set of compound plates that are then replicated for use in subsequent assays. Such a screening library will often represent a sizable portion of a corporate compound collection. Unless there is a dedicated effort to synthesize or purchase compounds suggested by some chemoinformatic strategy, there is little opportunity to follow such a sequential screening strategy. Although the application of any screening strategy could be started using such a library chosen for its diversity, there are often difficulties in following up on these data in a sequential manner because of the need to "cherry pick" out the suggested compounds for subsequent testing. Challenges facing this apparently simple operation include such minor aspects as compound availability, compound stability, and the resources to plate and track the newly ordered compound sets. To date there have been very few efforts to overcome these logistic issues *(65,66)*.

The other issue that arises is the quality of the screening data and the redundancy (or lack of it) present in such data sets. Although statistical methods have been applied to evaluate the quality of screening data *(67,68)*, these methods fail to reflect all the variability of screening data. One statistic that has gained widespread acceptance is the Z' value, which seeks to relate the variability between the positive and negative screening data and the size of the signal to give a signal value that relates to assay quality. **Figure 5** shows the intraday variability for four assays that have been run in our laboratory and the associated Z' values for these assays. It should be obvious that, although high throughput assays with large signal to noise and relatively small assay variability can be designed, the data variability is still usually much greater than assumed by most computational chemists. There are two major reasons for this:

1. The error associated with the data is not evenly distributed, being largest for data close to the activity cutoff point, making it even harder to associate active/inactive designations to compounds. **Figure 6** illustrates this by plotting the variability associated for each compound, tested in duplicate in one assay, versus the average activity for each compound. This point makes the comparison of different chemoinformatic methods difficult, as not only are different datasets used but that different methods for defining active/inactive cutoffs are used.
2. The second factor that contributes to this variability is that in most high throughput screens the compounds are usually only tested once, at a single concentration. Consequently, differences in compound concentration and purity will have a large effect on the accuracy of the assay data. The differences in compound concentration can be due to differences in compound preparation or compound stability in dimethylsulfoxide (DMSO). The concentration of the test compound can even be varied depending on the length of time the DMSO stock solution is exposed to the atmosphere, as DMSO can take up water *(69,70)*.

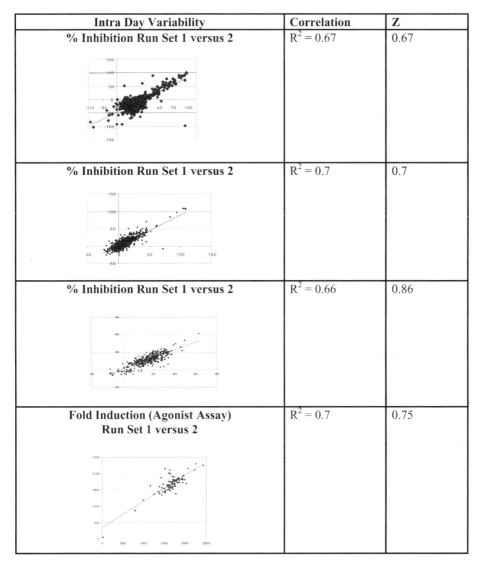

Intra Day Variability	Correlation	Z
% Inhibition Run Set 1 versus 2	$R^2 = 0.67$	0.67
% Inhibition Run Set 1 versus 2	$R^2 = 0.7$	0.7
% Inhibition Run Set 1 versus 2	$R^2 = 0.66$	0.86
Fold Induction (Agonist Assay) Run Set 1 versus 2	$R^2 = 0.7$	0.75

Fig. 5. Comparison of assay variability and Z'. This figure serves to highlight that, while assays with excellent Z' values can be developed, their reproducibility is still less than would be required for computational modeling. As discussed in the text, this is a function of single-point, single-concentration activity determinations

4.1. Issues Associated with the NCI Datasets

The most commonly used dataset for testing potential data mining packages is the NCI Tumor-Screening data set, which is publicly available

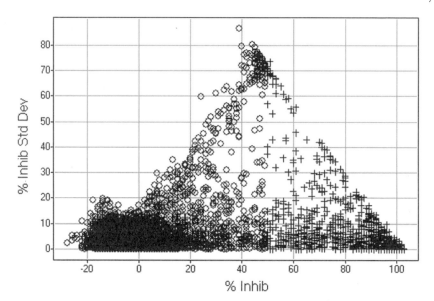

Fig. 6. Error structure of HTS results. This figure shows how the reproducibility of activity data varies with differences in activity. The circles represent compounds designated as inactive and crosses designate active compounds. From this figure it is obvious that assay variability is closest at the cutoff between active and inactive compounds.

(http://dtp.nci.nih.gov/webdata.html). Yet this dataset reports the activity of compounds tested with a dose response, not at a single concentration, and against a whole battery of cell lines. Another reason why this dataset does not accurately reflect the data quality usually generated by high throughput screens is that this compound collection has historically been acquired by expanding around compounds of interest and not designed for maximal diversity, as are many of the screening collections currently used in large pharmaceutical companies. **Figure 7** graphically displays the distribution of intramolecular similarities for four Pharmacia compound collections, three of which were designed to sample chemistry space as effectively as possible (the DT, BRO, and CAC libraries) and one that was accrued over time as compounds were obtained for

---

Fig. 7. *(see facing page)* Comparison of the intramolecular similarity distribution for four compound collections versus the NCI collection. This figure shows the intermolecular similarity (calculated using the Tanimoto similarity coefficient using ISIS fingerprint descriptors) between each compound in each library. The first panel shows how the NCI dataset contains many identical compounds (or salts of the same compound) that have been submitted for testing.

Library	Distribution of Inter Molecular Similarities	Statistics	
NCI		Mean	0.833
		St. Dev	0.133
		Upper 95% Mean	0.833
		Lower 95% Mean	0.832
His		Mean	0.828
		St. Dev	0.130
		Upper 95% Mean	0.829
		Lower 95% Mean	0.827
BRO		Mean	0.793
		St. Dev	0.123
		Upper 95% Mean	0.794
		Lower 95% Mean	0.792
CAC		Mean	0.773
		St. Dev	0.121
		Upper 95% Mean	0.774
		Lower 95% Mean	0.772
DTC		Mean	0.606
		St. Dev	0.095
		Upper 95% Mean	0.607
		Lower 95% Mean	0.604

internal projects (the HIS Library). Comparing the distribution of intermolecular similarities between these libraries it is apparent that the NCI and HIS compound collections contain many more similar compounds than the dissimilarity libraries. This introduces redundancy into the data so that structural features, common to related compounds, will have been tested multiple times, thus making any inference about the structural features present in these compounds more valid. In addition, the NCI dataset differs in the types of structures present from most pharmaceutical compound collections in that it has many more simple alkyl compounds lacking ring systems and many more natural products containing many large ring systems **(Fig. 8)**. This difference is probably due to the desire of pharmaceutical companies to populate their screening libraries with compounds that comply with heuristic rules such as the "Rule of Five," or rules to limit the number of rotatable bonds a compound should have *(71,72)*. From this discussion it has been shown that, although chemoinformatics is of great value in the analysis of screening data, the scarcity of actual screening data (with its associated errors and inadequacies) means that novel methods are rarely evaluated using primary screening data. It is possible, though, that this situation may change as the number of academic laboratories undertaking screening efforts increases. Already the availability of public databases of gene sequence information and small molecule and protein structures, and even databases of protein/ligand structures have played an important role in driving the development of software for analysis and prediction. There is an effort to develop such a public database of screening data which will surely help to stimulate the development of new data mining methods (http://iccb.med.harvard.edu/chembank/).

5. Summary

This chapter has outlined the ways in which chemoinformatics is being applied to HTS projects, from the earliest stages of library design and organization of the compounds into coherent groups to the final stage of identifying additional compounds similar to confirmed hits in order to develop rudimentary structure activity relationships. In essence chemoinformatics both lays the foundations for an "omics' screening strategy (by ensuring that a diverse representative group of compounds are screened) and then helps to refine and organize the data allowing hypotheses concerning the data to be generated, and then expanding the hypotheses by identifying compounds similar to hits of interest for further evaluation. This chapter has in addition highlighted the constraints that are inherent within screening data and how these constraints limit which chemoinformatic methods are of use and how such methods can be implemented.

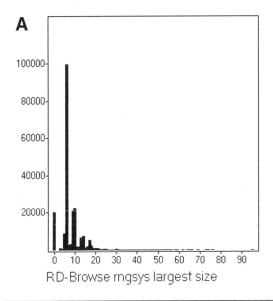

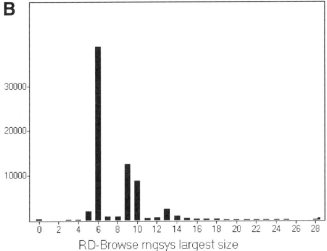

Fig. 8. Comparison of the different ring sizes present in the NCI with the Pharmacia CAC pharmaceutical library. (**A**) Histogram of the distribution of ring system size present in the NCI dataset. Note the approx 2000 compounds with no ring system and the large number of very large cyclic ring systems (larger than 30 and as large as 95, NCI compound # 683343). (**B**) By comparison the CAC library contains very few compounds with no cyclic system and the largest cyclic system is 28.

References

1. Kubinyi, H. (1999) Chance favors the prepared mind—from serendipity to rational drug design. *J. Recep. Signal Transduc. Research* **19,** 15–39.
2. Lepre, C. A. (2001) Library design for NMR-based screening. *Drug Discovery Today* **6,** 133–140.
3. Nienaber, V. L., Richardson, P. L., Klighofer, V., Bouska, J. L., Giranda, V. L., and Greer, J. (2000) Discovering novel ligands for macromolecules using x-ray crystallographic screening. *Nature* **18,** 1105–1108.
4. Su, A. I., Lorber, D. M., Weston, G. S., Baase, W. A., Mathews, B. W., and Shoichet, B. K. (2001) Docking molecules by families to increase the diversity of hits in database screens: computational strategy and experimental evaluation. *Proteins: Struc. Func. Genet.* **42,** 279–293.
5. Joseph-McCarthy, D. (1999) Computational approaches to structure-based ligand design. *Pharmacology Therapeutics* **84,** 179–191.
6. Frye, S. V. (1999) Structure-activity relationship homology (SARAH): a conceptual framework for drug discovery in the genomic era. *Chem. Biol.* **6,** R3–R7.
7. Butte, A. J., Tamayo, P., Slonim, D., Golub, T. R., and Kohane, I. S. (2000) Discovering functional relationships between RNA expression and chemotherapeutic susceptibility using relevance networks. *Proc. Natl. Acad. Sci. USA* **97,** 12,182–12,186.
8. Sills, M. A., Weiss, D., Pham, Q., Schweitzer, R., Wu, X., and Wu, J. J. (2002) Comparison of assay technologies for a tyrosine kinase assay generates different results in high throughput screening. *J. Biomol. Screen.* **7,** 191–214.
9. Caron, P. R., Mullican, M. D., Mashal, R. D., Wilson, K. P., Su, M. S., and Murcko, M. A. (2001) Chemgenomic approaches to drug discovery. *Current Opinion Chem. Biol.* **5,** 464–470.
10. Engels M. F., Wouters L., Verbeeck R., and Vanhoof G. (2002) Outlier mining in high throughput screening experiments. *J. Biomol. Screen.* **7,** 341–351.
11. Weinstein, J. N. (1998) Fishing expeditions. *Science* **282,** 628–629.
12. Spencer, R. W. (1997) Diversity analysis in high throughput screening. *J. Biomol. Screen.* **2,** 69–70.
13. Hann, M., Hudson, B., Lewell, X., Lifely, R., Miller, L., and Ramsden, N. (1999) Strategic pooling of compounds for high-throughput screening. *J. Chem. Inf. Comput. Sci.* **39,** 897–902.
14. Balkenhohl, F., van dem Bussche-Hunnefeld, C., Lansky, A., and Zechel, C. (1996) Combinatorial synthesis of small organic molecules. *Angew. Chem. Int. Ed.* **35,** 2288–2337.
15. Villar, H. O. and Koehler, R. T. (2000) Comments on the design of chemical libraries for screening. *Molecular Diversity* **5,** 13–24.
16. Lajiness, M. S. (1997) Dissimilarity-based compound selection techniques. *Perspect. Drug Disc, Des.* **7/8,** 65–84.
17. Ferguson, A. M., Patterson, D. E., Garr, C. D., and Underiner, T. L. (1996) Designing chemical libraries for lead discovery. *J. Biomol. Screen.* **1,** 65–73.

18. Doman, T. N., Cibulskis, J. M., Cibulskis, M. J., McCray, P. D., and Spangler, D. P. (1996) Algorithm5: A technique for fuzzy similarity clustering of chemical inventories. *J. Chem. Inf. Comput. Sci.* **36**, 1195–1204.

19. Schnur, D. (1999) Design and diversity analysis of large combinatorial libraries using cell-based methods. *J. Chem. Inf. Comput. Sci.* **39**, 36–45.

20. Nilakantan, R., Immermann, F., and Haraki, K. (2002) A novel approach to combinatorial library design. *Combi. Chem. High Through. Screen.* **5**, 105–110.

21. Xu., Y.-J. and Johnson, M. (2001) Algorithm for naming molecular equivalence classes represented by labeled pseudographs. *J. Chem. Inf. Comput. Sci.* **41**, 181–185.

22. Voigt, J. H., Bienfait, B., Wang, S., and Nicklaus, M. C. (2001) Comparison of the NCI open database with seven large chemical structural databases. *J. Chem. Inf. Comput. Sci.* **41**, 702–712.

23. Teig, S. L. (1998) Informative libraries are more useful than diverse ones. *J. Biomol. Screen.* **3**, 85–88.

24. Stanton, D. T., Morris, T. W., Roychoudhury, S., and Parker, C. N. (1999) Application of nearest neighbor and cluster analysis in pharmaceutical lead discovery. *J. Chem. Inf. Comput. Sci.* **39**, 21–27.

25. Schneider, G., Neidhart, W., Giller, T., and Schmid, G. (1999) "Scaffold-hopping" by topological pharmacophore search: a contribution to virtual screening. *Angew. Chem. Int. Ed.* **38**, 2894–2896.

26. Martin, Y. C., Kofron, J. L., and Traphagen, L. M. (2002) Do structurally similar molecules have similar biological activity? *J. Med. Chem.* **45**, 4350–4358.

27. Brown, R. D. and Martin, Y. C. (1996) Use of structure-activity to compare structure-based clustering methods and descriptors for use in compound selection. *J. Chem. Inf. Comput. Sci.* **36**, 572–584.

28. Brown, R. D. and Martin, Y. C. (1997) The information content of 2D and 3D structural descriptors relevant to ligand-receptor binding. *J. Chem. Inf. Comput. Sci.* **37**, 1–9.

29. Sheridan, R. P. and Kearsley, S. K. (2002) Why do we need so many chemical similarity search methods? *Drug Disc. Today* **7**, 903–911.

30. Holliday, J. D., Hu, C.-Y., and Willett, P. (2002) Grouping of coefficients for the calculation of inter-molecular similarity and dissimilarity using 2D fragment bit-strings. *Combi. Chem. High Through. Screen.* **5**, 155–166.

31. Morgan, J. N. and Sonquist, J. A. (1963) Problems in analysis of survey data and a proposal. *J. Am. Statist. Assoc.* **58**, 415–434.

32. Rusinko III, A., Farmen, M., Lambert, C. G., Brown, P. B., and Young, S. S. (1999) Analysis of a large structure/biology activity data set using recursive partitioning. *J. Chem. Inf. Comput. Sci.* **39**, 1017–1026.

33. Chen, X., Rusinko III, A., Tropsha, A., and Young, S. S. (1999) Automated pharmacophore identification for large chemical data sets. *J. Chem. Inf. Comput. Sci.* **39**, 887–896.

34. Jones-Hertzog, D. K., Mukhopadhyay, P., Keefer, C. E., and Young, S. S. (1999) Use of recursive partitioning in the sequential screening of G-protein-couples receptors. *J. Pharmacol. Toxicol.* **42**, 207–215.

35. Blower, P., Fligner, M., Verducci, J., and Bjoraker, J. (2001) On combining recursive partitioning and simulated annealing to detect groups of biologically active compounds. *J. Chem Inf. Comput. Sci.* **42**, 393–404.

36. Welch, W. J., Lam, R. L. H., and Young, S. S. (2002) Cell-based analysis of high throughput screening data for drug discovery, WTO 02/12568 A2.

37. Abt, M., Lim, Y. B., Sacks, J., Xie, M., and Young, S. S. (2001) A sequential approach for identifying lead compounds in large chemical databases. *Stat. Science* **16**, 154–168.

38. van Rhee, A. M., Stocker J., Printzenhoff, D., Creech, C., Wagoner, P. K., and Spear, K. L. (2001) Retrospective analysis of an experimental high-throughput screening data set by recursive partitioning. *J. Comb. Chem.* **3**, 267–277.

39. Godden J. W., Furr J. R., and Bajorath, J. (2003) Recursive median partitioning for virtual screening of large databases. *J. Chem. Inf. Comput. Sci.* **43**, 182–188.

40. Tong, W., Hong, H., Fang, H., Xie, Q., and Perkins, R. (2003) Decision forest: combining the predictions of multiple independent decision tree models. *J. Chem. Inf. Comput. Sci.* **43**, 525–531.

41. Miller, D. W. (2001) Results of a new classification algorithm combining K nearest neighbors and recursive partitioning. *J. Chem Inf. Comput. Sci.* **41**, 168–175.

42. Roberts, G., Myatt, G. J., Johnson, W. P., Cross, K. P., and Blower, P. E. (2000) LeadScope: software for exploring large sets of screening data. *J. Chem Inf. Comput. Sci.* **40**, 1302–1314.

43. Xu, Y. J. and Johnson, M. (2002) Using molecular equivalence numbers to visually explore structural features that distinguish chemical libraries. *J. Chem. Inf. Comput. Sci.* **42**, 912–926.

44. Nilakantan, R., Bauman, N., Haraki, K. S., and Venkataraghavan, R. (1990) A ring-based chemical structural query system: use of a novel ring-complexity heuristic. *J. Chem. Inf. Comput. Sci.* **30**, 65–68.

45. Labute, P. (1999) Binary QSAR: a new method for the determination of quantitative structure activity relationships. *Pac. Symp. Biocomput.*, pp. 444–455.

46. Klopman, G. (1984) Artificial intelligence approach to structure-activity studies. Computer automated structure evaluation of biological activity of organic molecules. *J. Am. Chem. Soc.* **106**, 7315–7318.

47. Klopman, G. (1998) The MultiCASE program II. Baseline activity identification algorithm (BAIA). *J. Chem. Inf. Comput. Sci.* **38**, 78–81.

48. ter Harr, E., Rosenkranz, H. S., Hamel, E., and Day, B. W. (1996) Computational and molecular modeling evaluation of the structural basis for tubulin polymerization inhibition by colchicine site agents. *Bioorg. Med. Chem.* **4**, 1659–1671.

49. Gao, H. (2001) Application of BCUT metrics and genetic algorithm in binary QSAR analysis. *J. Chem. Inf. Comput. Sci.* **41**, 402–407.

50. Gao, H., Lajiness, M. S., and Van Drie, J. (2002) Enhancement of binary QSAR analysis by a GA-based variable selection method. *J. Mol. Graph. Model.* **20**, 259–268.

51. Harper, G., Bradshaw, J., Gittins, J. C., Green, D. V. S., and Leach, A. R. (2001) Prediction of biological activity for high-throughput screening using binary kernel discrimination. *J. Chem. Inf. Comput. Sci.* **41**, 1295–1300.

52. Gao, H. and Bajorath, J. (1990) Comparision of binary and 2D QSAR analysis using inhibitors of human carbonic anhydrase II as a test case. *Mol. Div.* **4,** 115–130.
53. Maxwell, A. (1997) DNA gyrase as a drug target. *Trends Microbiol.* **5,** 102–109.
54. Wermuth, C. G. (2001) The SOSA approach, an alternative to high-throughput screening. *Med. Chem. Res.* **10,** 431–439.
55. Hopfinger, A. J. and Duca, J. S. (2000) Extraction of pharmacophore information from high-throughput screens. *Curr. Opin. Biotech.* **11,** 97–103.
56. Hecker, E. A., Duraiswami C., Andrea T. A., and Diller D. J. (2002) Use of catalyst pharmacophore models for screening of large combinatorial libraries. *J. Chem. Inf. Comput. Sci.* **42,** 1204–1211.
57. Tamura, S. Y., Bacha, P. A., Gruver, H. S., and Nutt, R. F. (2002) Data analysis of high-throughput screening results: application of multidomain clustering to the NCI anti-HIV data set. *J. Med. Chem.* **45,** 3082–3093.
58. Bacha, P. A., Gruver, H. S., Den Hartog, B. K., Tamura, S. Y., and Nutt, R. F. (2002) Rule extraction from a mutagenicity data set using adaptively grown phylogenetic-like trees. *J. Chem. Inf. Comput. Sci.* **42,** 1104–1111.
59. Andersson, P. M., Linusson, A., Wold, S., Sjostrom, M., Lundstedt, T., and Norden, B. (1999) Design of small molecule libraries for lead exploration. In *Molecular diversity in drug design*, Dean, P. M. and Lewis, R. A. (eds.), Kluwer Academic Publishers, pp. 197–220.
60. Brown, P. J., Smith-Oliver, T. A., Charifson, P. S., et al. (1997) Identification of peroxisome proliferator-activated receptor ligands from a biased chemical library. *Chem. Biol.* **4,** 909–918.
61. Schreyer, S. K., Parker, C. N., and Maggiora, G. M. (2004) Data Shaving—A Novel Strategy for Analysis of High Throughput Screening Data, *J. Chem. Inf. Comput. Sci.*, in press.
62. Xue, L., Stahura, F. L., Godden, J. W., and Bajorath, J. (2001) Fingerprint scaling increases the probability of identifying molecules with similar activity in virtual screening calculations. *J. Chem. Inf. Comput. Sci.* **41,** 746–753.
63. Brown, N., Willett, P., and Wilton, D. J. (2003) Generation and display of activity-weighted chemical hyperstructures. *J. Chem. Inf. Comput. Sci.* **43,** 288–297.
64. Bissantz, C., Folkers, G., and Rognan, D. (2000) Protein-based virtual screening of chemical databases. 1. Evaluation of different docking/scoring combinations. *J. Med. Chem.* **43,** 4759–4767.
65. Andersson, P. M., Sjostrom, M., Wold, S., and Lundstedt, T. (2001) Strategies for subset selection of parts of an in-house chemical library. *J. Chemometrics* **15,** 353–369.
66. Agrafiotis, D. K. and Rassokhin, D. N. (2001) Design and prioritization of plates for high-throughput screening. *J. Chem. Inf. Comput. Sci.* **41,** 798–805.
67. Zhang J.-H., Chung, T. D., and Oldenburg K. R. (1999) A simple statistical parameter for use in evaluation and validation of high throughput screening assays. *J. Biomol. Screen.* **4,** 67–73.
68. Zhang, J.-H., Chung, T. D. Y., and Oldenburg, K. R. (2000) Confirmation of primary active substances from high throughput screening of chemical and biological

populations: a statistical approach and practical considerations. *J. Comb. Chem.* **2,** 258–265.

69. Yurek, D. A., Branch, D. L., and Kuo, M. S. (2002) Development of a system to evaluate compound identity, purity, and concentration in a single experiment and its application in quality assessment of combinatorial libraries and screening hits. *J. Comb. Chem.* **4,** 138–148.

70. Humphrey, P. (2002) Studies on compound stability in DMSO, presented at the Sample Management Special Interest Group Meeting, September 24, 8th Annual General Meeting of The Society for Biomolecular Screening, The Hague, The Netherlands.

71. Lipinski, C. A. (2000) Drug-like properties and the causes of poor solubility and poor permeability. *J. Pharmacol. Toxicol. Methods* **44,** 235–249.

72. Veber, D. F., Johnson, S. R., Cheng, H.-Y., Smith, B. R., Ward, K. W., and Kopple, K. D. (2002) Molecular properties that influence the oral bioavailability of drug candidates. *J. Med. Chem.* **45,** 2615–2623.

73. Hagadone, T. R. (1992) Molecular substructure searching: efficient retrieval in two-dimensional structure databases. *J. Chem. Inf. Comput. Sci.* **32,** 515–521.

74. Lajiness, M. S. (2000) Using Enterprise Miner to explore and exploit drug discovery data. Published in the proceedings of the SAS Users Group International-SUGI 25 paper, 266–255.

5

Strategies for the Identification and Generation of Informative Compound Sets

Michael S. Lajiness and Veerabahu Shanmugasundaram

Abstract

Mounting pressures in pharmaceutical research necessitate ever increasing efficiency to lower cost and produce results. This is especially true in the realm of high-throughput screening (HTS) where large pharmaceutical companies historically test many hundreds of thousands of compounds in the search for new drug leads. As a result of this pressure the old mantra of "screen them all" is rapidly becoming a phrase of the past and the search for new, more efficient methods for discovering leads begins. This chapter will describe some of the methods, techniques, and strategies that have been implemented at Pharmacia that attempt to identify compounds that are likely to provide the most useful information so that one might discover solid leads rapidly.

Key Words: Prioritization; compound quality; structural diversity; consensus scoring; regularization; molecular complexity; structural alerts; biological promiscuity.

1. Introduction

The race to find the next blockbuster has never been more important in the pharmaceutical industry. The very existence of many companies may depend on the timely discovery of new chemical entities that can be developed into the next Celebrex® or Lipitor®. Adding to this is the need to reduce cost and increase shareholder value. Consequently, the productivity of the pharmaceutical industry has dramatically fallen short of its own expectations *(1)*.

1.1. Screening Everything is too Costly

Pharmaceutical companies house many hundreds of thousands to more than a million compounds in their corporate repositories. So as not to miss potentially interesting compounds in screening, a common strategy is to "screen them all."

From: *Methods in Molecular Biology, vol. 275:*
Chemoinformatics: Concepts, Methods, and Tools for Drug Discovery
Edited by: J. Bajorath © Humana Press Inc., Totowa, NJ

Given the cost of screening of up to $1/well or more, it doesn't take an accountant to figure out that the cost of screening the whole collection is very high. But do we need to test everything?

A well-known principle is that "similar compounds have similar activities." While not uniformly true, it still holds in enough cases that similarity searching is an accepted way of finding other interesting compounds based on a known lead or hit. Given the similarity principle and the rising costs in drug discovery and development, can we in good faith recommend screening everything as a cost effective way to discover need leads? We think not.

1.2. More Data Are Not Necessarily Better

"It's hard to see the forest for the trees" is an expression that most have heard. It's also one that relates a truism. Sometimes less is actually more.

Let's say you are a carpenter and are looking for a nice tree to cut down so you can build a cabinet. You walk to a 1-acre woods and, it being a small tract of land, you quickly choose a nice oak tree. Imagine if you were selecting a tree from a 10 square mile tract. You might be tempted to look and look and look for the best tree you could find. It may very well turn out that selecting a good tree from the 1-acre plot will move you faster to your goal of building a cabinet than looking at the larger tract and choosing the absolute best tree. It's all about how you utilize your search space.

There are often many results obtained during HTS that confuse and point scientists in the wrong direction. These false positives are due to many factors such as aggregation, metal chelation, insolubility, and reactive and unstable compounds. The sheer volume of data makes it hard to visualize the results and understand what the data are telling you. The fact is that many of these false leads can be avoided by intelligent treatment of the results.

1.3. A Typical HTS Problem

A typical problem encountered in HTS is when a biological assay identifies many thousands of compounds as being active. The sheer number of compounds makes it impossible to perform concentration–response experiments in a timely manner. A common practice in this situation is to raise the definition of activity. For example, one might have an initial list of 50,000 actives after screening 1,000,000 compounds (a 5% hit rate) and arbitrarily setting a percentage inhibition cutoff to 75% inhibition or higher may lower the number of hits to a more manageable size of 10,000. Even after such a reduction, the remaining compounds may still contain compounds that have rule-of-five scores over 2, $cLogP$'s over 7, or molecular weights greater than 800. In addition, the list may contain a large number of highly similar compounds. Clearly, there must be a better way to reduce the number of compounds while keeping the most interesting and informative compounds in the list.

1.4. What to Do?

Obviously, one could choose to ignore the issues mentioned above and just screen as many compounds as desired and selecting hits starting with the most active first. Another possibility is to filter the lists of hits based on other criteria. Yet another, more attractive possibility is to have a medicinal chemist review the list and eliminate the ones he/she doesn't like. However, there are two problems with this idea. First, there are not enough medicinal chemists available to review lists of thousands of compounds in a reasonable amount of time. The second problem is that medicinal chemists are inconsistent.

1.5. Medicinal Chemists are Inconsistent

In a recent study at Pharmacia it was found that medicinal chemists were inconsistent in the compounds they reject *(2)*. In addition, it was also observed that individual medicinal chemists don't consistently reject the same compounds! In this study, 13 experienced chemists reviewed the same list of 250 compounds that were previously rejected by a senior medicinal chemist. These 250 compounds were broken down into 23 lists. Each chemist reviewed from one to three lists. **Figure 1** contains a histogram that indicates how many compounds were consistently rejected. As one can see in this figure, only one compound was rejected from the 23 lists by all the 13 chemists. **Figure 2** illustrates how consistent the 13 medicinal chemists are to themselves when reviewing the same list of 250 compounds organized differently.

The obvious conclusion from the Pharmacia study is that chemists are inconsistent and cannot be relied upon to consistently select the same compounds to form informative sets of compounds. So, if chemists are biased, how can one consistently and intelligently create interesting and informative sets of compounds?

1.6. Computational Methods

One answer to this dilemma is to use computational methods to identify the most interesting and informative compounds to pursue. Several workers have devised rules to identify undesirable or desirable compounds *(3–12)*. These applications generally rely upon hard rules or structural criteria applied with limited focus to define interesting compounds. For example, the rule-of-five utilizes a score of 0–4 and is meant to assess bioavailability issues alone. Triage methods eliminate compounds that violate one or more of a variety of rules, which results in a limited set of compounds passing all filters. This is in some

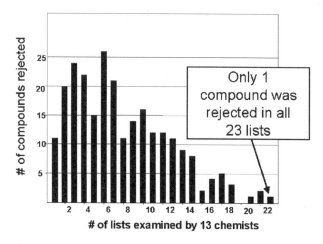

Fig. 1. The number of compounds consistently rejected by 13 chemists.

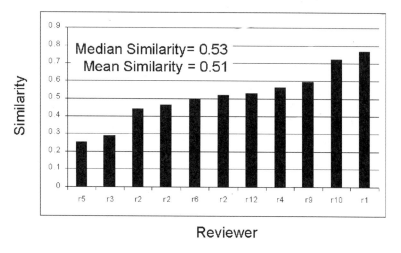

Fig. 2. Average consistency (similarity) of a chemist in rejecting the same compounds.

sense the best set of compounds. However, this set may contain many similar compounds and also may have excluded many interesting compounds that only violated a single criterion by a small amount. The problem with these approaches is that they ignore the fact that interesting compounds reside in a complicated multivariate space and by focusing on one or two parameters one can easily eliminate great lead compounds.

It is suggested in this chapter that it is better to use prioritization methods, which utilize a series of soft scores so that compounds with the most interesting profile rank higher and compounds with the least desirable profile rank lower.

2. Custom Prioritization Software

Custom software was developed to perform compound prioritization. The objective of this work was:

- Faster and more consistent decision making.
- Reprioritizing compounds rather than eliminating some of them completely from hit-lists.
- To encourage rapid interaction with medicinal chemists, not eliminate need for their opinion.

The software utilizes a wide variety of information contained in corporate databases to identify interesting compounds with lead-like features. These features of a compound are grouped into several categories and are combined to create scores that define fairly independent measures of a compound's suitability for follow-up evaluation. These scores are then combined to create a composite score that weights the features according to project team objectives.

One important result of this type of a score is that project teams are forced to address what makes a compound interesting. Another effect is that the resultant scores are unbiased and consistent. Needless to say, the software and scoring system evolves as more results become available and as the goals of the collaboration changes.

2.1. Score Components

There are four component scores that can be used to assess how informative and desirable a compound might be. These scores are as follows:

- *Q-score* Compound quality score based on molecular weight, biological promiscuity, and other data commonly accepted to measure lead-like properties of a compound.
- *B-score* Biological profile score based on potency, selectivity, and toxicity of a compound.
- *D-score* Dissimilarity score based on Tanimoto-like similarity among compounds in the "set." This will ensure that compounds from different structural classes are prioritized higher.
- *S-score* Similarity score based on Tanimoto similarity to selected desirable compounds.

It should be noted that the S-score will not be discussed any further in this chapter except to say that this score can be used to bias the prioritization toward particular compound classes. These scores are then combined into a *Composite-score*, which is a linear combination of the above scores with weights reflecting relative "worth" of each component.

2.2. Q-score or Quality Score

The Q-score is composed of a number of components. Some of these are listed below.

- Rule-of-five score.
- Molecular weight.
- $c$log$P$.
- Number of rings.
- Presence of a structural alert.
- Estimated solubility.
- Molecular complexity.
- Biological promiscuity.
- Other parameters.

Much has been written in the literature regarding the desirable levels of many of these features *(3–12)*. Owing to space and other limitations, we will briefly describe three of these features. These are biological promiscuity, molecular complexity, and estimated solubility.

2.2.1. Biological Promiscuity

Biological promiscuity is a term first suggested by Lajiness in 1998 to describe the tendency of a compound to be found active in multiple, unrelated assays. It is clearly related to Shoichets' notion of "pathological" compounds. Aggregation is one reason that compounds appear to be promiscuous *(13–16)*. The Biological Promiscuity Index (BPI) is essentially an empirical probability value and ranges from 0 to 1. The index relates the proportion of compounds exhibiting promiscuity (activity in multiple unrelated assays) given the number of assays that a particular compound has been tested in. To illustrate this, **Fig. 3** shows the relationship between the BPI and the number of nonantibiotic assays reporting a compound as active.

In general, antibiotic assays are not used in calculating biological promiscuity, because many compounds that are active against one species of bacteria are often active against many others. It should also be noted that these data were generated based on the vast collection of historical screening data accumulated at Pharmacia over the last 20 yr. Preliminary visual data analysis indicated that many compounds exhibiting high biological promiscuity are often compounds eliminated by chemists upon review. It is also interesting to note that these compounds are generally not identifiable by any other type of filter that the authors are aware of. Thus, it forms a valuable component in the creation of the quality score.

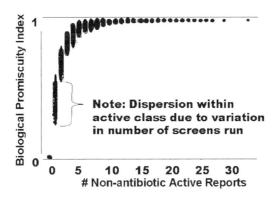

Fig. 3. Biological Promiscuity Index (BPI) versus the observed number of active assay reports.

2.2.2. Molecular Complexity

The authors feel that compounds need to be sufficiently complex in order to provide a significant level of information content. On the other hand, compounds that are too complex may be viewed as undesirable. A number of measures for characterizing molecular complexity have been developed over the years. Complexity has been defined in terms of size, elemental composition, topology, symmetry, and functional groups present in a molecule *(17,18)*. In the present work, we have applied a simple, chemically intuitive measure developed by Barone and Channon *(18)*. This approach is based on a simple additive model, where values are assigned to specific classes of molecular features such as the types of atoms and bonding patterns, and the number and types of rings. This is illustrated in **Eq. 2.1**:

$$C_{BC} = B_{rings} + B_{cnt} + B_{atom} \tag{2.1}$$

where the Barone–Channon complexity index C_{BC} is composed of a B_{rings} term, which is a "ring term," a B_{cnt} term, which accounts for atom connectivity/valency, and a B_{atom} term for atom types.

More explicitly,

$$B_{rings} = \sum_{i=1}^{N_{rings}} 6 \times R_i^{ringsize} \tag{2.2}$$

where $R_i^{ringsize}$ is the number of atoms in the ith ring

$$B_{cnt} = 3 \times N_{atoms}(1) + 6 \times N_{atoms}(2) + 12 \times N_{atoms}(3) + 24 \times N_{atoms}(4) \tag{2.3}$$

where N_{atoms} (v) is the number of atoms with connectivity/valency equal to $v = 1$, 2, 3, or 4, and

$$B_{atom} = 3 \times N_{carbon} + 6 \times N_{hetero} \tag{2.4}$$

where N_{carbon} is the number of carbon atoms and N_{hetero} is the number of hetero atoms in the molecule.

2.2.3. Estimated Solubility

The aqueous solubility of a compound is a very important molecular quality component. At Pharmacia, Gao et al. *(19)* have reported a method for estimating the aqueous solubility of organic compounds using a QSPR approach. Their analysis included 930 diverse compounds that were analyzed using principal component regression. The diverse compounds were selected using MACCS fingerprints and a BCUT chemistry space. The derived model had an r^2 of 0.92 and a q^2 of 0.91. The QSPR model was validated using 209 compounds not included in the training set and the absolute error for the test set was 0.40 log S_w. This model is readily available through Cousin/ChemLink, the chemoinformatics database system developed at Pharmacia.

2.2.4. Scoring Strategy

The strategy used to define the Q-score was to first define the components that would contribute to the score and the relative weights that should be assigned to each component. Q-score would then be calculated and a training set of compounds ranked. These results were reviewed and weights adjusted accordingly until deemed acceptable. Once the compounds were ranked acceptably, the resultant score was then transformed and regularized (a process described below) to obtain a normalized distribution ranging between 0 and 1.

A discrete-style scoring scheme is illustrated in **Fig. 4**, and **Fig. 5** contains an example that shows a linear-style scoring scheme. In either case, the net result is that one identifies a portion of the range of a particular feature such as molecular weight and assigns a score that is reflective of the desirability of that value.

Once all of the component scores are defined and calculated, one can then compute the Q-score by forming a linear combination of the components. For example, Q-score could be computed using the formula shown in **Eq. 2.5**:

$$Q - score = \frac{\sum_{i=1}^{n} a_i \times s_i}{\sum_{i=1}^{n} a_i} \tag{2.5}$$

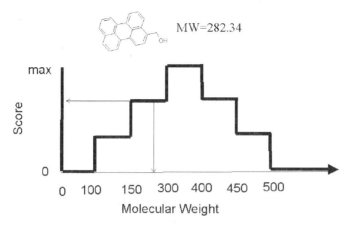

Fig. 4. Example of a discrete treatment of a component score.

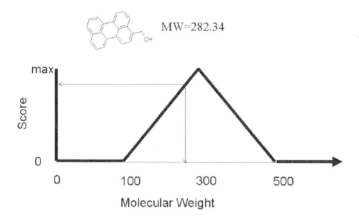

Fig. 5. Example of a continuous treatment of a component score.

where a_i = weight for component i, s_i = regularized score for component i, component i = molecular weight, cLog$P$, ROF score, . . . n components.

Note that weights may be either intrinsic or extrinsic. This means that one can build the weight into the range of the scores themselves or assign an explicit weight later if the components are all on the same scale. For example, the range of the scores used for the BPI could be from 0 to 50 and the range for molecular weight could be from 0 to 100. Thus, molecular weight would potentially have twice the weight of the BPI. It should be noted that in **Eq. 2.5** the numerator is divided by the sum of the weights. This is done, assuming the components themselves are in the range 0–1, so that the Q-score also ranges between 0 and 1.

2.3. B-score or Biological Score

The biological score is meant to reflect how well a compound performed in an assay or series of assays. In the case of HTS, one might have a single inhibition value in which case no sophisticated scoring needs to be done. In other cases a variety of IC_{50} or K_i values might be available that attempt to define potency, selectivity, and toxicity. Thus, one can envision a series of assays that result in IC_{50} or K_i values that reflect absolute potency, a selectivity ratio, and an efficacy/toxicity ratio. Often project teams are interested in compounds that are at or near the nanomolar level of potency. However, one might also desire far less activity or more selectivity versus a related target. Thus, a ratio of IC_{50}s might be appropriate to define selectivity. Also, if there is a corresponding toxicity endpoint, one could also envision a toxicity ratio. After suitable normalization and regularization, one could obtain a Potency score (PS), a Selectivity score (SS), and then a Toxicity score (TS). One then could construct a Biological score (BS) that combines the three as shown in **Eq. 2.6**:

$$B-score = \frac{\left((2 \times PS) + SS + 0.5 \times TS\right)}{3.5} \tag{2.6}$$

As was done for the Q-score, the numerator sum was divided by the sum of the weights so that the B-Score ranged between 0 and 1.

2.4. Important Features of Scores and Statistics

2.4.1. Normalization

The goal of the prioritization scheme is to design the scores so that the overall worst looking compounds are de-emphasized and the best looking compounds are moved toward the top of the list. Thus, it is important to ensure that the best and the worst compounds are clearly separated and that the vast bulk of the population is in the middle. The normal distribution is ideally suited for this and thus it is advantageous to transform our component scores into a normal-like distribution. EnterPrise Miner® from SAS Institute was used to do this as it has a *maximize normality* transformation built into it.

2.4.2. Regularization

Essentially what we are trying to do in this attempt at prioritization is to combine apples and oranges to make a tasty fruit salad! If the recipe called for equal proportions of apples, grapes, and watermelon one would NOT use 5 apples, 5 grapes, and 5 watermelons! Obviously such a fruit salad would be dominated by the watermelon since it is so much bigger. Thus, one needs to make sure that the scale of each of the components is adjusted so that one can purchase the right amount and make the best fruit salad possible. This process is sometimes called regularization and can be simply computed by the following formula shown in **Eq. 2.7**:

$$New\_value = \frac{(Old\_value - Min\_value)}{(Max\_value - Min\_value)} \tag{2.7}$$

Score or Diversity Score

The D-score is computed using the maximum dissimilarity algorithm of Lajiness *(20)*. This method utilizes a Tanimoto-like similarity measure defined on a 360-bit fragment descriptor used in conjunction with the Cousin/ChemLink system *(21)*. The important feature of this method is that it starts with the selection of a seed compound with subsequent compounds selected based on the maximum diversity relative to all compounds already selected. Thus, the most obvious seed to use in the current scenario is the compound that has the best profile based on the already computed scores. Thus, one needs to compute a "preliminary consensus score" based on the Q-score and the B-score using weights as defined previously. To summarize this, one needs to

- Compute the normalized and regularized component scores (B-score and Q-score)
- Compute the preliminary consensus score (e.g., Q-score + .5*B-score)
- Rank the compounds based on the preliminary score
- Choose the best scoring compound as the dissimilarity seed
- Compute the dissimilarity score and transform it appropriately

The intent of the diversity score is to ensure that methyl-ethyl-propyl-butyl compounds won't all rank near the top and that lower scoring (on other measures) compounds that are structurally novel will be evaluated more favorably.

2.6. Final Consensus

After all the individual scores have been computed and transformed appropriately, one can define the consensus score. This score should weight the various components according to the desires of the project team. For example, the Consensus Score (CS) could be define as:

$$CS = (2*Q\text{-score} + B\text{-score} + .5* D\text{-score}) \tag{2.8}$$

This function weights compound quality the highest followed by performance in relevant biological assays, followed by diversity. It is really not necessary to regularize this score but can be done to be consistent with the other scores. Many different weights can be used and will result in greater or lesser emphasis being placed on diversity, quality, or the biological profile.

Compound	Q_score	B_score	Consensus0	Order0	Dissim	Dissim order	Consensus	Final Order
NP-103930	0.92	0.9	0.91	1	0.94	1	0.92	1
PHA-0055 9017	0.94	0.81	0.88	3	0.47	114	0.74	2
PHA-0054 4900	1	0.74	0.87	4	0.45	145	0.73	3
PHA-0037 3741	0.92	0.76	0.84	8	0.47	112	0.72	4
NP-79732	0.86	0.65	0.76	27	0.61	30	0.71	5
PHA-0034 2321	0.89	0.79	0.84	7	0.42	195	0.7	6
PHA-0034 1332	0.97	0.74	0.86	5	0.38	313	0.7	7
NP-107491	0.92	0.65	0.78	15	0.52	61	0.7	8
NP-77675	0.89	0.72	0.8	12	0.46	135	0.69	9
PHA-0038 2149	0.76	0.78	0.77	20	0.49	84	0.68	10
PHA-0034 2488B	0.84	0.62	0.73	46	0.57	39	0.67	11
NP-48699	0.84	0.76	0.8	13	0.4	247	0.66	12
NP-36821	0.76	0.76	0.76	24	0.47	117	0.66	13
PNU-0058 341	0.76	0.61	0.69	115	0.59	32	0.65	14
PHA-0034 3274	0.72	0.64	0.68	139	0.6	31	0.65	15
PHA-0055 7761	0.84	0.82	0.83	10	0.3	719	0.65	16
PNU-0287 902	0.86	0.61	0.74	40	0.47	109	0.65	17

Fig. 6. Example of final consensus information.

As in the computation of all the scores, one needs to check to make sure that the rank-ordered compounds are reasonable. In the early stages of development of this prioritization method there was a great deal of adjustment to the scoring functions to match medicinal chemists' and project team members' opinions.

An example of a final consensus list can be seen in **Fig. 6**. In this figure one can see the Q-score and B-score and the computed preliminary consensus score. On the basis of the preliminary consensus, NP-103930 was chosen as the best compound and selected to be the dissimilarity seed. After the maximum dissimilarity calculation, the diversity score was input and the final consensus score was calculated. As one can see from this figure, the first compound in the preliminary run remains the best. The second compound from the preliminary run does not appear in this list as it was very similar to the NP-103930 and was de-prioritized and moved down the list accordingly. Also the 155th compound in the preliminary ranking moved up the 14th rank because it was considered as a structurally novel compound. This, we feel, illustrates the power of this approach. Compounds with the most desirable properties move up the list and compounds with less desirable properties move down the list.

2.7. Forming Priority Lists

Once the final consensus score has been calculated for all compounds, the lists were divided into smaller compound sets for convenience. In one particular example, the total set was split into 6 sets of approx 400 compounds each. This is illustrated in **Fig. 7**. Selected lists were then sent out for plating and subsequent testing.

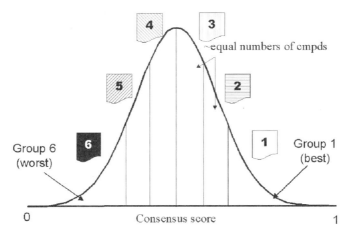

Fig. 7. Defining priority lists based on consensus scores.

3. Results

For a variety of reasons we are not able to show the detailed results as to how the method allowed us to identify interesting compounds more quickly. What we are able to show is the distribution of compounds relative to various component measures, which illustrates that for the vast majority of cases the top priority lists contain the best looking compounds and the lowest priority lists contain the worst looking compounds.

In this section the results of a prioritization in terms of component distributions will be given for a set of approx 2,400 compounds that were divided into 6 priority lists.

In **Figs. 8–10** one can see that the distribution of average potency, selectivity, and average efficacy/toxicity ratio is exactly as one would desire. One can conclude that list 1, the highest priority list, contains the most efficacious compounds based on the degree of testing performed so far.

Average Quality (based on Q-score) for each of the six lists is illustrated via histograms in **Fig. 11**. Clearly, list 1 contains the highest quality compounds and list 6 contains the worst in terms of compound quality.

Figures 12–14 indicate that the distributions of average molecular weight, average rule-of-five score, and average biological promiscuity have trends consistent with the goal of the priority lists.

However, in **Fig. 15**, the graphic clearly shows that list 1, the highest priority group, does not have the best estimated solubility. This might indicate that the weight assigned to estimated solubility was not as high as it could be to force the overall prioritization procedure to select compounds so as to make the average more in line with the desired prioritization. It should be pointed out,

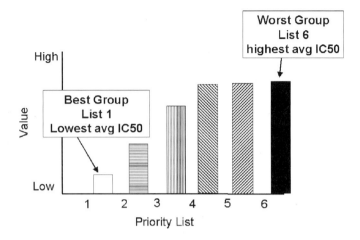

Fig. 8. Distribution of average IC50 grouped by priority list.

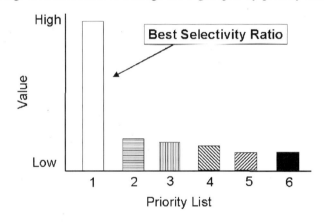

Fig. 9. Distribution of average selectivity grouped by priority list.

however, that there may be *no* way to adjust the weights so that all of the parameters will be distributed as desired.

Figure 16 shows that compounds with structural alerts, substructural features that are generally not wanted in drug candidates but may be acceptable in lead compounds, are pushed back into the fifth and sixth lists.

Somewhat surprisingly the lists contain compounds with structural diversity much in line with what was desired. What is plotted in **Fig. 17** is the distribution of similarity values between compounds contained in a priority list. Thus, lower similarity values reflect more diversity. Clearly, list 1 contains the most diverse compounds and lists 3 and 4 the least diverse. It should be pointed out that lists 5 and 6 both contain very diverse compounds, but these compounds were most likely placed into these groups due to poor scores in other areas.

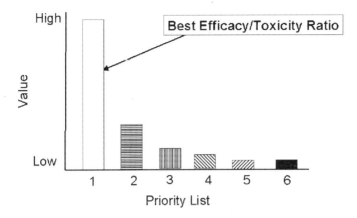

Fig. 10. Distribution of average efficacy/toxicity ratio grouped by priority list.

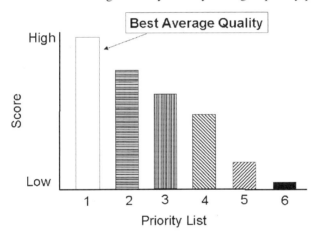

Fig. 11. Distribution of average quality grouped by priority list.

4. Summary and Conclusions

What has been described in this chapter is an approach where one prioritizes compounds for follow-up screening instead of filtering. One starts with a list of compounds ordered by some parameter such as percentage inhibition and then calculates scores that are reflective of various measures of desirability. These scores are combined into a consensus score and then are used to reprioritize the list so that compounds with desirable features are near the top of the list and less desirable compounds move near the bottom of the list. These compounds can be organized into groups to facilitate analysis. It is anticipated that this is a dynamic process and evolves as more experience is gained.

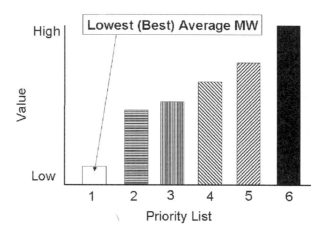

Fig. 12. Distribution of average Molecular Weight grouped by priority list.

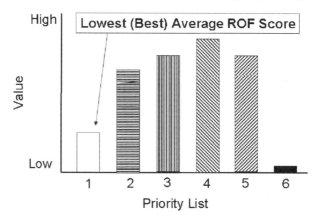

Fig. 13. Distribution of average Rule-of-Five score grouped by priority list.

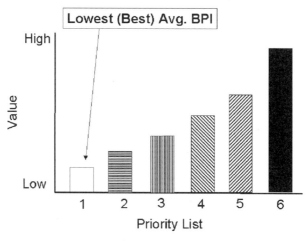

Fig. 14. Distribution of average biological promiscuity index grouped by priority list.

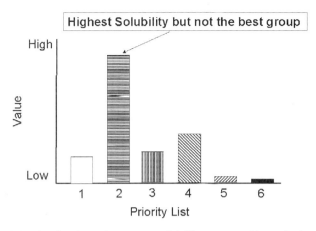

Fig. 15. Distribution of average solubility grouped by priority list.

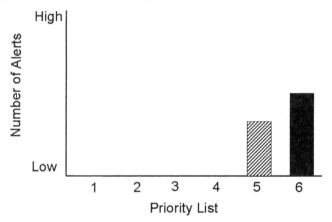

Fig. 16. Distribution of structural alerts grouped by priority list.

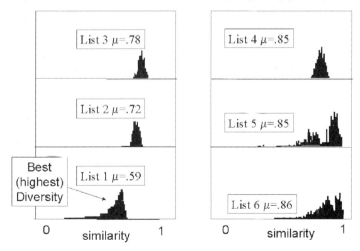

Fig. 17. Distribution of diversity grouped by priority list.

It seems clear that eliminating compounds from consideration based on one or two parameters is not ideal and that prioritizing compounds based on a more complete multivariate landscape of properties is more appropriate. Prioritization may not be as good as expert medicinal chemistry opinion, but it's cheaper, unbiased, more consistent, and more readily available.

Acknowledgments

The authors would like to thank Pharmacia colleagues Mary Lajiness, Chris Haber, Michele Kagey, Gerry Maggiora, Tom Doman, and Christian Parker for their efforts and input in the development of these ideas.

References

1. Drews, J. (2003) Strategic trends in the drug industry. *Drug Disc. Today* **8,** 411–420.
2. Lajiness, M. S. and Maggiora, G. M. (2004) How consistent are medicinal chemists in reviewing lists of compounds (manuscript in preparation).
3. Lipinski, C. A., Lombardo, F., Dominy, B. W., and Feeney, P. J. (1997) Experimental and computational approaches to estimate solubility and permeability in drug discovery and development settings. *Adv. Drug. Del. Rev.* **23,** 3–25.
4. Roche, O., Schneider, P., Zuegge, J., et al. (2002) Development of a virtual screening method for identification of "frequent hitters" in compound libraries. *J. Med. Chem.* **45,** 137–142.
5. Rishton, G. M. (1997) Reactive compounds and in vitro false positives in HTS. *Drug Disc. Today* **2,** 382–384.
6. Bikker, J. A., Dunbar, J. B., Bornemeier, D., Wild, D. J., Calvet, A., and Humblet, C. (2001) Needles in hayfields: strategies for rapid HTS triage analysis. *Abstracts of Papers of the ACS*, **222,** 50-CINF, Part 1 Aug 2001.
7. Muegge, I. (2003) Selection criteria for drug-like compounds. *Med. Res. Rev.* **23,** 302–321.
8. Egan, W. J., Walters, W. P., and Murcko, M. A. (2002) Guiding molecules towards drug-likeness. *Curr. Opin. Drug. Disc. Des.* **5,** 540–549.
9. Rishton, G. M. (2003) Nonleadlikeness and leadlikeness in biochemical screening. *Drug Disc. Today* **8,** 86–96.
10. Charifson, P. S. and Walters, W. P. (2002) Filtering databases and chemical libraries. *J. Comput.-Aided Mol. Design* **16,** 311–323.
11. Oprea, T. I. (2002) Current trends in lead discovery: Are we looking for the appropriate properties? *J. Comput.-Aided Mol. Design* **16,** 325–334.
12. Matter, H., Baringhaus, K. H., Naumann, T., Klabunde, T., and Pirard, B. (2001) Computational approaches towards the rational design of drug-like compound libraries. *Comb. Chem. HTS* **4,** 453–475.
13. McGovern, S. L., Caselli, E., Grigorieff, N., and Shoichet, B. K. (2002) A common mechanism underlying promiscuous inhibitors from virtual and high-throughput screening. *J. Med. Chem.* **45,** 1712–1722.

14. McGovern, S. L. and Shoichet, B. K. (2003) Kinase inhibitors: not just for kinases anymore. *J. Med. Chem.* **46,** 1478–1483.
15. McGovern, S. L., Helfand, B., Feng, B., and Shoichet, B. K. (2003) A specific mechanism for nonspecific inhibition. *J. Med. Chem.* **46,** 4265–4272.
16. Seidler, J., McGovern, S. L., Doman, T. N., and Shoichet, B. K. (2003) Identification and prediction of promiscuous aggregating inhibitors among known drugs. *J. Med. Chem.* **46,** 4477–4486.
17. Whitlock, H. W. (1998) On the structure of total synthesis of complex natural products. *J. Org. Chem.* **63,** 7982–7989.
18. Barone, R. and Channon, M. (2001) A new and simple approach to chemical complexity. Application to the synthesis of natural products. *JCICS* **41,** 269–272.
19. Gao, H., Shanmugasundaram, V., and Lee, P. H. (2002) Estimation of aqueous solubility of organic compounds with QSPR approach. *Pharm. Res.* **19,** 497–503.
20. Lajiness, M. S. (1997) Dissimilarity-based compound selection techniques. *Perspect. Drug Disc. Design* **7/8,** 65–84.
21. Hagadone, T. R. and Lajiness, M. S. (1993) Integrating chemical structures into an extended relational database system. *Proceedings of the 2nd international chemical structures in chemistry conference.* Warr, W. (ed.), Springer, Berlin, Germany, pp. 257–269.

6

Methods for Applying the Quantitative Structure–Activity Relationship Paradigm

Emilio Xavier Esposito, Anton J. Hopfinger, and Jeffry D. Madura

Abstract

There are several Quantitative Structure–Activity Relationship (QSAR) methods to assist in the design of compounds for medicinal use. Owing to the different QSAR methodologies, deciding which QSAR method to use depends on the composition of system of interest and the desired results. The relationship between a compound's binding affinity/activity to its structural properties was first noted in the 1930s by Hammett *(1,2)* and later refined by Hansch and Fujita *(3)* in the mid-1960s. In 1988 Cramer and coworkers *(4)* created Comparative Molecular Field Analysis (CoMFA) incorporating the three-dimensional (3D) aspects of the compounds, specifically the electrostatic fields of the compound, into the QSAR model. Hopfinger and coworkers *(5)* included an additional dimension to 3D-QSAR methodology in 1997 that eliminated the question of "Which conformation to use in a QSAR study?", creating 4D-QSAR. In 1999 Chemical Computing Group Inc. *(6)* (CCG) developed the Binary-QSAR *(7)* methodology and added novel 3D-QSAR descriptors to the traditional QSAR model allowing the 3D properties of compounds to be incorporated into the traditional QSAR model. Recently CCG released Probabilistic Receptor Potentials *(8)* to calculate the substrate's atomic preferences in the active site. These potentials are constructed by fitting analytical functions to experimental properties of the substrates using knowledge-based methods. An overview of these and other QSAR methods will be discussed along with an in-depth examination of the methodologies used to construct QSAR models. Also, included in this chapter is a case study of molecules used to create QSAR models utilizing different methodologies and QSAR programs.

Key Words: 2D-QSAR; traditional QSAR; 3D-QSAR; nD-QSAR; 4D-QSAR; receptor-independent QSAR; receptor-dependent QSAR; high throughput screening; alignment; conformation; chemometrics; principal components analysis; partial least squares; artificial neural networks; support vector machines; Binary-QSAR; selecting QSAR descriptors.

From: *Methods in Molecular Biology, vol. 275:*
Chemoinformatics: Concepts, Methods, and Tools for Drug Discovery
Edited by: J. Bajorath © Humana Press Inc., Totowa, NJ

1. Introduction

The underlying theory of Quantitative Structure–Activity Relationship (QSAR) is that biological activity is directly related to molecular structure. Therefore, molecules with similar structure will possess similar bioactivities for similar proteins/receptors/enzymes and the changes in structure will be represented through the changes in the bioactivities. The best general description of a QSAR model is

$$\text{Predicted Bioactivity} = a(\text{descriptor}_1) + b(\text{descriptor}_2) + \cdots + c \quad (1)$$

There are several QSAR methods to assist in the design of compounds for medicinal use and deciding the method to use depends on the system of interest. The origin of the concept of QSAR is a debated topic, with most agreeing *(9)* that QSAR as we know it today originated with the works of Hansch and Fujita *(3)* and Free and Wilson *(10)* in 1964. In 1988 Cramer and coworkers developed Comparative Molecular Field Analysis (CoMFA) *(4)*, which incorporates the three-dimensional (3D) aspects of the compound, specifically the electrostatic fields, into the QSAR model. CoMFA is a method of describing the 3D structure–activity relationships in a quantitative manner and is an improvement on traditional QSAR by taking into consideration 3D structures, steric regions, and the electrostatic nature of molecular substituents. CoMFA differs from traditional QSAR techniques because it is a representation of steric and electrostatic fields of the ligand on a 3D grid thus producing an image that can be viewed and compared *(4)*. There are two major points of contention with CoMFA, (1) the alignment and (2) the conformation of the molecules in the study. Following the development of CoMFA, the addition of 3D descriptors for traditional QSAR *(6)*, 4D-QSAR incorporating ensembles of molecular conformations *(5)*, Binary-QSAR *(7)*, and Probability Receptor Potentials *(8)* have been devised to aid in computer-aided drug design. This chapter is not meant to be the "holy grail" of QSAR, but an explanation of how each part of the QSAR process fits together and influences potential successes and failures, while also highlighting the benefits and pitfalls of the methods used to create the models.

The underlying process of creating a QSAR model is shown in **Fig. 1A**. The process starts by collecting the molecules of interest and calculating all possible descriptors. Next the significant descriptors are selected and a model is created. If the correct descriptors are selected, the model will produce good results when evaluated on the Test Set. Normally a poor model is constructed and a modified or new set of descriptors is chosen and the process is repeated. Once a good model is found, it is used to design novel compounds for the system of interest. Unfortunately this is all that is typically understood or seen when using a QSAR package such as QuaSAR *(6)*, CoMFA *(4)*, SOMFA *(11)*,

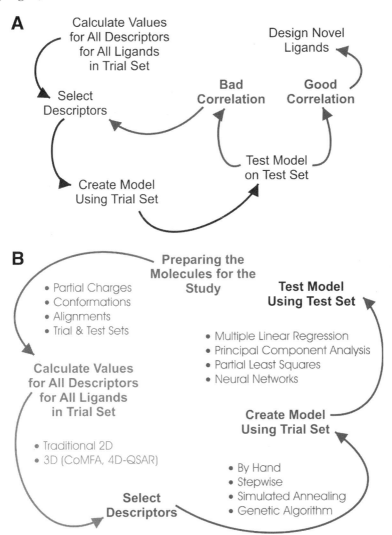

Fig. 1. General methodology of a QSAR Study. (**A**) Underlying process of creating and using a QSAR model. Molecules are collected and descriptors are calculated. The model is created using the Training Set and the model is then tested on the Test Set. If the model has a bad correlation to experimental values, the descriptor set is modified or a new set of descriptors is selected. Otherwise the model is dissected and novel ligands are designed using the information from the descriptor set. (**B**) Different methods of performing the same task in the creation of a QSAR model. At each point in the generation of a QSAR model there are several acceptable methods of calculating the descriptors (this is based on the type of QSAR study), selecting the descriptors, and creating the QSAR model.

or 4D-QSAR *(5)*. Each QSAR package has a unique method of calculating descriptors and a standard method for selecting descriptors and constructing the models. The backgrounds of these methods are typically glossed over in the user manuals. At each step in a QSAR study **(Fig. 1B)** there are different methods for performing the same task, specifically the selection of descriptors and creation of models. Preparing the molecules for the study appears straightforward except the number of choices for the different parameters can be baffling. During the initial setup of a QSAR study, there are no steadfast rules for implementing many of the parameters, only "rules-of-thumb." These rule-of-thumb parameters are the atomic partial charges, the molecular conformers, alignment of the molecules, and the composition of the Training and Test Sets. The previous parameters are key features used to monitor and indicate the outcome of a QSAR study.

2. QSAR Methodologies

The field of QSAR methodology is an ever-evolving field. This section highlights the different types of wide-ranging QSAR methodologies based on the concepts first proposed by Free, Wilson, Hansch, and Fujita, and how the changes in chemical structure affect the binding of compounds to receptors *(9)*. The discipline of QSAR originated when chemists noted a relationship between the structure of a compound and its activity. By the early-to-mid 1930s Hammett and others devised linear free energy relationships (LFER) between the influences of benzene polar substituents on side-chain reactions to form benzene derivatives.

The popularity of commercial programs such as Comparative Molecular Field Analysis *(4,12)* (CoMFA) and Catalyst *(13)* has limited both the evaluation and use of other QSAR methodologies. Often well-known issues associated with CoMFA and Catalyst have come to be viewed as shortcomings that simply are accepted as working limitations in a 3D-QSAR analysis. In this section we challenge this position and present 3D- and *n*D-QSAR methods that are able to overcome some of the issues associated with current mainstream 3D-QSAR application products.

Each QSAR package can be characterized by having a particular (a) method of calculating descriptors, (b) procedure for selecting descriptors, and (c) statistical algorithm for constructing the models. A common characteristic of 3D- and *n*D-QSAR methods is the creation of significantly more descriptors than molecules in the study, and the subsequent use of an adaptive search method [Evolutionary *(14)* and Genetic *(15)* Algorithms] or Support Vector Machines *(16)* (SVMs) to determine the best set of descriptors. The QSAR model is then constructed using a multivariate analysis *(17,18)* method such as principal component analysis *(19,20)* (PCA), principal component regression *(21)* (PCR), partial least squares *(22,23)* (PLS), or artificial neural networks *(24,25)* (ANN). This section briefly explains the general classification of QSAR methods.

There are two major points of contention common to all 3D-QSAR methodologies, the assignments of alignment and the conformation for the molecules in a study. The most common reason a 3D-QSAR model fails is that the non-bioactive conformation of the ligand is used in the QSAR study. Hopfinger *(26)* included the additional pseudo-dimension of an ensemble of conformations to the 3D-QSAR paradigm in 1980, thus creating the field of *n*D-QSAR. This additional dimension eliminated the question of "Which conformation to use in a QSAR study?" A qualitative 3D-QSAR method, Probabilistic Receptor Potentials *(8)*, calculates ligand atomic preferences in the active site. The potentials for PRP are constructed by fitting analytical functions to experimental properties of the substrates using knowledge-based methods. Another advance to the field of QSAR was the development of virtual high throughput screening (VHTS) methods such as the Binary-QSAR *(7)* methodology that allows the incorporation of QSAR methods into HTS and virtual 3D-pharmacophore screening *(27)*. These QSAR methods have been devised to assist in computer-aided drug design by contributing different information about how the ligand interacts with its potential receptor site.

The method for creating a QSAR model is generally automated. The user enters the parameters (molecules with partial atomic charges designated, alignment of molecules, Training and Test Sets, number of descriptors to be used in the model, the parameters for the selection of the descriptors, and the number of models to create) and the program creates a QSAR model. This is where QSAR studies with good intentions go bad. The user envisions the QSAR program as a "black-box" able to take this entire set of information and return novel drug compounds. Instead the user painstakingly sets all the parameters, the QSAR program calculates the descriptors, and depending on the maximum number of descriptors desired, creates a model using the Training Set as a template. To determine the validity of the model it is internally evaluated using the Training Set and externally tested on the Test Set. The selection of descriptors and creation of the best model is an iterative process and the QSAR program creates a myriad of models in the search for the optimal model. The program returns the best model or a collection of best models. The process described above is a generalization of the QSAR model creation scheme.

2.1. Receptor Independent (RI) QSAR

There are two types of QSAR studies, those that are interested in the common and diverse physicochemical characteristics from a selection of bioactive compounds and those that use the interactions between the ligands and the binding site. In this section the discussion will be focused on the most common type of QSAR study, Receptor Independent (RI). The main motivation in pursuing a RI-QSAR study is the lack of a well-defined receptor or receptor model. Commonly a RI-QSAR study utilizes one or several of the methodologies and applications discussed in the following sections.

2.1.1. Traditional (2D-) QSAR Methodology

The original method of conducting a QSAR study was to calculate physicochemical descriptors and construct a linear model of the important descriptors. This methodology for QSAR laid the groundwork for QSAR as it is known today and as shown in **Fig. 1A**. The descriptors used are easily recognizable features of the molecules; the number of double bonds, the number of hydrogen bond acceptors and donors, and the log of the octanol/water coefficient to name a few. The use of *ab initio*–based descriptors is also possible, such as the HOMO and LUMO energies of the molecules of interest. Yet for the simplicity that is traditional QSAR it too has drawbacks. The most notable is the difficulty in taking the important descriptors and modifying the compounds in the necessary manner. It can be argued that this is true for all methodologies of QSAR. But how does one increase the LUMO value of a compound? Recently, the addition of 3D descriptors has added to the pool of possible descriptors, yet they can be criticized in the same way. The program MOE-QuaSAR from CCG's computational suite MOE *(28)* is currently a good example of a traditional QSAR program. In this application the molecules are constructed and their physicochemical descriptors are calculated. Following the calculation of the descriptors, the important descriptors can be selected based on a contingency test that calculates the contingency coefficient, Cramer's *V*, the uncertainty coefficient and the correlation coefficient (R^2). Using the results of the contingency test can help eliminate descriptors that possess the same value for each molecule and highlight those that correlate well with the experimental bioactivities. Following the selection of the descriptions, the model is created and cross-validated. Depending on the validity of the model, descriptors are removed or added and the model is once again validated. Once a QSAR final model is completed, it can be used to evaluate novel compounds and aid in the construction of new drug-like compounds.

2.1.2. 3D-QSAR Methodology

The focus of 3D-QSAR is to identify and quantitatively characterize the interactions between the ligand and the receptor's active site. As the title of the field suggests, the main basis of the QSAR models are the molecules' 3D atomic (Cartesian) coordinates. The interactions between the atomic 3D coordinates and the receptor are correlated to the bioactivities producing a 3D-QSAR model. There are several methods to achieve the creation of QSAR models based on the atomic coordinates. The most widely known 3D-QSAR methodology is Comparative Molecular Field Analysis *(4)* (CoMFA) based on placing the ligands in a 3D grid and using a probe to map the surface of the ligand based on the ligand's interaction with the probe. Comparative Molecular Similarity Index Analysis *(29)* (CoMSIA) and Self-Organizing Molecular Field Analysis *(11)* (SOMFA) QSAR methodologies are based on the same methodology as CoMFA. The methodology of CoMSIA is based on aligning molecules using the SEAL *(30)* methodology, where molecules are aligned based on physicochemical properties mapped to individual atoms and using these properties to construct QSAR models. CoMSIA is similar in execution to CoMFA in the alignment of the molecules on a grid, the use of a probe, and partial least squares *(22)* (PLS) to construct the model, yet the interaction energies calculated by CoMSIA are the steric, electrostatic, hydrophobic, and hydrogen-bonding properties and not the Lennard-Jones and Coulombic potentials calculated in CoMFA. The probe's interaction with the ligand is calculated for each grid point including those inside the molecule's atomic van der Waals radius, eliminating the need for cutoffs as in CoMFA. These values are not direct measurements of similarity for the molecules of interest, but can be indirectly assessed (as measurements of similarity) through the similarity of each molecule in the dataset with a common probe placed at the grid points. When determining the similarity of the molecules of interest, the distance between the probe and the atoms of the molecule is considered using a functional form. Gaussian-type functions are used to define the distance dependence between the probe and the atoms of the molecule, thus removing the subjective cutoff limits and smoothing the distance-dependence energy well (compared to Lennard-Jones potential). The molecular data are analyzed using the CoMFA *(4)* PLS protocol *(29)*. Even with CoMSIA's similar methodology to CoMFA, the results obtained from each are significantly different. CoMFA's results show where and how (in 3D space) to modify the compounds to increase or decrease their ability to interact with the receptor. The results of a CoMSIA study express regions of the compound that prefer or dislike the presence of an identifiable group (substituent) with a specific physicochemical property *(29)*. Using fundamental molecular properties and "mean centered activity," SOMFA creates a QSAR model based on molecular shape and electrostatic potentials (ESP) *(11)*. 3D-QSAR methods that do not rely on a grid or alignment are Autocorrelation of Molecular Surfaces Properties (AMSP) *(31)*, Molecular Representation of Structures Based on Electron Diffraction *(32)* (3D-MoRSE), and Comparative Molecular Moment Analysis *(33)* (CoMMA). The methods of AMSP and 3D-MoRSE map the physical properties of the ligands to a van der Waals surface and individual atoms, respectively. The physical properties are transformed into a vector of equal length for all the ligands in the study, eliminating the problem of molecular alignment. CoMMA removes the alignment issue by calculating molecular moments and uses them as descriptors to construct a QSAR model. The qualitative method of Probabilistic Receptor Potentials (PRP) *(8)* is able to predict the type of receptor atom most likely to interact with the ligand thus providing an approximation of the type of atoms in the active site. The technique of 3D-QSAR is built on methods that take into consideration the 3D structure of the molecules and their inherent physical properties (with respect to how the ligand will interact with the receptor) to construct a QSAR model. All of these methods are receptor independent (RI); the models are created without any firm knowledge of the composition or 3D structure of the receptor.

None of the QSAR methodologies mentioned in this section are useful if the 3D structures of the ligands are incorrectly constructed. In small QSAR studies it is possible to build the ligands by hand; in a large QSAR study, that is, using ligands extracted from a large proprietary database, the need to construct the ligands quickly and accurately from the molecular information within the database is essential. The need for a method to construct the 3D structures comes from how the ligands are encoded in the database. Commonly the molecules are stored in 2D strings of variables; Connection Format, SMILES strings, or analogous formats are used to facilitate viewing of the database and to reduce the storage size of the databases. The ability to convert a 2D string of variables into its 3D molecular structure greatly increases productivity and enables the scientist to computationally explore the compounds. Thus, the ability to accurately construct molecules from 2D strings is of great importance. The program CORINA *(34)* developed by Sadowski et al. was determined *(35)* to be the most suitable program for converting 2D structures to 3D representation.

The methodology of 3D-QSAR can be robust for constructing QSAR models utilizing the structure of the compounds and how they will interact with the receptor; however, there are several open questions that can complicate any application of this paradigm. The first and most prominent question is "Which conformation of the molecule should be used?" This problem is considered *(36)* a leading cause of generating non-significant QSAR models, specifically those created with 3D-QSAR methods (CoMFA, CoMSIA, and SOMFA). The next question is "How to align the molecules?" The alignment of the molecules might seem rather straightforward from the standpoint of a simple visual comparison of ligand chemical structures, but alignment becomes a complex problem within the context of "good receptor binders" binding in different orientations, or modes, than "poor binders." Thus, a clear and unbiased method of aligning the molecules for the study is needed such as SEAL *(30)*, FlexS *(37)*, Superposition of 3D-Structures *(38)*, or FlexAlign *(39)*. The optimal general way of minimizing the alignment problem is to create multiple alignment schemes focusing on different regions of the molecules. This leads to the question, "Can QSAR models be improved using alignment schemes based on physicochemical methods such as SEAL *(30)*, FlexS *(37)*, Superposition of 3D-Structures *(38)*, or FlexAlign *(39)*?" The method of CoMMA frees itself from the issue of alignment, yet it has not overcome the problems associated with bioactive conformations and the appropriate atomic partial charge. AMSP and 3D-MoRSE eliminate the problems of alignment through the mathematical transformation of the 3D molecular structures into vectors. These methods also break new ground in the ability to create nonlinear models using ANNs. CoMSIA is restrained by alignment and conformation issues yet uses different molecular interactions as descriptors, thus surpassing CoMFA. SOMFA is closest in methodology to CoMFA in respect to the use of grids but is not as statistically rigorous. SOMFA does, however, endure the same traditional 3D-QSAR methodology impediments. All of these methods, when conditions are optimal (molecular conformations, alignment, and partial charges) will produce good QSAR models. In the creation of 3D-based QSAR models it is key to remember the importance of proper alignment and conformation of the compounds in the study.

2.1.3. nD-QSAR Methodology

The methodology of *n*D-QSAR adds to the 3D-QSAR methodology by incorporating unique physical characteristics, or a set of characteristics, to the descriptor pool available for the creation of the models. The methods of Eigen-Value Analysis *(40)* (EVA) and 4D-QSAR *(5)* are examples of using unique physical characteristics in the creation of a QSAR model. 4D-QSAR uses an ensemble of molecular conformations to aid in the creation of a QSAR. The EVA-QSAR method uses infrared spectra to extract descriptors for the creation of the QSAR model.

The *n*D-QSAR methods attempt to overcome the downfalls of most of the 3D-QSAR methods through the use of additional physical properties and/or degrees of freedom in building the QSAR models. The use of 4D-QSAR eliminates the issue of what conformation and alignment to use through the sampling of multiple conformations and alignment schemes, thus constructing optimal QSAR models. The EVA method has removed the alignment and conformation issues that have plagued most of the 3D- and *n*D-QSAR methods yet falls prey to the problem of how to extract useful information from a model constructed with PLS.

2.2. Virtual High Throughput Screening (VHTS)

The ability to use the developed QSAR model to screen compound libraries is an attractive prospect, yet is difficult to implement. Two types of compound libraries can be considered; those composed of analogous compounds (compounds constructed from a main scaffold with many different possible substituents) and those composed of molecules with little molecular structure similarity (company/supplier/research group libraries of compounds). There are VHTS methods to accommodate each of these cases individually. Binary-QSAR *(7,41)* has the ability to screen large libraries of diverse compound makeup to aid in the preparation of future HTS experiments. The implementation of virtual 3D-pharmacophore screening *(27)* is better suited for the examination of a library of compounds devised from a common scaffold.

2.3. Receptor-Dependent (RD) QSAR

Traditionally, QSAR methods are used to aid in the design of novel compounds without a 3D structure of the receptor. The field of receptor-dependent (RD) QSAR is used for a QSAR study when the 3D structure of a binding site is known and can be implemented once an initial compound (analog, pharmacophore, scaffold) is bound. RD-QSAR is used to gather binding and interaction energies, as descriptors, from the interaction between the analog and the receptor. These descriptors cannot be determined without the receptor and can improve the ability of a QSAR model created using receptor-independent descriptors. An initial compound does not need to be docked (through simulations) to the receptor if a solved 3D structure of the receptor complexed with the compound (or similar compound) is available.

There are two methods that have the ability to create QSAR models using information derived either from a theoretical active site [5D-QSAR *(42)*] or from a solved or modeled binding site [FEFF-3D-QSAR *(43)*]. The methodology of 5D-QSAR is similar to 4D-QSAR (creation of an ensemble of conformations) plus the mimicking of the induced fit of the ligand during binding to the receptor site. The FEFF-3D-QSAR methodology treats the energy terms in the force field used to estimate the thermodynamics of the ligand–receptor binding process as descriptors in the development of a "QSAR force field" for the particular ligand-class/receptor system.

The use of receptor-dependent (RD) QSAR adds to the QSAR model through the inclusion of ligand–receptor interactions. 5D-QSAR is unique because it mimics the binding site of the receptor (constructed from experimental data or random placement of physicochemical properties) to aid in the construction of an optimal QSAR model and to aid in the construction of a pharmacophore, yet is also alignment dependent. The FEFF 3D-QSAR method is a true RD-QSAR method using the solved 3D structure of the receptor in the calculation of ligand–receptor interaction values.

Although ADMET-QSAR methodologies are traditionally not considered RD methods, a pseudo-receptor may be needed to extract relevant ADMET descriptors about the system that is not grasped exclusively from the intramolecular solute test molecule descriptors. Through the implementation of Membrane Interaction (MI) QSAR *(44)* (a RD-based method) the extraction of significant descriptors deduced from interactions between the ligand and a membrane ("receptor") is possible, thus leading to a more significant ADMET-QSAR model. MI-QSAR differs from other ADMET-QSAR applications through the inclusion of an assumption and a specific set of descriptors in its methodology. MI-QSAR is a receptor-dependent QSAR method assuming that the phospholipid regions of the cell membrane represent the "receptor" *(44)*. The MI-QSAR specific descriptors are measures of interaction between the compounds of interest and the cell membrane and a set of membrane–solute intermolecular properties. These descriptors can be further classified into solute aqueous dissolution and solvation descriptors, solute–membrane interaction descriptors, and general intramolecular solute descriptors. The MI-QSAR method is receptor-based, requiring a 3D structure or model of the receptor and is usually constructed as a monolayer from the phospholipids that comprise the cell membrane of the system of interest. The determination of the best placement for the solute molecule (compound of interest) in the monolayer is by placing the compound (with the solute molecule's most polar region oriented toward the headgroup region) at three different depths (locations with respect to the phospholipid monolayer), in the headgroup region, in the center region of the aliphatic chains, and in the tail region of the aliphatic chains. Molecular dynamics simulations (MDSs) are performed at body temperature with only a single solute molecule in the monolayer for each simulation. Separate MDSs need to be performed for each compound; the individual solute molecule is systematically placed at one of the three positions as described above and molecular dynamics is performed. At the completion of all the MDSs, the most favorable orientation and locations of each compound in the monolayer is determined based on energetics *(44)*.

3. Preparing Molecules for a QSAR Study

Before starting the actual QSAR study, it is imperative to have the molecules properly configured with respect to bioactivities, partial charges and force fields, conformation, alignment, and Training and Test Set construction. These topics at times seem trivial, however, once the QSAR study is undertaken, the importance of these concepts will become more apparent. Often questions regarding "Which partial charges were used?," "Which force field was implemented?," "Was the *active* conformation used?," "How were the molecules aligned?," "Which molecules comprised the Training Set?" will be asked. The alignment and conformation of molecules are primary issues when performing a 3D-QSAR study since these methods are grid-based and rely on the comparison of molecular interactions (ligand–probe/receptor). The molecules must be properly aligned for a study to be effective, because poorly aligned molecular sets create poor models. The models are then created based on spatial arrangement of the molecules; the space not occupied by any of the molecules in the study cannot be interpreted *(36)*. Finally the conformation of the aligned molecules, bent or high-energy conformations, such as those observed in the transition state or bound conformations of a ligand, will not be explored if the conformation of the molecule was derived using a geometry optimization program, individual ligand X-ray structure or by local minima conformational search methods.

3.1. Bioactivity Data

The bioactivity data can be considered the most sensitive external information for a QSAR study. Depending on how the experimental study was conducted, an investigator can have bioactivity data in the form of K_d, K_i, relative binding affinity (RBA), or IC_{50} values. These are valid ways of reporting how well a molecule interacts with a protein; the best bioactivity measure is K_d for a QSAR study. K_d values are the preferred bioactivity measure because it is a value of how well a ligand binds to and activates the protein with respect to the concentration of ligand that dissociates from a known concentration of protein. K_i is the measure of ligand needed to inhibit the protein. RBA is the value of a molecule's binding affinity divided by the binding affinity of a known (commonly the native ligand) ligand for the protein. The RBA for the known ligand is one. Ligands that bind better to the same protein will have an RBA <1 and ligands which do not bind as well will have an RBA >1. The RBA values are a method of comparing bioactivities of the same ligand binding to protein homologs or isozymes and should not be used in the construction of QSAR models. The bioactivity data reported in IC_{50} values relate to the amount of ligand needed to bind or incapacitate 50% of the proteins or cells. This is a popular method of reporting bioactivity data; the values reported can vary from lab-to-lab because IC_{50} values are dependent on the concentrations and ratios used to perform the experiments.

3.1.1. Transforming the Bioactivities

A standard assumption in QSAR studies is that the models describing the data are linear. It is from this standpoint that transformations are performed on the bioactivities to achieve linearity before construction of the models. The assumption of linearity is made for each case based on theoretical considerations or the examination of scatter plots of experimental values plotted against each predicted value where the relationship between the data points appears to be nonlinear. The transformation of the bioactivity data may be necessary if theoretical considerations specify that the relationship between the two variables (descriptors and bioactivities) is nonlinear, yet the model is being fit by a linear method. Assuming the relationship between the original variables and bioactivities was nonlinear, the transformation of the bioactivities converts the relationship between the variables to a linear relationship. Another reason to transform the bioactivities is based on evidence gathered by examining the residuals from the fit of a linear regression model between the original and predicted bioactivities. The main advantage of transforming data is to guarantee linearity, to achieve normality, or to stabilize the variance. Several simple nonlinear regression relationships can be made linear through the appropriate transformations.

3.1.1.1. LOG OF THE BIOACTIVITIES

The simplest and most common method of transforming *(45)* bioactivity data is to take the log or negative log of the bioactivities to reduce the range of the data. The logarithmic transformation is useful when the bioactivities being analyzed possess a large standard deviation compared to the mean; this is especially apparent when the bioactivities have a large range (for example the range 0 to 1000 with most of the values occurring between 0 and 100). The use of a logarithmic transformation has the added effect of dampening variability, reducing asymmetry, and removing heteroscedasticity, when the error variance is not constant over all the bioactivity values *(45)*.

3.1.1.2. CENTERING AND SCALING

The practice of centering and scaling the bioactivities and descriptors is to reduce the dimension of the data (range of the values) because the shifting or scaling of data does not affect correlations. Subtracting the mean of the values (μ) from each value (x_i) centers the data. The centered data only sets the mean of the values to zero and does not reduce the range of the values. Scaling the data (standardizing) performs the reduction in range and is performed separately for the bioactivities and the descriptors. The standardized value (z) is determined from the difference of x_i from μ and divided by the standard deviation (σ) of all the x_i values:

$$z = \frac{x_i - \mu}{\sigma} \tag{2}$$

$$\sigma = \sqrt{\frac{\sum_{i=1}^{n}(x_i - \bar{x})^2}{n-1}} \tag{3}$$

3.1.1.3. BINDING FREE ENERGY (ΔG)

The conversion of binding affinities (bioactivities) to binding free energies is the scaling of the natural log (ln) of the bioactivities. This is accomplished using the equation:

$$\Delta G = -RT \ln(\text{Bioactivity}) \qquad (4)$$

where R is the gas constant (1.987×10^{-3} kcal mol^{-1} K^{-1}) and T is the temperature in Kelvin at which the binding affinities were experimentally performed. The result is bioactivities, normally, expressed kilocalories per mole (kcal/mol).

3.2. Chiral Centers

The chirality of a molecule can have a direct impact on its ability to bind to the receptor. In traditional QSAR studies the "handedness" of a molecule's chiral center(s) is not important unless 3D-Traditional descriptors are being used. For 3D and nD-QSAR methodologies where the shape (geometry) of the molecule is used to create the model, the chirality can have a significant impact on the experimental bioactivities and will have an impact on the QSAR model. When compiling the molecules for a QSAR study, make certain that chiral compounds have bioactivities that are chiral-specific. If a 3D or nD-QSAR model is created using chiral molecules yet the bioactivities are for a racemic mixture, the model can be flawed. The main reasoning for the correct chirality is that bioactivities can be directly affected by the chirality of a molecule. Using a racemic mixture of a compound to determine the binding affinity leaves the questions "Which chiral orientation is the bioactive molecule?" and "Is one enantiomer preventing the other from binding?" For example, a 50/50 racemic mixture of a compound is synthesized, tested, and demonstrates an average bioactivity for its system. What the experimentalist might not know is whether the R or S is the more bioactive. Also, is one of the racemates preventing the other from efficiently performing the desired task? These questions cannot be answered until the individual R and S enantiomers bioactivities are known. It is also possible that both R and S molecules have the same bioactivity, yet this assumption cannot be made without definitive experimental results.

The creation of a descriptor that takes into consideration the number of chiral centers, their location in the molecule, and how their handedness affects the bioactivities is needed. Through the use of a descriptor of this nature, when a QSAR program is presented with the correct information (bioactivities for individual enantiomers and correctly constructed molecules), it will be able to construct QSAR models that incorporate chirality.

3.3. Force Fields and Partial Charges

When first posed with the question "Which force field or partial charges to use?" a typical reply might be, "Partial charges derived from semiempirical or *ab initio* calculations," but after some thought and consideration these might not be a wise choice. There will be instances when force fields and partial charges might not be a primary factor in a QSAR study, but these parameters can have a significant impact on the values of the descriptors regardless of the QSAR methodology used. The choice of a specific force field for assigning atomic partial charges and radii to the molecules is effective because the force fields are highly characterized and the partial charges, atomic radii, and bonding information are a complete set. The compound's atomic partial charges, atomic radii, and bond and dihedral angles can be set using a common force field such as Merck Molecular Force Fields *(46–52)* (MMFF), Assisted Model Building with Energy Refinement *(53,54)* (AMBER), Saccharides and Sugars *(55)* (PEF95SAC), Optimized Potentials for Liquid Simulations *(56–61)* (OPLS), Chemistry at HARvard Macromolecular Mechanics *(62–68)* (CHARMM), and Engh–Huber *(69)*. Other methods of determining partial charges are the use of Partial Equalization of Orbital Electronegativity *(70)* (PEOE), commonly referred to as Gasteiger Partial Charges, or Full Equalization of Orbital Electronegativity *(71)* (FEOE), also referred to as Electrostatic Energy Minimization partial charges (EEM), that can be combined with the above-mentioned force fields. In the pursuit of accurate input for a QSAR study, it is tempting to use a geometry-optimization program, such as Gaussian98 *(72)*, MOPAC *(73,74)*, or GAMESS *(75)*, to determine the partial charges and conformation of the ligand, yet this is not needed. The atomic partial charges determined by geometry-optimization programs are relatively correct; however, the partial charges are dependent on the conformation of the ligand. During the binding of the ligand to the protein, the conformation of the ligand can change drastically depending on the forces imposed upon it from the receptor. The advantage of using a force field such as MMFF is that the partial charges, radii, bond lengths, and torsions are derived from a large set of computationally determined data along with a large number of crystallographically determined molecules, thus any errors are averaged out. The MMFF was parametrized using more than 20 chemical families for the core parametrization and contains many combinations of functional groups *(46)*. Originally designed for molecular dynamics MMFF has been modified *(52)* and re-released to incorporate a complete set of parameters for energy minimization.

3.4. Molecular Conformation

A conformation is the different special arrangement of a ligand's atoms that result from rotation about a single bond; a specific conformation is a conformer. Unlike constitutional isomers, different conformations cannot be isolated because they quickly interconvert, yet there are several computational methods to determine the possible conformations a molecule may possess. The energy of a conformer plotted against its torsional angle(s) can be based on a single or double dihedral angle rotation. The single-bond (dihedral) rotation plots illustrate the fluxuation in the molecule's potential energy with respect to bond rotation. The lowest point on the plot corresponds to the "local" minima for a particular configuration with respect to the rotatable bonds. Plotting energy versus the double dihedral angles will create a potential energy surface displaying the energy landscape of the system, specifically the energy barriers between local minima conformers **(Fig. 2)**.

The conformation of the molecules being studied has an influential role in a 3D-QSAR study. The conformation of a molecule affects the volume and surface area, which are now being incorporated as 3D descriptors into traditional QSAR methods. The main issue is "How will the conformation of the molecule resemble the active site/binding pocket?" If the conformation of the molecule used in a CoMFA study is not similar to the conformation assumed by the ligand when bound to the protein, the study and resulting model will be of no use. When performing a QSAR study of any type, the ligands need to assume the bound conformation. This leaves those wishing to use 3D-QSAR in a quandary of "Which conformation to use?" The use of a molecule's gas-phase-optimized conformation after a random conformational search is plausible yet is not advisable. Studies by Nicklaus et al. *(76)* and Vieth et al. *(77)* provide insight on how to arrive at the assumed bound conformation of a ligand. These authors agree that the use of an isolated crystal structure or global energy minimum conformation calculated in a vacuum of the ligand is an erroneous practice owing to crystal packing effects and lack of molecular interactions, respectively *(76,77)*. Vieth et al. *(77)* also noted that certain atoms (anchor atoms) in the ligand are more responsible for binding the ligand to the active site than others. In addition Vieth et al. *(77)* realized a similarity in the position of anchor atoms between geometry-optimized low-energy solution structures and the active-site conformations. It is understood that, when a ligand binds, the receptor may change the detailed solution structure of the ligand *(76)*; however, it is the premise that a majority of these changes take place in regions of ligands that contribute little to binding *(77)*.

In searching for the best conformation it is important to determine all conformations efficiently because a molecule's physicochemical and biological properties are usually dictated by the conformation of the molecule. The molecular conformation is of great importance for drug design because the conformer of the "global" minima is usually not the bound conformation of a molecule. Thus, the desire to find the lowest-energy (geometry-optimized) structure is not profitable and usually not the preferred conformations for use in the QSAR study. Discussed below are several methods to determine different conformations of a molecule that are useful when determining clusters of

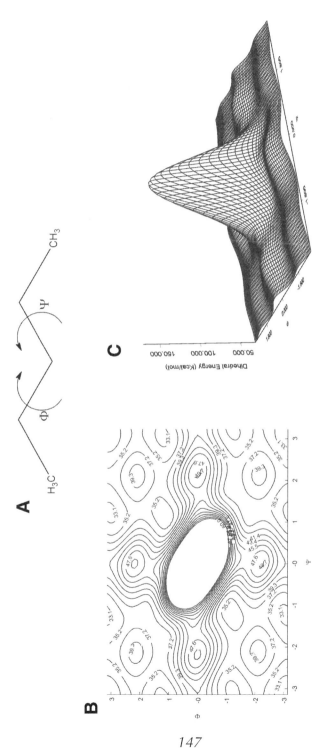

Fig. 2. Dihedral energy exploration of pentane. (A) Pentane (C_5H_{12}) molecule with two dihedral bonds (rotatable bonds). (B) 2D contour plot of the energy landscape for pentane. (C) 3D contour plot of the energy landscape of pentane. The large circle and peak in the center of the plots (B) and (C), respectively, are the result of carbons 1 and 5 in close proximity ($\Phi \approx 57$, -57, $\psi \approx -57$, 57).

147

different molecular conformations for use in 3D-QSAR studies. Molecular dynamics is not discussed as a method of determining conformations because it traditionally only finds structures for a given local minima; for more information on molecular dynamics, the reader is directed to books by Frenkel and Smit *(78)*, Field *(79)*, and Leach *(80)*. The question of "Which conformation to use?" can easily be determined by using the conformer of a ligand, or similar compound, bound to the receptor derived through X-ray crystallographic or multidimensional NMR methods. These methods are currently used to determine the conformation of the ligands when bound to the receptor; however, if high-quality information about the receptor and ligand interactions is known, it is questionable if QSAR is the best method to design novel drugs. Given this experimentally derived information it is advisable to consider docking and receptor-dependent QSAR methods to explore possible ligand–receptor interactions. Excellent reviews of docking methodology and procedures are given by Murcko *(81)* and Muegge and Rarey *(82)*. An in-depth and early review on the search for small and medium-sized molecule conformations is provided by Leach *(80,83)*.

3.4.1. Systematic Conformation Search

The purpose of a systematic conformation search is to generate a database of practical conformations consisting of local minima, and low-energy and high-energy structures. A systematic search generates molecular conformers by methodically rotating molecular bonds by predetermined increments. Creating a collection of conformations in this manner can lead to a combinatorial headache because the number of conformations to be generated is determined by

$$Number\ of\ Conformations = \prod_{i=1}^{N} \frac{360}{\theta_i} \qquad (5)$$

where N is the number of bonds to be rotated and θ_i is the incremental value which the bond is rotated in degrees. This provides the ability to determine all of the possible conformations, but the desire to make the search for all probable conformations efficient is ever present. To make this and other conformational search methods efficient, molecules with non-bonded atomic van der Waals interactions greater than a user-specified value are discarded.

The algorithm for the systematic conformation search starts with a minimized molecule. The rotatable bonds are selected along with the rotation increment and all possible conformations are created. At this point the search is terminated or each of the proposed conformations is energy minimized according to predefined parameters. After the database of conformers is finalized, each structure is compared to all the other structures through superimposition. Two conformers are considered equivalent if their RMSD value based on atomic positions, when compared to each other, is less than the user-defined value.

3.4.2. Perturbation-Based Conformational Search Methods

The search for different conformations of a molecule can be performed quickly using a search algorithm based on the perturbation of either the Cartesian coordinates *(84)* or rotatable bonds *(6)*. The rapid incremental pulse search (RIPS) method was developed by Ferguson and Raber *(84)* to generate conformations by randomly perturbing the position of each atom in the molecule by a small amount followed by energy minimization to generate a new conformer. The stochastic conformation search method *(6)* is drawn from the concept of RIPS yet is based on the random rotation of bonds, including the bonds of rings, instead of the perturbation of Cartesian coordinates.

The RIPS conformational search starts by perturbing all of the atoms' X, Y, and Z coordinates by plus or minus the perturbation value (usually 2 Å or less) the sign (±) is randomly assigned. Next the molecule is energy minimized to a user-defined RMS gradient requirement. After each molecule is minimized, a check is preformed for a duplicate conformation existing in the conformer list. If the current structure is a new conformation, it is added to the list and the failure count (number of times a conformation that exists in the conformer list is repeated) is set to zero. A duplicate conformer is discarded and the failure count is increased by one. The search is considered complete once the number of failures has reached the user-defined values.

Stochastic conformation searches start with a minimized molecule followed by the random inversion of chiral centers and the identification of rotatable bonds. The rotatable bonds are rotated on a uniform distribution and all the atoms' 3D coordinates are perturbed by plus or minus the perturbation value (usually 2 Å or less) with the sign (±) randomly assigned as in the RIPS method. After random rotation and perturbation, the molecule is energy minimized until the RMS gradient requirement is reached. A check is performed for a duplicate conformation existing in the conformer list; if the conformation is an "original," it is added to the conformer list and the failure count is reset to zero, but if the conformer is a duplicate, the failure count increases by one and the duplicate is discarded. The algorithm again randomly rotates the bonds and perturbs the Cartesian coordinates of the atoms and continues the search for new conformations. The molecular conformation search is complete once the failure limit is reached.

These methods are best when determining conformers in local minima on the potential energy surface. The number of rotatable bonds the molecule of interest possesses dictates the failure limit value; accordingly, molecules with few rotatable bonds require a lower failure value than molecules with many rotatable bonds. The minimization performed in the systematic and perturbation-based conformational search methods ensure that the conformers found lie in local potential energy minima. These methods of conformation searching are powerful tools for locating conformational minima of flexible molecules containing chiral centers and can be coupled to 4D-QSAR.

3.5. Molecular Alignment

The alignment of molecules for a 3D-QSAR–based study is crucial. Improper or incorrect alignment of the molecules can create models providing little information relating to the main orientation of the molecule in the active site. A study by Lemmen and Lengauer *(36)* noted three serious limitations for molecular alignment with respect to 3D-QSAR methodology. The first limitation for molecular alignment is the compounds of interest must bind at the same binding site of the same receptor and possess similar binding modes. The second limitation relates to the aligned molecules; any 3D space not occupied by the compounds cannot be considered (used) in the construction of the QSAR model. If substituents of the compounds are able to explore conformational space, the QSAR model will not take into consideration these different conformations of a molecule's functional groups. The final limitation relates to 3D-QSAR models being constructed with the low-energy conformations of the compounds being studied. The conformations of the compounds are most likely not the bound conformation of the molecules *(76,77)* as would be observed in the binding site. Using the low-energy conformers will result in a 3D-QSAR model being constructed from the least probable conformations. As mentioned above the ligands must bind to the receptor site at the same location and preferably derive the same conformation to construct an effective 3D-QSAR model. The alignment of molecules is the process of aligning two or more molecules (different conformation of the same molecule or different molecules with similar scaffolds/analogs) in 3D space to optimally superimpose specific atoms upon each other based on distances. The difference between the molecules is measured using a root mean square deviation (RMSD):

$$\text{RMSD} = \sqrt{\frac{\sum_{i=1}^{N_{atoms}} \left([x,y,z]_A - [x,y,z]_B\right)^2}{N_{atoms}}} \tag{6}$$

where $[x,y,z]_A$ and $[x,y,z]_B$ are the coordinates of atoms A and B, respectively, and N_{atoms} is the number of atoms being aligned. The goal of molecular alignment is to minimize the distance between the selected atoms by reorienting the molecules in 3D space. The alignment of molecules can be thought of as aligning two or more molecules based on atomic nuclei position and using a simple super-imposition method of reducing the RMSD value by keeping either the molecules rigid or allowing molecular flexibility to improve the alignment. The use of atomic nuclei distance reduction is a common method of aligning molecules and can be based on the physicochemical properties of the molecules.

3.5.1. FlexAlign

Using physical properties and a scoring function, molecules can be aligned by mapping the localized physical properties to an individual atom *(30)*. Flex-Align *(39)*, an alignment application in MOE *(6)* and derived from work by Kearsley and Smith *(30)*, is a stochastic search method that explores the con-formational space of a molecular dataset and aligns the molecules based on physical properties. FlexAlign utilizes an algorithm that allows rotation about single bonds, inversion of chiral centers, and translation and rotation of atoms in space to determine a better alignment. The different molecular conforma-tions are created through rapid incremental pulse searches *(84)* (RIPS), and the molecules can be aligned based on a single or collection of physical properties [e.g., acid/base, aromaticity, exposure, H-bond acceptor, H-bond donor, hydrophobicity, log*P* (octanol/water partition), molar refractivity, partial charge, and volume] *(39)*. The flexible alignments are ranked using a probability den-sity function scoring function.

A flexible molecular alignment starts with the selection of the physical prop-erties for alignment, the parameters for the conformational search protocol, and the molecular conformer creation and minimization settings. Using the RIPS conformational search methodology, random rotation of bonds, and inversion of chiral centers are followed by energy minimization to create "new" conforma-tions of the molecules, this and other methods of molecular conformation deter-mination are discussed below. Once minimized, the molecules are held rigid and aligned using a similarity function that is minimized with respect to the atomic coordinates using the equation *(39)*:

$$\text{Similarity Function} = -kT \times \log F + U \qquad (7)$$

where $-kT$ is approx 0.6 kcal/mol, F is the similarity measure derived from the atomic coordinates, and U is the average potential energy of the system (mole-cules). The MOE–FlexAlign alignment search terminates once the user-defined number of consecutive failed attempts to generate a new molecular configuration based on the initial parameters is reached. The user-defined value for the max-imum number of failed attempts is dependent on the system of interest. The alignment method of FlexS *(37)* by Lemmen et al. is a similar process, yet uses similar molecular fragments for the alignment of the molecules.

3.5.2. Field Fit

The method of "Field Fit" from CoMFA *(4)* is similar to MOE–FlexAlign *(6,30,39)* because it is used to increase field similarity within a series of molecules. Field Fit determines the optimal alignment for the molecules of interest by minimizing the RMSD with respect to the six rigid body degrees of freedom and/or any user-specified torsion angles. The RMSD function for this method is the sum of steric and electrostatic interaction energies averaged across all the lattice points between the molecule of interest and a template molecule. For example, the alignment of molecule A to B, where B is the template molecule, using Field Fit is similar to the above method of MOE–FlexAlign. The process begins with the minimization of the RMSD between the two molecules by modifying the position and/or torsion angles of molecule A. To keep portions of molecule A from extending past the boundary of the lattice, a steric repulsion term is implemented. Once molecule A is aligned with molecule B, it is minimized using the original force field parameters. Molecule A is considered aligned with the template when the individual atoms move no more than 0.2 Å after a minimization step and when successive energy function evaluations vary less than 1%. This method is only useful if the minimized structure is expected to closely resemble the active site conformation and starting geometry since the steric and electrostatic fields will be moved with the molecule.

3.5.3. Three-Point Alignment

The most common molecular alignment method is based on aligning three atoms in the molecule. First a common scaffold of the molecules in the study is determined followed by dividing the scaffold into three sections based on the longest plane with at least three atoms in each section; sections can overlap if care is taken when selecting atoms. Next three non-hydrogen atoms are selected from each section, ensuring the selected atoms encompass the range of the section. In creating the alignment schemes, the exploration of the entire topology of the molecules is crucial to locate the correct alignment. In a small molecule there is a possibility of sections overlapping, yet in larger molecules the number of possible alignment schemes becomes daunting.

The small molecule is divided into three sections (**Fig. 3A**) consisting of the benzene ring (the head), the ethyl-bromide (the middle), and the dimethyamine (the tail). A similar molecule (**Fig. 3B**) is divided into three sections with the head and tail sections overlapping the middle section. The overlap is due to the structural composition of the molecule; it has a defined head and tail (six-member aromatic rings) and the middle consisting of one carbon. To remedy this problem the scaffold is divided into overlapping sections consisting of the rings for the head and tail and the middle consisting of the lone carbon and a

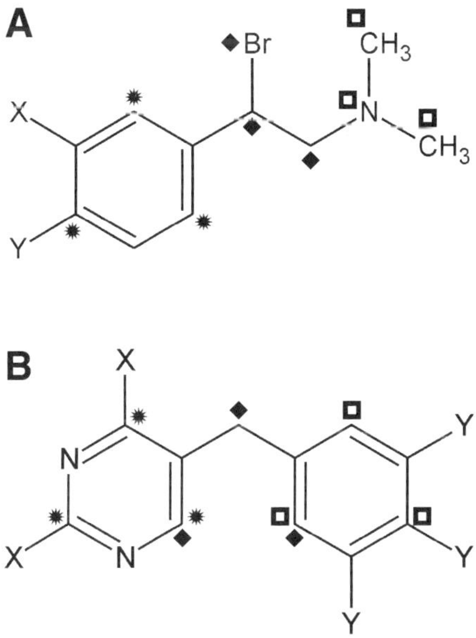

Fig. 3. Examples of three-point alignment schemes. (**A**) The core of the molecules used in the case study with alignment scheme denoted as used for the 4D-QSAR portion. There are three distinct regions for alignment (head = *, middle = ◆, tail = ◻). In (**A**) the scaffold (analog) has distinct head, middle, and tail regions making the division of the molecule simple. The molecule in **B** is considerably more complex (due to its symmetry) to divide into three sections. The molecule is similarly in size to the molecule in **A**, yet is divided into three overlapping sections for alignment (head = *, middle = ◆, tail = ◻).

portion of the head and tail rings (**Fig. 3B**). The atoms considered for the alignment are then numbered and the alignment schemes are constructed. Typically, alignment schemes are based solely on the head, middle, and tail of the scaffold with additional alignments constructed to explore the importance of alignment schemes based on a combination of atoms from the head, middle and tail.

3.5.4. The Alignment and Binding Modes of the Ligands

Molecular alignments are most often selected to align portions of the ligands of similar chemical structures (scaffolds) to emphasize regions of similarity in the set of molecules of interest. But what, if using different alignment schemes, (a) better QSAR models were created?, or, (b) the atoms important for binding (anchoring atoms) were identified?, or it was found that some molecules bind in different orientation compared to others? As has been discussed previously, the alignment of the molecules for a 3D-QSAR study can play a major role in the quality and information obtained from a QSAR study.

The concept of using different alignments to determine the binding mode or anchoring atoms is not a novel idea, yet the ability to implement it is far from trivial. Two different methodologies are associated with these concepts. The concept of predicting the binding mode for a group of molecules can be considered a more difficult task. The binding mode is the conformation, orientation, and location the molecule(s) occupies in the binding site, and for some biological systems certain molecules will bind in different poses compared to other molecules. The difference in binding modes can be the result of the drug-like compound's potency, substituents, or scaffold. To make this concept straightforward, the discussion will focus on a theoretical set of compounds with experimentally determined 3D structures to check the predictive ability of the QSAR models and the configuration (alignment) of the compounds in the binding site. For instance, if a set of 10 compounds, based on an quinoline ring scaffold, are examined and their bioactivities for a receptor measured, it can be argued owing to their somewhat symmetrical scaffold, and the position of substituents, that this set of compounds could bind in different orientations (dependent on the location of the nitrogen in the quinoline ring system) based on location of similar substituents. These multiple modes of binding could only be definitively determined using experimental techniques (X-ray diffraction and NMR) to solve the 3D structure of the orientation of the ligand in the binding site. The question being asked is "What makes this set of compounds important?" Is it the scaffold or the substituents? Or is it a combination of the two? The correct answer is the combination of the two, because the scaffold is "holding" (positioning) the substituents in a specific configuration (pattern) for the binding site. The process of determining which orientation the scaffold possesses with respect to the binding site is dictated by the receptor's desire for specific interactions. For example, molecules with a quinoline scaffold can be similar in shape and substitution to each other. The question of "Which binding mode each will possess with respect to the receptor?" is an intriguing question, yet is it relevant if the two compounds reflect similar binding affinities? If the binding affinities are similar, then the scaffold is little more than a holder for the substituents and there are different binding modes. Yet, if the binding affinities are different, it can be argued that the scaffold is imparting a substantial effect on the orientation of the ligand in the binding site.

Another aspect of the molecules to examine is their physicochemical properties. A possible major contributor to ligands binding in different orientations is their physicochemical properties mapped to their surface. Consider molecules that are symmetrical with respect to their physicochemical properties mapped to their molecular surface. The molecule might be asymmetrical based on structure, yet symmetrical when examining physical properties. In cases such as these, there is the possibility that, when one molecule binds, the binding site it is in one orientation with a "good" bioactivity, and when the other binds, it is at a considerable less bioactivity due in part to it binding in the opposite orientation as a result of the more favorable physicochemical properties of the ligand aligning with specific regions of the binding site.

Identifying anchoring atoms *(77)* is a less complex process than characterizing multiple binding modes because only the alignment of the molecules, and not, specifically, their orientation to other (with respect to different binding modes) ligands is involved. In determining the atoms that are important for binding the ligand (small organic molecule) to the binding site, several alignment schemes need to be devised that explore different binding mode possibilities, yet allow for statistically sound QSAR models. Using the example of three-atom alignment, a series of molecules are aligned in a manner that emphasizes the location of specific substituents in 3D space. An excellent example is the construction of 10 alignments for a set of compounds bound to the same receptor with varying bioactivities. The molecules are flexible with their scaffolds varying slightly in structure, while retaining a similar shape. Determining which atoms of the scaffold are important for binding can provide information regarding regions of the ligands' scaffold that interact with the binding site (regions not to modify) and those with substituents that interact with the binding site (regions acceptable to modify). By constructing alignment schemes that align regions or specific atoms, the preferred anchor atoms can be deduced based on the quality of the QSAR model constructed.

An important consideration in a QSAR study is to determine if the molecules align in the same orientation when bound. If they do, that is great, and less work is required. But if the molecules align in different (binding) orientations, finding the correct set of alignments can prove difficult. The ability to construct several (to many) different alignment schemes that encompass the different possible alignments is not simple, yet the ability to discover many poor alignments is simple. In addition, the ability to construct the needed number of QSAR models that would encompass every permutation of the possible different binding modes can quickly become overwhelming. To test and validate this methodology, a series of compounds bound to a common receptor with bioactivities and the solved 3D structures illustrating the orientation of the ligands in the binding site is needed.

The method used to align molecules is still an area of contention. Applications like MOE–FlexAlign *(30,39)* and FlexS *(37)* are used to help discover different alignment configurations or to ensure that user bias has not entered the alignment scheme. Methods like MOE–FlexAlign and CoMFA's Field Fit *(4)* are useful if one knows the bioactive conformation or if the molecules of interest are very rigid, yet the only proven method of aligning molecules for QSAR studies is through the design and implementation of different alignment schemes or experimental results.

3.6. Training and Test Set Creation

At first glance the Training Set (also referred to as Trial Sets) and Test Set appear as two collections of randomly chosen molecules, yet they are key components of a QSAR study. The Training Set is used to "build" and "train" the model and the Test Set is used to "test" the effectiveness of the model. In practice the Training Set is considerably larger, approx 75% of the total number of molecules in the study, than the Test Set. There are cases when the number of molecules available for a QSAR study is low (≤ 10), hindering the ability to create Training and Test Sets. In these cases all the molecules are used in the Training Set and several different model-validation methods are used to test the predictive ability of the model. A QSAR model is created by the minimization of the overall squared error of the data presented. From this basis it is best to have a Training Set representative of the overall population, with the major concern being bias toward one outcome. For instance, a model is created using a Training Set consisting of 85% "bad" compounds with the model evaluated on a series of novel molecules; if the molecules are truly "good," the model will be unable to predict whether a molecule is a "good" or "poor" binder. The best method of obtaining sound QSAR models is to have an even representation of the molecules of interest in the Training Set used to create the models.

The method of creating Training and Test Sets that are representative of the population is to choose molecules that represent all the molecules of interest based on molecular structure and bioactivity. The Molecular-Structure-Based Training Set is designed to represent all the scaffolds (basic molecular structure) of the molecules in the study throughout the bioactivity range. For example, assuming the molecules of interest are populated with molecules ranging from "good" to "bad," one can proceed to construct the "perfect" Training Set. The number of molecules in the Training Set is determined (approx 75% of the total molecules in the study) and the molecules are separated into groups based on their scaffolds. The molecules are placed in a table and ordered based on bioactivities. The molecules can be color-coded base on scaffold type to ease in the selection of different scaffold type (if more than one is present). The table is then divided into three sections based on binding affinity values: low, middle, and high. Dividing the largest bioactivity by three and using the 1/3 and 2/3 values as division points can aid in determine these regions or one can simply divide the compounds into three numerically equal sections. With the table prepared, the extraction of the molecules for the Training Set can begin through an iterative process starting at the top of the table. Molecules from the low, middle, and high regions with the same scaffold type are selected and placed into the Training Set. This process is done again for a different scaffold type and repeated until the Training Set is full. It is advantageous to "randomly" select specific scaffold types from the regions so the Training Set is a complete sample of the population and prevents selecting molecules from just the low or high end of a section. In a perfect case the remaining molecules should also be representative of the population and will comprise the Test Set.

4. Calculating the Descriptors

In a QSAR study the descriptors are the chemical characteristics of a molecule in numerical form. There are different types of descriptors based on the method of QSAR being employed. In traditional QSAR the descriptors are based on 2D aspects of the compounds (single numerical values based on physicochemical properties of the compounds). The calculation of traditional descriptors is fast and straightforward and can also translate a 3D feature of a molecule into a single numeric value. Some descriptors are based on atomic partial charges; thus, there is the need to use the force fields and partial charges available in the QSAR programs. Determining the partial charges for the molecules using a quantum mechanics program such as GAMESS *(75)*, Gaussian98 *(72)*, or MOPAC *(73,74)* is also feasible; in addition, the use of these programs can also yield *ab initio*–based descriptors. The descriptors calculated in 3D-QSAR methods differ from traditional QSAR descriptors because 3D-QSAR descriptors are typically shape-based or calculated using electrostatic potentials representing the molecules as felt by the receptor *(85)*.

Traditional 2D-QSAR descriptors are generally considered to be the characteristics of a molecule, as a chemist would perceive the molecules. The molecules are described by their physical properties, subdivided surface area *(86)*, atom counts and bonds, Kier and Hall connectivity and kappa shape indices *(87,88)*, adjacency and distance matrix descriptors *(89–92)*, pharmacophore features *(6)*, and partial charge. Further complicating matters are 3D traditional QSAR descriptors that are internally dependent (conformation-based) and externally dependent (alignment-based), thus emphasizing the need for correct conformation and alignment. Even single value 3D descriptors based on potential energy values, surface area, volume, and molecular shape are conformationally sensitive. The conformation and alignment of the molecules are crucial when calculating descriptors because the binding orientation and conformation of the compounds in most QSAR investigations are not known.

5. Determining the Best Model from an Extensive Descriptor Set

The determination of the best set of descriptors for a QSAR model can be a daunting task, especially when a large number of descriptors have been calculated. Choosing several descriptors out of many to construct an effective QSAR model is not a trivial matter. Selection of descriptors, creation of models, and evaluation of the model's effectiveness by hand is a time-consuming proposition and not very efficient. Consider a Training Set consisting of 300 descriptors and the desire for a model with 15 or fewer descriptors. The number of possible models to construct and test is 8.11×10^{24}. Even building and testing a billion QSAR models daily, using brute force, would take 2.2×10^{13} yr to complete all possible combinations landing one in the center of Levinthal's paradox *(93)*. The number of possible combinations of models can be calculated using the equations:

$$\binom{m}{r} = \frac{m!}{r!(m-r)!} \tag{8}$$

$$^{m}C_{r} = \frac{m!}{1!(m-1)!} + \frac{m!}{2!(m-2)!} + \cdots + \frac{m!}{r!(m-r)!} \tag{9}$$

where **Eq. 8** is the basic formula for determining the number of combinations given a specific number of descriptors, and **Eq. 9** is the formula for determining the total number of combinations up to a specific number of descriptors. The variable m is the total number of descriptors and r is the number of descriptors for the model.

Several methods have been developed to aid in the selection of descriptors to create a QSAR model. The use of brute computational force to test every possible combination of the above problem is wasteful. Methods such as the Stepwise Searches *(45)*, Simulated Annealing *(94)*, and Genetic Algorithms *(15)* are ways of dealing with this enormous problem. These methods are used in conjunction with linear and nonlinear models methods (multiple linear regression, principal component analysis, principle component regression, partial least squares, and artificial neural networks) to determine if the descriptors chosen constitute a "good model." The process of selecting the best descriptors for a model is an iterative process where the model is created using the selected descriptors and based on the Training Set followed by validation of the model. It is commonly thought that selecting the descriptors and creating the model is one step; in this chapter, this process is separated into its two components.

5.1. Reduction of Redundant Descriptors

Before an attempt to create a model is undertaken, it is necessary to remove descriptors with values of no use. This is accomplished first by removing descriptors with values missing for any of the molecules in the study. Next, the descriptors are checked for variation in values; descriptors where a constant value is present for all structures in the dataset are discarded. Once the non-contributing descriptors are removed, the one-parameter correlation values (Pearson's) and the squared correlation coefficient (t-test) values are calculated for each descriptor. Descriptors are removed if they do not meet the following criteria: the squared correlation coefficient or the t-value less than a user-defined minima and high intercorrelation between descriptors. Intercorrelation between descriptors is present if descriptor A is highly correlated (based on a user-defined correlation value) with descriptor B, and descriptor B possesses a higher correlation coefficient with the experimental binding affinity than descriptor A. Using these methods one is able to remove non-contributing descriptors from the QSAR model.

5.2. Forward and Backward Model Creation

The selection of the descriptors can happen in a forward or backward manner. A model created using the forward method starts with one descriptor followed by the addition of descriptors to the model until the model meets the specifications of the user. Models created in the backward method start with all the possible descriptors; descriptors are taken away as they are deemed unnecessary. It is safe to assume that most QSAR models are created using the forward method due to the sheer number of descriptors and the desire for only a few in the model. Models can be pruned using the backward method; specifically, once the model is created, the user wants to reduce the number of descriptors yet keep the same level of validity for the model.

5.3. Stepwise Searches

A similar method of selecting descriptors by hand for the QSAR model is the Stepwise Method Search *(45)*. This iterative improvement method searches for the optimum QSAR model starting from a known configuration. Each component (descriptor) of the model is rearranged in turn until an improved configuration compared to the last is found. This new configuration then becomes the current system for improvement and the process is continued until no further improved QSAR models are found. The iterative improvement of the system is done by searching coordinate space (different possible models) for rearrangement steps leading to better $R2^2$ values, similar to energy-minimization techniques. This method of searching for QSAR models has the tendency to find "okay models" but not the "best model" due to the nature of the landscape being searched. To perform a robust search of the landscape when using the Stepwise Search Method it is advantageous to start with several random original configurations in an attempt to find the optimal configuration, thus the possibility of finding the "best" model is increased.

A Stepwise Search starts with arranging the descriptors based on their one-parameter correlation value with respect to the molecule's bioactivity in descending order. Next all two-parameter correlations are calculated until no correlations with an R^2 value above a user-defined value has been found. A predetermined number of best pairs (two-parameter correlations) selected to continue in the search for an effective QSAR model. Each of the remaining descriptors (not highly correlated to the remaining descriptors based on a user-defined R-value) are used to create the next group of models. It is evident that this is a computationally intensive method that is similar to choosing descriptors by hand, yet the computer does all of the work. Owing to the method of initially selecting descriptors for the QSAR model, a Stepwise Search has the potential to overlook groups of descriptors (descriptors that individually correlate poorly) that correlate well to the bioactivities.

5.4. Simulated Annealing (SA)

A move forward in the selection of descriptors is the method of Simulated Annealing (94) (similar to Stepwise Searching) used to find the solution of a complex problem with many incorrect solutions at a minimal computational cost. This method comes from annealing, the physical process of heating a solid and letting it slowly cool to form a perfect crystal lattice. This experiment leads to the discovery of the minimum free energy of the solid. The crystal can become defective and trapped in a local minimum instead of a perfect crystal structure at the global minimum if the cooling happens too quickly. Simulated Annealing has been implemented by combinatorial optimization; the search for an optimal model starts with an initial model at a very high temperature. The temperature is reduced with each successive cycle to simulate the annealing process (95). The reduction of the temperature at the beginning of each cycle allows the model to gradually cool producing a perfect model in the *global minima* of the landscape.

To simulate the annealing process each state is accepted or rejected probabilistically using a modified Monte Carlo method (96). The random configurations are chosen using the probability function $\exp(-R^2/kT)$, thus weighting each configuration equally. The implementation of SA in the selection of QSAR models is similar to its use in other computational areas. The criterion for the R^2 value is increased for each cycle and the composition of the model is changed for each step. After each modification to the model, the change in the coefficient of determination (R^2) of the system is calculated, and if the new R^2 value is greater than the previous, then the new model is accepted. The change in the model is accepted probabilistically if the new R^2 value is less than the previous R^2. The probabilistic accepting of the model is based on the selection of a random number, ζ, between 0 and 1; if $\zeta < \exp(-R^2/kT)$, the new

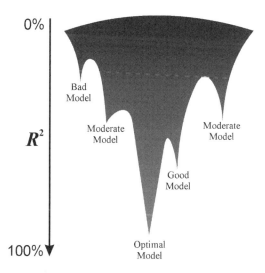

Fig. 4. Representation of simulated annealing for the selection of descriptors for a QSAR model. The potential well represents all possible models and as the value of R^2 increases (low R^2 values at the top and high R^2 values at the bottom of the Y axis), the number of models decreases.

configuration is accepted and if $\zeta > \exp(-R^2/kT)$, the configuration is rejected and the original model is once again the starting point. The system average is recalculated for new models, whereas if the model retains an old configuration, the average is not calculated. Through Simulated Annealing the model explores the various valleys of the energy landscape **(Fig. 4)**.

The method of simulated annealing is more advanced than the Stepwise Search Method and through the use of multiple starting points (different initial models) a more thorough exploration of possible models can be performed. The downfall of Stepwise Searching and Simulated Annealing is also their strong point; they are very good at exploring a small landscape with several descriptors, yet they are not suited for large number of descriptors. It is because of these constraints that evolutionary programs (such as genetic algorithms) have become more prevalent in the search for the optimal model.

5.5. Genetic Algorithms (GA)

Following the biological processes of gene mutation and rearrangement Genetic Algorithms (GA) *(15)* are an artificial intelligence technique utilizing stochastic search algorithms to model natural phenomena *(97)*. GAs perform a multidirectional search and evolve the population of possible solutions through mutations and crossovers. In each generation there are "good" and "bad" solu-

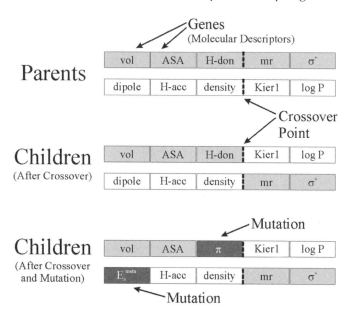

Fig. 5. Representation of a genetic algorithm for the selection of descriptors for a QSAR model. The model is commonly referred to as a gene and is encoded with different descriptors. Two **Parents** creating two **Children** is a *crossover* of genetic information (descriptors). The genes of an individual can *mutate*, introducing random changes in the model. Crossover and mutation are can occur independent of each other.

tions; the "good" solutions evolve to the next generation as the "bad" solutions die in a process that is similar to natural selection.

In the area of QSAR model creation, the models of a GA are constructed of genes that are encoded with different molecular descriptors **(Fig. 5)**. The first step in a genetic algorithm is the creation of a population of QSAR models corresponding to the number of individuals determined by the user. Iterative looping creates a number of evaluation models, forming the generations. The model generation contains different evolutionary levels used in the following order to determine if a model survives. The fitness is the correlation (R^2) between the experimentally determined binding affinities and the ability of the model to predict the experimental values. The selection process determines which individuals (models) get to reproduce or perish and is based on the model's fitness. Models with a "good" correlation to the experimental values (high R^2 value, good fitness) are allowed to reproduce, models with average correlation stay the same, and models with "bad" correlations expire. The exchange of information between models is done through a crossover where genes (molecular descriptors) from two parents produce two children allowing the parents to pass on. A crossover is the selection of genes (descriptors) from the parents to construct a child randomly composed of the parents' descriptors *(98)* as is common in biological systems. The process of a crossover also occurs by breaking the parents into two (or more) sections and swapping the genetic information to produce two complete children; this can occur at a single point **(Fig. 5)**, or at multiple points. The random changing of descriptors in a model is done through mutation, and can happen anywhere in the model, introducing random ensembles of descriptors. Crossover and mutation occur randomly throughout the population adding to the possibility of a better model being discovered; crossover and mutation do not have to occur concurrently. Elitist selection is the preservation of the strong individuals based on fitness. A user-defined value determines the number of preferred individuals that directly proceed into the next generation without modification *(97)*. A review of GAs applied to different fields of computational chemistry can be found in separate works by Devillers *(99)* and Clark *(100)*.

The QSAR methodology of 4D-QSAR (a RI-, RD-, and VHTS *n*D-QSAR method) implements a genetic algorithm into its descriptor selection process. In the following section the methodology of 4D-QSAR is discussed along with the genetic function approximation method *(101)* as employed in 4D-QSAR model building.

5.5.1. Genetic Algorithm Implemented in 4D-QSAR

Traditional and 3D-QSAR methodologies have three inherent limitations:

1. How to assign the active conformation to each ligand?
2. How to align the ligands?
3. How to subdivide each ligand molecule into pharmacophore sites with respect to intermolecular receptor interactions *(5)*?

Hopfinger et al. *(5)* developed 4D-QSAR analysis which incorporates conformational and alignment freedom into the development of a 3D-QSAR model and can be viewed as the evolution of molecular shape analysis, also developed by Hopfinger *(26,102)* in the early 1980s.

4D-QSAR *(5)* is unique in that it uses a grid to determine the regions in 3D space that are important for binding, yet it does not use a probe or interaction energies to construct the QSAR model like CoMFA. The reference grid cell is constructed to accommodate the largest compound of the study and usually has a grid spacing (resolution) of 1.0 Å. Next, a combination of the seven different interaction pharmacophore elements (IPEs) *(5)* is selected to determine how the compounds are partitioned into their specific atom/region types during analysis. The third step is to construct the conformational ensemble profile (CEP) *(5)* for each compound in the study using molecular dynamics simulations (MDSs), thus alleviating the question of "What is the active conformation?" The CEP does not contain all of the molecules sampled during the MDS calculations, only the conformations selected based on a Boltzmann distribution. The different alignment schemes are devised next, and are constructed based on three-atom-alignment methods. The alignments are constructed to explore the entire topology of the compounds of the study, keeping in mind that the regions with substitution are of most interest.

Following the construction of the CEP, the grid cell occupancy descriptors (GCODs) are calculated based on the selected IPEs for each conformation stored in the respective CEP *(43)*. This is accomplished by placing each conformation in the reference grid cell based on the alignment scheme being explored. As each conformation for a specific compound is aligned in and with the reference grid *(43)*, the thermodynamic probability of each grid cell occupied by an atom is recorded noting its IPE. In step six the grid occupancy data are reduced using the same method as CoMFA [Partial least squares regression analysis *(21)*], yet it differs from CoMFA by including all grid cells occupied (at least once) in the initial model. CoMFA uses a distance cutoff to determine if the potential field at a specific grid point should be included in the creation of a model *(4)*. The data fit between the GCODs and the bioactivities (ΔG) is determined using partial least squares (PLS) regression analysis *(21)* creating a new set of descriptors. The number of grid cells to be analyzed can be further reduced by excluding GCODs that were only occupied by atoms twice. Following the data reduction the top 200 GCODs plus any user-included descriptors are used to construct the 4D-QSAR model *(43)*. In addition to the GCODs, additional externally determined physicochemical properties can be incorporated into the 4D-QSAR model (creating a fifth dimension) to improve the final model. The descriptors are selected using a modified genetic function approximation *(101)* (GFA) and the 4D-QSAR model is created using multiple linear regression *(43)* (MLR). The eighth step of 4D-QSAR is the option to repeat steps four through seven for additional alignment schemes.

The Genetic Function Approximation (GFA) methodology is a combination of a genetic algorithm *(15)* and the multivariate adaptive regression splines algorithm *(103)* (MARS). The main purpose of the MARS algorithm is to create spline-based regression models using a minimal number of features (descriptors), yet is a computationally intensive method and constructs models in a stepwise fashion. The main issue of constructing QSAR models using stepwise searches (as discussed above) is that the method is not sufficiently adaptive to select groups of descriptors that will predict well as a group, yet poorly as individuals. The genetic algorithm replaces the stepwise search method of MARS enabling the initial random selection of descriptors and construction of models from the top performing sets of descriptors. This transformation to a QSAR model creation method is carried out by replacing the traditionally binary string of variables *(15)* with strings of basis functions (sets of descriptors) *(103)*. The GFA methodology is a more robust method of determining a QSAR model than other methods which may incorporate a type of stepwise search methods. The benefits occur through the construction of multiple models, testing the "full" model instead of "partial" models on the Training Set, the ability to find combinations of basis functions that take advantage of correlations between a set of descriptors and the bioactivities, resistance to overfitting the model using a "lack of fit" (LOF) *(103)* function, and the ability to control the number of descriptors in the final models (smoothness of fit). The lack of fit function is:

$$LOF = \frac{LSE}{\left(1 - \frac{c + dp}{n}\right)^2} \tag{10}$$

In the LOF equation (**Eq. 10**) the least squared error (LSE) is defined in **Eq. 29**. The values composing the denominator are the number of basis functions (c) (sets of descriptors) in the model, the user-definable smoothing factor (d), the total number of features contained in all the basis functions (p), and the number of molecules in the Training Set (n). The benefit of using LOF vs LSE is evident. To decrease the LSE value a common practice is to increase the number of basis functions (c), yet this is not a sound practice. The addition of more descriptors than necessary to a QSAR model (in the hopes of decreasing the LSE and increasing the R^2) creates a generalized model. Taking the same system and monitoring the predictive ability of the model with the LOF, the addition of descriptors will decrease the LSE value, yet increase the LOF value. The increasing of the LOF value indicates a reduction in the predictive ability of the model and withstands overfitting.

QSAR model analysis is made possible through the generation of several plausible 4D-QSAR models. The ninth step examines all the models created and reports the "top" model with respect to the alignment of interest. Reporting the best model is good, but the top 10 models could prove more useful. By exploring multiple models it can be determined if other important GCODs exist and may be possible to construct better models using this information, forming a composite model or a *manifold* 4D-QSAR model *(43)*. The construction of multiple QSAR models from the same descriptor pool allows for statistical analysis of the GCODs used to construct the QSAR model. Step 10 proceeds by identifying the low-energy conformations of each molecule's CEP. These low-energy conformations are evaluated (one at the time) using the best 4D-QSAR model. *The low-energy conformation of the molecule with the highest predicted bioactivity using the 4D-QSAR model and the affiliated alignment is*

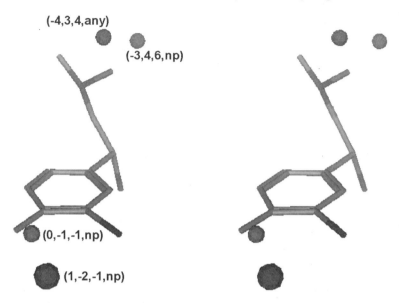

Fig. 6. The spheres corresponding to positive interaction pharmacophore element (IPE) represent regions that will be beneficial to the QSAR model. The sphere corresponding to negative IPEs indicate the region(s) where the particular IPE will degrade the QSAR model.

then defined as the bioactive conformation for the molecule. A unique bioactive conformation can thus be assigned to each molecule considered as an intrinsic part of doing 4D-QSAR analysis. 4D-QSAR also permits the prediction of the loss in bioactivity due to the loss in ligand conformational entropy upon binding to the receptor.

The graphical representation of a 4D-QSAR model consists of the significant descriptors in space (a 3D pharmacophore) along with their attributes (increase or decrease specific physicochemical properties). **Figure 6** best illustrates the graphical interpretation of a 4D-QSAR model, specifically for a molecule from the Case Study **(Subheading 8.)**. 4D-QSAR also overcomes the issue of 3D-QSAR models being created based on static molecular spatial arrangements (rigid molecules), meaning that the space unoccupied by any of the molecules in the study cannot be interpreted *(36)* and used in the creation of the model. 3D-QSAR methodologies such as CoMFA do not take an ensemble of molecular conformations into consideration; the models are based solely on the molecular volumes of the *probable* bioactive conformations. 4D-QSAR is able to overcome this hurdle and hypothesize the bioactive conformation of the compounds in the active site thus creating QSAR models based on bioactively favorable conformations. The combination of the active conformation with an optimal alignment can be used in additional drug-design applications such as pharmacophore construction or other 3D-QSAR methods.

Bioactivity = log (1/c) = 8.82 (−4, 3, 4, *any*) + 8.48 (−3, 4, 6, *np*)

$$+ -1.34 \ (0, -1, -1, np) + 15.13 \ (1, -2, -1, np)$$

$$+ 6.45$$

$$n = 22 \quad R^2 + 0.84 \quad Q^2 = 0.88 \quad LSE = 0.05 \quad LOF = 0.19$$

4D-QSAR does not solve the issues related to alignment, but alignments can be rapidly sampled so that, effectively, a 4D-QSAR model can be optimized as a function of alignment. The constructed 4D-QSAR model can also be implemented as a 3D-pharmacophor screening tool. The construction of QSAR models that can be interpreted in terms of pharmacophore requirements, but also used to screen libraries of compounds (usually analogs) efficiently (correctly and quickly), can be of great utility. In the creation of a 3D-QSAR model to be implemented as a VHTS, it is necessary for the model to include not only the "favorable" space occupied by the molecules of the Training Set, but also the space not available to the molecules during binding due to steric hindrance imposed by the receptor *(27)*. This pharmacophore-based method of VHTS can be realized using QSAR models constructed from 4D-QSAR analysis *(5,43)*.

There are two possible application strategies for the use of 4D-QSAR models as a VHTS. The first is to take a collection of (manifold) 4D-QSAR models and create a consensus 4D-QSAR model. The consensus model is evaluated for each molecule using all of the individual 4D-QSAR models:

$$\langle \Delta G[c] \rangle = \sum_i \Delta G_i [c] W_i \qquad (11)$$

The consensus binding free energy ($<\Delta G[c]>$), in this particular case **Eq. 11**, for each compound is the summation of the product of the predicted binding free energy (ΔG) of each compound ($[c]$) for each model (i) and a relative significance (W_i, weighting factor). The relative significance value can be calculated using several different methods, yet the most reasonable is to divide the coefficient of determination (R^2) for the current model by the sum of all the R^2's for all the models of interest (**Eq. 12**):

$$W_i - \frac{R_i^2}{\sum_j R_j^2} \qquad (12)$$

Another way to form a VHTS from several 4D-QSAR models is to use all the distinct grid cell occupancy descriptors (GCODs) and the bioactivity (ΔG) values of the training set. This simple method of constructing a VHTS-QSAR model is likely to suffer from overfitting the data, but is useful in a VHTS context because it contains the relevant GCODs found for the Training Set and will create a VHTS model that is unambiguous.

Once the VHTS model is constructed from the 4D-QSAR models its application is straightforward, and similar to how novel compounds are evaluated in 4D-QSAR analysis. The library of compounds is evaluated by performing molecular dynamic simulations (MDSs), aligning the molecules based on the alignment rules for each of the 4D-QSAR models, determining the GCOD values defined in the VHTS model and predicting the compounds bioactivity using the regression equations of the 4D-QSAR models. There is a misconception that if enough descriptors (traditional 2D-QSAR descriptors) are calculated a valid QSAR/VHTS model will be constructed by selecting the important descriptors from the descriptor pile through the use of data-reduction techniques. The QSAR/VHTS model deduced from a myriad of descriptors is then considered apt in the screening of an arbitrary virtual library. In actuality a QSAR model should consist of as few descriptors as possible, but a VHTS model can contain more descriptors than its QSAR counterpart, creating a robust VHTS model. QSAR and VHTS models created with a bogus conformation and/or alignment can lead to models of low quality even if the models were constructed with the optimal descriptors.

The benefits of using 4D-QSAR models for VHTS arise from the use of GCODs. Each GCOD defines a specific location in 3D space relative to the molecules in the training set (other GCODs) and the alignment of the molecules. 4D-QSAR VHTS models are able to predict binding affinities of molecules beyond the values used to construct the VHTS model; demonstrating the models' predictive ability. However, this predictive capacity can only be accomplished if the molecules of the virtual library do not extend beyond the concatenated 3D space sampled by the molecules of the training set.

6. Methods to Develop QSAR Models

Once the descriptors are selected, the QSAR model is created allowing the prediction of bioactivities. The QSAR model has the general form of **Eq. 1**, and is developed using each molecule (the Training Set) in the study. The values for the descriptors (descriptor$_x$) are a specific physicochemical value for the compound and the coefficients and constant (in this case a and b, and c, respectively) are set values derived to create models capable of reproducing the experimental biological activities. A simple way of thinking about the creation of a QSAR model is the correlating of molecular descriptors to the bioactivities. Next, the model is used to predict the bioactivities of the molecules used to create the model (Training Set) as a method of internally checking the QSAR model for usefulness. If the model is deemed useful, it is tested against novel compounds. There are several regression methods for determining the coefficients and constant for the generalized QSAR model. Traditionally, multiple linear regression (MLR) is used to determine these values, with recent implementation of methods such as principal component analysis (PCA) *(19,20)*, partial least squares (PLS) *(21)*, and artificial neural networks (ANN) *(104)* to accommodate the large amount of data produced by 3D, nD-QSAR methods and large numbers of traditional QSAR descriptors. The creation of the model is not an additive process; creating a model using two descriptors with single R^2 values of 0.45 and 0.36, with respect to the bioactivities, will not yield a model with an R^2 of 0.81.

The types of problems capable of being solved with the following regression methods are defined by the manner in which each of the regression methods works. The basic premise is that a method is given input variables (bioactivities and descriptors) and in turn the method produces output variables (coefficients and a constant). These methods work best when information about the system of interest is known and inferences can be made about the problem being solved. This can only be done if there is confidence that a relationship exists between the known input data and the unknown output data before these methods are utilized; if there is no relationship, then the model will be useless.

6.1. Linear Regression

The original method of correlating binding affinities with the molecular descriptors is multiple linear regression (MLR) and through this correlation the QSAR model is created. The process of fitting a model to a set of points using a straight line is LR. This was one of the first statistical methods used to create the coefficients and constant for models in traditional QSAR studies. The model is then used to predict the bioactivities of the molecules used to create the model. The predicted values are compared to the experimental values through least squares fitting, and the model that performs the best at reproducing the experimental values is used to predict the bioactivities of novel compounds. This method is straightforward, and it uses two assumptions: (a) the errors in the predicted values are substantially greater than the errors in the known values and (b) the standard deviations in all of the predicted values are similar. These assumptions state that the predicted values will never be as exact as the experimental values and the error for the predicted values will be the same.

An easy way to visualize a linear equation is with one variable as in simple linear regression. An example of the one-variable linear regression equation is between the dependent variable (a bioactivity value) and an independent variable (the descriptor coefficient) and is expressed:

$$\hat{y} = b_0 + b_1 x_1 \tag{13}$$

$$b_1 = \frac{S_{xy}}{S_{xx}} \tag{14}$$

$$S_{xy} = \sum xy - \frac{\left(\sum x\right)\left(\sum y\right)}{n} \tag{15}$$

$$S_{xx} = \sum x^2 - \frac{\left(\sum x\right)^2}{n} \tag{16}$$

$$b_0 = \frac{1}{n}\left(\sum y - b_1 \sum x\right) \tag{17}$$

where b_0 and b_1 are fixed numbers (y intercept and slope respectively), x_1 is the independent variable, and $\hat{y}$ is the dependent variable. Given a set of data points it is possible to draw several straight lines through these points; therefore, a method to choose the best straight line is needed. The least squares criterion is the line that best fits the data points and is determined using the sum of the errors squared *(SSE)*, the sum of the square difference between the actual values and the predicted values. The line with the lowest *SSE* is chosen as the straight line for the data and is termed "the model." The least squares criterion only gives the properties of the regression line for a set of data and does not tell how to determine the coefficients and constants for this regression line.

6.2. Coefficient of Determination and Linear Correlation Coefficient

Once a model is created and has predicted the bioactivities of the Training Set, the effectiveness of the model needs to be evaluated. The coefficient of determination (r^2) is a descriptive measure of the model's ability to make predictions. The r^2 value is the percentage reduction gained in the total squared error by using the model to predict the y values instead of the average y values. The r^2 can also be interpreted to explain the percentage of total variation in the experimental y values, the coefficient of determination. As mentioned above, the *SSE* is used to choose which model will be reported, yet this value also measures the chance variation within the sample and the "error" denotes the experimental error, *SSE*. The quantitative measure of the total error produced is the total sum of squares *(SST)* and is the sum of the difference between the actual value and the mean of the actual values squared. The total amount of squared deviation explained by the regression line is the regression sum of squares *(SSR)*, which is the sum of the squares of the difference between the predicted values and the mean of the actual values:

$$SSE = \sum (y - \hat{y})^2 \tag{18}$$

$$SST = \sum (y - \bar{y})^2 \tag{19}$$

$$SSR = \sum (\hat{y} - \bar{y})^2 \tag{20}$$

$$r^2 = 1 - \frac{SSE}{SST} \tag{21}$$

$$r^2 = \frac{SSR}{SST} \tag{22}$$

Calculating r^2 using these methods (**Eqs. 21** and **22**) will yield incorrect values, especially if the slope of the data deviates from a value of 1.0; instead, it is best to square the linear correlation coefficient (**Eq. 23**), discussed below, to calculate the coefficient of determination.

It is important to know the effectiveness of the model for predicting values; however, it is also important to know the strength of the linear relationship between the two variables (known and predicted) being studied. This is achieved using the linear correlation coefficient (Pearson's product moment correlation coefficient), r, as a descriptive measure for the strength of the linear relationship (straight line) between the two variables:

$$r = \frac{\sum xy - \left(\sum x\right)\left(\sum y\right)/n}{\sqrt{\left(\sum x^2 - \left(\sum x\right)^2/n\right)\left(\sum y^2 - (y)^2/n\right)}} = \frac{S_{xy}}{\sqrt{S_{xx}S_{yy}}} \tag{23}$$

Multiple linear regression is an extension of simple linear regression; the difference being more than one independent variable (descriptor) is used in the prediction of the dependent variable:

$$\hat{y} = b_0 + b_1 x_1 + \cdots + b_k x_k \tag{24}$$

$$\hat{y} = b_0 + b_1 x_1 + b_2 x_2 + b_3 x_3 \tag{25}$$

The same principles and techniques used for simple linear regression are used for MLR, yet the ability to calculate the regression values by hand is lost. Another change between SLR and MLR is the coefficient of determination, denoted as R^2 instead of r^2 and the linear correlation coefficient, denoted as R instead of r.

6.3. Creating Models from Uncorrelated Descriptors: Chemometrics

When searching for possible descriptors for a traditional QSAR study, it is common practice to calculate all of the available descriptors, in some instances more than 300 descriptors including descriptors calculated from outside methods.

Constructing the model using all the calculated descriptors is feasible, but this leads to overgeneralized models. The problem of "many descriptors" is further compounded when using 3D and *n*D-QSAR methodology where thousands of descriptors are calculated. The end results of calculating all possible descriptors for traditional QSAR and the data returned from 3D-QSAR methods are tables containing many columns (descriptors) and few rows (molecules, bioactivities).

In 3D and *n*D-QSAR methodologies it is common to have more descriptors than molecules in a study owing to the nature of the descriptors (interaction energies between a probe and a molecule on a 3D grid, ensembles of molecular conformations, IR spectrum peaks, and induced fit models). This normally would be considered a problem, except in projection methods of creating a model where the large number of relevant variables helps create a better model *(105)*. This concept of using more variables to construct a better model is similar to finding an average; the more samples collected results in a more relevant average and thus a more precise prediction can be made from the models. The methods discussed below are able to handle situations of this nature and were specifically devised to construct models from variables appearing to have no correlation.

Chemometrics is the field of model creation based on indirect measurements to determine the properties (bioactivities in the case of QSAR) of compounds that are difficult to determine through direct measurements (traditional LR or MLR methods) *(106,107)*. Articles discussing chemometric methods and techniques can be found in reviews by Wold and Sjöström *(105)*, and a series of reviews by Lavine *(106,107)*. The series of reviews by Lavine discuss the developments in the chemometric field and highlights the advancement of chemometrics in different disciplines. Books that give excellent in-depth information on different multivariate methods along with PCA are by Manly *(17)* and by Grimm and Yarnold *(18)*. In addition, a book by Chatterjee et al. *(45)* discusses regression techniques and methodology with well-defined examples. An in-depth review discussing the use and processes of artificial neural networks is by Schneider and Wrede *(108)* along with a book by Zupan and Gasteiger *(25)*, which contains examples and ANN applications in chemistry and drug design. Another machine-learning method of constructing QSAR models is support vector machines (SVMs) *(16,109)*. SVMs is an extension of artificial neural networks (ANN) allowing nonlinear models to be created, which are less likely to experience overfitting as compared to ANN models, yet are suitable for screening compounds in a HTS methodology.

6.3.1. Principal Component Analysis (PCA)

Principal component analysis *(19,20)* is used to create correlated descriptors from existing descriptors as the dimensionality of a descriptor set is reduced to create QSAR models. Principal component analysis is a method capable of reducing the number of variables needed to create a QSAR model by taking the selected descriptors and transforming them to orthogonal principal components. The model is created using only enough principal components (PC) to reproduce the vital variance of the original descriptors. The enticing reason for using PCA in creating QSAR models is the ability to create compact and accurate models and minimizing the loss of information from the original data (descriptors). The greater the number of PCs the greater the ability for the model to recreate the original data (bioactivities) based on the same descriptors. PCA is an internal analysis method dealing with the variances and covariances of the selected molecular descriptors (elements of the vector) and has no relationship to a different set of descriptors *(110)*. The goal of multivariate regression is to replace the entire set of descriptors with a set of new variables that are compact and correlated.

After the important descriptors have been selected, they are reduced into principal components creating the QSAR model becoming the "new" descriptors of the model. The first component will contain the most information (variance) about all the descriptors used to create the model. PCA works the best when there are several dozen correlated descriptors and several principal components can effectively embody the QSAR model. PCA will not work if the original descriptors are uncorrelated and it is not guaranteed to return a compact set of components from a large set of original descriptors.

Using PCA it is possible to describe the location and shape of the N-space data cloud (the model) for a given set of compounds, where N is the number of independent variables (PCs) used to create the PCA model. The location and shape of the data cloud are constructed by translating the descriptors to the origin through mean-centering, followed by rotating it about the origin. The translation and rotation of the descriptors are performed to create the latent variables (principal components). A latent variable is the principal axis, more specifically the axis with the greatest variance. The rotation of the first principal component of the model orients the axis along the longest dimension through the data set. The first PC's axis is held fixed and the following PC axes are determined orthogonal to each other and are termed latent variables. There are times when all the data are retained, yet this is not typically the case. Traditionally only the first couple of PCs are used because they contain a majority of the important information from the descriptors used to create the model. Creating a model using PCA from four descriptors constructs a model with four principal components; most of the variance of the original descriptors will be explained in the first two or three PCs. The justification for using the first few PCs to construct a model is that the first few PCs are the most significant and the remaining PCs are considered nonessential to the model. Error is removed from the model through the retention of the optimal number of PCs.

Using all of the PCs in a model will explain the entire variance, yet this is unnecessary because the first several will likely explain a significant amount of the variance (approx 80%) and using all of the PCs can add error to the predictive quality of the model. The first PC contains more information and variance about the original descriptors than the second PC, and the second PC contains more information and variance than the third PC and so forth. The optimal number of PCs can be determined in a stepwise addition method, by adding PCs to the model until the predictive ability of the model plateaus or decreases. The maximum number of PCs for the model is the number of PCs before its decline of predictive power. This same method can be applied in a backward stepwise search by starting with all the PCs and removing PCs until the model is constructed. Another method of PC selection is through the use of cross-validation. The optimal number of descriptors for model creation and cross-validation will be discussed below. The main use of PCA in QSAR is the construction of models and data reduction, yet it can also be used to detect outlier molecules in the Training Set. The removal of an outlier from the Training Set, for that specific model, can yield an improved model.

The strength of PCA is the ability to take more than the optimal number of descriptors (that appear to be uncorrelated) and construct latent variables that are internally correlated yet uncorrelated to each other. The best feature of PCA is the ease of determining which of the original descriptors are most important.

6.3.2. Partial Least Squares (PLS)

Exceeding PCA in ability to handle large number of descriptors is partial least squares (21), but is extended to datasets containing many more descriptors than bioactivities, essentially more columns than rows. The relationship of PLS to PCA is that the PCs are constructed from the original descriptors, which have been modified twice before creating the PLS model. PLS attempts to discover several latent models (linear combinations of molecular descriptors) that best correlate with the bioactivities. Like any method of analysis, overfitting is a problem and is kept in check by using cross-validation. The most notable feature of PLS is its ability to correctly create a model when presented with strongly collinear descriptors (input data) and missing input data values (descriptors and bioactivities).

The methodology of PLS is derived from principal component regression (PCR), which is PCA with multiple regression performed on the latent variables created by PCA. PCR works by exploiting the nonexistent correlation between latent variables and the data of the first few PC axes. PLS differs from PCA by performing regression on the new latent variables PLS has created from the PCs of PCR. The latent variables of PLS are selected to satisfy three criteria simultaneously. The new variables need to be highly correlated to the bioactivities (dependent variables); this is key for good model creation. The latent variables must model a significant amount of the variance contained in the descriptors (independent variables); this is based on the concept of the components with the smallest percentage of error will contain the greatest variance *(21)*. The error referred to in this section is not the usual error expected when taking a physical measurement or performing a calculation, but refers to any feature not typical of the molecules as a full set. The new variables must also be uncorrelated with respect to each other to minimize the redundancy of information between the variables; the minimization of information redundancy reduces the number of variables needed to construct a model. The model created in PLS uses latent variables formed by rotating the data set in N-space, with the number of variables in the regression equal to the number of PLS components retained. Preprocessing of the initial descriptors and bioactivities, discussed earlier, is required to remove false correlations between descriptors (independent variables) not typical of the entire set of molecules and the bioactivities (dependent variables).

The reduction of latent variables is an effective method to reduce the number of possible models, yet in PLS, variable reduction is not needed. The reduction of the number of variables in traditional regression techniques will lead to models with improved predictive ability and, in the case of PLS, a model that is easier to understand. The attempts to reduce the number of variables for PLS have only resulted in simpler models that fit the Training Set better yet do not have the predictive abilities of the complete PLS model *(111)*. The reduction of latent variables with respect to the descriptors is possible with no apparent decrease in the model's ability to predict bioactivities, yet the remaining descriptor-based variables are considered to be more important before reduction and thus introduces bias *(111)*.

Once a PLS model is constructed, the predictive ability of the model is of main interest. For each component of the model constructed, the percentage of the variance explained for the bioactivities and descriptors (dependent and independent variables, respectively) is reported. The percentage of variance explained by the components is represented as the %y and %x score. The %y score relates to the percentage of variance between the bioactivity-derived latent variables and the descriptor-based latent variables. A high %y value shows that the model is reliable for a prediction yet does not ensure good predictions. Guaranteeing a good prediction relies on the percentage of the model based on the descriptor-based latent variables data instead of error. As with any model-building technique, the more variables added, the lower the error. The maximum number of variables (descriptors, latent variables) for a QSAR model is reached as more latent variables are added and the model's ability to better predict bioactivity values is not significantly increased. The increase in the R^2 value is minimal (approx 2%) and possibly decreases as more descriptors are added to the model. The process of adding variables until the predictive ability of the model plateaus or decreases along with taking into consideration the percentage variance explained are common methods of performing PLS regression. The strength of PLS lies in its ability to determine a new set of uncorrelated latent variables in *N*-space rotation. PLS attempts to explain as much of the variance in the independent-variable matrix (the molecules with their corresponding descriptors) and in the dependent-variable matrix (the molecules' bioactivities) based on uncorrelated latent variables. In this attempt to explain the variance, the PLS axes are rotated away from the principal component axes thus maximizing only the variance explained in the independent-variable matrix. Another strong point of PLS is its ability to take a large set of descriptors and reduce them to a minimal set of latent variables and create a model with exceptional predictive capability. An added benefit of PLS with respect to MLR is its ability to analyze several response variables simultaneously and use non-precise data that can cause problems for MLR and QSAR methodologies. Taking into consideration the benefits of PLS, the main drawback is the format of the variables returned. The variables are abstract and awkward to decipher because they are based on values derived from principal components, thus making the modification of physicochemical properties difficult.

6.3.2.1. PLS Implemented in Comparative Molecular Field Analysis (CoMFA)

The QSAR package Comparative Molecular Field Analysis (CoMFA) *(4)* is a method allowing the exploration of a molecule's physical properties similar to how the active site would "feel" the molecule *(85)*. CoMFA possesses four essential parts:

1. Construction of a grid around the aligned molecules.
2. Placement of a probe at each of the grid points and calculating interaction energies.
3. Utilization of Partial Least Squares (PLS) *(22)* regression to reduce the data set and create the QSAR model.
4. Displaying the results as isosurfaces.

These four components may appear trivial by themselves, but combining them results in a dynamic method to create a QSAR model. Unfortunately, these main components of CoMFA are more complicated than a quick glance might suggest.

CoMFA is based on interactions between a molecule and a probe; traditionally, the probe has the properties consistent with a van der Waals sp^3 carbon and a charge of +1.0. The interactions calculated between the probe and the molecules of interest are steric (van der Waals 6–12) and electrostatic (Coulombic with a $1/r$ dielectric) energies *(4)*. The CoMFA process starts by constructing a 3D grid large enough to surround the largest molecule in the series by several angstroms with grid spacing typically of 1.0 Å. The probe is then place at each grid point and an interaction energy calculation is performed. The data gathered are placed in a table for data analysis and the QSAR model is created employing PLS.

To extract a suitable QSAR model from the disproportionate data table, with underdetermined character resulting from many more columns than rows, the PLS method developed by Wold and colleagues *(22)* is used. This is made possible because the units of all the independent variables (grid point interaction values) are the same (kcal/mol). In CoMFA the PLS is utilized in a manner that rotates the PLS solution back into the original data space to generate a traditional QSAR equation. The CoMFA QSAR equation contains coefficients for each column in the data table along with two coefficients for each grid point, and thus can be drawn in 3D space. The interaction energies are represented as color-coded surfaces to aid in how and where to improve the molecule to achieve better binding.

In CoMFA, as in most 3D-QSAR methodology, the alignment of the molecules is a main issue because the relative interaction energies strongly depend on the relative molecular position. The choice of molecular conformation and alignment is usually left to the discretion of the user, yet CoMFA possesses the ability to determine a suitable alignment through, "Field Fit," discussed below. The main difference between CoMFA and traditional QSAR is the implementation of a graphical output in addition to the QSAR model. CoMFA constructs a traditional QSAR model, but its strength is the ability to graphically display the output of the probe–molecule interaction. These CoMFA coefficient contour maps are surfaces surrounding the grid points where the QSAR model strongly associates changes in the molecule–probe interaction values with a change in bioactivities. The surfaces surround grid points where the scalar products of the QSAR model's coefficient and the standard deviation of all values in the corresponding column of the data table are higher or lower than a user-specified value. The surfaces are color-coded depending on the direction and magnitude of the differential interactions. The blue or cyan contours exhibiting regions where more steric bulk is "good" and should increase the ability of the molecule to bind, whereas contours that are red or yellow represent regions where less steric bulk is "good."

The methodology of 3D-QSAR appears and is a robust method of constructing QSAR models, but there are several issues, discussed below in detail, that complicate this methodology. The first and most prominent question is "Which conformation of the molecules to use?" This problem is considered *(36)* a leading cause to incorrect QSAR models, specifically those created with 3D-QSAR methods such as CoMFA. The next issue is "How to align the molecules?" The alignment of the molecules might seem rather straightforward from a visual standpoint, but consider the concept of molecules that are "good binders" and can bind in a different orientation or mode than the poorly binding molecules. Thus, a clear and unbiased method of aligning the molecules for the study is needed. The final trouble spot of 3D-QSAR methodology is related to alignment, where the overall alignment of the Training and Test Sets might bias the creation and validation of the model. This is due to the Training Set containing good and poor binding compounds, yet they are misaligned. The models created have the possibility of being biased toward an inactive compound if too much emphasis is placed on the poor-binding compounds in the overall alignment. The only method of overcoming the alignment issue is to create multiple alignment schemes focusing on different regions of the molecules.

6.3.3. Artificial Neural Networks (ANN)

Continuing the theme of computational methods mimicking biological processes is artificial neural networks *(104)*, a method of forming linear and nonlinear models. This method is used to model complex functions and was developed in research concerning artificial intelligence. As mentioned in the case of QSAR Training and Test Sets, it is imperative that the learning sets are representative of the entire population. Once presented with the Training Set, the ANN uses a training algorithm(s) to learn the structure of the data and constructs the model.

ANN's are proficient at extracting nonlinear functions from a given dataset. Artificial neural networks are able to learn from examples and acquire their own "knowledge" (induction), to generalize, provide flexible nonlinear models of input/output relationships, and, similar to PLS, to cope with noisy data and accept incomplete datasets. There are two main types of ANN's, "supervised" and "unsupervised." Supervised neural networks (SNN), also referred to as adaptive bidirectional associative memory (ABAM), require that every molecule in the QSAR Training Set has an experimentally determined binding affinity. ABAMs possess the ability to associate patterns, thus learning patterns and applying them to novel datasets to find relationships between what were originally considered unrelated patterns. Unsupervised neural networks (UNN) are able to automatically identify clusters of important chemical characteristics from a set of descriptors. The characteristic(s) being searched for need to be carefully calculated because the selection of appropriate descriptors is crucial for clustering. This method can be considered a hybrid method because of its ability to extract important molecular descriptors (with no knowledge of core essential characteristics) and to create a generalized model. The use of UNNs is primarily for preliminary assessment of a descriptor set because UNNs are able to create an overview of the variation between the descriptors and bioactivities. In QSAR methods utilizing artificial neural networks a SNN is used

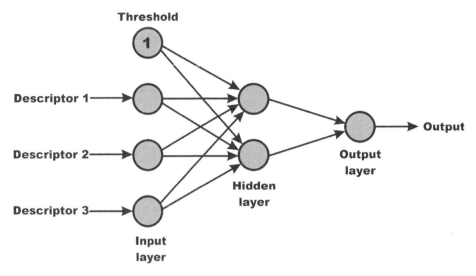

Fig. 7. Artificial neural network model. Bioactivities and descriptor values are the input and a final model is the output. Numerical values enter through the input layer, pass through the neurons, and are transformed into output values; the connections (arrows) are the numerical weights. As the model is trained on the Training Set, the system-dependent variables of the neurons and the weights are determined.

because the binding affinities are known whereas an UNN would be used to screen a library of compounds where only a handful of compounds have experimental binding affinities, thus removing the need for a Training and Test Set.

Unlike PCA, PCR, and PLS, artificial neural networks can be easily described due to their biological origin. The base components of an ANN are the formal neurons and connections between the neurons (**Fig. 7**). All ANNs are constructed in layers and the simplest ANN contains only two layers of neurons, the input and output layers. There are several traditional ANN configurations possible from simple to complex depending on the number of layers and method of connecting the neurons. A layer is defined as the connection between two neurons on different layers. The most common type of ANN used in molecular modeling, the fully connected feed-forward networks, is designed with each neuron in one layer connected to all the neurons in the following layer with no intralayer connections existing *(108)*. Numerical input values are passed through the neurons and are transformed into output values; the connections between neurons symbolize numerical weights. During network development (training phase) the system-dependent variables of the neurons and the weights connecting the neurons are determined.

A drawback of using SNNs in the creation of QSAR models is their inability to determine the important descriptors. It is for this reason that SNNs usually employ a search method, such as a step-wise search, simulated annealing, or genetic algorithm *(112–114)* to select the descriptors for a model. SNNs are used to develop models that correctly associate the inputs (compounds and selected descriptors to the bioactivities) in a manner to determine if other compounds possess good or bad bioactivities or help create a receptor-specific compound. As mentioned before the molecules from the Training Set are used to create a model able to reproduce the binding affinities of the Training Set compounds expecting the model will be able to correctly predict if novel compounds are good or bad binders.

A neural network works by first "training" on the known data values (Training Set) and is then tested on an unknown set of data (Test Set). The ANN is trained by taking in the known data, putting it through the network, comparing the output to the original data, and modifying the weights of the connections between the neurons based on the errors between the original values and the output. A more precise take on how ABAM neural networks create a model starts with the reformatting of the data into a vector that is passed onto the hidden-layer neurons. The input neurons of the SNN and UNN are identical and pass the data to the next layer in the network without performing any calculations on the data and are thus are referred to as "fan-out units." As the data are iteratively passed between the neurons of the hidden layers, the weighted values on the connections are adjusted until the output values equal the original input. Once the model is created, it can be validated on the Test Set. The original data from the Training Set is passed into the network with the weighted values arbitrarily set. The output values are compared to the initial values using the root mean square of the errors. The output is then used as input, the weighted values are adjusted, and the output is compared to the original data again. This loop continues until the output has converged to the original Training Set values within a set tolerance. The neural network learns the pattern of the data in the training period through iterative adjustment of the weighted values between the interconnecting nodes. The network is then able to make quantitative predictions for novel patterns, such as determining the bioactivities of a novel set of compounds. The construction of the ANN can vary, depending on the accuracy of the fit desired, by adjusting the number of layers and neurons. In general, the number of weighted values should be less than the number of molecules in the Training Set to reduce the likelihood of overfitting *(108)*. By monitoring the creation of the model through periodic testing against a Test Set provides the ability to prevent overfitting by stopping the training of the network before full convergence has occurred on the Training Set along with gaining useful information about the creation of the model. Poor performance of the model on the Test Set can point to inadequacies in the descriptors chosen, a bad neural network design, or a poorly constructed Training Set.

Artificial neural networks are especially adept at modeling functions for which the linear model approximations are poor, creating a model from a Training Set in a similar method to how QSAR models are created. The ANN models are developed from learning datasets (Training Sets) compiled by the user. The use of an ANN simplifies the solving of complex statistical problems by requiring the user to possess a basic understanding of statistics (to select and prepare the data), Artificial neural networks (to select the type of ANN), and how to interpret the results.

6.3.4. Support Vector Machines (SVMs)

Another chemometric method of constructing a QSAR is support vector machines and can be considered an improvement on artificial neural networks. SVMs are created by dividing the descriptor space into two parts, separating the known active and nonactive compounds into the positive and negative half-space, respectively *(115)*. SVMs are used to construct QSAR models because they offer stability and simple geometric interpretation, the correlations between the descriptors are assumed to be zero, and a kernel *(109)* is used to construct nonlinear models. A kernel is a subset of the elements from one set (a group) that a function maps onto an identity element of another set. Support vector machine QSAR models can be constructed using active learning; a method were the data set grows each round and the Test Set is selected by the SVM algorithm *(115)*. A SVM-driven QSAR model cannot predict the bioactivity of a compound, it can only predict where a compound will be active or nonactive.

In the simplest form an SVM plots two different physicochemical properties for a series of compounds and separates the active and inactive compounds using a hyperplane. There are infinite number of hyperplanes that can be constructed between the two sets of compounds *(116)*, yet the most desirable hyperplane is the one with the largest margin between the active and inactive compounds. The margins are considered a "region of uncertainty" and compounds from the Training Set do not occupy this region, yet molecules for the Test Set are able to reside in this region *(115)*. The small number of compounds that populate the edge of the active and inactive margins are termed support vectors (SVs). The SVs flanking the hyperplane are the most difficult to categorize due to their sharing of similar descriptor space. The most robust hyperplanes are those with large separation between the active and inactive compounds. The SVM QSAR model (and all SVMs in general) are constructed using a large-scale quadratic programming problem *(117)* (**Fig. 8**). The bioactivities for the compounds of the Training and Test Sets are predicted using the distance the compounds fall from the hyperplane. The distance an active

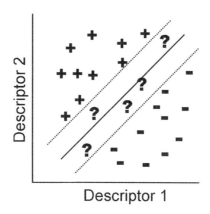

Fig. 8. Representation of a support vector machine. There are three different compounds in this simplified SVM representation. The plus (+) symbols represent active, the minus (–) symbols represent nonactive, and the question mark (?) symbol represents undetermined compounds. The solid line in the hyperplane and the dotted lines represent the maximum margin as defined by the support vectors.

compound resides from the hyperplane is not correlated to its potency, and this has been shown by Warmuth et al. *(115)*.

The active learning method of constructing a decision tree is an intriguing method of iteratively determining the QSAR model, selecting compounds that will strengthen the model. Traditionally, a QSAR model is constructed from a predetermined set of compounds and then tested on a set of unobserved compounds. The model constructed would be constructed without any interim feedback other than the cross-validation obtained after the model is constructed. This is one advantage of several QSAR models being constructed, as in 4D-QSAR *(5,101)*. Other than constructing several QSAR models, the only way to improve the model is to iteratively search for the best set of descriptors or select the Training Set. In the active learning method of constructing a QSAR model, the models utilize the same set of descriptors and iteratively select the compounds to construct the Training Set. This method rapidly improves the QSAR model *(115)*, yet this optimization requires advanced knowledge of the physicochemically relevant descriptors. The benefit of utilizing active learning to construct the QSAR models is the ability to construct robust models; yet, if a static set of compounds are used as the Training Set, then the performance of the model will be diminished.

The most beneficial aspect of SVMs are their ability to construct high-dimensional models (including nonlinear models) without overfitting when presented with a large number of descriptors and are not adversely affected by experimental (in determining the bioactivities or calculating the descriptors) error.

QSAR models created with SVMs are best utilized in Binary QSAR applications to determine if compounds are bioactive for the system of interest as is the case with high throughput screening. The Binary QSAR method of Binary-QuaSAR *(7,41)* of the Chemical Computing Group, Inc., is the best example of a Binary QSAR application, and is provided with the software suite MOE *(28)*.

6.3.5. Binary-QuaSAR

An approach to scanning libraries of possible lead compounds is Binary-QSAR *(7,41)*; a method that is based on and can be incorporated into HTS. Through the use of HTS it is possible to perform millions of physical experiments in a relatively short time span, yet there are two issues keeping it from reaching its full potential; time and money *(7)*.

With the inception of Binary-QSAR *(7)* the creation of a methodology utilizing the error-prone bioactivities of HTS as input for a QSAR study was created. Binary-QSAR is useful in determining the priority of compounds for future HTS experiments; designing focused combinatorial libraries, screening a virtual database of compounds, and predicting the activity of products in a reaction pathway. Binary-QSAR examines the structure and bioactivity of compounds and establishes a probability distribution function to determine if novel compounds are either "active" or "inactive." Traditionally QSAR methods fit the model to the experimental data, but Binary-QSAR creates a QSAR model using large-scale probabilistic and statistical deductions *(7)*. The predictive Binary-QSAR models are not created by interpolation, but are based on generalizations substantiated by HTS experimental data. By examining past experiments and weighing the alternatives, the Binary-QSAR program provides information for the possible next step or set of experiments in a study.

The main basis for QSAR methodology is the small structural changes of compounds correlated to the changes in binding affinity, yet compounds in screening libraries traditionally do not share similar scaffolds *(7)*. It is the basic principle of QSAR that prevents analyzing the HTS data by traditional QSAR methods. Binary-QSAR incorporates molecular descriptors and bioactivities expressed in a "binary fashion" (active or inactive) in conjunction with a training set to calculate the probability distribution for active and inactive compounds. Traditionally, QSAR methods base the worth of the QSAR model on the coefficient of determination (R^2) and squared error between the experimental and predicted bioactivities. Instead of using MLR, PCA, PCR, PLS, or ANN, Binary-QSAR uses a nonlinear method to create the model without adjusting the parameters of the model to lower the squared error. The Binary-QSAR model is then used to predict whether novel compounds in a test set are active or inactive, or can be used to screen libraries of compounds for the next set of HTS experiments.

Using Binary-QSAR allows for the quick creation of QSAR models in contrast to models created with artificial neural network because a training phase is not required. This allows Binary-QSAR to efficiently process the large datasets common in HTS experiments and construct a model. Binary-QSAR is a valuable tool in the screening of combinatorial and company molecular databases as seen by the work of Gao et al. *(118)*, Stahura et al. *(119)*, and Gao *(120)*. Binary-QSAR can assign a probability to whether a compound will be active for a particular test set; however, it cannot inform the chemist how to modify the lead compounds to improve their activity. The methodology of Binary-QSAR is best used to complement other methods of drug discovery and is not a true QSAR methodology. The use of Binary-QSAR to highlight possible lead compounds is legitimate and can precede conventional QSAR methods to optimize lead compounds.

6.4. Overfitting a Model

Creating a QSAR model (or any model) is a delicate balance; not enough descriptors and the model will not contain the important features of the molecules of interest, yet a model with too many descriptors will yield a generalized model. Creation of an over generalized model is called overfitting, and exists when the model has become too generalized for the Training Set and its ability to predict the bioactivities of new molecules decreases or is absent. Overfitting is a common problem and occurs in two different manners. The basic type of overfitting occurs when too many descriptors are chosen. When selecting the descriptors to use for the model, choosing all the descriptors available should theoretically create a model able to predict the bioactivities of the Training Set with 100% accuracy, yet this model is not able to effectively predict the bioactivity values for the Test Set. For optimum model creation only several descriptors need to be selected. The rule-of-thumb for the optimal number of descriptors in a QSAR model is that the number of descriptors should equal one-sixth to one-third the number of molecules in the Training Set. The second method of overfitting is related to ANN, where the model has overtrained on the Training Set as discussed above. Here the model is too specific and can only accurately predict the bioactivities of molecules either in the Training Set or molecules derived from the molecules in the Training Set.

6.5. Validation of QSAR Models

Regardless of the methods used to create the descriptors and construct the equation for the models, there is a need to validate the model by comparing the predicted bioactivities with the Experimental Bioactivities. Using the data that created the model (an internal method) or using a separate data set (an external method) can help validate the QSAR model. To determine if the model can be considered a "good model," there are several internal validation methods available to validate the QSAR model. The methods of least squares fit (R^2), cross-validation (q^2) *(80,121,122)*, chi (χ), root-mean-squared error (RMSE), and scrambling *(111,114)* are internal methods of validating a model. The best method of validating a model is an external method, such as evaluating the QSAR model on a Test Set of compounds. These are statistical methodologies used to ensure the models created are sound and unbiased. A poor model can do more harm than good, thus confirming the model as a "good model" is of utmost importance. Although considering a model is good based on its R^2 value with respect to the Training Set is one method, it is best to validate the model using a process that rigorously tests the model or does not fully depend on the data used to construct the model.

6.5.1. Least Squares Fit

The most common internal method of validating the model is least squares fitting as mentioned above. This method of validation is similar to linear regression and is the R^2 for the comparison between the predicted and experimental binding affinities. An improved method of determining R_2 is the robust straight-line fit, where data points with a large departure from the central data points (essentially data points a specified standard deviation away from the model) are given less weight when calculating the R^2. An alternative to this method is the removal of outliers (compounds from the Training Set) from the dataset in an attempt to optimize the QSAR model and is only valid if strict statistical rules are followed.

6.5.2. Cross-Validation

A common method of internally validating a QSAR model is cross-validation (CV, Q^2, q^2, or jack-knifing) used to measure a model's predictive ability and draw attention to the possibility a model has been overfitted. It is typical for the values of R^2 to be larger than the q^2 values, yet overfitting of the model is usually suspected if the R^2 value from the original model is significantly larger (25%) than the q^2 value *(80)*. Cross-validation values are considered more characteristic of the predictive ability of the model. Thus, CV is considered a measure of goodness of prediction and not fit in the case of R^2. The process of CV begins with the removal of one or a group of compounds (n_v), which becomes a Temporary Test Set, from the Training Set (n). A CV model is created from the remaining data points (n_c) using the descriptors from the original model, and tested on the removed molecules (n_v) for its ability to correctly predict the bioactivities. In the leave-one-out (LOO) method of CV, the process of removing a molecule ($n_v = 1$), and creating and validating the model against the individual molecules is performed for the entire Training Set. Once complete, the mean is taken of all the q^2 values and reported. The data utilized in obtaining q^2 is an augmented Training Set of the compounds (data points) used to determine R^2. The method of removing one molecule from the Training Set is considered to be an inconsistent method (121,122); selection of a larger set of data to create a CV model and validating the model against a single compound is inconsistent. A more correct method is leave-many-out (LMO), where a group of compounds (n_v = many) is selected for validation of the CV model. This method of cross-validation is especially useful if the Training Set used to create the model is small (≤ 20 compounds) or if there is no Test Set. The equation for cross-validation is

$$q^2 = 1 - \frac{\text{PRESS}}{\sum_{i=1}^{n}(y_i - \bar{y}_{obs})^2} \tag{26}$$

$$\text{PRESS} = \sum_{i=1}^{n}(\hat{y}_i - y_i)^2 \tag{27}$$

where the $\hat{y}_i$ is the data value(s) not used to construct the CV model. PRESS is the predictive residual sum of the squares and is calculated in the same manner as SSE (Eq. 17).

6.5.3. Fit of the Model

Additional examination of the model's fit is performed through the comparison of the experimental and predicted bioactivities and is needed to statistically ensure that the models are sound. The methods of chi (χ) and root-mean squared error (RMSE) are performed to determine if the model possesses the predictive quality reflected in the R^2. The use of RMSE shows the error between the mean of the experimental values and predicted activities. The chi value exhibits the difference between the experimental and predicted bioactivities:

$$\chi = \sqrt{\frac{\sum_{i=1}^{n}(y_i - \hat{y}_i)^2}{n}} \tag{28}$$

$$LSE \text{ or } \chi^2 = \frac{\sum_{i=1}^{n}(y_i - \hat{y}_i)^2}{n} \tag{29}$$

$$RMSE = \sqrt{\frac{\sum_{i=1}^{n}(\hat{y}_i - \bar{y})^2}{n}} \tag{30}$$

where y_i and $\hat{y}_i$ are the experimental and predicted bioactivity, respectively, for an individual compound in the Training Set, $\hat{y}$ is the mean of the experimental bioactivities, and n is the number of molecules in the set of data being examined. Large chi or RMSE values (≥ 0.5 and 1.0, respectively) reflect the model's poor ability to accurately predict the bioactivities even when a large R^2 value (≥ 0.75) is returned. These methods of error checking can also be used to aid in creating models and are especially useful in creating and validating models for nonlinear data sets, such as those created with ANN.

6.5.4. "Scrambling" Models

Even through the use of the previous validation methods one is concerned with the possibility that the original QSAR model is a chance occurrence. The creation of a Scrambled Model *(111,114)* is a unique method of checking the descriptors used in the model because the bioactivities are randomized ensuring the new model is created from a bogus data set. The basis for this method is to test the validity of the original QSAR model and to ensure that the selected descriptors are appropriate. The process of changing the bioactivities, through redistribution of bioactivities or random assignment of integers, is employed to yield proof that given different bioactivity values a model created using the same set of descriptors will produce a bad model. These new models (Scram-models) are created using the same descriptors as the original model, yet the bioactivities are changed. After each Scram-model is created, validation is performed using the methods mentioned earlier. To ensure that the Scram-models are truly random, the process of changing the bioactivities can be repeated and as each new Scram-model is created its R^2 and q^2 values recorded. The recorded analysis values are compared against the original R2 and q2 values for the original model. Each time the R2 and q2 values of the Scram-model are substantially lower further enforces that the true QSAR model is sound. The basis of using this method is to validate the original QSAR model because the Scam-models are created using the original descriptors and bogus bioactivities. The model would be in question if there was a strong correlation ($R^2 > 0.50$) *(42)* between the randomized bioactivities and the predicted bioactivities, specifically that the model is not responsive to the bioactivities.

Internal methods of validation are good; the true test of how a QSAR model will perform is demonstrated when presented with compounds not used to create the model (Test Set). At this point in a QSAR study possessing a Test Set is crucial. It can be argued that the use of CV to obtain a mean q^2 value is similar to possessing a Test Set, yet the models created within a CV analysis are augmented versions of the full Training Set. The creation of a QSAR model using a truncated Training Set can lead to problems if the Training Set is small or a poor sample of the population and therefore does not contain all of the compounds of interest. The Test Set, as mentioned earlier, should be well representative of the overall set of molecules and bioactivities to test the strength of the model.

7. Using the QSAR Model

After performing the steps to create a reliable QSAR model the question of "What to do with the model?" now exists. The biggest hurdle to overcome is visualizing the model. The model is not the predicted bioactivity values of the compounds but the line through the data points created by the model, similar to the linear regression line plotted when performing a least squares fit. The overall goal of QSAR is to design new drugs with better bioactivities and possessing fewer side effects than their predecessors. The QSAR model can be used to screen large libraries of possible drugs, yet this method is only fruitful if the library contains compounds structurally related to the molecules used to construct the model. A more practical method is to examine the QSAR model and modify the compounds based on the physicochemical properties, and is possible if the physical properties are easy to understand. In performing a Traditional QSAR study most of the descriptors are 2D and are straightforward to visualize, yet problems arise when trying to implement modifications based on 3D descriptors. The new classes of descriptors, specifically 3D molecular features and *ab initio* calculated properties, are useful descriptors but in the same respect difficult to visualize and modify. For example, the trend of increasing LUMO energy correlates to better binding molecules. At first this may appear simple, increase the LUMO energy value and get a better binding compound, yet how is the LUMO energy increased? The situation of increasing LUMO energy is not as trivial as modifying a molecule to possess a more negative charge in a specific region or make the molecule bulkier. This is an example of what is meant by "creating a usable QSAR model," a model that can be easily dissected (contains components the chemist knows how to modify). In the same respect the method used to create a model can make the deciphering of the model more difficult. Using Traditional QSAR to calculate the descriptors and creating the model with PLS best demonstrate an example of the method of model creation causing problems. The model was constructed from 2D descriptors yet was created with PLS; PLS creates models with new latent variables derived from latent variables resulting from principal components. Using simple-to-analyze descriptors and constructing a model with a complex regression method (such as PLS) creates a convoluted model that is not easy to evaluate for physical meaning. Thus, determining what impact specific descriptors possess has become difficult due to the method of model creation.

The method of taking apart a QSAR model is worthwhile, but the "holy grail" of QSAR is the ability to create a model, insert the desired bioactivity, and create a molecule based on the coefficients of the descriptors. The methodology of Inverse QSAR *(123,124)* is the process of developing a compound based on a chosen bioactivity. The goal is to design novel compounds possessing the ability to bind to a specific protein at a specified bioactivity. The problem is developing a QSAR model, which lends itself to this kind of manipulation. Traditional QSAR models are open to this kind of interpretation because the descriptors are typically well-defined physicochemical properties, i.e., number of atoms, ionized atoms, functional groups, and so forth. The remaining issue is where to place or remove these substituents. Inverse QSAR and the examination of QSAR models becomes difficult when the descriptors are 3D in nature or intangible thus making it difficult to add or subtract from these properties. Because of the added benefits and difficulties in deciphering the descriptors of 3D-based methodologies such as CoMFA, SOMFA, and 4D-QSAR, the program highlights the regions of the molecule where to modify the current compounds to create regions of differing physicochemical properties. The ability of programs to illustrate the location and manner of the modifications does not solve the problem of how to modify 3D descriptors relative to physicochemical properties such as volume, surface area, charge distribution, and dipole moment.

The information also provided by the quality and type of descriptors based on alignment can also add significant insight about the system of interest. Through the use of multiple alignment schemes (as implemented in 4D-QSAR) it is conceivable that the probable binding mode of a set of ligands can be discerned. Using the most reasonable alignment scheme (based on statistically sound QSAR model) can lead to information regarding which atoms are the most important for binding and the probable binding mode of the ligands in the binding site.

8. Comparison of Selected QSAR Methodologies

A case study composed of *meta-* and *para*-di-substituted *N,N*-dimethyl-α-bromophenethylamines molecules and bioactivities from papers by Graham and Karrar *(125)* and Hansch et al. *(126,127)* along with several QSAR packages were used to compare traditional (2D), 3D, and 4D methodologies in addition to different methods of selecting descriptors and QSAR model creation. Traditional QSAR methods of creating models, such as MLR, PCA, PCR, and PLS based on 2D descriptors were performed using QuaSAR from CCG *(6)*, and software from Jay Ponder *(128)* at Washington University, St. Louis, MO, USA. 3D-QSAR methodology was explored using SOMFA2 *(11)* from W. Graham Richards *(11)* group. Using 4D-QSAR *(5)* the role of the conformation in creating a QSAR model and extract the bioactive conformation was explored. This case study is intended to be a comparison between the different

QSAR methodologies, not to determine which is best. Instead, it is being used to explore the different methods, techniques, and results obtained from each of the methods. The standard steroid data set of Cramer et al. *(4)* was not used because the molecules of the dataset are rigid making alignment simpler and would not be of interest in a QSAR method that uses molecular conformations to create of the model. This set of molecules was chosen because there is a known Traditional QSAR model and the possibility of adding to the model through 3D- and 4D-QSAR methodologies is attractive. In addition MOE's QuaSAR *(6)* was used to discover new descriptors and construct QSAR models implementing PCA. 3D-QSAR methods were explored using SOMFA2 *(11)* that utilizes PLS to construct the QSAR models. 4D-QSAR *(5)* was used to create the QSAR model based on an ensemble of molecular conformations through the use of descriptors selected using GFA and models created utilizing PLS. Validation employing the LOO and LMO methodologies was used along with the Scramble method to validate the models.

8.1. Preparing the Molecules

It was mentioned earlier that the molecular partial charges and conformation along with the methods used to construct the Training and Test Sets were important. In this case study the authors have constructed several molecular sets (based on partial charges) and different Training and Test Sets composition to investigate these effects on the construction and validity of QSAR models. The molecules in this test case are *meta-* and *para-*di-substituted *N,N*-dimethyl-α-bromophenethylamines (**Table 1**). All molecules were built in MOE *(6)* and assigned Gasteiger *(70)* or MMFF *(46–52)* partial charges and minimized using the MMFF. Two sets of molecules were constructed, one set of molecules with Gasteiger partial charges and another set with MMFF partial charges for use in the 3D-QSAR portion of the case study. The differing partial charges will be examined using SOMFA2 to explore the effects that partial charges have on determining QSAR models, specifically, the construction of QSAR models based on electrostatic potentials. The molecules were exported using the SVL *(28,129)* code written in house to export to the SOMFA molecular file format and 4D-QSAR molecular file format.

The molecules examined in this case study are in **Table 1** along with the original, sequential, reverse sequential, and random bioactivities. The purpose of the sequential and reverse sequential bioactivities is to demonstrate the power of incorrectly constructed scramble models. The sequential and reverse sequential bioactivities also demonstrate that a good R^2 value can be found, yet the model is poor based on large chi and RMSE values. The molecules were purposely ordered from poor to good binders based on the $\log(1/c)$ values *(2)*.

Table 1
Molecules and Bioactivities used in Case Study

	meta (X)	para (Y)	Original bioactivities log(1/c) (2)	Sequential bioactivities	Reverse sequential bioactivities	Random bioactivities
Hu01	H	H	7.46	22	1	13
Hu02	F	H	7.52	21	2	12
Hu03	H	F	8.16	20	3	4
Hu04	Cl	H	8.16	19	4	10
Hu05	Cl	F	8.19	18	5	8
Hu06	Br	H	8.30	17	6	15
Hu07	I	H	8.40	16	7	2
Hu08	Me	H	8.46	15	8	22
Hu09	Br	F	8.57	14	9	18
Hu10	H	Cl	8.68	13	10	17
Hu11	Me	F	8.82	12	11	16
Hu12	H	Br	8.89	11	12	19
Hu13	Cl	Cl	8.89	10	13	1
Hu14	Br	Cl	8.92	9	14	7
Hu15	Me	Cl	8.96	8	15	5
Hu16	Cl	Br	9.00	7	16	14
Hu17	Me	Br	9.22	6	17	6
Hu18	H	I	9.25	5	18	21
Hu19	H	Me	9.30	4	19	3
Hu20	Me	Me	9.30	3	20	11
Hu21	Br	Br	9.35	2	21	20
Hu22	Br	Me	9.52	1	22	9

There is one chiral center in this set of molecules that has been set to be the *R* configuration. A search of the literature has been unfruitful in an attempt to determine the correct chirality of this carbon, yet none of the QSAR studies *(125–127,130)* or experimental papers mentions the chiral orientation. This method of arbitrarily setting the chirality is not correct. The only reason the authors can assume this is the correct chirality is because all the molecules have been set to the same chirality and this is a case study examining different QSAR methodologies. If this was a true QSAR study, this assumption could not be undertaken.

The initial set of molecules used the lowest-energy structure (conformation) determined from a systematic conformational search of the most bioactive compound. This low-energy conformation was used as a scaffold to build all of the molecules of this case study. This is a poor method of determining the conformation of a set of molecules for a 3D-QSAR study (in the case of SOMFA2), yet once the 4D-QSAR study is complete and the presumed bioactive conformation is known, the SOMFA2 study can be repeated to determine if the conformation was a true issue. In studies where all the molecules share the same common scaffold, the conformation used can be considered less of an issue, such as the case with the compounds used in this study. It is feasible that the conformation of these compounds might not be of importance for creating a valid QSAR model because the only structural changes occur on the benzene ring. The conformational ensemble profile (CEP) for each molecule was constructed using the molecular dynamics simulation package in 4D-QSAR. The molecular dynamics simulation for each molecule was calculated in the gas phase at 310 K for 100,000 steps with a time step of 0.001 ps (1 fs) with a conformation extracted every 100 time steps. The alignment of the molecules in this case study is not an issue for the 3D-QSAR (SOMFA2) study because the molecules contain the same scaffolds. This is not the case for the 4D-QSAR portion of the study, the alignment schemes are important because different molecules can possess different bioactive conformations (when compared to each other). Ten different alignment schemes (Alignment 7 of **Table 5**) have been devised using the method of three-point alignment to explore the topology of the molecules.

The manner in which the Training and Test Sets are constructed can have one of the biggest impacts on the ability of the QSAR method to create a valid model as can be seen from the original CoMFA paper *(4,85)*. In this case study the authors have devised six different Training and Test Set combinations (**Table 2**). The first Training Set (named **All**) contains all the molecules, thus there is no Test Set to validate the model and the authors rely entirely on cross-validation, chi, and RMSE values and the Scramble method to determine if a model is sound. The Training and Test Sets (**Bioheavy** and **Biolite**) were constructed by placing the six *most* and six *least* bioactive compounds in the Test Set, respectively. These two Training and Test Sets were devised to illustrate the importance of selecting a diverse set of molecules (based on bioactivities and structure) to construct and test the model. The next groups of Training Sets (named **Test01** and **Test02**) are based on the Molecular-Structure-Based Training

Table 2
Composition of the Training and Test Sets for the Case Study[a]

Molecules	All	Bioheavy	Biolite	Test01	Test02	Test random
Hu01	#	♦	#	♦	#	#
Hu02	#	♦	#	#	♦	#
Hu03	#	♦	#	#	#	#
Hu04	#	♦	#	#	#	#
Hu05	#	♦	#	#	♦	#
Hu06	#	♦	#	#	#	#
Hu07	#	#	#	♦	#	♦
Hu08	#	#	#	#	#	♦
Hu09	#	#	#	♦	#	#
Hu10	#	#	#	#	♦	♦
Hu11	#	#	#	#	#	#
Hu12	#	#	#	#	#	#
Hu13	#	#	#	♦	#	♦
Hu14	#	#	#	#	#	#
Hu15	#	#	#	#	♦	#
Hu16	#	#	#	#	#	#
Hu17	#	#	♦	#	#	#
Hu18	#	#	♦	♦	♦	#
Hu19	#	#	♦	#	#	#
Hu20	#	#	♦	#	#	#
Hu21	#	#	♦	♦	#	♦
Hu22	#	#	♦	#	♦	♦

[a]# = Training Set and ♦ = Test Set.

Set method of designing Training and Test Sets. The sixth Training Set (named **Random**) was constructed by randomly selecting molecules for the Training Set with the remainder becoming the Test Set. Statistical analysis of the predicted bioactivities was performed in Microsoft Excel 97 unless so noted.

8.2. Traditional QSAR Methodologies Results: MOE QuaSAR (6) and QSAR (128)

This part of the case study was broken into two sections, the original descriptor set (2,125,127) (Hansch descriptors) and a new set of descriptors calculated in MOE (6) (MOE descriptors). The MOE Descriptors were calculated for molecules assigned Gasteiger (70) partial charges in the MMFF (46–52). The new descriptor set is constructed of three properties. The water accessible surface area (ASA) calculated using a radius of 1.4 Å for a water molecule and the volume (vol) determined from the van der Waals surface area determined using a grid with 0.75 Å spacing *(6)*. In calculating of ASA and vol, the surface area is a polyhedral representation of each atom *(6)*. The log of the octanol/water partition coefficient [Log*P* (o/w)] includes implicit hydrogens and is based on a linear-atom-type model *(131)*, parametized using 1847 molecules and an $R^2 = 0.931$ and RMSE = 0.393 *(6)*. The values for the descriptors used in this portion of the case study can be found in **Table 3**.

The models were created from the predetermined sets of descriptors and constructed with MLR, PCA, PCR, and PLS. A correlation matrix **(Table 4)** contains the pairwise *R* values for the bioactivities compared to the Hansch and MOE descriptors. There is a strong correlation between the original bioactivities and the sequential and reverse sequential bioactivities, –97 and 97, respectively. This is due to the method that the sequential and reverse sequential bioactivities were assigned. The molecules were ordered based on the log(1/*c*) from smallest to greatest and the sequential and reverse sequential values were assigned based on this feature as seen in **Table 1**. The comparison of the original bioactivities to the random bioactivities returns a correlation coefficient of 1, demonstrating that a correlation is nonexistent. A correlation between the Hansch lipophilicity parameter (π) and MOE descriptors [ASA, vol, log*P* (o/w)] is evident, with coefficients of 96, 95, and 97, respectively. The relationship of all the descriptors to the Random Bioactivities shows little correlation when compared to the descriptors correlation to the original bioactivities.

Regardless of the method used to construct the model (MLR, PCA, PCR, or PLS) the QSAR models constructed were relatively the same with respect to the descriptor set. There were discrepancies between the cross-validation values ($\Delta Q^2 \approx 0.04$) being attributed to the method used to create the model. Through the examination of **Tables 3** and **4** an understanding of the physicochemical properties that are important to increase or decrease binding can be achieved.

Analysis of the Hansch descriptors illustrates that increasing the lipophilicity property for this series of compounds will increase the bioactivity in a more dramatic fashion than increasing the Tafts steric parameter. Increasing the water accessible surface area (MOE descriptor) will increase the bioactivity of the compounds. But there is more than just adding lipophilicity and water accessible surface area to the molecules to increase binding affinity. A comparison of the substituents to the bioactivities illustrates that the bulkier X and Y groups increase bioactivity in conjunction with atomic partial charge distribution of the substituents.

8.3. 3D-QSAR Results: SOMFA (11)

Using SOMFA2 *(11)*, QSAR models were constructed based on shape and electrostatic potential [Gasteiger *(70)* and MMFF *(46–52)* partial charges] for

Table 3
The Hansch and MOE Descriptors Used in the Traditional QSAR Portion of the Case Study[a]

	Hansch Descriptors			MOE Descriptors		
	π	σ^+	E_s^{meta}	ASA	vdW Volume	$logP$ (o/w)
Hu01	0.00	0.00	1.24	405.6450	202.9219	2.836
Hu02	0.13	0.35	0.78	412.0307	203.7656	3.026
Hu03	0.15	−0.07	1.24	412.4412	205.0313	2.989
Hu04	0.76	0.40	0.27	430.2373	218.1094	3.465
Hu05	0.91	0.33	0.27	435.0059	220.6406	3.616
Hu06	0.94	0.41	0.08	445.6125	232.4531	3.671
Hu07	1.15	0.36	−0.16	451.0489	237.0938	4.063
Hu08	0.51	−0.07	0.00	435.6399	223.1719	3.171
Hu09	1.09	0.34	0.08	448.9601	233.7188	3.822
Hu10	0.70	0.11	1.24	430.2698	217.2656	3.428
Hu11	0.66	−0.14	0.00	439.7979	226.1250	3.322
Hu12	1.02	0.15	1.24	446.7925	229.9219	3.634
Hu13	1.46	0.51	0.27	451.6472	234.5625	4.055
Hu14	1.64	0.52	0.08	464.1606	245.9531	4.261
Hu15	1.21	0.04	0.00	454.6609	235.8281	3.761
Hu16	1.78	0.55	0.27	465.8516	246.7969	4.261
Hu17	1.53	0.08	0.00	467.6037	249.3281	3.967
Hu18	1.26	0.14	1.24	453.8200	233.2969	4.026
Hu19	0.52	−0.31	1.24	435.4634	217.2656	3.134
Hu20	1.03	−0.38	0.00	457.4708	241.7344	3.467
Hu21	1.96	0.56	0.08	478.5604	259.0313	4.467
Hu22	1.46	0.10	0.08	467.4184	249.3281	3.967

[a]The π, σ^+, and E_s^{meta} values were experimentally determined, and the ASA, vdW and $logP$ (o/w) were determined in MOE. [π = lipophilicity parameter; σ^+ = Hammett constant for benzylic cations; E_s^{meta} = Tafts steric parameter; ASA = water accessible surface area; vol = van der Waals volume; $logP$ (o/w) = log of the octanol/water partition coefficient.]

the six model types. The molecules were placed on a 25 × 25 × 25 cubic grid with 0.5 Å grid spacing as suggested by Robinson et al. *(11)*.

These settings proved to be adequate for the models constructed based on the molecular shape and original bioactivities (# R^2 ≈ 0.77, Q^2 ≈ 0.58, ♦ R^2 ≈ 0.80). The models show that by increasing the bulk of the molecules at the *meta* substituent and reducing the bulk at the *para* would create molecules with better bioactivities. The original bioactivities and partial charge-based models of MMFF

Table 4
**Pairwise Correlation Coefficients for the Bioactivities and Descriptors
Used in the Traditional QSAR Case Study[a]**

log (1/c)	100									
Sequential bioactivity	−97	100								
Reverse sequential bioactivity	97	−100	100							
Random bioactivity	1	−2	2	100						
π	72	−71	71	−1	100					
σ^+	−15	15	−15	3	51	100				
E_s^{meta}	23	21	−21	13	−52	−27	100			
ASA	83	−82	82	4	96	30	−58	100		
vol	78	−77	77	5	95	32	−63	99	100	
logP (o/w)	61	−59	56	−1	97	63	−49	90	89	100

[a]The π, σ^+, and E_s^{meta} values were experimentally determined, and the ASA, vdW and logP (o/w) were determined in MOE. [π = lipophilicity parameter; σ^+ = Hammett constant for benzylic cations; E_s^{meta} = Tafts steric parameter; ASA = water accessible surface area; vol = van der Waals volume; logP (o/w) = log of the octanol/water partition coefficient.]

(# $R^2 \approx 0.17$, $Q^2 \approx 0.03$, ♦ $R^2 \approx 0.14$) and Gasteiger (# $R^2 \approx 0.23$, $Q^2 \approx 0.08$, ♦ $R^2 \approx 0.28$) resulted in poor models. These values do not include Training Set R^2, Q^2, or Test Set R^2 values since the models were built using the Bioheavy and Biolite Training and Test Sets; these models skew the bioactivity data in unrealistic manners. The visual examination of ESP models (constructed with Gasteiger or MMFF atomic partial charges) denoted two differing models based on the *meta* and *para* regions of substitution. The model created using Gasteiger partial charges suggested better binding molecules would possess more positive charge in the region of the *meta* (X) substituent and more negative charge in the region of the *para* (Y) substituent. This was contradicted by the MMFF partial charge model that suggests molecules with more negative charge in the region of the *meta* (X) substituent and more positive charge in the region of the *para* (Y) substituent will bind better. This is a conundrum; the R^2 values are poor yet the models display information that is expected. The question posed at this point is "Which set of partial charges is correct?" Both sets of partial charges are well respected, yet, when examining the partial charge for the fluorine, chlorine, bromine, and the methyl group substituents, it was noted that the partial charge for the halides was more negative for the molecules assigned the MMFF partial charges than those assigned Gasteiger partial charges. This discrepancy was further investigated using quantum mechanical calculations for all the molecules in the case study, with the exception of the two molecules containing iodine because iodine is not included in the basis set chosen. A single point calculation

Table 5
Alignment Schemes of *N,N*-dimethyl-α-bromophenethylamines for 4D-QSAR

Alignment 1	✻	✻	✻	Alignment 6	◆	◆	□
Alignment 2	✻	✻	◆	Alignment 7	□	□	□
Alignment 3	✻	✻	□	Alignment 8	✻	□	□
Alignment 4	◆	◆	◆	Alignment 9	◆	□	□
Alignment 5	✻	◆	◆	Alignment 10	✻	◆	□

was performed in Gaussian98 **(72)** for each molecule using density functional theory, specifically Becke's three parameter hybrid method **(132)** (B3LYP) with Lee, Yang, and Parr's correlation function **(133)** and the LANL2DZ basis set **(134–137)**. The single point calculations proved that the methyl group attached to the benzene ring exhibits a negative charge and the halide atoms are more positive than the methyl group. Taking these findings into consideration the ESP model created with the Gasteiger partial charges is considered correct. The models created using the Bioheavy, Biolite, and Random Bioactivities Training and Test Sets produced the expected results. The Bioheavy and Biolite models produced good R^2 and poor chi and RMSE values. The Scramble model further validated that the models are valid.

This portion of the case study demonstrated that partial charges could be incorrect for certain chemical systems. Quantum mechanical calculations were only used to determine which model was correct not to perform the actual calculations. Several of the models were re-evaluated (data not shown) using PM5 partial charges determined in MOPAC2002 *(74)*. The results were similar to the R^2 values determined using Gasteiger partial charges.

8.4. nD-QSAR Results: 4D-QSAR

The results of the 4D-QSAR study are the most interesting due to the proposed steric and interaction-based descriptors. One of the main differences between this method and the others examined is the use of multiple alignment schemes to determine the best alignment based on Q^2 values and the utility of the models produced. The alignments explored in this case study are displayed in **Table 5**.

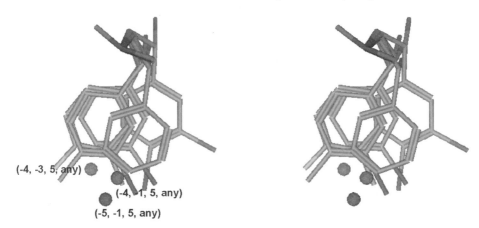

Fig. 9. Spinning. Four N,N-dimethyl-α-bromophenethylamines ligands were aligned by their ethylamines (tail) as denoted in Alignment 7 of **Table 5**. Alignments that do not take into consideration the substituted regions of interest can lead to poor alignments providing dis-informative 3D-QSAR models. It is for this reason that many alignment schemes are tested to elucidate the one that will render the most useful model.

The alignments are three-atom alignments as discussed above. In this portion of the case study only the actual bioactivities were examined to test the ability of 4D-QSAR to produce usable 3D-QSAR models, and not to examine the effects of different sets of bioactivity data. 4D-QSAR is more complex than the other QSAR packages examined in this case study based on the amount of data that is produced and the possibility of user error. The tradeoff between the complexity of the software and the information gained about the system of interest is immense. The strong point of 4D-QSAR is the methodology's ability to predict the bioactive conformation and return several (manifold) models for the user's examination. In using 4D-QSAR one develops a respect for the power of the model-generating methods; in several cases, QSAR models with excellent Q^2 values (0.879 in this example) were constructed from what can be considered a poor alignment (Alignment 7) as illustrated in **Fig. 9** and **Eq. 31**. The results from the 4D-QSAR analysis were imported into MOE *(28)* using SVL *(28,129)* code written in house.

$$\log(1/c) = 10.25(-5,-1,5,any) - 8.22(-4,-3,5,any) - 5.44(-4,-1,5,any) + 9.17$$

$$N = 22 \quad R^2 = 0.912 \quad Q^2 = 0.879 \quad LSE = 0.027 \quad LOF = 0.077$$

(31)

The alignments of the molecules of interest bring to light another phenomenon: spinning. Spinning is the effect that different conformations have on the alignment of a group of similar molecules. The three atoms that are aligned will occupy the same plane and the rest of the molecules are able to sample the remaining 3D space. In QSAR the main basis of the methodology is the comparison of like compounds that differ by several key locations and compare these differences with the bioactivities. When aligning the molecules of a study, it is important to examine all possible alignments and keep the important functional groups in the same location. When the molecules are aligned by what can be considered unimportant regions, spinning of the important regions can occur. Important information about the system is lost and misleading models are created. In the same respect poor alignments can lead to an unimportant physicochemical feature being considered important. This is the main reason why selecting an alignment based on Q^2 and R^2 is dangerous if the alignments examined truly walk the entire topology of the molecules of interest. Looking at the 10 proposed alignments, it is obvious that Alignments 1 and 2 are the most important because they keep the functional groups of interest in relatively the same location. The best 4D-QSAR models based on the requirement of a maximum of three descriptors for Alignment 1 with no Test Set (All) are Models 2 (**Eq. 32**) and Model 4 (**Eq. 33**):

$$\log(1/c) = 6.41(3,-1,-1,any) + 0.59(0,2,4,any) + 0.85(0,4,1,any) + 7.59$$
$$N = 22 \quad R^2 = 0.827 \quad Q^2 = 0.755 \quad LSE = 0.053 \quad LOF = 0.136 \tag{32}$$

$$\log(1/c) = -4.24(3,-3,-2,any) + 0.54(0,2,4,any) + 0.94(0,4,1,any) + 8.76$$
$$N = 22 \quad R^2 = 0.816 \quad Q^2 = 0.749 \quad LSE = 0.057 \quad LOF = 0.145 \tag{33}$$

The only difference between these two models is the first descriptor. Given the location and disparity between the descriptors, both can be considered false; bringing attention to a region that is not important to the model. In Model 2 the descriptor adds to the model, yet in Model 4 the descriptor subtracts from the model. Most striking is that the descriptors are separated by 2.24 Å as illustrated in **Fig. 10** and more than 6 Å from either of the other descriptors at the substitution locations of interest. The two descriptors at positions (0, 2, 4, *any*) and (0, 4, 1, *any*) at the *meta* and *para* substituent locations of the benzene ring are the most important of those displayed. The descriptors represent steric properties because they will accept any type of heavy atom at those two locations; the addition of a heavy atom at either of these two locations will improve the bioactivity of a compound from the series.

The use of *manifold* models as an aid to gauge the important descriptors of a 4D-QSAR model is an intriguing proposition. Methods such as CoMFA and SOMFA provide the user with a single, graphical QSAR model from which to harvest usable information. Traditional QSAR results are better, providing a model that can be dissected, but if an automated method was employed to

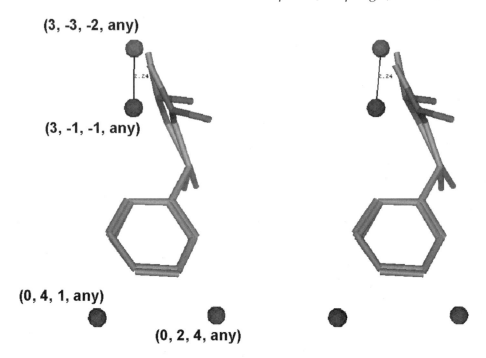

(3, -3, -2, any)

(3, -1, -1, any)

(0, 4, 1, any)

(0, 2, 4, any)

Fig. 10. Case study nD-QSAR methods: 4D-QSAR. Two models (Models 2 and 4) are compared for Alignment 1. The only difference between the models is the two erroneous descriptors near the ethylamine of the compound. These two descriptors $(3, -1, -1, any)$ and $(3, -3, -2, any)$, for Models 2 and 4, respectively, provide misleading results.

select descriptors, it may be difficult to add and subtract descriptors to modify the QSAR model. With 4D-QSAR one is not able to add descriptors at will, but instead the program provides a user-determined number of top models. In this case study it was requested that the top 10 models be reported for evaluation. **Figure 11** shows three 4D-QSAR models for Alignment 2 with varying number of descriptors. In Models 1 **(Fig. 11A)**, 6 **(Fig. 11B)**, and 8 **(Fig. 11C)**, the number of descriptors were four, two, and three, respectively. There was one descriptor between Models 1 and 8 with a common location $(0, -1, -1, np)$ and Models 6 and 8 with both common location and IPE atom type $(-1, -1, -1, any)$. Alignment 2 is able to keep the substituents of interest in the same general region, and provide useful 4D-QSAR models. The information pro-

---

Fig. 11. *(see facing page)* Manifold 4D-QSAR models. Three separate models are illustrated for the same set of compounds for Alignment 2. The models are ordered based on Q^2 values with (A) being the best (0.767) and (C) the worst (0.619).

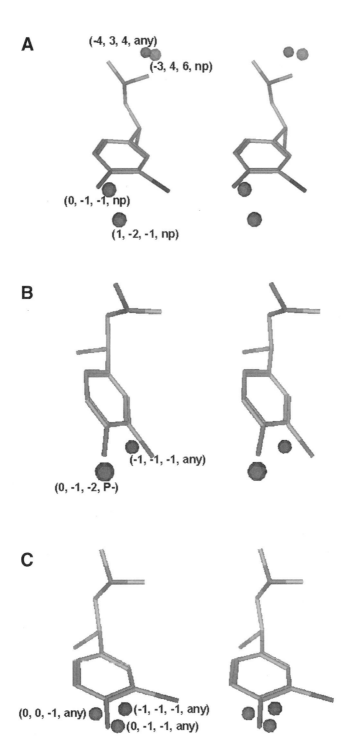

vided by the three 4D-QSAR models of Alignment 2 is interesting because of the ability to watch the model grow in number of descriptors and at the same time decrease in its ability to predict bioactivities. The 3D model presented by 4D-QSAR for Alignment 1 is the most informative, yet is not able to provide what type of atoms to place at the (0, 2, 4, *any*) and (0, 4, 1, *any*) positions. This further refinement of Alignment 1 would have to come from the user's chemical intuition given the composition of the data set or further probing with the 4D-QSAR software. In either respect, the ability of this method to correctly predict the $\log(1/c)$ values (bioactivities) is impressive.

8.5. Summary

From the above methods of constructing QSAR models several important parameters can be realized. The composition of the Training and Test Sets play an important role in the ability of the model to predict the bioactivities of the known and novel compounds. The methods used to set up the molecules, specifically the partial charges, can have a large impact on the information extracted from the model. The type of QSAR model to construct (traditional, 3D, nD) will dictate the type of information gathered from the model.

The construction of the Training and Test Sets can have a significant impact on the ability of the model. In the traditional QSAR portion, Bioheavy models were able to adequately predict the original bioactivities for the Training and Test Set for the Hansch (# $R^2 = 0.86$, $Q^2 = 0.78$, ♦ $R^2 = 0.58$) and MOE (# $R^2 = 0.79$, $Q^2 = 0.69$, ♦ $R^2 = 0.66$) descriptors. This was not the case when the Biolite models were confronted with the same task. The Biolite models were unable to predict the original bioactivities for the Test Sets even though the models were able to predict the bioactivities for the Training Set: Hansch descriptors (# $R^2 = 0.91$, $Q^2 = 0.86$, ♦ $R^2 = 0.00$) and MOE Descriptors (# $R^2 = 0.84$, $Q^2 = 0.77$, ♦ $R^2 = 0.09$).

The atomic partial charges used in the 3D-QSAR portion of the case study brings to the forefront the question of "What caused the bad models?" There are several possibilities for the poor results. The grid could have been too small, thus inducing error. Additional models were constructed using grid spacing of 1.0 Å and Gasteiger and MMFF partial charges. Similar results were produced for models with low R^2 values and visually acceptable models. It is possible that the atomic partial charges need to be more exact for SOMFA to work correctly, yet similar models were constructed when PM5 partial charges were implemented. When examining the SOMFA authors' initial paper *(11)*, there was no mention of the R^2 values obtained from ESP models. This fact alone could point to concept that SOMFA is only able to inform how to improve the molecules (from visual inspection of the model) and is not able to predict the bioactivities of the molecules in the Training or Test Sets.

The results of the 4D-QSAR case study are interesting and provide large amounts of data about the system of interest, and, unlike static 3D-QSAR methods (CoMFA and SOMFA), 4D-QSAR is able to provide the exact locations of statistically important interaction pharmacophore elements. The ability of this method to overcome the question of "What conformation to use?" and predict the bioactive conformation is impressive and a major reason to use the software. Yet it is the ability to construct *manifold* models and examine several models for the same alignment that is the true benefit of this method. Add to the list the ability to determine the best alignment scheme (based on statistical and experimental results) and this method will provide more information than one could imagine. This abundance of information is key when troubleshooting results that are not in agreement with current beliefs.

The information gathered from each of the QSAR methodologies informs the researcher on how to modify the molecules to improve binding, yet in different ways. The models created using traditional QSAR noted that increasing the amount of water accessible surface area would improve binding along with increased lipophilicity. These are physical properties that can be increased, but the location on the molecules is not known, yet can be inferred to be the region of the substituents. The models received from 3D- and *n*D-QSAR methodologies show where to make the changes and to what extent. The ability to visualize the model interacting with the molecule is important and gives the chemist the ability to visualize the possible changes to the molecule. All the methods explored in this review are valid methods of determining a QSAR model; it all depends on the type of information desired.

9. Conclusion

This chapter has discussed the main methods of performing a QSAR study beginning with the set up of the molecules, the different methods of selecting descriptors, the ways of constructing a QSAR model, and validating and interpreting the model. The goal of this chapter was to inform about the different methods employed in common QSAR packages.

The implementation of 3D- and *n*D-QSAR methodologies has added a wealth of information with regards to the understanding of how small organic molecules interact with biological molecules and macromolecules. The reason these methods are not always able to adequately reproduce bioactivity values is not a break down in the underlying QSAR philosophy, but that the SAR to be studied is at times more complex, or less-defined, than can be reliably handled by current QSAR methodologies. The addition of molecular simulations (molecular dynamics) to 3D-QSAR modeling, for example, will enable the calculation of more pertinent physicochemical properties (descriptors) for the 3D-QSAR-descriptor pool, thus making 3D- and *n*D-QSAR more powerful and reliable.

As has been discussed, there are several key steps to keep in mind when performing a QSAR study. They may seem minor details or trivial, yet all are important for obtaining a usable final model. From the molecules chosen for the Training and Test Sets to the number of descriptors used to create the model, all aspects of how the model was created are valuable in assessing the worthiness of the model or determining where errors may have occurred in construction of the model. The following are questions to ask when performing a QSAR study:

1. Are the bioactivity values binding affinities, K_d values, RBAs, or IC_{50} values?
2. Do any of the molecules have chiral centers?
3. If there are chiral centers, are the bioactivities chiral specific?
4. What type of force field and atomic partial charges are being implemented?
5. Which conformation of each molecule in the study is being used?
6. How were the conformations of the molecules determined?
7. Are the Training and Test Sets representative of the molecular population?
8. Is the QSAR methodology appropriate for the desired use of the QSAR model?
9. Will the descriptors chosen for the model be easily manipulated?
10. How was the model constructed?
11. How thoroughly was the QSAR model validated?
12. Will the model be used on similar novel molecules in comparison to the original scaffolds?

Asking these questions about any QSAR study should reduce the chances of constructing a poor model and gain insight to how the model was created. This does not guarantee that the model will work to the user's desire; it only ensures the plausibility that the model was created soundly. It cannot be stressed enough that a model capable of reproducing the bioactivities for the Training and Test Set can still fail when presented with novel compounds.

The key to any successful QSAR study is attention to detail. Special care needs to be taken not to bias the results in any manner and be aware that a small indiscretion with the preparation of the molecules or bioactivities at the beginning of the study can lead to a large issue at the end. Remember that QSAR is based on statistics, and like any science based on an art, it can be fickle.

References

1. Shorter, J. (1998) Linear free energy relationships (LFER). In *Encyclopedia of computational chemistry.* P. von Ragué Schleyer (ed.). John Wiley & Sons, Chichester, Vol. 2, pp. 1487–1496.
2. Kubinyi, H. (1998) Quantitative structure-activity relationships in drug design. *Encyclopedia of computational chemistry*, P. von Ragué Schleyer (ed.), John Wiley & Sons, Chichester, Vol. 3, pp. 2309–2320.

3. Hansch, C. and Fujita, T. (1964) ρ-σ-π analysis. A method for the correlation of biological activity and chemical structure. *J. Am. Chem. Soc.* **86,** 1616–1626.

4. Cramer III, R. D., Patterson, D. E., and Bunce, J. D. (1988) Comparative molecular field analysis (CoMFA). 1. Effect of shape on binding of steriods to carrier proteins. *J. Am. Chem. Soc.* **110,** 5959–5967.

5. Hopfinger, A. J., Wang, S., Tokarski, J. S., et al. (1997) Construction of 3D-QSAR models using the 4D-QSAR analysis formalism. *J. Am. Chem. Soc.* **119,** 10,509–10,524.

6. Chemical Computing Group Inc. (2001) Molecular Operating Environment. 1010 Sherbrooke Street West, Suite 910, Montreal, Quebec, H3A 2R7, Canada. http://www.chemcomp.com.

7. Labute, P. (2001) Binary QSAR: A new technology for HTS and UHTS data analysis. *J. Chem. Comput. Grp.*, http://www.chemcomp.com/feature/htsbqsar.htm.

8. Labute, P. (2001) Probabilistic receptor potentials. *J. Chem. Comput. Grp.*, http://www.chemcomp.com/feature/cstat.htm.

9. van de Waterbeemd, H. (ed.) (2001) Newsletter. http://www.qsar.org/news/QSAR oct2001.pdf.

10. Free, S. M., Jr. and Wilson, J. W. (1964) A mathematical contribution to structure-activity studies. *J. Med. Chem.* **7,** 395–399.

11. Robinson, D. D., Winn, P. J., Lyne, P. D. and Richards, W. G. (1999) Self-organizing molecular field analysis: a tool for structure-activity studies. *J. Med. Chem.* **42,** 573–583. SOMFA is available at http://bellatrix.pcl.ox.ac.uk/downloads/.

12. Tripos Inc. (2003) SYBYL. 1699 South Hanley Road, Saint Louis, MO 63144, USA. http://www.tripos.com.

13. Accelrys Inc. (2003) Insight II. 9685 Scranton Road, San Diego, CA 92121-3752. http://www.accelrys.com.

14. Clark, D. E. (2000) Evolutionary algorithms in molecular design. *Methods and principles in medicinal chemistry,* Mannhold, R., Kubinyi, H., and Timmerman, H. (eds.), Wiley-VCH, Vol. 8, Weinheim, Federal Republic of Germany.

15. Holland, J. H. (1975) *Adaptation in natural and artificial systems.* Ann Arbor, MI.

16. Cristianini, N. and Shawe-Taylor, J. (2000) *An introduction to support vector machines and other kernel-based learning methods.* Cambridge University Press, Cambridge, UK, and New York, NY.

17. Manly, B. F. J. (1994) *Multivariate statistical methods. A primer.* Chapman and Hall, New York.

18. Grimm, L. G. and Yarnold, P. R., Eds. (1995) *Reading and understanding multivariate statistics.* American Psychological Association, Washington, DC.

19. Pearson, K. (1901) On lines and planes of closest fit to a system of points in space. *Philosophical Mag.* **2,** 557–572.

20. Hotelling, H. (1933) Analysis of a complex of statistical variables into principal components. *J. Educat. Psychol.* **24,** 417–441, 498–520.

21. Glen, W. G., Dunn, W. J., III, and Scott, D. R. (1989) Principal components analysis and partial least squares regression. *Tetrahedron Comput. Meth.* **2,** 349–376.

22. Lindberg, W., Persson, J.-Å., and Wold, S. (1983) Partial least-squares methods for spectrofluorimetric analysis of mixtures of humic acid and ligninsulfonate. *Anal. Chem.* **55,** 643–648.
23. Dunn III, W. J., Wold, S., Edlund, U., and Hellberg, S. (1984) Multivariate structure-activity relationships between data from a battery of biological tests and an ensemble of structure descriptors. *Quant. Struct.-Act. Relat.* **3,** 131–137.
24. Gasteiger, J. and Zupan, J. (1993) Neuronale Netze in der Chemie. *Angew. Chem.* **105,** 510–536.
25. Zupan, J. and Gasteiger, J. (1999) *Neural networks in chemistry and drug design.* Wiley-VCH, Weinheim, Federal Republic of Germany.
26. Hopfinger, A. J. (1980) A QSAR investigation of dihydrofolate reductase inhibition by Baker triazines based upon molecular shape analysis. *J. Am. Chem. Soc.* **102,** 7196–7206.
27. Hopfinger, A. J., Reaka, A., Venkatarangan, P., Duca, J. S., and Wang, S. (1999) Construction of a virtual high throughput screen by 4D-QSAR analysis: application to a combinatorial library of glucose inhibitors of glycogen phosphorylase *b*. *J. Chem. Inf. Comput. Sci.* **39,** 1151–1160.
28. Chemical Computing Group Inc. (2002) Molecular Operating Environment. 1010 Sherbrooke Street West, Suite 910, Montreal, Quebec, H3A 2R7, Canada. http://www.chemcomp.com.
29. Klebe, G., Abraham, U., and Mietzner, T. (1994) Molecular similarity indices in a comparative analysis (CoMSIA) of drug molecules to correlate and predict their biological activity. *J. Med. Chem.* **37,** 4130–4146.
30. Kearsley, S. K. and Smith, G. M. (1990) An alternative method for the alignment of molecular structures: maximizing electrostatic and steric overlap. *Tetrahedron Comput. Meth.* **3,** 615–633.
31. Wagener, M., Sadowski, J., and Gasteiger, J. (1995) Autocorrelation of molecular surface properties for modeling corticosteriod binding globulin and cytosolic Ah receptor activity by neural networks. *J. Am. Chem. Soc.* **117,** 7769–7775.
32. Schuur, J. H., Selzer, P., and Gasteiger, J. (1996) The coding of the three-dimensional structure of molecules by molecular transforms and its application to structure-spectra correlations and studies of biological activity. *J. Chem. Inf. Comput. Sci.* **36,** 334–344.
33. Silverman, B. D. and Platt, D. E. (1996) Comparative molecular moment analysis (CoMMA): 3D-QSAR without molecular superposition. *J. Med. Chem.* **39,** 2129–2140.
34. Sadowski, J. and Gasteiger, J. (1993) From atoms and bonds to three-dimensional atomic coordinates: automatic model builders. *Chemical Rev.* **93,** 2567–2581.
35. Sadowski, J., Gasteiger, J., and Klebe, G. (1994) Comparison of automatic three-dimensional model builders using 639 x-ray structures. *J. Chem. Inf. Comput. Sci.* **31,** 1000–1008.
36. Lemmen, C. and Lengauer, T. (2000) Computational methods for the structural alignment of molecules. *J. Comput.-Aided Mol. Des.* **14,** 215–232.

37. Lemmen, C., Lengauer, T., and Klebe, G. (1998) FlexS: a method for fast flexible ligand superposition. *J. Med. Chem.* **41,** 4502–4520.

38. Handschuh, S., Wagener, M., and Gasteiger, J. (1998) Superposition of three-dimensional chemical structures allowing the conformational flexibility by a hybrid method. *J. Chem. Inf. Comput. Sci.* **38,** 220–232.

39. Labute, P. (1999) Flexible alignment of small molecules. *J. Chem. Comput. Grp.* http://www.chemcomp.com/feature/malign.htm.

40. Heritage, T. W., Ferguson, A. M., Turner, D. B., and Willett, P. (1998) EVA: a novel theoretical descriptor for QSAR studies. *Persp. Drug Disc. Des.* **9/10/11,** 381–398.

41. Labute, P. (1998) QuaSAR-Binary: a new method for the analysis of high through-put screening data. http://www.netsci.org/Science/Compchem/feature21.htm.

42. Vedani, A. and Dobler, M. (2002) 5D-QSAR: the key for simulating induced fit? *J. Med. Chem.* **45,** 2139–2149.

43. Venkatarangan, P. and Hopfinger, A. J. (1999) Prediction of ligand-receptor binding free energy by 4D-QSAR analysis: application to a set of glucose analogue inhibitors of glycogen phosphorylase. *J. Chem. Inf. Comput. Sci.* **39,** 1141–1150.

44. Kulkarni, A. S., Han, Y., and Hopfinger, A. J. (2002) Predicting Caco-2 cell permeation coefficients of organic molecules using membrane-interaction QSAR analysis. *J. Chem. Inf. Comput. Sci.* **42,** 331–342.

45. Chatterjee, S., Hadi, A. S., and Price, B. (2000) *Regression analysis by example.* Wiley-Interscience, New York.

46. Halgren, T. A. (1996) Merck molecular force field. I. Basis, form, scope, parameterization, and performace of MMFF94. *J. Comput. Chem.* **17,** 490–519.

47. Halgren, T. A. (1996) Merck molecular force field. II. MMFF94 van der Waals and electrostatic parameters for intermolecular interactions. *J. Comput. Chem.* **17,** 520–552.

48. Halgren, T. A. (1996) Merck molecular force field. III. Molecular geometries and vibrational frequencies for MMFF94. *J. Comput. Chem.* **17,** 553–586.

49. Halgren, T. A. and Nachbar, R. B. (1996) Merck molecular force field. IV. Conformational energies and geometries for MMFF94. *J. Comput. Chem.* **17,** 587–615.

50. Halgren, T. A. (1996) Merck molecular force field. V. Extension of MMFF94 using experimental data, additional computational data, and empirical rules. *J. Comput. Chem.* **17,** 616–641.

51. Halgren, T. A. (1999) MMFF VI. MMFF94s option for energy minimization studies. *J. Comput. Chem.* **20,** 720–729.

52. Halgren, T. A. (1999) MMFF VII. Characterization of MMFF94, MMFF94s, and other widely available force fields for conformational energies and intermolecular-interaction energies and geometries. *J. Comput. Chem.* **20,** 730–748.

53. Weiner, S. J., Kollman, P. A., Case, D. A., et al. (1984) A new force field for molecular mechanical simulation of nucleic acids and proteins. *J. Am. Chem. Soc.* **106,** 765–784.

54. Cornell, W. D., Cieplak, P., Bayly, C. I., et al. (1995) A second generation force field for the simulation of proteins, nucleic acids, and organic molecules. *J. Am. Chem. Soc.* **117,** 5179–5197.

55. Fabricius, J., Engelsen, S. B., and Rasmussen, K. (1997) The consistent force field. 5. PEF95SAC: optimized potential energy function for alcohols and carbohydrates. *J. Carbohydr. Chem.* **16,** 751–772.

56. Jorgensen, W. L. and Tirado-Rives, J. (1988) The OPLS potential function for proteins. Energy minimizations for crystals of cyclic peptides and crambin. *J. Am. Chem. Soc.* **110,** 1657–1666.

57. Maxwell, D. S., Tirado-Rives, J., and Jorgensen, W. L. (1995) A comprehensive study of the rotational energy profiles of organic systems by *ab initio* MO theory, forming a basis for peptide torsional parameters. *J. Comput. Chem.* **16,** 984–1010.

58. Jorgensen, W. L., Maxwell, D. S., and Tirado-Rives, J. (1996) Development and testing of the OPLS all-atom force field on conformational energetics and properties of organic liquids. *J. Am. Chem. Soc.* **118,** 11,225–11,236.

59. Jorgensen, W. L. and McDonald, N. A. (1998) Development of an all-atom force field for heterocycles. Properties of liquid pyridine and diazenes. *J. Mol. Struct. (Theochem.)* **424,** 145–155.

60. McDonald, N. A. and Jorgensen, W. L. (1998) Development of an all-atom force field for heterocycles. Properties of liquid pyrrole, furan, diazoles, and oxazoles. *J. Phys. Chem. B* **102,** 8049–8059.

61. Rizzo, R. C. and Jorgensen, W. L. (1999) OPLS all-atom model for amines: resolution of the amine hydration problem. *J. Am. Chem. Soc.* **121,** 4827–4836.

62. Brooks, B. R., Bruccoleri, R. E., Olafson, B. D., States, D. J., Swaminathan, S., and Karplus, M. (1983) CHARMM: a program for macromolecular energy, minimization, and dynamics calculations. *J. Comput. Chem.* **4,** 187–217.

63. Roux, B. (1990) Theoretical study of ion transprot in the gramicidin A channel. Harvard University, Cambridge, MA.

64. Stote, R. H. and Karplus, M. (1995) Zinc binding in proteins and solution: a simple but accurate nonbonded representation. *PROTEINS: Structure, Function, and Genetics* **23,** 12–31.

65. MacKerell, Jr., A. D. (1995) Molecular dynamics simulation analysis of a sodium dodecyl sulfate micelle in aqueous solution: decreased fluidity of the micelle hydrocarbon interior. *J. Phys. Chem.* **99,** 1846–1855.

66. Schlenkrich, M., Brickmann, J., MacKerell Jr., A. D., and Karplus, M. (1996) An empirical potential energy function for phospholipids: criteria for parameter optimization and application. In *Biological membranes: a molecular perspective from computational and experiment*, Merz Jr., K. M. and Roux, B. (eds.), Birkhäuser, Boston, 31–81.

67. Feller, S. E., Yin, D., Pastor, R. W., and MacKerell Jr., A. D. (1997) Molecular dynamics simulation of unsaturated lipid bilayers at low hydration: parameterization and comparison with diffraction studies. *Biophys. J.* **73,** 2269–2279.

68. MacKerell Jr., A. D., Bashford, D., Bellott, M., et al. (1998) All-atom empirical potential for molecular modeling and dynamics studies of proteins. *J. Phys. Chem. B* **102,** 3586–3616.

69. Engh, R. A. and Huber, R. (1991) Accurate bond and angle parameters for x-ray protein structure refinement. *Acta Crystallograph. A* **A47,** 392–400.

70. Gasteiger, J. and Marsili, M. (1980) Iterative partial equalization of orbital electronegativity—a rapid access to atomic charges. *Tetrahedron* **36,** 3219–3228.

71. Mortier, W. J., Van Genechten, K., and Gasteiger, J. (1985) Electronegativity equalization: application and parametrization. *J. Am. Chem. Soc.* **107,** 829–835.

72. Frisch, M. J., Trucks, G. W., Schlegel, H. B., et al. (1998) Gaussian 98, Revision A.9, Gaussian Inc., Pittsburgh, Pennsylvaina. http://www.gaussian.com.

73. Stewart, J. J. P. (1996) Applications of localized molecular orbitals to the solution of semiemperical self consistent field equations. *Int. J. Quantum Chem.* **58,** 133–146.

74. Fujitsu Limited (Stewart, J.J.P.). (1999) MOPAC 2002. Tokyo, Japan. http://www.cachesoftware.com/.

75. Schmidt, M. W., Baldridge, K. K., Boatz, J. A., et al. (1993) GAMESS. *J. Comput. Chem.* **14,** 1347–1363.

76. Nicklaus, M. C., Wang, S., Driscoll, J. S., and Milne, G. W. A. (1995) Conformational changes of small molecules binding to proteins. *Bioorganic Med. Chem.* **3,** 411–428.

77. Vieth, M., Hirst, J. D., and III, C. L. B. (1998) Do active site conformations of small ligands correspond to low free-energy solution structures? *J. Comput.-Aided Mol. Des.* **12,** 563–572.

78. Frenkel, D. and Smit, B. (1996) *Understanding molecular simulation.* Academic, New York.

79. Field, M. J. (1999) *A practical introduction to the simulation of molecular systems.* Cambridge, University Press, New York.

80. Leach, A. R. (2001) *Molecular modelling: principles and applications.* Pearson Education Limited, Harlow, England.

81. Murcko, M. A. (1997) Recent advances in ligand design methods. In *Reviews in computational chemistry,* Lipkowitz, K. B. and Boyd, D. B. (eds.), Wiley-VCH, New York, Vol. 11, pp. 1–66.

82. Muegge, I. and Rarey, M. (2001) Small molecule docking and scoring. In *Reviews in computational chemistry,* Lipkowitz, K. B. and Boyd, D. B. (eds.), Wiley-VCH, New York, Vol. 17, pp. 1–60.

83. Leach, A. R. (1991) A survey of methods for searching the conformational space of small and medium-sized molecules. In *Reviews in computational chemistry,* Lipkowitz, K. B. and Boyd, D. B. (eds.), VCH Publishers, New York, Vol. 2, pp. 1–55.

84. Ferguson, D. M. and Raber, D. J. (1989) A new approach to probing conformational space with molecular mechanics: random incremental pulse search. *J. Am. Chem. Soc.* **111,** 4371–4378.

85. Kubinyi, H. (1998) Comparative molecular field analysis (CoMFA). In *Encyclopedia of computational chemistry*, von Ragué Schleyer, P. (ed.), John Wiley & Sons Inc., Chichester, Vol. 1, pp. 448–460.

86. Wildman, S. A. and Crippen, G. M. (1999) Prediction of physiochemical parameters by atomic contributions. *J. Chem. Inf. Comput. Sci.* **39**, 868–873.

87. Hall, L. H. and Kier, L. B. (1977) The nature of structure-activity relationships and their relation to molecular connectivity. *Eur. J. Med. Chem.* 12–Chim. Therap. *4, 307–312.*

88. Hall, L. H. and Kier, L. B. (1991) The molecular connectivity chi indexes and kappa shape indexes in structure-property modeling. In *Reviews in Computational Chemistry*, Lipkowitz, K. B. and Boyd, D. B. (eds.), VCH Publishers, Inc., New York, Vol. 2, pp. 367–422.

89. Wiener, H. (1947) Structural determination of paraffin boiling points. *J. Am. Chem. Soc.* **69**, 17–20.

90. Balaban, A. T. (1979) Five new topological indices for the branching of tree-lite graphs. *Theor. Chim. Acta* **53**, 355–375.

91. Balaban, A. T. (1982) Highly discriminating distance-based topological index. *Chem. Phys. Lett.* **89**, 399–404.

92. Petitjean, M. (1992) Applications of the radius-diameter diagram to the classification of topological and geometrical shapes of chemical compounds. *J. Chem. Inf. Comput. Sci.* **32**, 331–337.

93. Levinthal, C. (1969) How to fold graciously. *Mossbauer Spectroscopy in Biological Systems*, Allerton House, Monticello, IL, University of Illinois Press.

94. Kirkpatrick, S., Gelatt, C. D., and Vecchi, M. P. (1983) Optimization by simulated annealing. *Science* **220**, 671–680.

95. Aarts, E. H. L. (1989) *Simulated annealing and Boltzmann machines: a stochastic approach to combinatorial optimization and neural computing.* Wiley, New York.

96. Metropolis, N., Rosenbluth, A. W., Rosenbluth, M. N., Teller, A. H., and Teller, E. (1953) Equation of state calculations by fast computing machines. *J. Chem. Phys.* **21**, 1087–1092.

97. Michalewicz, Z. (1994) *Genetic algorithms + data structures = evolution programs.* Springer-Verlag, New York.

98. Parrill, A. L. (2000) Introduction to evolutionary algorithms. In *Evolutionary algorithms in molecular design*, Clark, D. E. (ed.), Wiley-VCH, Weinheim, Federal Republic of Germany, Vol. 8, pp. 1–13.

99. Devillers, J. (ed.) (1996) *Genetic algorithms in molecular modeling.* Academic Press, London.

100. Clark, D. E., Ed. (2000) *Evolutionary algorithms in molecular design. Methods and Principles in Medicinal Chemistry.* Wiley-VCH, Weinheim, Federal Republic of Germany.

101. Rogers, D. and Hopfinger, A. J. (1994) Application of genetic function approximation to quantitative structure-activity relationships and quantitative structure-property relationships. *J. Chem. Inf. Comput. Sci.* **34**, 854–866.

102. Hopfinger, A. J. (1981) Inhibition of dihydrofolate reductase: structure-activity correlations of 2,4-diamino-5-benzylpyrimidines based upon molecular shape analysis. *J. Med. Chem.* **24**, 818–822.

103. Friedman, J. [November 1988 (reviscd August 1990)] Multivariate adaptive regression splines, technical report number 102. Laboratory for Computational Statistics, Department of Statistics, Stanford University, Stanford, CA.

104. Rosenblatt, R. (1959) The perceptron: a probabilistic model for information storage and organization in the brain. *Psychol. Rev.* **65**, 386–408.

105. Wold, S. and Sjöström, M. (1998) Chemometrics, present and future success. *Chemometrics and Intelligent Laboratory Systems* **44**, 3–14.

106. Lavine, B. K. (1998) *Chemometrics. Anal. Chem.* **70**, 209R–228R.

107. Lavine, B. K. (2000) *Chemometrics. Anal. Chem.* **72**, 91R–97R.

108. Schneider, G. and Wrede, P. (1998) Artificial neural networks for computer-based molecular design. *Prog. Biophys. Mol. Biol.* **70**, 175–222.

109. Müller, K.-R., Mika, S., Rätsch, G., Tsuda, K., and Schölkopf, B. (2001) An introduction to kernel-based learning algorithms. *IEEE Trans. Neural Net.* **12**, 181–201 http://mlg.anu.edu.au/raetsch/ps/review.pdf.bz2 or http://mlg.anu.edu.au/raetsch/ps/review.ps.gz.bz2.

110. Kshirsagar, A. M. (1972) *Multivariate analysis.* Marcel Dekker, Inc., New York.

111. Wold, S., Sjöström, M., and Eriksson, L. (1998) Partial least squares projections to latent structures (PLS) in chemistry. In *Encyclopedia of computational chemistry*, von Ragué Schleyer, P. (ed.), John Wiley & Sons, Chichester, Vol. 3, pp. 2006–2021.

112. So, S.-S. and Karplus, M. (1996) Evolutionary optimization in quantitative structure-activity relationship: an application of genetic neural networks. *J. Med. Chem.* **39**, 1521–1530.

113. So, S.-S. and Karplus, M. (1996) Genetic neural networks for quantitative structure-activity relationships: improvements and application of benzodiazepine affinity for benzodiazepine/$GABA_A$ receptors. *J. Med. Chem.* **39**, 5246–5256.

114. Yasri, A. and Hartsough, D. (2001) Toward an optimal procedure for variable selection and QSAR model building. *J. Chem. Inf. Comput. Sci.* **41**, 1218–1227.

115. Warmuth, M. K., Liao, J., Rätsch, G., Mathieson, M., Putta, S., and Lemmen, C. (2003) Active Learning with support vector machines in the drug discovery process. *J. Chem. Inf. Comput. Sci.* **43**, 667–673.

116. Ivanciuc, O. (2002) Support vector machine idetification of the aquatic toxicity mechanism of organic compunds. *Internet Electronic Journal of Molecular Design and BioChem Press* **1**, 157–172(http://www.biochempress.com/av01_0157.html and ftp://biochempress.com/iejmd_2002_1_0157.pdf).

117. Burbidge, R., Trotter, M., Holden, S., and Buxton, B. (2001) Drug design by machine learning: support vector machines for pharmaceutical data analysis. *Computers and Chemistry* **26**, 4–15 (http://stats.ma.ic.ac.uk/rdb/pubs/aisb00rbmt-final.pdf).

118. Gao, H., Williams, C., Labute, P., and Bajorath, J. (1999) Binary quantitative structure-activity relationship (QSAR) analysis of estrogen receptor ligands. *J. Chem. Inf. Comput. Sci.* **39,** 164–168.

119. Stahura, F. L., Godden, J. W., Xue, L., and Bajorath, J. (2000) Distinguishing between natural products and synthetic molecules by descriptor Shannon entropy analysis and binary QSAR calculations. *J. Chem. Inf. Comput. Sci.* **40,** 1245–1252.

120. Gao, H. (2001) Application of BCUT metrics and genetic algorithm in binary QSAR analysis. *J. Chem. Inf. Comput. Sci.* **41,** 402–407.

121. Shao, J. (1993) Linear model selection by cross-validation. *J. Am. Stat. Assoc.* **88,** 486–494.

122. Besalú, E. (2001) Fast computation of cross-validated properties in full linear leave-many-out procedures. *J. Math. Chem.* **29,** 191–204.

123. Tropsha, A., Zheng, W., and Cho, S. J. (1996) *Application of topological indices in rational design of combinatorial chemical libraries.* Book of Abstracts, 211th ACS National Meeting, New Orleans, LA, March 22–28, American Chemical Society: Washington, DC.

124. Cho, S. J., Zheng, W., and Tropsha, A. (1998) Rational combinatorial library design. 2. Rational design of targeted combinatorial peptide libraries using chemical similarity probe and the inverse QSAR approaches. *J. Chem. Inf. Comput. Sci.* **38,** 259–268.

125. Graham, J. D. P., and Karrar, M. A. (1963) Structure-action relations in *N,N*-dimethyl-2-halogenophenethylamines. *J. Med. Chem.* **6,** 103–107.

126. Hansch, C. and Lien, E. J. (1968) An analysis of the structure-activity relationship in the adrenergic blocking activity of the β-haloalkylamines. *Biochem. Pharmacol.* **17,** 709–720.

127. Unger, S. H. and Hansch, C. (1973) On model building in structure-activity relationships. A reexamination of adrenergic blocking activity of β-halo-β-arylakylamines. *J. Med. Chem.* **16,** 745–749.

128. Ponder, J. (1999) QSAR. Dept. of Biochemistry & Molecular Biophysics, Box 8231, Washington University School of Medicine, 660 South Euclid Avenue, St. Louis, Missouri 63110, USA. (Available from http://dasher.wustl.edu/.)

129. Labute, P. and Santavy, M. (2000) SVL: The scientific vector language. *J. Chem. Comput. Grp.* http://www.chemcomp.com/feature/svl.htm.

130. Cammarata, A. (1972) Interrelationship of the regression models used for structure-activity analyses. *J. Med. Chem.* **15,** 573–577.

131. Chemical Computing Group, Inc. (Labute, P.). (1998) MOE logP(Octanol/Water) model. 1010 Sherbrooke Street West, Suite 910, Montreal, Quebec, H3A 2R7, Canada (http://www.chemcomp.com).

132. Becke, A. D. (1993) Density-functional thermochemistry. III. The role of exact exchange. *J. Chem. Phys.* **98,** 5648–5652.

133. Lee, C., Yang, W., and Parr, R. G. (1988) Development of the Colle-Salvetti correlation-energy formula into a functional of the electron density. *Phys. Rev. B* **37,** 785–789.

134. Dunning, T. H., Jr. and Hay, P. J. (1977). *Modern theoretical chemistry*, Schaefer III, H. F. (ed.), Plenum Press, New York, Vol. 3, pp. 1–27.

135. Hay, P. J. and Wadt, W. R. (1985) *Ab initio* effective core potentials for molecular calculations. Potentials for the transition metal atoms Sc to Hg. *J. Chem. Phys.* **82**, 270–283.

136. Wadt, W. R. and Hay, P. J. (1985) *Ab initio* effective core potentials for molecular calculations. Potentials for main group elements Na to Bi. *J. Chem. Phys.* **82**, 284–298.

137. Hay, P. J. and Wadt, W. R. (1985) *Ab initio* effective core potentials for molecular calculations. Potentials for K to Au including the outermost core oribitals. *J. Chem. Phys.* **82**, 299–310.

7

3D-Log*P*

An Alignment-Free 3D Description
of Local Lipophilicity for QSAR Studies

Jérôme Gomar, Elie Giraud, David Turner, Roger Lahana, and Pierre Alain Carrupt

Summary

The major hurdle to overcome in the development of 3D-QSAR models using steric, electrostatic, or lipophilic "fields" is related to both conformation selection and subsequent suitable overlay (alignment) of compounds. Therefore, it is of some interest to provide a conformationally sensitive lipophilicity descriptor that is alignment-independent. In this chapter we describe the derivation and parametrization of a new descriptor called 3D-Log*P* and demonstrate both its conformational sensitivity and its effectiveness in QSAR analysis. The 3D-Log*P* descriptor provides such a representation in the form of a rapidly computable description of the local lipophilicity at points on a user-defined molecular surface.

Key Words: 3D-QSAR; hydrophobicity; lipophilicity; 3D-Log*P*; conformation-dependent lipophilicity; alignment-independent 3D descriptor; molecular lipophilicity potential (MLP); ADME-related descriptor.

1. Introduction

From a historical point of view, the research axes of the pharmaceutical industry have shifted away from acute and more toward chronic pathology solutions. The drug discovery technologies have evolved in parallel because the cost of the research linked to the failure rate has increased with the complexity of the pathology of interest. As a consequence, in order to enhance research

---

*This chapter is dedicated to the memory of Jean-Luc Fauchère who recently passed away.

From: *Methods in Molecular Biology, vol. 275:*
Chemoinformatics: Concepts, Methods, and Tools for Drug Discovery
Edited by: J. Bajorath © Humana Press Inc., Totowa, NJ

efficacy, the current discovery processes integrate at an early stage more and more data deriving from the in vivo pharmacokinetic behavior of drug candidates, as measured by absorption, distribution, metabolism, and excretion (ADME) experiments. There is, therefore, a great deal of interest in the effective modeling of these parameters.

ADME-related properties of compounds have been shown partly to depend upon the passive distribution properties of drug candidates and partly onto the partitioning characteristics of the drugs, inherent in their lipophilicity. The optimization of these characteristics is thus of critical importance in the preclinical and clinical phases of a drug development program. Indeed, the chosen compound is quite often not the most potent candidate but rather the one that has the optimum balance of suitable potency, safety, pharmacokinetics (PK), drug–drug interaction, and manufacturing cost. In order to decrease the length of the lead optimization process, it would be helpful to be able to find solutions to both the potency and the ADME profiling issues. In practical terms, the possibility of modeling several activities of the compounds screened on the basis of an unique description will ease the fine tuning of all these observables. From this point of view, lipophilicity is a molecular property of great importance, because it is related both to the pharmacokinetic properties of a drug candidate and, in more structurally local terms, to the molecular recognition process with respect to a specific protein target.

Lipophilicity is a molecular property experimentally determined as the logarithm of the partition coefficient ($\log P$) of a solute between two non-miscible solvent phases, typically *n*-octanol and water. An experimental $\log P$ is valid for only a single chemical species, while a mixture of chemical species is defined by a distribution, $\log D$. Because $\log P$ is a ratio of two concentrations at saturation, it is essentially the net result of all intermolecular forces between a solute and the two phases into which it partitions *(1)* and is generally pH-dependent. According to Testa et al. *(1)* lipophilicity can be represented (**Fig. 1**) as the difference between the hydrophobicity, which accounts for hydrophobic interactions, and dispersion forces and polarity, which account for hydrogen bonds, orientation, and induction forces:

Lipophilicity = hydrophobicity – polarity

More recently, the concept of the molecular lipophilicity potential (MLP), initially introduced by Audry and coworkers *(2)*, has attracted increasing attention. The method involves mapping the local lipophilicity at points in 3D space around a chemical compound through the use of a parametrized fragmental system coupled to an empirical distance function. Despite the absence of any physical basis for the distance-dependent functions introduced, and the difficulties inher-

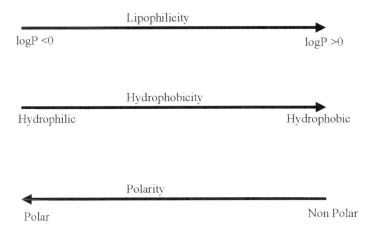

Fig. 1. The conventions of empirical MLP.

ent in the use of the atomic log P_{oct} contributions, this process is analogous to force-field calculations of electrostatic potential at points around a structure.

The studies of Audry *(2)*, Fauchère et al. *(3)*, and Furet et al. *(4)* have demonstrated the ability of the MLP to describe qualitatively the 3D distribution of lipophilicity over all the different parts of a molecular surface. New methods for displaying *(5)* and analyzing *(6)* lipophilic/hydrophilic properties on molecular surfaces have also been published. For example, the binding of arylpiperazines to the 5-HT$_{1A}$ receptor was successfully modeled for a set of molecules using comparative molecular field analysis (CoMFA) 3D-QSAR to which a lipophilic potential had been added *(7,8)*. The HINT program *(9)* also utilizes MLP calculations in a similar manner. Moreover, Volsurf descriptors *(10)*, extensively used to model PK properties, have been found relevant in modeling the interactions involved in ligand receptor binding *(11)*. In addition, MLP calculations have been shown to be sensitive to conformational effects *(7,12)* when sampling conformational space *(13)*. The major hurdle to overcome in the development of 3D-QSAR models using steric, electrostatic, or lipophilic "fields" is related to both conformation-selection and subsequent suitable overlay (alignment) of compounds. It is, therefore, of some interest to provide a conformationally sensitive lipophilicity descriptor that is alignment-independent. The 3D-Log*P* descriptor provides such a representation in the form of a rapidly computable description of the local lipophilicity at points on a user-defined molecular surface. In this chapter we describe the derivation and parametrization of this new descriptor and demonstrate both its conformational sensitivity and its effectiveness in QSAR analysis.

The chapter is divided into three sections: the first part is concerned with the derivation of 3D-Log*P* descriptor and the selection of suitable parameters for the computation of the MLP values. This study was performed on a set of rigid molecules in order, at least initially, to avoid the issue of conformation-dependence. In the second part, both the information content and conformational sensitivity of the 3D-Log*P* description was established using a set of flexible acetylated amino acids and dipeptides. This initial work was carried out using log *P* as the property to be estimated/predicted. However, it should be made clear that, while the 3D-Log*P* descriptor can be used for the prediction of log *P*, this was not the primary intention behind its the development. Rather, as previously indicated, the rationale for this work was the development of a conformationally sensitive but alignment-free lipophilicity descriptor for use in QSAR model development. The use of log *P* as the property to be estimated/predicted enables one to establish the extent of information loss, if any, in the process used to transform the results of MLP calculations into a descriptor suitable for use in QSAR analyses.

The final part of the chapter is devoted to a demonstration of the effectiveness of the 3D-Log*P* approach as a descriptor in QSAR analysis through the modeling and prediction of pIC_{50} values for a set of 49 structurally diverse HIV-1 protease inhibitors taken from the literature *(14)*.

2. Material and Methods

2.1. Software and Hardware

For analysis of conformational flexibility the TSAR® (Oxford Molecular Ltd., Oxford, UK, now part of Accelerys, San Diego, CA, USA) package was used. Molecular modeling was performed using Sybyl software (Tripos Associates, St. Louis, MO, USA) version 6.5. The calculation of the 3D-Log*P* descriptor is implemented as a standalone program and also as a new module, LipoDyn, in the Synt:em in-house (not commercially available) program MultiDyn *(15)*. PLS and other statistical analysis was performed using SIMCA–P 7.01 software and experimental design was carried out using MODDE 4.0 (both packages are provided by Umetri AB, Umeâ, Sweden). All software was run on an SGI Origin 200 except the SIMCA/MODDE packages, which were run on a PC under Windows 95.

2.2. Descriptor Calculation

The derivation of the 3D-Log*P* descriptor requires a suitable 3D space for the calculation of the molecular lipophilicity potential and validated MLP parameters.

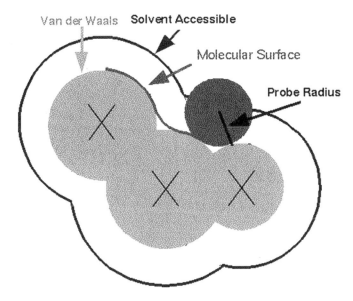

Fig. 2. Molecular surface definition.

2.2.1. Molecular Surface

The *Molecular Surface* (MS) first introduced by Richards *(19)* was chosen as the 3D space where the MLP will be calculated. MS specifically refers to a molecular envelope accessible by a solvent molecule. Unlike the solvent accessible surface *(20)*, which is defined by the center of a spherical probe as it is rolled over a molecule, the MS *(19)*, or Connolly surface *(21)* is traced by the inward-facing surface of the spherical probe (**Fig. 2**). The MS consists of three types of "faces," namely "contact," "saddle," and "concave reentrant," where the spherical probe touches molecule atoms at one, two, or three points, simultaneously. Calculation of molecular properties on the MS and integration of a function over the MS require a numerical representation of the MS as a manifold $S(M_k, n_k, ds_k)$, where M_k, n_k, ds_k are, respectively, the coordinates, the normal vector, and the area of a small element of the MS. Among the published computational methods for a triangulated MS *(22,23)*, the method proposed by Connolly *(21,24)* was used because it provides a numerical presentation of the MS as a collection of dot coordinates and outward normal vectors. In order to build the 3D-log*P* descriptor independent from the calculation parameters of the MS, the precision of the MS area computation was first estimated as a function of the "point density" and the "probe radius" parameters. When varying the point density from 2 to 20 points/Å^2 in steps of 1.0 Å^2, and the probe radius from 1.3 to 1.8 Å with a 0.1 Å step, the precision of the computed area was of the order of 5%, for each of the probes used. All further calculations were carried out with a density of 9 points/Å^2 and a probe radius of 1.4 Å, a combination which was found to be a good compromise between accuracy and computational efficiency.

2.2.2. Molecular Lipophilicity Potential (MLP) Calculations

The MLP is expressed by the following general equation:

$$MLP_k = \sum_{i=1}^{N} f_i \ fct(d_{ik}) \tag{1}$$

where k = label of the given point on the molecular surface, i = fragment label, N = total number of fragments in the molecule, f_i = lipophilic constant for fragment i, fct = distance function, and d_{ik} = distance between fragment i and space point k.

The function $fct(d)$ has no physical basis. According to Heiden (**6**), it should fulfill only two conditions: it should be smooth and continuous and have finite values for $d < d_{\text{cut-off}}$. The value of $d_{\text{cut-off}}$ should be larger than the van der Waals radius of any atom in the molecule under consideration. In the program LipoDyn, the Ghose and Crippen parameters (**18**) as well as the Broto and Moreau parameter set (**16**) are implemented, with the the exponential function used by Fauchère ($\exp(-d)$) (**3**), the hyperbolic function defined by Audry $1/(1 + d)$ (**2**) and the parameterized Fermi distance function used by Testa and coworkers (**1**).

$$\frac{1 + \exp(-ab)}{1 + \exp(a(d - b))}.$$

For each molecule, MLP values were calculated at every k point on the molecular surface.

2.2.3. Derivation from MLP Calculations

The main idea of the 3D-Log$P$ descriptor approach is to sample the molecular surface and then to sum the area of those points with similar MLP values. The 3D-Log$P$ descriptor proposed here is a vector V with NBINS elements each element of which V_i is the sum of the area of all surface elements whose MLP lies between two arbitrary discrete values. The number of bins to be used was chosen after experimentation with various values and 200 was found to be appropriate here, because it allowed the population of the bins with a significant number of area elements for both hydrophilic (MLP < 0) and hydrophobic (MLP > 0) surfaces. However, other values for NBINS may be more suitable in particular cases. In order to simplify things, in the following description it is assumed that 200 bins are to be used. First, the MLP values calculated on the chosen molecular surface are computed as integers to save memory space:

$$MLPsc(k) = INT(MLP(k)) \qquad (2)$$

where k = index for points on the molecular surface.

Second, the coordinates of the vector V are computed according to the following convention:

$$V_i = \sum_{j \,/\, MLPsc(j)+100\,=\,i} dS(j) \qquad i = 1, 200 \qquad (3)$$

The first NBINS/2 coordinates of the vector V correspond to the hydrophilic surface (MLP < 0), while the remaining coordinates correspond to the hydrophobic surface (MLP > 0). Thus, for each compound, the 3D-Log$P$ offers a fixed number of 200 descriptors allowing its use in 3D-QSAR studies.

2.2.4. Visualization of MLP

In order to visualize the results of MLP calculations for a given set of parameters and molecules, a LipoDyn output file for the molecular surface can be color-coded by the MLP values and displayed in VRML 2.0 format *(25)*. The surface triangulation is carried out, after descriptor generation, using the program detri *(26)* which provides a robust 3D Delaunay triangulation coupled to a randomized incremental flip algorithm (**Fig. 3**).

2.2.5. Dataset 1 for MLP Validation

The first dataset consisted of 91 rigid compounds (mono- and di-substituted benzenes, polycyclic aromatic hydrocarbons, cyclic amides, and pyrazole and imidazole derivatives) selected from the WDI on the basis of a count of the number of rotatable bonds computed using TSAR®; none of the 91 structures had rotatable bonds. The structures are listed in **Table 1** together with their experimental log P_{oct} values, which cover a range from –2.17 to +6.5; the values were retrieved from the SRC web site *(27)*.

2.2.6. Dataset 2 for 3D-LogP Validation

The second dataset consists of 50 *N*-acetyl peptide amides (**Table 2**); these peptides have un-ionizable side chains and have previously been studied by Buchwald and Bodor *(28)*. The three-dimensional structures of the di-peptides were built using the force field and partial charges of Kollman *(29)* as implemented in Sybyl 6.5.3. The initial random starting conformations were energy minimized *in vacuo*. For all calculations described herein, the dielectric of the medium was set to unity and the electrostatic cut-off distance was set to 16 Å. For each molecule, the Sybyl Genetic Algorithm–based conformational search,

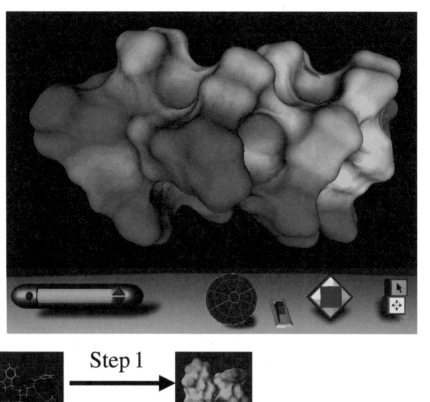

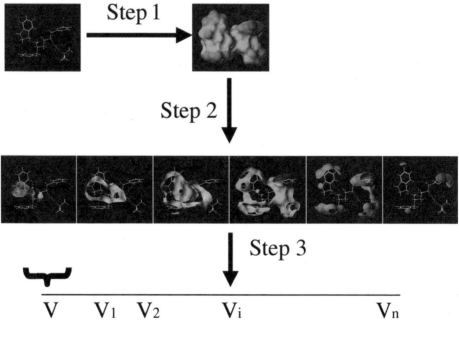

Step 1

Step 2

Step 3

$$\underbrace{}_{V} \quad V_1 \quad V_2 \quad\qquad V_i \qquad\qquad\qquad V_n$$

$$V_i = \sum_{j \,/\, MLP(j)+100=i} dS(j)$$

which operates in dihedral angle space, was used to determine the peptide geometries. The initial population was set to 300, the number of generations to 10,000, and the duplicate window to 60.0 degrees. The conformation with the lowest energy obtained from the conformational analysis was then used for descriptor calculation.

2.2.7. Dataset 3 for QSAR Studies

A third dataset was built in order to demonstrate that the descriptor is relevant for estimating binding affinity in a QSAR analysis. This last dataset contains 49 HIV-1 protease inhibitors, the 3D coordinates of which were those used by Pastor et al. *(30)*. It has the four transition-state isosteres—hydroxyethylene, hydroxyethylamine, statine, and a symmetrical diol. The X-ray structures of molecules numbered 1 and 3–34 have been reported *(31)*, whereas molecules numbered 35–50 were modeled on the crystallographic structure of the complex of HIV-1 protease with L-689,502 solved at 2.25 Å resolution *(32)*. The binding affinity is expressed as pIC_{50} values.

2.2.8. PLS Regression Analysis and Orthogonal Signal Correction

2.2.8.1. PLS REGRESSION

The relationship between the observable variables Y and the computed 3D-Log$P$ descriptor matrix X for each of the three dataset compounds was determined using the Partial Least Squares Projection to Latent Structures (PLS) method *(33,34)* as implemented in SIMCA–P 7.01. PLS modeling consists of simultaneous projections of both the X and Y spaces on low-dimensional hyper-planes *(35)*. Since PLS is a projection method, it can handle co-linear data having many more descriptor variables than observations *(N)*, as long as the resulting components are few compared to N. The criterion used to determine the number of significant PLS components is leave-group-out (LGO) cross-validation and we used seven group CV as recommended in the literature *(36)*. Group membership in LGO is random and, in order to avoid chance effects, the procedure is repeated 200 times and the optimal number of PLS components selected from these results *(36)*.

2.2.8.2. ORTHOGONAL SIGNAL CORRECTION (OSC)

Descriptor matrix coordinates can be preprocessed using the recently developed filtering technique *(37)* known as OSC, which is also implemented in

---

Fig. 3. *(top photo)* MLP-based representation of the lipophilicity. On the VRML surface yellow represents the hydrophobic surface, blue the hydrophilic surface.

Fig. 4. *(top photo)* 3D-Log$P$ calculation procedure.

Table 1

Chemical Structures, CAS Number, and Experimental log P_{oct} Values for the Set of 91 Rigid Molecules

ID	structure	CAS	logPoct exp	ID	structure	CAS	logPoct exp
1		288-13-1	0.26	11		110-86-1	0.65
2		3469-69-0	1.7	12		75-19-4	1.72
3		461-89-2	-0.59	13		66-71-7	1.78
4		315-30-0	-0.55	14		91-22-5	2.03
5		6714-29-0	-0.25	15		71-43-2	2.13
6		288-32-4	-0.08	16		287-92-3	3
7		119-65-3	2.08	17		275-51-4	3.2
8		56-55-3	5.76	18		591-50-4	3.25
9		66-97-7	1.67	19		91-20-3	3.3
10		491-38-3	1.38	20		260-94-6	3.4

Table 1 *(continued)*

ID	structure	CAS	logPoct exp	ID	structure	CAS	logPoct exp
21		95-50-1	3.43	31		85-01-8	4.46
22		106-46-7	3.44	32		129-00-0	4.88
23		119-64-2	3.49	33		206-44-0	5.16
24		58-89-9	3.72	34		218-01-9	5.5
25		319-85-7	3.78	35		92-24-0	5.76
26		319-84-6	3.8	36		50-32-8	5.97
27		90-13-1	3.9	37		5103-73-1	6.08
28		86-73-7	4.18	38		76-44-8	6.1
29		281-23-2	4.24	39		192-97-2	6.44
30		120-12-7	4.45	40		309-00-2	6.5

Table 1 *(continued)*

ID	structure	CAS	logPoct exp	ID	structure	CAS	logPoct exp
41		120-72-9	2.14	51		68-94-0	-1.11
42		288-88-0	-0.58	52		72-20-8	5.2
43		87-41-2	0.8	53		1024-57-3	4.98
44		244-63-3	3.17	54		298-46-4	2.45
45		496-16-2	2.14	55		90-47-1	3.39
46		57-13-6	-2.11	56		85-41-6	1.15
47		54-95-5	0.14	57		4425-23-4	2
48		523-50-2	2.08	58		91-56-5	0.83
49		91-64-5	1.39	59		108-94-1	0.81
50		82-05-3	4.81	60		86-74-8	3.72

Table 1 *(continued)*

ID	structure	CAS	logPoct exp	ID	structure	CAS	logPoct exp
61		59-49-4	1.16	71		96-48-0	-0.64
62		110-89-4	0.84	72		106-51-4	0.2
63		60-57-1	5.4	73		84-65-1	3.39
64		51-21-8	-0.89	74		123-75-1	0.46
65		66-22-8	-1.07	75		26232-35-9	2.4
66		123-33-1	-0.84	76		461-72-3	-1.69
67		616-45-5	-0.85	77		135-67-1	3.85
68		1820-81-1	-0.35	78		696-07-1	0.04
69		85-44-9	1.6	79		108-86-1	2.99
70		130-15-4	1.71	80		68367-52-2	0.78

(continued)

Table 1 *(continued)*

ID	structure	CAS	logPoct exp	ID	structure	CAS	logPoct exp
81		51-17-2	1.32	87		18356-28-0	-1.11
82		109-99-9	0.46	88		69-89-6	-0.73
83		67-52-7	-1.47	89		110-91-8	-0.86
84		57-24-9	1.93	90		51-20-7	-0.21
85		110-85-0	-1.5	91		110-88-3	-0.43
86		69-93-2	-2.17				

SIMCA 7.01. OSC is based on PLS and involves the reduction of the weighting of variables not correlated to the Y response; as a consequence, OSC removes some of the "noise" in the X description. The 3D-Log$P$ coordinates modified by the OSC mathematical transformation are highly correlated with the initial coordinates, which reduces the impact of this transformation on model interpretation. Moreover, coupling OSC filtering with PLS modeling has the advantages that it diminishes the model coefficients of irrelevant descriptors thus simplifying model interpretation and it may also lead to models with a better predictive ability *(38,39)*.

3. Results

3.1. Use of Back Calculation of log P_{oct} Values for Parameter Evaluation

The solvent accessible surface has been widely used for calculating the MLP *(7)*, because it should represent how the molecule is perceived by its

Table 2

Experimental and Estimated log $P_{oct/water}$ Values for a Set of 49 Acetylated Amino Acids and Dipeptides

Sequence	Log P octanol/water	
	Observed	Calculated
Ac-Ala-NH2	−1.47	−1.24
Ac-AlaAla-NH2	−2	−1.36
Ac-AlaLeu-NH2	−0.54	−0.53
Ac-AlaVal-NH2	−1.13	−0.86
Ac-Asn-NH2	−2.41	−2.15
Ac-AsnIle-NH2	−1.43	−1.24
Ac-AsnVal-NH2	−1.85	−1.79
Ac-Cys-NH2	−0.29	−0.35
Ac-Gln-NH2	−2.05	−2.19
Ac-GlnLeu-NH2	−1.32	−1.39
Ac-GlnPhe-NH2	−1.14	−1.25
Ac-GlnVal-NH2	−1.85	−1.76
Ac-Gly-NH2	−1.76	−1.44
Ac-GlyLeu-NH2	−0.78	−0.80
Ac-GlyPhe-NH2	−0.56	−0.55
Ac-GlyVal-NH2	−1.33	−0.79
Ac-Ile-NH2	−0.03	−0.35
Ac-IleAsn-NH2	−1.41	−1.04
Ac-Leu-NH2	−0.04	−0.49
Ac-LeuAsn-NH2	−1.3	−1.43
Ac-LeuIle-NH2	0.68	0.40
Ac-LeuVal-NH2	0.26	−0.17
Ac-Met-NH2	−0.47	−0.87
Ac-MetPhe-NH2	0.42	−0.80
Ac-Phe-NH2	0.04	−0.08
Ac-PheGln-NH2	−1.03	−0.94
Ac-PheGly-NH2	−0.5	−0.58
Ac-PhePhe-NH2	1.19	0.82
Ac-PheVal-NH2	0.43	0.18
Ac-Pro-NH2	−1.34	−1.26
Ac-Ser-NH2	−1.87	−2.00
Ac-SerPhe-NH2	−0.79	−1.04
Ac-SerVal-NH2	−1.53	−1.58
Ac-Thr-NH2	−1.57	−1.64
Ac-ThrIle-NH2	−0.86	−0.36

(continued)

Table 2 *(continued)*

| | Log P octanol/water | |
Sequence	Observed	Calculated
Ac-ThrVal-NH2	−1.25	−0.99
Ac-Trp-NH2	0.42	0.46
Ac-Tyr-NH2	−0.79	−0.77
Ac-TyrLeu-NH2	0.32	0.19
Ac-TyrPhe-NH2	0.54	0.41
Ac-TyrTyr-NH2	−0.16	0.04
Ac-TyrVal-NH2	−0.2	−0.24
Ac-Val-NH2	−0.61	−0.77
Ac-ValAla-NH2	−1.14	−0.81
Ac-ValGln-NH2	−1.82	−1.62
Ac-ValVal-NH2	−0.32	−0.41
Ac-IleVal-NH2	0.16	0.07
Ac-TrpVal-NH2	0.73	0.87
Ac-MetVal-NH2	−0.28	−0.46

environment. However, this approach is restricted by definition to the very local environment of the molecule studied, such as, for example, the first hydration layer of a compound. The selection of the MS as an appropriate surface for computing MLP values was tested by back-calculating log P_{oct} values and comparing them to the original experimental values. At the same time the distance functions and parameters were evaluated and compared.

In order to back-calculate log P_{oct} for each molecule, the guidelines proposed by Testa et al. *(1)* have been followed. Two parameters, $\sum MLP^+$ and $\sum MLP^-$, the total of positive and negative MLP values, respectively, were calculated using various combinations of atomic parameters and distance functions, for the set of 91 rigid structures. The best log P_{oct} re-predictions (**Fig. 5**) are obtained using the Fermi distance function and the Broto and Moreau parameters:

$$\log \ P = 2.12 \cdot 10^{-3} \sum MLP^+ + 0.53 \cdot 10^{-3} \sum MLP^- - 0.29$$
$$n = 91; \quad r^2 = 0.83; \quad q^2 = 0.82; \ s = 0.95; \ F = 215$$

(4)

This combination of parameters was found to be the most relevant, although it is accepted that these results are likely to be dataset-dependent.

One of the limitations of current log P_{oct} prediction techniques is in the accuracy of the atomic fragmental system used. The weaknesses of the atomic fragmentation systems of Ghose and Crippen or of Broto and Moreau have been

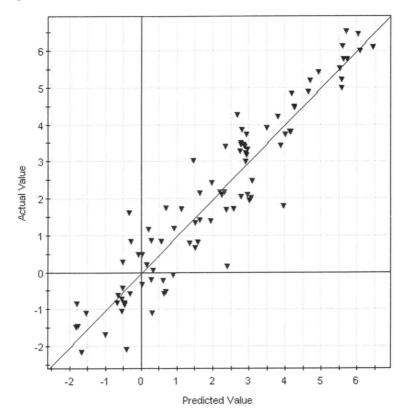

Fig. 5. Estimation of log P_{oct} using MLP calculation with the atomic fragmental system of Ghose and Crippen and the Fauchère distance function on the 91 selected WDI rigid molecules.

discussed previously *(45)*. For example, in the Ghose and Crippen system *(17)*, the carbon atoms in an ether functionality group are considered as polar atoms and the oxygen as nonpolar. Moreover, the fragmental constant of polar hydrogens seems to be overestimated. Indeed, the polarity associated with polar hydrogens is principally due to their ability to form hydrogen bonds. However, this feature only weakly influences the log P_{oct} coefficient, as illustrated in the solvatochromic equations characterizing log P_{oct}, where the coefficient of H-bond donating acidity α of the solutes *(46)* has a low significance. The fact that this system works so well in QSAR studies might be due to the importance of the hydrogen bond donors in biological media. In any case, the commercial programs CLOGP or KOWWIN are recognized solutions, because the accuracy of their estimations is within the experimental error range of 0.4 (*see* **Table 3**).

Table 3

**Statistics Reported by Using Syracuse Research
Corporation's Experimental Log P_{oct} Database**

	n	r^2	SD
KOWWIN	10331	0.94	0.47
CLOGP	7250	0.96	0.3

3.2. QSPR-Based Estimation of log P_{oct} for the Amino Acid/Dipeptide Dataset

Dataset 2 was used for two different analyses. In the first we determined whether the 3D-Log$P$ description could be used in combination with regression-based techniques to effectively model a chosen end-point, in this case log P_{oct}. In the second analysis, the log P_{oct} repredicted by using the 3D-log$P$ vector are shown to be conformation dependent for the di-peptide GlnPhe. The conformational sensitivity of the descriptor is thus demonstrated.

3.2.1. Regression Analysis

Each of the columns of the descriptor matrix was initially autoscaled to zero mean and unit variance to give each vector element equal importance prior to analysis. PLS regression analysis was applied in order to predict log P_{oct} values. The best log P_{oct} re-predictions were obtained by using the Fermi distance function, the Ghose and Crippen set of parameters, and a two-significant-component PLS model selected on the basis of leave-seven-out cross-validation procedure repeated 200 times with fitted $r^2 = 0.87$ and a mean q^2 of 0.81 (*see* **Fig. 6**). We also investigated the possibility that the predictive capacity of the model was a chance effect through data-scrambling analysis. The Y values are randomly permuted a number of times and a cross-validated QSAR model computed for each permutation. Nine hundred permuted models were computed, which gave the resulting r^2 intercepts of 0.25 and the q^2 intercepts of –0.18. The results from the permutation tests suggest that the predictive capacity of the PLS model is not a chance effect.

The prediction of the partition properties of peptide molecules is difficult, owing to their conformational flexibility, and the possible presence of multiple intramolecular hydrogen bonds and ionizable groups. Richards and coworkers *(40–42)* were the first to consider explicitly the effects of the population of accessible conformational minima in both phases. These types of calculation are, however, computationally intensive. The introduction of the solvent-accessible surface area in the prediction of log P_{oct} for steric isomers *(43,44)* also constitutes a promising approach.

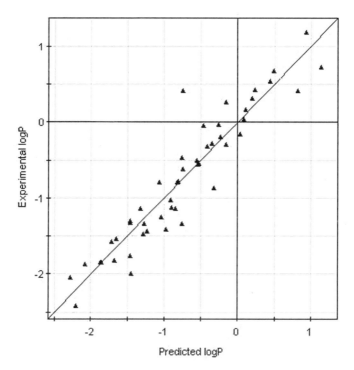

Fig. 6. Prediction of log P_{oct} values of a set of 49 acetylated amino acids and di-peptides.

3.2.2. Conformational Sensitivity

A key question with regard to QSAR applications is the sensitivity of the 3D-Log$P$ description with respect to molecular conformation. A systematic sampling of the conformational space of the di-peptides clearly showed that the range of the log P_{oct} estimations is greater than the standard deviation of the estimation in the dipeptide data set. For example, a systematic conformational search was performed on the dihedral angles of the di-peptide GlnPhe. By using the grid search function in the AMBER 4.1 force field, a set of 1296 energy-minimized conformations was generated with phi and psi values varied in steps of 60°. The mean of the log P_{oct} values for the different conformations of GlnPhe is −1.42, with a standard deviation of 0.14. Because the estimated log P_{oct} value for the energy-minimized GlnPhe di-peptide is equal to −1.19 ± 0.085, the conformational dependence of 3D-Log$P$ method is clearly shown. One advantage of the 3D-Log$P$ descriptor lies in its duality, whereby it can be applied to the estimation of log P_{oct} but can also be used as a QSAR descriptor, as will be demonstrated below.

3.3. HIV-1 Protease Inhibitors—Evaluation by 3D-LogP-QSAR

The second important point of this chapter is to evaluate the use of local lipophilicity information in 3D-QSAR studies. For that purpose, we used a set of 49 HIV-1 protease inhibitors that has been widely used in the 3D-QSAR literature.

3.3.1. Analysis Without Prediction Set

To set up a baseline, we first mimicked the study that has been conducted by Holloway by building a model on the whole dataset of 49 structures. With regard to the 3D-log$P$ descriptor, we found that the best combination of parameters for this particular dataset was the use of the Ghose and Crippen atomic parameters combined with the Fauchère distance function. We then preprocessed this raw description by filtering out all the 3D-log$P$ variables having less than 0.1 of variance. We ended up with a 3D-log$P$ description matrix of 76 variables that we used for all our regression model building.

The PLS model built on this 49•76 matrix showed interesting statistics (*see* **Table 4**). However, by looking more closely at the variation in importance of our 76 description vectors, we realized that most of them did not contribute to the explanation of the overall pIC50 variance. To overcome this issue, we decided to apply the OSC filtering technique to the 49•76 matrix. We expected this transformation to identify the most relevant subset of the 3D-log$P$ description by removing the "noise." The modified 3D-log$P$ description matrix resulted in a single OSC component retaining slightly more than 67% of the original variance. As expected, the OSC transformation led to a dramatic decrease of the number of 3D-log$P$ vectors used to build the PLS model. Indeed, more than 50% of them were removed by the OSC transformation and the resulting PLS model exhibited a clearly improved q^2 ($q^2 = 0.95$) over the value obtained without the OSC filtering. The OSC filtering also helped us to remove irrelevant information as reflected by the SDEP value we obtained ($SDEP_{CV} = 0.30$) and the fact that none of the molecules were predicted with an absolute prediction error value greater than 0.70 log units. Interestingly, by comparing our statistics with those previously published, we found the PLS model based on the 3D-log$P$ description to be at least as predictive, without having to remove any structure (*see* **Table 4**).

To further evaluate the ability of our 3D-log$P$ description to model the HIV dataset, we used different ways to design training sets and test sets. By doing so, we expected to have a better idea of the real predictive ability of the 3D-log$P$–based PLS model. For the first design, we reproduced the split training/test sets published by Holloway and for the second one we applied a

(text continues on page 252)

Table 4
Predictive Power and Robustness of the PLS Models on the HIV Data Set

No	Structures	Observed	Calculated						Predicted				
			No Prediction Set	Working Set					Prediction Set				
				WS 3.1	WS 3.2	WS 3.3	WS 3.4		PS 3.1	PS 3.2	PS 3.3	PS 3.4	
MM01		9.6021	9.52128	9.67507						9.526389	9.52128	9.52128	
MM03		8.1135	8.49268	8.60727	8.61641						8.49268	8.49268	
MM04		9.7212	9.67769	9.60032	9.53871							9.67769	9.67769

(continued)

235

Table 4 (continued)

No	Structures	Observed	Calculated						Predicted			
			No Prediction Set	Working Set					Prediction Set			
				WS 3.1	WS 3.2	WS 3.3	WS 3.4	PS 3.1	PS 3.2	PS 3.3	PS 3.4
MM05		9.585	9.54954	9.44919	9.70998						9.54954	9.54954
MM06		9.6383	9.21021	9.16337	9.32885						9.21021	9.21021
MM07		9.2218	9.11327	9.42525						9.231151	9.11327	9.11327

236

No	Structures	Observed	Calculated						Predicted			
			No Prediction Set	Working Set					Prediction Set			
				WS 3.1	WS 3.2	WS 3.3	WS 3.4		PS 3.1	PS 3.2	PS 3.3	PS 3.4
MM08		9.5376	9.43556	9.92853		9.43556				9.427544		9.43556
MM09		9.5086	9.75977	9.64809	9.85208						9.75977	9.75977
MM10		9.5686	9.70385	9.62284	9.79198						9.73385	9.70385

(continued)

237

Table 4 (*continued*)

No	Structures	Observed	No Prediction Set	Calculated — Working Set				Predicted — Prediction Set			
				WS 3.1	WS 3.2	WS 3.3	WS 3.4	PS 3.1	PS 3.2	PS 3.3	PS 3.4
MM11		5.5325	5.64846	5.54272	5.71656					5.64846	5.64846
MM12		9.7959	10.0249	10.1546	10.1882					10.0249	10.0249
MM13		7.5607	7.23959	7.42708	7.29127					7.23959	7.23959

238

No	Structures	Observed	Calculated						Predicted			
			No Prediction Set	Working Set					Prediction Set			
				WS 3.1	WS 3.2	WS 3.3	WS 3.4		PS 3.1	PS 3.2	PS 3.3	PS 3.4
MM14		9.1427	8.92455	8.96303						9.288795	8.92455	8.92455
MM15		8.266	8.97425	8.92147		8.97425				8.822011		8.97425
MM16		9.2757	9.26379	9.21432	9.34214						9.26379	9.26379

(continued)

239

Table 4 *(continued)*

No	Structures	Observed	Calculated						Predicted			
			No Prediction Set	Working Set					Prediction Set			
				WS 3.1	WS 3.2	WS 3.3	WS 3.4	PS 3.1	PS 3.2	PS 3.3	PS 3.4
MM17		9.6021	9.01118	9.04717	9.09882					9.01118	9.01118
MM18		9.7696	9.74443	9.77696		9.74443			9.339221		9.74443
MM19		6.9431	7.13188	7.13668	7.05723	7.13188					7.13188

No	Structures	Observed	No Prediction Set	Calculated				Predicted			
				Working Set				Prediction Set			
				WS 3.1	WS 3.2	WS 3.3	WS 3.4	PS 3.1	PS 3.2	PS 3.3	PS 3.4
MM20		8.0209	8.00622	7.81056		8.00622			8.264937		8.00622
MM21		7.4653	7.42943	7.55027	7.37341					7.42943	7.42943
MM22		6.1612	6.62208	6.52955	6.60611					6.62208	6.62208

(continued)

Table 4 *(continued)*

No	Structures	Observed	Calculated						Predicted			
			No Prediction Set	Working Set					Prediction Set			
				WS 3.1	WS 3.2	WS 3.3	WS 3.4		PS 3.1	PS 3.2	PS 3.3	PS 3.4
MM23		6.7932	6.42925	6.20521	6.47032						6.42925	6.42925
MM24		7.1785	6.61714	6.75522						6.721797	6.61714	6.61714
MM25		6.6728	6.83172	6.8529						6.839004	6.83172	6.83172

242

No	Structures	Observed	Calculated					Predicted			
			No Prediction Set	Working Set				Prediction Set			
				WS 3.1	WS 3.2	WS 3.3	WS 3.4	PS 3.1	PS 3.2	PS 3.3	PS 3.4
MM26		6.9144	7.00545	6.97256	7.15953					7.00545	7.00545
MM27		9.1549	8.94296	8.87309	9.10746					8.94296	8.94296
MM28		9.7447	9.53835	9.53553	9.75865					9.53835	9.53835

(continued)

243

Table 4 *(continued)*

No	Structures	Observed	Calculated						Predicted			
			No Prediction Set	Working Set					Prediction Set			
				WS 3.1	WS 3.2	WS 3.3	WS 3.4		PS 3.1	PS 3.2	PS 3.3	PS 3.4
MM29		7.3925	7.68948	7.53999	7.57264	7.68948						7.68948
MM30		4.5229	4.71824	4.73964	4.79355	4.71824						4.71824
MM31		6.8861	7.16186	7.40008		7.16186	7.16186			7.351424		

244

No	Structures	Observed	Calculated						Predicted			
			No Prediction Set	Working Set					Prediction Set			
				WS 3.1	WS 3.2	WS 3.3	WS 3.4		PS 3.1	PS 3.2	PS 3.3	PS 3.4
MM32		6.8356	7.09712	7.01618	6.97945		7.09712				7.09712	
MM33		10.000	9.54446	9.51534	9.53448						9.54446	9.54446
MM34		7.4134	6.82687	6.94136						7.005641	6.82687	6.82687

(continued)

245

Table 4 (continued)

No	Structures	Observed	Calculated						Predicted			
			No Prediction Set	Working Set					Prediction Set			
				WS 3.1	WS 3.2	WS 3.3	WS 3.4		PS 3.1	PS 3.2	PS 3.3	PS 3.4
MM35		6.2299	6.25446						6.295794	6.575991	6.25446	6.25446
MM36		9.1612	9.65801		9.37122	9.65801	9.65801		10.094749			
MM37		6.2457	5.91148		5.75055	5.91148	5.91148		5.807993			

246

No	Structures	Observed	No Prediction Set	Calculated				Predicted			
				Working Set				Prediction Set			
				WS 3.1	WS 3.2	WS 3.3	WS 3.4	PS 3.1	PS 3.2	PS 3.3	PS 3.4
MM38		8.8861	8.79293		8.88654			8.778541		8.79293	8.79293
MM39		10.222	10.0489			10.0489	10.0489	9.834761	9.98735		
MM40		5.8965	6.38677		6.10747			6.658533		6.38677	6.38677

(continued)

247

Table 4 (*continued*)

No	Structures	Observed	No Prediction Set	Calculated Working Set				Predicted Prediction Set			
				WS 3.1	WS 3.2	WS 3.3	WS 3.4	PS 3.1	PS 3.2	PS 3.3	PS 3.4
MM41		9.6383	9.96519			9.96519	9.96519	9.11167	9.189701		
MM42		8.2676	8.35813		8.12613		8.35813	7.722494		8.35813	
MM43		10.267	10.1797		9.98563			9.317187		10.1797	10.1797

248

| No | Structures | Observed | Calculated | | | | | | Predicted | | |
| | | | No Prediction Set | Working Set | | | | PS 3.1 | Prediction Set | | |
				WS 3.1	WS 3.2	WS 3.3	WS 3.4		PS 3.2	PS 3.3	PS 3.4
MM44		7.2774	7.24593		6.87364	7.24593		7.400203			7.24593
MM45		5.1675	5.033		4.92905	5.033	5.033	5.222603			
MM46		5.5229	5.51431		5.58965	5.51431		5.886484			5.51431

(continued)

249

Table 4 (continued)

No	Structures	Observed	Calculated						Predicted			
			No Prediction Set	Working Set					Prediction Set			
				WS 3.1	WS 3.2	WS 3.3	WS 3.4		PS 3.1	PS 3.2	PS 3.3	PS 3.4
MM47		8.1163	8.064		7.82987				8.19309		8.064	8.064
MM48		6.6402	6.95968		6.94074				7.224765		6.95968	6.95968
MM49		5.3279	5.16601						5.268966	5.818124	5.16601	5.16601

250

No	Structures	Observed	Calculated						Predicted			
			No Prediction Set	Working Set					Prediction Set			
				WS 3.1	WS 3.2	WS 3.3	WS 3.4		PS 3.1	PS 3.2	PS 3.3	PS 3.4
MM50		5.8617	5.84363						5.964676	5.838982	5.84365	5.84363

Table 5

Summary of the 3D-QSAR Analysis Results for the 49 HIV-1 Protease Inhibitors Using the 3D-Log*P* Descriptor and Statistical Comparison with the Comparative Binding Energy Analysis *(50)* (COMBINE)

Model	Number of TS molecules	Number of variables	Number of latent variables	r^2	q^2	$SDEP_{CV}$	$SDEP_{ex}$
COMBINE No PS	48[a]	54	2	0.91	0.81	0.66	—
COMBINE TS1	32[a]	47	2	0.90	0.73	0.69	0.59
3D-LogP No PS	49	76	2	0.97	0.95	0.30	—
3D-LogP TS 3.1	33	76	2	0.95	0.91	0.33	0.49
3D-LogP TS 3.2	33	76	3	0.97	0.93	0.29	0.34
3D-LogP TS 3.3	15	76	2	0.94	0.87	0.46	0.71
3D-LogP TS 3.4	8	76	2	0.95	0.86	0.45	1.14

[a]MM30 excluded.

classical "random" selection. Finally, the following two designs were implemented to better investigate the robustness of our proposed model by drastically reducing the number of molecules, i.e. information, used in the training set to predict the remaining HIV-1 protease inhibitors.

3.3.2. Design 1

Following the work of Merck researchers *(31)*, the HIV dataset was split into two parts. The 33 inhibitors numbered 1 and 3–34 were assembled to form the Training Set 3.1 (TS 3.1), the remaining 12 selected by Holloway et al. *(27)* formed the Prediction Set 3.1 (PS 3.1). The PLS model computed on the training set gave a model with the following statistics (**Table 5** and **Fig. 8**): $r^2 = 0.95$; $q^2 = 0.91$; $SDEP_{CV} = 0.33$; $SDEP_{ex} = 0.49$. Again, our 3D-log*P*–based PLS model performed on the test set as well as previously published models ($SDEP_{ex} = 0.49$) and better if we consider that we did not have to remove any compound to obtain such results.

3.3.3. Design 2

In the second approach we used the information contained in the whole dataset of 49 molecules to build a training set using a classical "random" method. Every third compound was withdrawn from the list of compounds sorted by increasing activity, thus creating a prediction set of 16 molecules (Prediction Set PS 3.2) and a training set of 33 molecules (Training Set TS 3.2). The PLS-OSC model computed with this reduced training set retained its efficiency of prediction (**Table 5**;

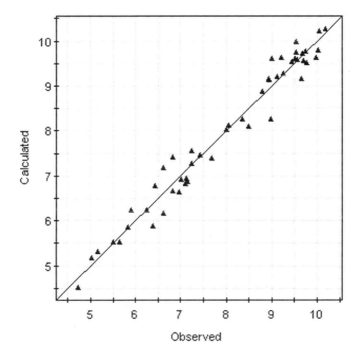

Fig. 7. HIV-1 protease inhibitors relationship between observed and predicted log pIC$_{50}$ values.

$r^2 = 0.97$; $q^2 = 0.93$; SDEP$_{CV} = 0.29$; SDEP$_{ex} = 0.34$). **Figure 9** shows that the model predicts all the compounds quite well, and that the prediction residuals are evenly distributed. The average residual on the test set TS 3.2 is of 0.20 log units and the most poorly predicted molecule is the compound MM49 that is over-predicted by less than 0.9 log units.

3.3.4. Designs 3 and 4

In the last two procedures, we tried to estimate the real predictive power and the robustness of our model. We used experimental design techniques to create the split training and testing sets. In our case, we based this split on the D-optimality criterion. This criterion allows the selection of a few molecules within a constrained situation, optimally spanning the multivariate regression space of interest *(47)* and permits the handling of discrete objects like molecular structures *(48)*. D-optimal designs also ensure maximization of the information matrix and, consequently, the independence, significance, and robustness of the calculated model's coefficients *(49,50)*. All the selected designs were built in the principal property (PP) space of the PLS model (using the MODDE 4.0 software). First, 15 molecules were selected using D-optimal design to form the

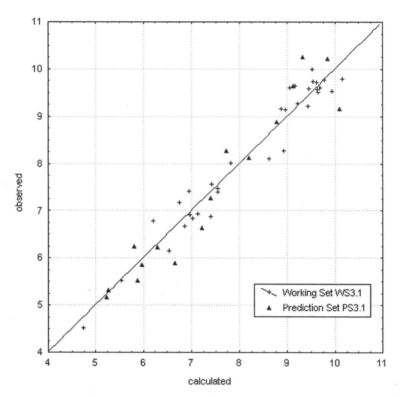

Fig. 8. HIV-1 protease inhibitors relationship between observed and predicted log pIC$_{50}$ values for design 1.

training set TS 3.3; the remaining 34 formed the prediction set PS 3.3. A second more drastic selection was made leading to the training set TS 3.4 consisting of only eight compounds. The remaining 41 formed the prediction set PS 3.4. In both cases the internal and external predictive performance of the derived models (q^2 and SDEP) highlights the robustness and the predictive ability of our 3D-Log$P$–based PLS approach **(Table 5)**. Indeed, the 3D-log$P$ model, based on 15 molecules, exhibits statistics that are comparable to Holloway's model, which was based on 33 molecules. Our second model, based on eight molecules, confirms that it is possible to use an extremely small training set and still have an average error of prediction that is less than one log unit (SDEP$_{ex}$ = 1.14). We summarized the observed and calculated inhibitory activities in **Table 4** and the PLS-OSC statistics in **Table 5**.

Some other studies have taken a more conventional approach in which the structure of the protease is a key part of the process leading to a statistical model. In this respect a feature of HIV-1 protease that must be considered is the

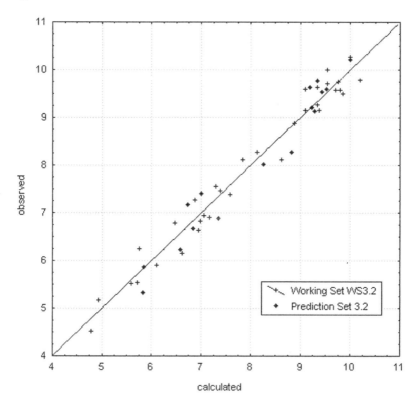

Fig. 9. HIV-1 protease inhibitors relationship between observed and predicted log pIC$_{50}$ values for design 2.

symmetrical nature of the enzyme. In the X-ray structures of the complexes between the enzyme and inhibitors, some ligands are observed *(32)* to bind in the active site both in an N→C and a C→N orientation with respect to the flaps, which, in their closed H-bonded form, introduce the asymmetry and hence the direction marker. A COMBINE analysis, carried out by Pastor et al. *(30)*, took into account both orientations of the docked ligand. Although the model obtained was reasonably successful at matching the inhibitory activities with the interaction energies, the process was complex and computationally intensive, largely because of the requirement for estimating the atomic partial charges of the ligand either by continuum electrostatics calculations or by charge interpolation. The statistical quality of this COMBINE model is comparable with the 3D-Log*P* model we have proposed *(see* **Table 5**). An alternative CoMFA model employing experimentally determined alignment rules for HIV protease inhibitors representing five different transition state isosteres, was proposed by Waller and coworkers *(51,52)*. The difficulty with these CoMFA-based studies *(53)* is that multiple alignment is needed to construct predictive models and that steric and electrostatic interactions alone do not take explicit account of the effects of solvation and lipophilicity, two factors which are known to strongly influence the free energy of binding. The 3D-Log*P* descriptor, which treats local lipophilic character explicitly, may add valuable information to the steric and electrostatic field approach implemented in procedures such as CoMFA. Furthermore, the predictive ability of our approach is comparable to the CoMFA models without the requirement for structural alignment.

4. Conclusions

3D-Log*P* is a macroscopic, thermodynamic metric. It is related to the partition properties of molecular ensembles, having its origins at the microscopic level in explicit hydrophobic and polar intermolecular interactions. When applied to sets of flexible molecules, the quality of the partition coefficient estimations is comparable to other published methods. When this descriptor is used in the context of QSAR, the requirement for structural alignment disappears, which is a major advantage compared to CoMFA, for example. In the case of structurally diverse compounds, the structural alignment of molecular sets of interest, and the orientation of the entire set of superimposed molecules relative to a 3D grid *(53)* constitute a limitation of this class of methods. In contrast, using the 3D-Log*P* descriptor, the ranking of different HIV-1 protease inhibitors can be obtained solely by using information extracted from the ligand conformations.

Finally, the 3D-Log*P* descriptor may be used for the 3D screening of virtual molecular conformation libraries wherein the selection of candidate molecules might not only be driven by pharmacophoric but also by physicochemical constraints. Similarly, we anticipate that the 3D-Log*P* descriptor will also become useful for the design of chemical libraries in which the description of the conformational space is taken into account in the description of the constituent molecules. We are currently enhancing the descriptor by implementing the last atom type classification system proposed by Wildman and Crippen *(54)*.

Acknowledgments

We wish to thank Prof. Tony Rees, Prof. Robert Brasseur, and Dr. Lennart Eriksson for discussion and enthusiastic support. We are very grateful to Prof. Federico Gago (Departemento de Farmacologica, Universidad de Alcalà, Madrid, Spain) for providing the HIV data set and thank also Jacques Duret and Tuan Do (Tripos Inc., France) for software support.

References

1. Testa, B., Carrupt, P. A., Gaillard, P., Billois, F., and Weber, P. (1996) Lipophilicity in molecular modeling. *Pharm. Res.* **13,** 335–343.

2. Audry, E., Dubost, J. P., Colleter, J. C., and Dallet, P. (1986) A new approach to structure-activity relations: the molecular lipophilicity potential. *Eur. J. Med. Chem.* **21,** 71–72.

3. Fauchere, J. L., Quarendon, P., and Kactterer, L. (1988) Estimating and representing hydrophobicity potential. *J. Mol. Graph.* **6,** 203–206.

4. Furet, P., Sele, A., and Cohen, N. C. (1988) 3D molecular lipophilicity potential profiles: a new tool in molecular modeling. *J. Mol. Graph.* **6,** 182–189.

5. Croizet, F., Langlois, M. H., Dubost, J. P., et al. (1990) Lipophilicity force field profile: an expressive visualization of the lipophilicity molecular potential gradient. *J. Mol. Graph.* **8,** 149–53.

6. Heiden, W., Moeckel, G., and Brickmann, J. (1993) A new approach to analysis and display of local lipophilicity/hydrophilicity mapped on molecular surfaces. *J. Comput.-Aided Mol. Design* **7,** 503–514.

7. Gaillard, P., Carrupt, P. A., Testa, B., and Boudon, A. (1994) Molecular lipophilicity potential, a tool in 3D-QSAR. Method and applications. *J. Comput.-Aided Mol. Design* **8,** 83–96.

8. Gaillard, P., Carrupt, P. A., Testa, B., and Schambel, P. (1996) Binding of arylpiperazines, (aryloxy)propanolamines and tetrahydropyridyl-indoles to the 5-HT$_{1A}$ receptor: contribution of the molecular lipophilicity potential to three-dimensional quantitative structure-activity relationship models. *J. Med. Chem.* **39,** 126–134.

9. Kellogg, G.E., Semus, S.F., Abraham, D.J. (1991) HINT: a new method of empirical hydrophobic field calculation for CoMFA. *J. Comput. Aided Mol. Des.* **5,** 545–542.

10. Cruciani, G., Pastor, M., and Guba, W. (2000) Volsurf: a new tool for the pharmacokinetic optimization of lead compounds. *Eur. J. Pharm. Sci.* **11,** 29–39.

11. Filipponi, E., Cruciani, G., Tabarrini, O., Cecchetti, V., and Fravolini, A. (2001) QSAR study and Volsurf characterization of anti HIV quinolone library. *J. Comput. Aided Mol. Des.* **15,** 203–217.

12. Gaillard, P., Carrupt, P. A., and Testa, B. (1994) The conformation-dependent lipophilicity of morphine glucuronides as calculated from their molecular lipophilicity potential. *Bioorg. Med. Chem. Lett.* **4,** 737–742.

13. Hudson, B. D., George, A. R., Ford, M. G., and Livingstone, D. J. (1992) Structure-activity relation ships of pyrethroid insecticides. Part 2. The use of molecular dynamics for conformation searching and average parameter calculation. *J. Comput-Aided Mol. Design* **6,** 191–201.

14. Perez, C., Pastor, M., Ortiz, A. R., and Gago, F. (1998) Comparative binding energy analysis of HIV-1 protease inhibitors: incorporation of solvent effects and validation as a powerful tool in receptor based drug design. *J. Med. Chem.* **41,** 836–852.

15. Grassy, G., Yasri, A., Sans, P., Armbruster, A. M., Lahana, R. and Fauchere, J. L. (1997) Molecular dynamics simulations as a tool to investigate the three-dimensional diversity of peptide and pseudopeptide libraries. In *Computer-assisted lead finding and optimization. Current tools for medicinal chemistry*, Van de Waterbeemd, H., Testa, B., and Folkers, G. (eds.), Wiley-VCH, Basel, pp. 209–222.

16. Broto, P., Moreau, G., and Vandycke, C. (1984) Molecular structures: perception, autocorrelation descriptor and SAR studies. System of atomic contributions for the calculation of the n-octanol/water coefficients. *Eur. J. Med. Chem.* **19,** 61–65.
17. Ghose, A. K. and Crippen, G. M. (1986) Atomic physicochemical parameters for three-dimensional-structure-directed quantitative structure-activity relationships. 1. Partition coefficients as a measure of hydrophobicity. *J. Comp. Chem.* **7,** 565–577.
18. Ghose, A. K. and Crippen, G. M. (1987) Atomic physicochemical parameters for three-dimensional-structure-directed quantitative structure-activity relationships. 2. Modeling dispersive and hydrophobic interactions. *J. Chem. Inf. Comput. Sci.* **27,** 21–35.
19. Richards, F. M. (1977) Areas, volumes, packing and protein structure. *Annu. Rev. Biophys. Bioeng.* **6,** 151–176.
20. Lee, B. and Richards, F. M. (1971) The interpretation of protein structures: estimation of static accessibility. *J. Mol. Biol.* **55,** 379–400.
21. Connolly, M. L. (1983) Solvent-accessible surfaces of proteins and nucleic acids. *Science* **221,** 709–713.
22. Vorobjev, Y. N. and Hermans, J. (1997) SIMS: computation of a smooth invariant molecular surface. *Biophys. J.* **73,** 722–732.
23. Zauhar, R. J. (1995) SMART: a solvent-accessible triangulated surface generator for molecular graphics and boundary element applications. *J. Comput.-Aided Mol. Des.* **9,** 149–159.
24. Connolly, M. L. (1993) The molecular surface package. *J. Mol. Graph.* **11,** 139–141.
25. Hartman, J. and Wernecke, J. (eds.) (1996) *The VRML 2.0 handbook. Building moving worlds on the web*, Addison-Wesley Publishing Company, Inc., Reading, MA.
26. Edelsbrunner, H. and Mucke, E. (1994) Three dimensional alpha shapes. *ACM Trans. Graphics* **13,** 43–72.
27. http://esc_plaza.syrres.com/interkow/logkow.htm.
28. Buchwald, P. and Bodor, N. (1998) Octanol-water partition: searching for predictive models. *Curr. Med. Chem.* **5,** 353–380.
29. Weiner, S. J., Kollman, P. A., Case, D. A., et al. (1984) A new force field for molecular mechanical simulation of nucleic acids and proteins, *J. Am. Chem. Soc.* **106,** 765–784.
30. Pastor, M., Perez, C., and Gago, F. (1997) Simulation of alternative binding modes in a structure-based QSAR study of HIV-1 protease inhibitors. *J. Mol. Graph. Model.* **15,** 364–371.
31. Holloway, M. K., Wai, J. M., Halgren, T. A., et al. (1995) *A priori* prediction of activity for HIV-1 protease inhibitors employing energy minimization in the active site. *J. Med. Chem.* **38,** 305–317.
32. Thompson, W. J., Fitzgerald, P. M., Holloway, M. K., et al. (1992) Synthesis and antiviral activity of a series of HIV-1 protease inhibitors with functionality tethered to the P1 or P1′ phenyl substituents: X-ray crystal structure assisted design. *J. Med. Chem.* **35,** 1685–1701.

33. Wold, S. (1995) PLS for multivariate linear modeling. In *Chemometric methods in molecular design*, van de Waterbeemd, H. (ed.), VCH Verlagsgesellshaft mbH, Weinheim, pp.195–218.

34. Kubinyi, H., Ed. (1993) *3D QSAR in drug design theory: methods and applications*, Escom Science, Leiden, pp.523–550.

35. Haaland, D. M. and Thomas, E. V. (1988) Partial least-squares methods for spectral analyses. 1. Relation to other quantitative calibration methods and the extraction of qualitative information. *Anal. Chem.* **60**, 1193–1202.

36. Wakeling, I. N. and Morris, J. J. (1993) A test of significance for partial least squares regression. *J. Chemomet.* **7**, 291–304.

37. Wold, S., Antti, H., Lindgren, F., and Ohman, J. (1998) Orthogonal signal correction of near-infrared spectra. *Chemom. Intell. Lab. Syst.* **44**, 175–185.

38. Sjoblom, J., Svensson, O., Josefson, M., Kullberg, H., and Wold, S. (1998) An evaluation of orthogonal signal correction applied to calibration transfer of near infrared spectra. *Chemom. Intell. Lab. Syst.* **44**, 229–244.

39. Andersson, P. M., Sjöström, M., and Lundstedt, T. (1998) Preprocessing peptide sequences for multivariate sequence-property analysis. *Chemom. Intell. Lab. Syst.* **42**, 41–50.

40. Richards, N. and Williams, P. B. (1994) Conformation dependent partition coefficient calculations. *Chemical Design Automation News* **9**, 20–25.

41. Richards, N., Williams, P. B., and Tute, M. (1991) Empirical methods for computing molecular partition coefficients. I. Upon the need to model the specific hydration of polar groups in fragment based approaches. *Int. J. Quant. Chem.* **18**, 299–316.

42. Richards, N., Williams, P. B., and Tute, M. (1992) Empirical methods for computing molecular partition coefficients. II. Inclusion of conformational flexibility within fragment based approaches. *Int. J. Quant. Chem.* **44**, 219–233.

43. Iwase, K., Komatsu, K., Hirono, S., Nakagawa, S., and Moriguchi, I. (1985) Estimation of hydrophobicity based on the solvent accessible surface area of molecules. *Chem. Pharm. Bull.* **33**, 2114–2121.

44. Masuda, T., Jikihara, T., Nakamura, K., Kimura, A., Takagi, T., and Fujiwara, H. (1997) Introduction of solvent-accessible surface area in the calculation of the hydrophobicity parameter log P from an atomistic approach. *J. Pharm. Sci.* **86**, 57–63.

45. Carrupt, P.A., Testa, B., and Gaillard, P. (1997) Computational approaches to lipophilicity: methods and applications. In *Reviews in computational chemistry*, Lipkowitz, K. B. and Boyd, D. B., (eds.), Wiley-VCH, John Wiley and Sons, Inc., New York, pp.241–315.

46 Steyaert, G., Lisa, G., Gaillard, P., et al. (1997) Intermolecular forces expressed in 1,2-dichloroethane-water partition coefficients. *J. Chem. Soc. Faraday Trans.* **93**, 401–406.

47. de Aguiar, P. F., Bourguignon, B., Khots, M. S., Massart, D. L., and Phan-Than-Luu, R. (1995) D-optimal designs. *Chemometrics Intell. Lab. Sys,* **30**, 199–210.

48. Giraud, E., Luttmann, C., Lavelle, F., Riou, J. F., Mailliet, P., and Laoui, A. (2000) Multivariate data analysis using D-optimal designs, partial least squares and

response surface modeling. A directional approach for the analysis of farnesyl transferase inhibitors. *J. Med. Chem.* **43,** 1807–1816.

49. Clementi, S., Cruciani, G., Baroni, M., and Skagerberg, B. (1991) Selection of informative structures for QSAR studies. *Pharmacochem. Lib.* **16,** 217–226.

50. Baroni, M., Clementi, S., Cruciani, G., Kettaneh, N., and Wold, S. (1993) D-optimal designs in QSAR. *Quant. Struct. Act. Relat.* **12,** 225–231.

51. Oprea, T. I., Waller, C. L., and Marshall, G. R. (1994). Three dimensional quantitative structure-activity relationship of human immunodeficiency virus (I) Protease inhibitors. 2. Predictive power using limited exploration of alternate binding modes. *J. Med. Chem.* **37,** 2206–2215.

52. Waller, C. L., Oprea, T. I., Giolitti, A., and Marshall, G. R. (1993) Three-dimensional QSAR of human immunodeficiency virus (I) protease inhibitors. 1. A COMFA study employing experimentally-determined alignement rules. *J. Med. Chem.* **36,** 4152–4160.

53. Cho, S. J. and Tropsha, A. (1995) Cross-validated R2-guided region selection for comparative molecular field analysis (COMFA): A simple method to achieve consistent results. *J. Med. Chem.* **38,** 1060–1066.

54. Wildman, S. A. and Crippen, G. M. (1999) Prediction of physicochemical parameters by atomic contirbutions. *J. Chem. Inf. Comput. Sci.* **39,** 868–873.

8

Derivation and Applications of Molecular Descriptors Based on Approximate Surface Area

Paul Labute

Abstract

Three sets of molecular descriptors that can be computed from a molecular connection table are defined. The descriptors are based on the subdivision and classification of the molecular surface area according to atomic properties (such as contribution to log$P$, molar refractivity, and partial charge). The resulting 32 descriptors are shown (a) to be weakly correlated with each other; (b) to encode many traditional molecular descriptors; and (c) to be useful for QSAR, QSPAR, and compound classification.

Key Words: Biological activity; molecular descriptor; QSAR; QSPR; molecular surface area; chemistry space.

1. Introduction

The pioneering work of Hansch and Fujita *(1)* and Leo *(2)* was an attempt to describe biological phenomena in a "language" consisting of a small set of experimentally determined physical molecular properties, in particular, log$P$ (octanol/water), pK_a, and molar refractivity. The fundamental concept was that (at least for analog series) differences in biological activity (or other properties) can be described by linear combinations of these few molecular properties (or "descriptors"). This concept is the basis of the fields of Quantitative Structure Activity Relationships (QSAR) and Quantitative Structure Property Relationships (QSPR). Abraham and Platts *(3)* also use a few experimentally determined molecular properties to describe a wide variety of chemical phenomena. The descriptors used include volume, hydrogen bond acidity, hydrogen bond basicity, and molar refractivity. The Hanch, Leo, and Abraham descriptors can be

From: *Methods in Molecular Biology, vol. 275:*
Chemoinformatics: Concepts, Methods, and Tools for Drug Discovery
Edited by: J. Bajorath © Humana Press Inc., Totowa, NJ

considered as "high quality," because they are experimentally determined. Naturally, experimentally determined descriptors are cumbersome for use for large collections of molecules owing to the time and effort required to determine them. For this reason, equally high-quality *calculated* descriptors have been an active area of research.

Calculated descriptors have generally fallen into two broad categories: those that seek to model an experimentally determined or physical descriptor (such as Clog$P$ or CpK_a) and those that are purely mathematical [such as the Kier and Hall connectivity indices *(4)*]. Not surprisingly, the latter category has been heavily populated over the years, so much so that QSAR/QSPR practitioners have had to rely on model validation procedures (such as leave-k-out cross-validation) to avoid models built upon chance correlation. Of course, such procedures are far less critical when very few descriptors are used (such as with the Hansch, Leo, and Abraham descriptors); it can even be argued that they are unnecessary.

It seems reasonable to assume that a few "high-quality" descriptors are more useful than hundreds of "low-quality" descriptors. High-quality descriptors are not restricted to experimentally determined descriptors. Higher levels of theory have been used to construct few but widely applicable descriptors *(5)* suggesting that "chemistry space" is relatively low dimensional. Putting it another way, *the dimensionality of chemistry space is likely related to the quality of the descriptors making up each dimension.*

In the present work, we will use a relatively low level of theory to derive 32 weakly correlated molecular descriptors, each based on the subdivision and classification of the molecular surface area according to three fundamental properties: contribution to Clog$P$, molar refractivity, and atomic partial charge. The resulting collection will be shown to have applicability in QSAR, QSPR, and compound classification. Moreover, the derived 32 descriptors linearly encode most of the information of a collection of "traditional" mathematical descriptors used in QSAR and QSPR.

2. Methods

2.1. The Approximate van der Waals Surface Area

The surface area of an atom in a molecule is the amount of surface area of that atom not contained in any other atom of the molecule (*see* **Fig. 1**). If we assume that the shape of each atom is a sphere with radius equal to the van der Waals radius, we obtain the van der Waals surface area (VSA) for each atom. The sum of the VSA of each atom gives the molecular VSA.

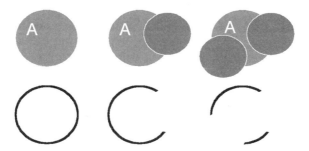

Fig. 1. Assuming spherical atoms, the surface area of atom A is the amount of surface area not contained in other atoms. The depictions are a 2D analogy in which an atom's exposed surface area is represented by its exposed perimeter. Each lower diagram depicts the exposed perimeter of atom A in each upper diagram.

The boundary surface of a region in space is an important physical quantity. The integral of a field in the region is related by the fundamental theorem of calculus to an integral over its boundary surface. A surface integral can be approximated by summing quantities associated with a subdivision of the surface into patches. In the present work, the surface patches are taken to be the (approximate) exposed surface area of atom in a molecule.

Consider two spheres A and B with radii r and s, respectively, and centers separated by a distance d. The amount of surface area of sphere A not contained in sphere B, denoted by V_A, is given by

$$V_A = \begin{cases} 4\pi r^2 - \pi r d^{-1}[s^2 - (r-d)^2] & \text{if } |r-s| < d < r+s \\ 4\pi r^2 & \text{otherwise} \end{cases} \tag{1}$$

The case of more than two spheres is more complicated, because a portion of sphere A may be contained in several other spheres. However, we will neglect this complication (in the hope that the error introduced will not be large). Thus, we approximate the VSA for sphere A with n neighboring spheres B_i with radii s_i and at distances d_i as

$$V_A = 4\pi r^2 - \pi r \sum_{i=1}^{n} \frac{s_i^2 - (r-d_i)^2}{d_i} \delta(|r-s_i| < d_i < r+s_i) \tag{2}$$

where the generalized delta function, $\delta(P)$, adopts a value of 1 if the condition P is satisfied and 0 otherwise. This formula is similar to the pairwise approximations used in approximate overlap volume calculations and approximate surface area calculations for generalized Born implicit solvent models (*6*). In a molecule of n atoms each with van der Waals radius R_i, let B_i denote the set of all atoms bonded to atom i. Neglect the effect of atoms not related by a bond and define the VSA for atom i, denoted by V_i, to be

$$V_i = 4\pi R_i^2 - \pi R_i \sum_{j \in B_i} \frac{R_j^2 - (R_i - d_{ij})^2}{d_{ij}} \tag{3}$$

$$d_{ij} = \min\{\max\{| R_i - R_j |, b_{ij}\}, R_i + R_j\}\}$$

where b_{ij} is the ideal bond length between atoms i and j. The approximate VSA for each atom can be calculated from connection table information alone assuming a dictionary of van der Waals radii and ideal bond lengths. In the present work the radii are derived from MMFF94 *(7)* with certain modifications for polar hydrogen atoms. The ideal bond length b_{ij} between atoms i and j was calculated according to the formula $b_{ij} = s_{ij} - o_{ij}$, where s_{ij} is a reference bond length taken from MMFF94 parameters that depends on the two elements involved and o_{ij} is a correction that depends on the bond order: 0 for single, 0.15 for aromatic, 0.2 for double, and 0.3 for triple. Finally, the approximate VSA for an entire molecule is just the sum of the V_i for each atom i in the molecule. The VSA of a molecule varies less than 2% between conformations. The approximate VSA is accurate to within 10% of a three-dimensional calculation and is independent of conformation (*see* **Fig. 2**).

Thus, we have defined V_i, the contribution of atom i to the approximate VSA of a molecule. This contribution is reasonably accurate and has the advantage that it can be calculated using just connection table information and much more rapidly than the 3D VSA contribution. The approximate molecular VSA is very much a 2-½D descriptor: it is (highly correlated to) a conformation independent 3D property that requires only 2D connection information.

2.2. Subdivision of the VSA with Binary Atomic Properties

A polar surface area approximation can be calculated by summing the V_i contribution of each polar atom in a molecule. A hydrophobic surface area approximation can be calculated by V_i contribution of each hydrophobic atom in a molecule. More generally, for a given binary property B_i (such as "is polar" or "is aromatic" or "is acceptor") for each atom i in a molecule, an approximate surface-area based descriptor can be calculated with

$$B\_VSA = \sum_i V_i \delta(B_i). \tag{4}$$

Surface-area-based descriptors tend to be more useful than simple atom counts because they take connectivity into account (and also, because of the surface integral motivation). For example, surface-area-based descriptors can

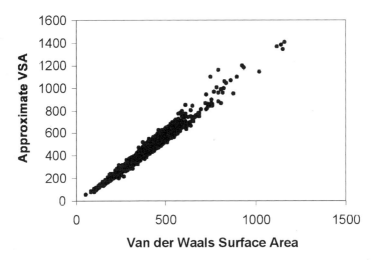

Fig. 2. A scatter plot of the approximate VSA for approx 2000 small molecules versus their VSA calculated with a high-density dot counting method using 3D coordinates of a conformation of each molecule. The correlation has an r^2 of 0.97 with a relative error was less than 10%. Most of the errors occurred for the larger molecules and in molecules with many atoms in fused ring systems.

distinguish hexane from cyclohexane because the surface areas are different. Indeed, for alkanes, the surface areas of each carbon atom with different heavy-atom coordination numbers will be different. With the described 2D approximation, surface-area-based descriptors of alkanes will reduce to branching-factor descriptors.

This surface area classification notion naturally can be extended to other properties. For example, a collection of pharmacophore-type VSA descriptors can be calculated by summing the V_i contribution of each in a molecule of a specific type. For example, if the atom classes are "donor," "acceptor," "polar," "hydrophobe," "anion," and "cation," then six VSA descriptors can be calculated such that for any given molecule the sum of the six descriptors is the VSA of the entire molecule and each descriptor is the VSA of all atoms one of the six classes. Such descriptors can be used for rough pharmacophore-based similarity measures.

2.3. Subdivision of the VSA with General Atomic Properties

We turn now to non-binary properties of each atom in a molecule. Suppose that for each atom i in a molecule we are given a numeric property P_i. Our fundamental idea is to create a descriptor consisting of the sum of VSA contributions of each atom with P_i in a specific range $[u,v)$. (The expression $[u,v)$

denotes the half closed interval $\{x : u \leq x \leq v\}$.) More precisely, we define the quantity P_VSA(u,v) to be

$$P\_VSA(u,v) = \sum_i V_i \delta(P_i \in [u,v)) \tag{5}$$

where V_i is the atomic contribution of atom i to the VSA of the molecule. We now define a set of n descriptors associated with the property P as follows:

$$P\_VSA_k = \sum_i V_i \delta(P_i \in [a_{k-1}, a_k)) \quad k = 1,2,...n \tag{6}$$

where $a_0 < a_k < a_n$ are interval boundaries such that $[a_0, a_n)$ bound all values of P_i in any molecule. **Figure 3** is an example of the calculation of a hypothetical set of descriptors from a chemical structure. Each VSA-type descriptor can be characterized as *the amount of surface area with P in a certain range*. If, for a given set of n descriptors, the interval ranges span all values, then the sum of the n descriptors will be the VSA of the molecule. Therefore, these VSA-type descriptors correspond to a subdivision of the molecular surface area.

Wildman and Crippen's recent methods *(8)* for calculating log$P$ (octanol/water) and molar refractivity (MR) provide a good basis for VSA analogs of log$P$ and MR, because these methods were parametrized with atomic contributions in mind. Both methods assign a numeric contribution to each atom in a molecule. Interval boundaries can be obtained by gathering statistics on a large database of 44,000+ small organic compounds [say from the Maybridge *(9)* catalog]. Interval boundaries are chosen so that the resulting intervals are equally populated over the database (resulting in non-uniform width boundaries). Such a procedure leads to 10 descriptors for log$P$ and 8 descriptors for MR. For the Maybridge catalog, the respective interval boundaries for log$P$ are ($-\infty$, -0.4, -0.2, 0, 0.1, 0.15, 0.2, 0.25, 0.3, 0.4, ∞) and the interval boundaries for MR are (0, 0.11, 0.26, 0.35, 0.39, 0.44, 0.485, 0.56, ∞). Alternatively, uniform interval boundaries can be used; for example, the Gasteiger (PEOE) method *(10)* of calculating partial charges require approx 14 uniform-interval descriptors: ($-\infty$, -0.3, -0.25, -0.20, -0.15, -0.10, -0.05, 0, 0.05, 0.10, 0.15, 0.20, 0.25, 0.30, ∞).

We have thus defined three sets of molecular descriptors:

- SlogP_VSA$_k$ (10) intended to capture hydrophobic and hydrophilic effects;
- SMR_VSA$_k$ (8) intended to capture polarizability;
- PEOE_VSA$_k$ (14) intended to capture direct electrostatic interactions.

Each of these descriptor sets is derived from, or related to, the Hansch and Leo descriptors with the expectation that they would be widely applicable. Taken together the VSA descriptors define, nominally, a $10 + 8 + 14 = 32$ dimen-

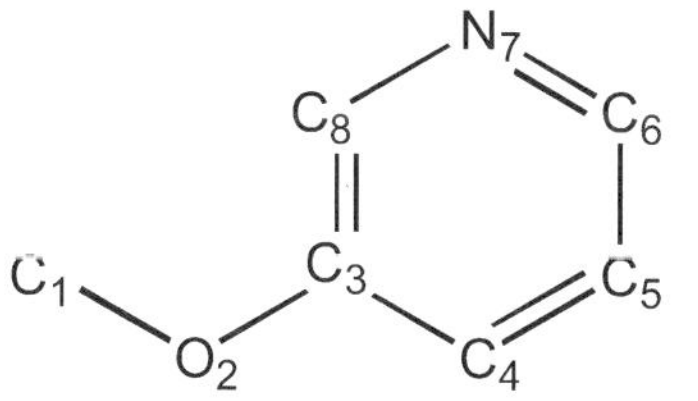

$$P_1°=°2.4 \quad V_1°=°9.2$$
$$P_2°=°1.2 \quad V_2°=°6.3$$
$$P_3°=°4.5 \quad V_3°=°2.2$$
$$P_4°=°5.9 \quad V_4°=°4.5$$
$$P_5°=°5.7 \quad V_5°=°4.5$$
$$P_6°=°3.1 \quad V_6°=°4.4$$
$$P_7°=°0.2 \quad V_7°=°4.6$$
$$P_8°=°3.9 \quad V_8°=°4.4$$

$$D_1 = P\_VSA(0,2) = V_2+V_7 = 6.3 + 4.6 \quad = 10.9$$

$$D_2 = P\_VSA(2,3) = V_1 \quad = 9.2$$

$$D_3 = P\_VSA(3,4) = V_6+V_8 = 4.4 + 4.4 \quad = 8.8$$

$$D_4 = P\_VSA(4,5) = V_3 \quad = 2.2$$

$$D_5 = P\_VSA(5,6) = V_4+V_5 = 4.5 + 4.5 \quad = 9.0$$

Fig. 3. The calculation of a hypothetical set of five VSA descriptors $D_1, \ldots, D_5$ based upon a property P. The chemical structure consists of eight atoms each with the given property value P_i and VSA contribution V_i.

sional chemistry space (less two dimensions because all three sets for a particular molecule sum to the molecular VSA).

2.4. Weak Correlation of Descriptors

The orthogonality of a set of molecular descriptors is a very desirable property. Classification methodologies such as CART *(11)* (or other decision-tree methods) are not invariant to rotations of the chemistry space. Such methods may encounter difficulties with correlated descriptors (e.g., production of larger decision trees). Often, correlated descriptors necessitate the use of principal components transforms that require a set of reference data for their estimation (at worst, the transforms depend only on the data at hand and, at best, they are trained once from some larger collection of compounds). In probabilistic methodologies, such as Binary QSAR *(12)*, approximation of statistical independence is simplified when uncorrelated descriptors are used. In addition, descriptor transformations can lead to difficulties in model interpretation. At first, it would appear that these descriptors would be highly correlated since they are derived from only three property types. However, this is not the case. **Figure 4** presents the results of a correlation analysis conducted on a database of approx 2,000 small molecules.

Among the SMR_VSA descriptors (rows/cols 25–32), the largest r value was 0.6 ($r^2 = 0.36$), which appeared once; the remaining pairs exhibited r values less than 0.27 ($r^2 = 0.07$), so SMR_VSA descriptors are, for the most part, weakly correlated with each other. Among the SlogP_VSA descriptors (rows/cols 15–24), the largest r value was 0.42 ($r^2 = 0.18$), which appeared once; the remaining pairs exhibited r values less than 0.27 ($r^2 = 0.07$), so the logP descriptors are, for the most part, weakly correlated with each other. Among the PEOE_VSA descriptors (rows/cols 1–14), the largest r value was 0.65 ($r^2 = 0.42$), so the PEOE_VSA descriptors are, for the most part, weakly correlated with each other. In the full correlation matrix, the intercorrelation between the descriptors generally is weak; however, seven r values are larger than 0.7 ($r^2 = 0.49$). At first glance, the sets seem to exhibit higher correlation than in the intraset cases. However, it must be remembered that for a given molecule each PEOE_VSA, SlogP_VSA, and SMR_VSA descriptor collection sums to the VSA of the molecule; hence, there two less dimensions than the nominal $14 + 10 + 8 = 32$. The correlation results strongly suggest that the VSA descriptors are weakly correlated with each other. As a consequence, we expect that methodologies such as Binary QSAR, CART, Principal Components Analysis, Principal Components Clustering, Neural Networks, k-means Clustering, etc., to be more effective (when measured over many problem instances).

2.5. Encoding of Traditional Descriptors

The SlogP, SMR, and PEOE_VSA descriptors have rich information content and can be used in place of many traditional descriptors *(13–17)*. **Figure 5** presents the results of a collection of 64 linear models each of which approximates a traditional descriptor as a linear combination of the VSA descriptors (trained on approx 2,000 small molecules). Out of the 64 descriptors, 32 showed an r^2 of 0.90 or better and 49 had an r^2 of 0.80 or better, and 61 showed an r^2 of 0.5 or better. Descriptors related to flexibility are poorly modeled. In particular, the Lipinksi parameters logP, acceptor count, donor count, and molecular weight are

---

Fig. 4. *(see facing page)* The full correlation matrix of r values (in unsigned percent) between the PEOE_VSA descriptors (rows/cols 1–14), SlogP_VSA descriptors (rows/cols 15–24), and SMR_VSA descriptors (rows/cols 25–32). The values can be converted to r^2 by dividing by 100 and squaring.

	1	2	3	4	5	6	7	8	9	10	11	12	13	14	15	16	17	18	19	20	21	22	23	24	25	26	27	28	29	30	31	32
1:	10	10	2	8	7	13	13	43	15	2	13	7	25	5	0	4	24	35	23	37	11	1	54	27	22	1	9	21	12	41	43	42
2:	10		19		16	11	2	23	14	7		4	9	29	21	5	28	49	12	27	12		20	2	17	28	3	42	11	23	50	16
3:	2	19		21	30			1	27		4	11	5	43	54	12	31	8		4		44	20	4	16	46	9	48	43	18	8	2
4:	8		21		26	9	16	8	20	5		24	31	26	41	37	25	4				14	12	0		19	47	11	40	14	0	4
5:	7	16	30	26		8	9	4	7	1		11	42	53	76	15	52	0	6	2	5	11	8	5	34	19	20	50	38	3	0	4
6:	13	11		9	8		2		20		7		61	17		31	46	3	34		24	12	9	4	37	65	7	11	6	1	8	22
7:	13	2		16	9	2		23	11								4	1		2	5		9	21	62	12	15	13	38	10	8	
8:	43	23	1	8	4		23			8	8	65	42				11	15	30	20	11	16	15	8	31	5	5	25	6	25	1	5
9:	15	14	27	20	7	20	20			3	11	19	61			20		6			22	29	26	39	7	22	13	4	15	43	22	45
10:	2	7		5	1			8	3		5	4	17	21	19	20	7	4	30	20	11	56	26	19	8	2	2	0	0	64	9	14
11:	13		4			7		8	11			1	8	3	4	3	6	7	2	4	3	12	10	23	5	27	2	1	3	10	7	19
12:	7	4	11	24	11	4	22	9	24	5	1		6	4	5	23	6	4	6	2	24	4	12	9	9	4	7	17	0	22	1	9
13:	25	9	5	31	42	61	65	42	19	4	8	6		23	67	27	69	4	40	5		20	20	22	20	15	11	46	11	-3	0	2
14:	5	29	43	26	53	17				4	3	4	23		32	69	39	1	0	6	21	6	14	3	4	36	14	42	42	-4	18	19
15:	0	21	54	41	76					2	4	5	67	32		27	74	15	5	2	10	14	2	51	78	71	24	65	57	10	2	10
16:	4	5	12	37	15	31			20	3	3	23	27	69	27		14	4	6	7	4	16	3	27	36	51	14	46	23	4	7	2
17:	24	28	31	25	52	46	4	11		7	6	6	69	39	74	14		4	13	4	21	16	14	3	27	29	20	10	22	10	0	
18:	35	49	8	4	0	3	1	15	6	4	7	4	4	1	15	4	4		15	11	10	22	6	27	1	4	15	46	11	7	19	2
19:	23	12			6	34		30		30	2	6	40	0	5	6	13	15		3	14	10	14	8	30	15	23	10	30		90	31
20:	37	27	4		2		2	20	11	20	4	2	5	1	2	7	4	11	3		10	10	10	11	23	9	23	3	4	7	12	1
21:	11	12			5	21	31	11	22	11	5	24		21	10	4	21	10	14	10		9	8	21	12	1	7	20	21	6	20	8
22:	1		44	14	11	12		16	29	56		4	20	6	16	16	14	22	10	10	9		6	16	1		8	60	11	10	6	36
23:	54	20	20	12	8	9	23	15	26	26	10	12	20	14	2	3	14	6	14	10	8	6		25	20	60	12	3	27	13	20	22
24:	27	2	4	0	5	4	20	8	39	19	23	9	22	3	51	27	3	27	8	10	14	16	6		18	21	9		18	71	10	
25:	22	17	16		34	5	62	31	7	8	5	9	20	36	71	36	27	1	30	23	12	1	14	25		1	20	10	21	55	13	83
26:	1	28	46	34	19	12		5	22	3	27	4	15	14	24	51	29	4	15	23	1		3	2	1		60	3	4	10	9	3
27:	9	3	9	19	65	5	15	5	13	2	7	11	25	14	24	14	20	15	2	8	4	8	11	8	20	60		3	12	9	3	17
28:	21	42	48	11	50	7	13	25	4	2	1	17	15	46	65	7	46	10	23	8	21	60	55	10	18	21	3		12	6	11	15
29:	12	11	43	40	38	3	6	6	15	0	3	0	11	42	57	12	22	7	4	22	10	11	4	13	1	9	12	12		11	3	13
30:	41	23	18	14	3	1	1	25	42	5	10	22	13	14	10	2	71	90	22	2	10	71	55	10	20	6	27	6	11		12	12
31:	43	50	8	0	0	8	10	22	9	7	0	0	18	-4	2	7	0	19	12	10		12	4	83		3		12	3	12		8
32:	42	16	2	4	4	22		5	14	19	9	2	10	19	10	2		2	31	1	8	36	2		22	1	17	15	13	13	8	

Name	r^2	Name	r^2	Name	r^2	Name	r^2
Chi0 [a]	0.99	Chi0v_C [a]	0.97	b_ar [h]	0.89	B_1rotN [i]	0.78
Kier1 [a]	0.99	KierA1 [a]	0.97	Kier2 [a]	0.89	B_double [h]	0.77
Vdw_area [b]	0.99	a_hyd [d]	0.96	vsa_pol [c]	0.89	B_rotN [i]	0.77
Vdw_vol [b]	0.99	a_nC [e]	0.96	vsa_acc [c]	0.88	A_ICM [f]	0.73
Vsa_hyd [c]	0.99	a_nH [e]	0.96	diameter [m]	0.87	vsa_don [c]	0.73
a_count [e]	0.98	a_nO [e]	0.95	VadjEq [f]	0.87	KierFlex [a]	0.69
a_heavy [e]	0.98	b_heavy [h]	0.95	a_nN [e]	0.86	balabanJ [l]	0.61
a_IC [f]	0.98	Chi1_C [a]	0.95	KierA2 [a]	0.86	A_nP [e]	0.60
apol [g]	0.98	Chi1v_C [a]	0.95	radius [m]	0.86	Kier3 [a]	0.57
b_count [h]	0.98	SlogP [j]	0.95	VdistMa [f]	0.86	A_nCl [e]	0.56
Chi0v [a]	0.98	a_acc [d]	0.94	weinerPath [n]	0.85	KierA3 [a]	0.55
Chi1 [a]	0.98	Chi1v [a]	0.94	weinerPol [n]	0.84	A_nS [e]	0.53
SMR [j]	0.98	Weight [k]	0.93	VadjMa [f]	0.82	B_1rotR [i]	0.50
b_single [h]	0.97	a_aro [e]	0.91	VdistEq [f]	0.82	density [b]	0.49
bpol [g]	0.97	a_don [d]	0.91	vsa_other [c]	0.82	B_rotR [i]	0.48
Chi0_C [a]	0.97	zagreb [o]	0.91	a_nF [e]	0.80	B_triple [h]	0.46

Fig. 5. The r^2 correlation coefficients for linear models of traditional descriptors as a function of the 32 VSA descriptors. Notes: (a) connectivity and kappa shape indices (4); (b) van der Waals surface area, volume, and density; (c) vsa_hyd, vsa_don, etc., refer to van der Waals surface areas of hydrophobic, H-bond donor atoms, etc.; (d) a_hyd, a_don, and a_acc refer to the number of hydrophobic, H-bond donor, and H-bond acceptor atoms; (e) a_count, a_heavy, a_nC, a_nH, etc., refer to element counts; (f) element and graph adjacency matrix entropy; (g) sum of *CRC Handbook* atomic and bond polarizabilities; (h) b_count, b_heavy, etc., are the number of bonds, aromatic, single double, and triple bonds; (i) total and fractional rotatable bonds; (j) log$P$ (octanol/water) and molar refractivity; (k) molecular weight; (l) Balaban's J index (13); (m) graph extents (14); (n) Wiener indices (17); (o) the Zagreb index.

270

all modeled with an r^2 better than 0.91. These results suggest that the 32 VSA descriptors encode much of the information contained in most of the 64 popular descriptors and can replace them. The use of many descriptors in a particular QSAR/QSPR situation can often lead to chance correlation. In general, it is preferable to use a relatively small, fixed collection of descriptors across many problem instances to reduce the likelihood of chance correlations notwithstanding the existence of methods to automatically select the appropriate descriptors from a large pool *(18)*. The use of a fixed collection of descriptors reduces the reliance on validation methods to identify spurious models (e.g., leave-one-out or *k*-fold cross-validation).

3. Applications

3.1. Quantitative Structure–Property Relationships

We now consider some applications of the presented VSA descriptors to the quantitative modeling of molecular properties. **Figure 6** presents the results of the linear modeling of the free energy of solvation *(19)* of a small molecule and the boiling point of a small molecule using only the described VSA descriptors. The r^2 in both cases was better than 90% and better than 88% on a leave-100-out validation test. **Figure 6** also presents the results of the linear modeling of the blood-brain barrier permeability *(20)* (r^2 of 0.83) and the solubility in water *(21)* of small molecules (r^2 of 0.75). The presented models are not intended to be definitive models of the properties. What is noteworthy is that the same set of descriptors that were used throughout. This strongly suggests that "chemistry space" defined by the VSA descriptors would find utility in chemical diversity and ADME assessment studies in which a compound is mapped to a 32-dimensional vector (of VSA descriptors), which is then used as a surrogate for comparision with other molecules (similarly mapped) when clustering compounds.

3.2. Quantitative Structure–Activity Relationships

It has been argued *(22)* the "traditional" descriptors such as log*P*, pK_a, and MR are more relevant to drug transport or pharmacokinetics than to receptor affinity. However, one says that a descriptor is strongly related to a particular property when effective QSPR models of the property have been made using the descriptor. Failure to produce a QSAR/QSPR model using a descriptor is *not*, in general, evidence of a lack of relevance. The relevance of descriptors must be evaluated either from theoretical considerations or long-term empirical success. Indeed, recent work *(23)* has suggested that the underlying atomic contributions to partial charge, molar refractivity, and log*P* *are* relevant to receptor affinity. The VSA descriptors represent a hydrophobicity, polarizabil-

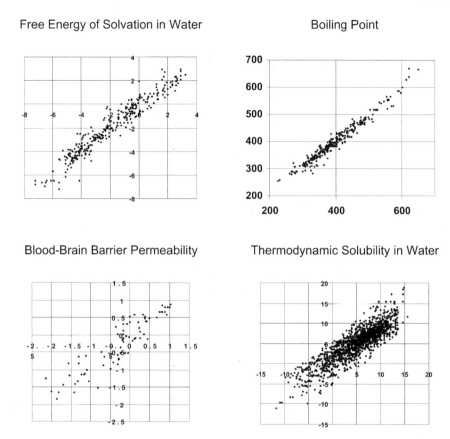

Fig. 6. Calculated (*y*-axis) and experimental (*x*-axis) molecular properties. Top Left: free energy of solvation in kcal/mol for 291 small organic molecules. Top Right: boiling points (in Kelvin) of 298 small organic molecules. Bottom Left: the log concentration ratio between the blood and brain for 75 compounds. Bottom Right: the solubility in water of 1438 small organic compounds (units are log concentration ratios).

ity, and electrostatic profile of a particular molecule, and these properties are indeed relevant to receptor affinity and ligand recognition. It is an added advantage that the underlying properties used in the definition of the VSA descriptors are possibly relevant to drug transport or pharmacokinetics.

One might fear that the "traditional" descriptors are "whole molecule" properties that cannot distinguish the details of important substructural differences. It is difficult to quantify the wholism of a descriptor. A qualitative definition might be that a "whole molecule" property is one in which small bioisosteric

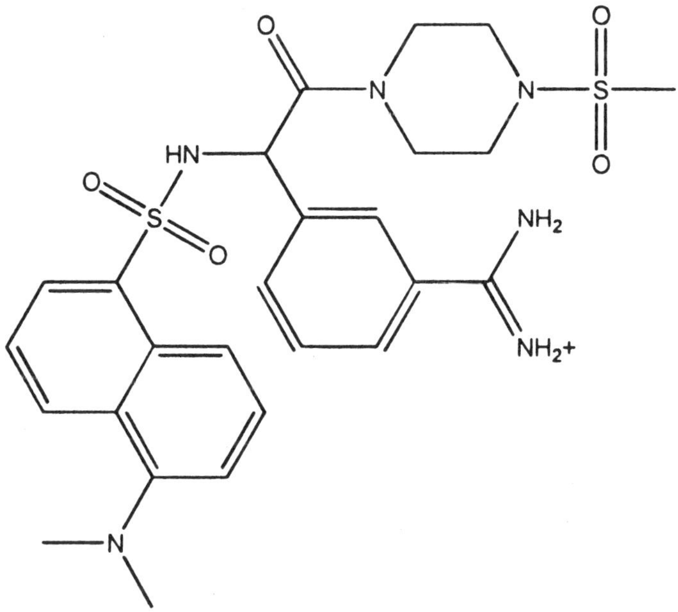

Fig. 7. A representative structure from a series of 72 compounds each of which was assayed against thrombin, trypsin, and factor Xa.

modifications to the structure lead to large changes in the descriptor value. It is interesting to note that BCUT *(24)* values [extensions of Burden *(25)* numbers derived from graph adjacency or distance matrix eigenvalues] are likely to exhibit far more wholism than more group-additive properties (such as log$P$ and free energy of solvation). Nevertheless, BCUT values have shown utility in QSAR/QSPR studies *(26)* and diversity work. Descriptors such as HOMO and LUMO energies are very wholistic and even these have been used successfully in QSAR work. The atomic VSA contributions are sensitive to connectivity and the properties considered (log$P$, MR, and charge) are sensitive to the chemical context of each atom. Moreover, each of the VSA descriptors is fundamentally additive in nature, which suggests a more reductionist than wholist character. The high correlations seen when modeling other descriptors such as number of nitrogens, number of oxygens, and number of aromatic atoms support this reductionist assertion.

We now consider some applications of the VSA descriptors to receptor affinity modeling. **Figure 7** depicts a typical structure of a series of 72 compounds each of which has been assayed against each of thrombin, trypsin, and factor Xa *(27)*. The PEOE_VSA, Slog$P$_VSA, and SMR_VSA descriptors were calculated for each structure and a principal components linear regression was calculated for each receptor, i.e., for each receptor the experimental pK_i was modeled with a linear combination of VSA descriptors. For each activity model, descriptors with small (normalized) coefficients were discarded. Using the remaining descriptors a principal components regression was calculated. For thrombin, a 10-descriptor model using PEOE_VSA$_{1,2,5,8,10,11,12}$ and SlogP_VSA$_{1,5,9}$ resulted in an r^2 of 0.65 with an RMSE of 0.61 pK_i (*see* **Fig. 8** left); the leave-one-out cross-validated r^2 was 0.54 with an RMSE of 0.70 pK_i. For trypsin, a 9-descriptor model using PEOE_VSA$_{1,8,11,12}$, SlogP_VSA$_{0,3,4,8}$, and SMR_VSA$_5$ resulted in an r^2 of 0.72 with an RMSE of 0.47 pK_i (*see* **Fig. 8** middle); the leave-one-out cross-validated r^2 was 0.62 with an RMSE of 0.54 pK_i. For factor Xa, a 15-descriptor model using PEOE_VSA$_{1,2,8,9,12,14}$, SlogP_VSA$_{5,7,8,10}$, and SMR_VSA$_{3,4,5,6,8}$ resulted in an r^2 of 0.69 with an RMSE of 0.35 pK_i (*see* **Fig. 8** right); the leave-one-out cross-validated r^2 was 0.52 with an RMSE of 0.45 pK_i. These results suggest that the VSA descriptors can distinguish the relatively small differences in a congeneric series of compounds. It should be noted that these models are not intended to be definitive; they are intended to show the applicability of the VSA descriptors to receptor affinity modeling.

The automation of physical experiments through robotics to effectively perform hundreds of thousands or millions of experiments in a short time has opened the door to a large-scale approach to drug discovery. High-throughput screening (HTS) and combinatorial chemistry offer access to a huge set of candidate structures; however, time and economic considerations require a selection of only a subset of this vast space for physical testing. Unfortunately, most people (if not all) find it very difficult to interpret all of the HTS data when effecting a focused combinatorial library design. HTS QSAR is an alternative to human inspection of HTS data. In this alternative, a set of HTS results are considered to be "understood" if an effective QSAR model can be constructed (by effective, we mean statistically significant). The activity of new compounds (for example, in a proposed library) can be predicted with the model. The PEOE_VSA descriptors have been used quite successfully in several HTS QSAR attempts *(28)* using the Binary QSAR method. Accuracy levels of 40–70% have been routinely observed on active compounds on datasets with hit rates well below 1% (inactives usually exhibit >90% accuracy). It is hoped that the SlogP_VSA and SMR_VSA descriptors will improve the accuracy levels (although the PEOE_VSA accuracy levels still resulted in significant enrichment when compared to the hit rate).

Data from HTS often has a relatively high error or noise content and provides a very low precision activity measure, often binary ("pass–fail"). This effectively makes linear activity modeling impossible and classification-based QSAR methods must be employed. The database of 455 compounds, each active against one

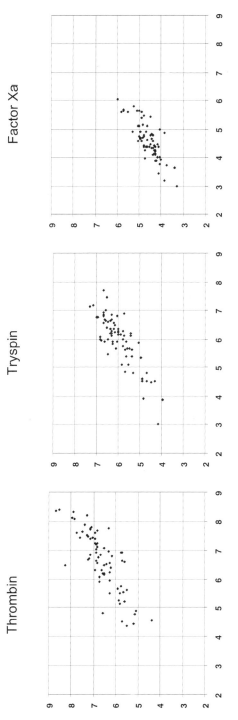

Fig. 8. Experimental (x-axis) and calculated (y-axis) pK_i values for a series of 72 compounds. The calculated values are linear models using the VSA descriptors.

of seven receptors, described in Xue et al. *(29)*, serves as a test set for compound classification. The database consisted of seven fairly congeneric classes:

    Class 1: Serotonin receptor ligands
    Class 2: Benzodiazepine receptor ligands
    Class 3: Carbonic anhydrase II inhibitors
    Class 4: Cyclooxygenase-2 (Cox-2) inhibitors
    Class 5: H3 antagonists
    Class 6: HIV protease inhibitors
    Class 7: Tyrosine kinase inhibitors

Binary QSAR is a probabilistic classification methodology based on Bayesian inference in which no regression procedure is used. A training set is used to model the probability Pr(active | molecule), which is the probability of observing an activity value of 1 given a particular molecule (as opposed to an activity value of 0). A total of seven Binary QSAR models were made from the VSA descriptors calculated from 455 compounds as follows. Model i was trained on a dataset consisting of "active" molecules (those that were active against the receptor of class i) and "inactive" molecules (those that were not active against the receptor of class i). The Binary QSAR model was constructed from these descriptors in an effort to predict membership in class i. The accuracy of prediction and the p value (probability of a chance occurrence) for each model was found to be:

    Class 1:   **98.7%** $p = 0.003$
    Class 2:   **96.7%** $p = 0.043$
    Class 3:   **96.5%** $p = 0.290$
    Class 4:   **98.7%** $p = 0.001$
    Class 5:   **98.7%** $p = 0.014$
    Class 6:   **98.7%** $p = 0.012$
    Class 7:   **99.1%** $p = 0.002$

Each of the models exhibited high accuracy and all but one (class 3: carbonic anhydrase II inhibitors) exhibited high significance in the χ-squared significance test. A similar classification model was built using the CART methodology with similar but lower accuracy. The results suggest that the collection of VSA descriptors define a "chemistry space" that could be put to good use in a chemoinformatics, chemical diversity, or HTS data analysis context.

4. Summary

We have derived three sets of (easily calculated) molecular descriptors based on atomic contributions to log$P$, molar refractivity, and atomic partial charge. The individual descriptors were found to be weakly correlated with each other (over a suitably large collection of compounds). Moreover, the chemistry space determined by the new descriptors was capable of expressing (as linear combinations) traditional QSAR/QSPR descriptors. Reasonably good QSAR/QSPR models of boiling point, free energy of solvation in water, water solubility, receptor class, and activity against thrombin, trypsin, and factor Xa were built using only these descriptors. The procedure used to derive these VSA descriptors can be applied to properties other than logP, MR, and partial charge. Although only atom-type based models of these properties were used, the methodology does not preclude the use of higher levels of theory.

References

1. Hansch, C. and Fujita,T. (1964) ρ-σ-π analysis. A method for the correlation of biological activity and chemical structure. *J. Am. Chem. Soc.* **86,** 1616–1626.
2. Leo, A., Hansch, C., and Church, C. (1969) Comparison of parameters currently used in the study of structure-activity relationships. *J. Med. Chem.* **12,** 766–771.
3. Abraham, M. H. and Platts, J. A. (2001) Hydrogen bond structural group constants. *J. Org. Chem.* **66(10),** 3484–3491.
4. Hall, L. H. and Kier, L. B. (1991) The molecular connectivity chi indices and kappa shape indices in structure-property modeling. In *Reviews of computational chemistry*, Boyd, D. B. and Lipkowitz, K. (eds.), Vol. 2.
5. Klamt, A. and Schuurmann, G. (1993) COSMO: a new approach to dielectric screening in solvents with explicit expressions for the screening energy and its gradient. *J. Chem. Soc. Perkin Trans.* **2,** 799–805.
6. Wodak, S. J. and Janin, J. (1980) Analytical approximation to the solvent accessible surface area of proteins. *Proc. Natl. Acad. Sci. USA* **77,** 1736–1740.
7. Halgren, T. A. (1996) MMFF94: The Merck force field. *J. Comp. Chem.* **17(5),** 490–512.
8. Wildman, S. A. and Crippen, G. M. (1999) Prediction of physicochemical parameters by atomic contributions. *J. Chem. Inf. Comput. Sci.* **39(5),** 868–873.
9. Maybridge Chemical Company Ltd., Cornwall, PL34 OHW England. URL: www.maybridge.co.uk.
10. Gasteiger, J. and Marsali. M. (1980) Iterative partial equalization of orbital electronegativity—a rapid access to atomic charges. *Tetrahedron* **36,** 3219–3225.
11. Breiman, L., Friedman, J., Olshen, R. A., and Stone, C. J. (1984) *Classification and regression trees*. Wadsworth Inc.
12. Labute, P. (1999) Binary QSAR: a new method for quantitative structure activity relationships. *Proceedings of the 1999 Pacific Symposium*, World Scientific Publishing, Singapore.
13. Balaban, A. T. (1979) Five new topological indices for the branching of tree-like graphs. *Theor. Chim. Acta* **53,** 355–375.
14. Petitjean, M. (1992) Applications of the radius-diameter diagram to the classification of topological and geometrical shapes of chemical compounds. *J. Chem. Inf. Comput. Sci.* **32,** 331–337.

15. Pearlman, R. S. and Smith, K. M. (1998) Novel software tools for chemical diversity. *Perspectives Drug Discovery Design* **9,** 339–353.
16. Todeschini, R., Lasagni, R., and Marengo, E. (1994) New molecular descriptors for 2D and 3D structures. Theory. *J. Chemometrics* **8,** 263–272.
17. Wiener, H. (1947) Structural determination of paraffin boiling points. *J. Am. Chem. Soc.* **69,** 17–20.
18. Rogers, D. and Hopfinger, A. J. (1994) Application of genetic function approximation to quantitative structure-activity relationships and quantitative structure-property relationships. *J. Chem. Inf. Comput. Sci.* **34,** 854–866.
19. Viswanadhan, V. N., Ghose, A. K., Singh, U. C., and Wendoloski, J. J. (1999) Prediction of solvation free energies of small organic molecules: additive-constitutive models based on molecular fingerprints and atomic constants. *J. Chem. Inf. Comput. Sci.* **39,** 405–412.
20. Luco, J. M. (1999) Prediction of the brain-blood distribution of a large set of drugs from structurally derived descriptors using partial least squares (PLS) methodology. *J. Chem. Info. Comput. Sci.* **36,** 396–404.
21. Syracuse Research Corporation, 6225 Running Ridge Road, North Syracuse, NY 13212 (URL:www.syrres.com).
22. Pearlman, R. S. and Smith, K. M. (1999) Metric validation and the receptor-relevant subspace concept. *J. Chem. Inf. Comput. Sci.* **39,** 28–35.
23. Crippen, G. M. (1999) VRI: 3D QSAR at variable resolution. *J. Chem. Inf. Comput. Sci.* **20,** 1577–1585.
24. Pearlman, R. S. and Smith, K. M. (1998) Novel software tools for chemical diversity. *Perspectives Drug Discovery Design* **9,** 339–353.
25. Burden, F. R. (1989) Molecular identification number for substructure searches. *J. Chem. Inf. Comput. Sci.* **29,** 225–227.
26. Stanton, D. T. (1999) Evaluation and use of BCUT descriptors in QSAR and QSPR studies. *J. Chem. Inf. Comput. Sci.* **39,** 11–20.
27. Bohm, M., Sturzebecher, J., and Klebe, G. (1999) Three-dimensional quantitative structure-activity relationship analyses using comparative molecular field analysis and comparative molecular similarity indices analysis to elucidate selectivity differences of inhibitors binding to trypsin, thrombin and factor Xa. *J. Med. Chem.* **42,** 458–477.
28. Labute, P. (1998,1999) *Unpublished work.*
29. Xue, L., Godden, J., Gao, H., and Bajorath, J. (1999) Identification of a preferred set of molecular descriptors for compound classification based on principal component analysis. *J. Chem. Inf. Comput. Sci.* **39,** 699–674.

9

Cell-Based Partitioning

Ling Xue, Florence L. Stahura, and Jürgen Bajorath

Abstract

Partitioning techniques are widely used to classify compound sets or databases according to specific chemical or biological criteria. Partitioning is conceptually related to, yet algorithmically distinct from, conventional clustering methods and is particularly suitable for efficient processing of very large compound sets. Currently, some of the most popular partitioning approaches in the chemoinformatics field involve dimension reduction of initially defined chemistry spaces and creation of subsections of low-dimensional space for molecular classification. These subsections are often called cells. Original chemical reference spaces are generated through selection of various descriptors of molecular structure and properties. Principles and methodological aspects of dimension reduction of chemical spaces and compound partitioning in low-dimensional space are described herein.

Key Words: Biological activity; chemical features; chemical space; cluster analysis; compound databases; dimension reduction; molecular descriptors; molecule classification; partitioning algorithms; partitioning in low-dimensional spaces; principal component analysis; visualization.

1. Introduction

Clustering or partitioning methods are among the preferred computational approaches for the analysis of compound databases or libraries *(1–4)*. Typically, cluster analysis or partitioning of molecular datasets is carried out in order to select representative or diverse compound subsets or identify compounds with topologically similar structures, similar molecular properties, or biological activity. These classification techniques require the definition of chemical reference spaces, which is usually facilitated through the selection of multiple chemical descriptors *(5,6)*. The basic premise of clustering and partitioning is that molecules that are close to each other in chemical space and occur in the same cluster or partition are similar in terms of their chemical properties and/or bio-

From: *Methods in Molecular Biology, vol. 275:*
Chemoinformatics: Concepts, Methods, and Tools for Drug Discovery
Edited by: J. Bajorath © Humana Press Inc., Totowa, NJ

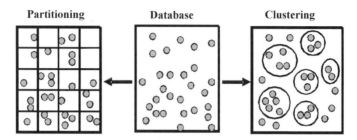

Fig. 1. Clustering versus partitioning. In cluster analysis, compounds (gray dots) are grouped together based on the calculation of pairwise intermolecular distances in chemical space. By contrast, partitioning methods subdivide chemical space into sections into which compounds fall based on their calculated descriptor coordinates.

logical activity. Regardless of the specifics of cluster algorithms, clustering generally involves the calculation of intermolecular distances in chemical space so that compounds that are close to each other can be grouped into clusters. This process requires pairwise distance comparisons in order to establish similarity relationships. Thus, when compound databases grow, the application of conventional clustering techniques becomes increasingly difficult and, at some point, computationally infeasible. On the other hand, when applying partitioning algorithms, a computed multidimensional grid, or coordinate system, is superposed onto the chemical reference space. Corresponding descriptor values are calculated for each compound and determine the absolute coordinates of these molecules in this space. Generation of a grid involves the definition of subsections of chemical space, which in turn permits the identification of molecules with similar positions based on their coordinate vectors and alleviates the need for computationally expensive pairwise molecular distance comparisons (*4*). This makes partitioning a particularly attractive approach for the analysis of increasingly large compound databases. Principal differences between clustering and partitioning are illustrated in **Fig. 1**.

2. Methods

In the following, we will describe methodological details of partitioning in low-dimensional chemistry spaces, which is currently one of the most popular adaptations of partitioning algorithms for compound classification and selection. In addition, statistically based partitioning methods, for example, recursive partitioning, a decision tree method (*7*), are also widely used in chemoinformatics and drug discovery research (*see also* **Note 1**).

Table 1
Molecular Descriptor Categories[a]

Descriptor category	Dimensionality
Topological descriptors	
Connectivity indices	2D
Physical property descriptors	
Molecular weight	1D
van der Waals volume	3D
Atom and bond counts	
Number of hydrogen bond acceptors	2D
Surface area descriptors	
van der Waals hydrophobic surface area	3D
Charge descriptors	
Total negative partial charge	2D
Positively charged molecular surface area	3D

[a]Commonly used molecular descriptor types are listed. For each category, one or two representative examples are given. Dimensionality refers to the molecular representation (molecular formula, 2D drawing, or 3D conformation) from which the descriptors are calculated (adapted from **ref. 4**).

2.1. Molecular Descriptors and Chemical Space Representation

Since the definition of chemical reference spaces very much depends on the choice of molecular descriptors, we begin the description with a brief overview of some commonly used types of descriptors, as summarized in **Table 1**.

The table shows a number of representative descriptor types (there are many more) that can be used to define chemical spaces. Each descriptor adds a dimension (with discrete or continuous value ranges) to the chemical space representation (e.g., selection of 18 descriptors defines an 18-dimensional space). Axes of chemical space are orthogonal only if the applied molecular descriptors are uncorrelated (which is, in practice, hardly ever the case).

2.2. Low-Dimensional Chemical Space and Dimension-Reduction Techniques

Once *n*-dimensional chemical reference space has been defined, the descriptors' values are calculated for all compounds in a dataset, thereby assigning a coordinate vector to each molecule. In principle, partitioning analysis could proceed in *n*-dimensional space, but it is often attempted to reduce its dimensionality in order to generate a low-dimensional representation. What are the advantages of operating in low-dimensional spaces? First, through dimension reduction, descriptor correlation effects can be reduced or eliminated and orthogonal axes can be generated. This prevents drastic distortions of chemical reference space and makes it possible to limit the number of generated partitions and control their occupany. Furthermore, dimension reduction methods often allow visual analysis of compound distributions in approximate three-dimensional reference spaces, which is often crucial for a chemical interpretation of partitioning calculations.

How is dimension reduction of chemical spaces achieved? There are a number of different concepts and mathematical procedures to reduce the dimensionality of descriptor spaces with respect to a molecular dataset under investigation. These techniques include, for example, linear mapping, multidimensional scaling, factor analysis, or principal component analysis (PCA), as reviewed in **ref. 8**. Essentially, these techniques either try to identify those descriptors among the initially chosen ones that are most important to capture the chemical information encoded in a molecular dataset or, alternatively, attempt to construct new variables from original descriptor contributions. A representative example will be discussed below in more detail.

2.3. Generation of Cells

After generating a low-dimensional space representation, each coordinate axis is divided into data intervals of defined size, a process which is often called binning and for which a number of different algorithms have been developed *(9)*. The number of bins set on the axes ultimately determines the number of subsections that are produced in chemical space, which critically influences the classification of near neighbors as either similar or not (*see also* **Note 2**). Subsections obtained by binning are generally called cells, and the basic assumption of partitioning analysis is that compounds populating the same cell are similar in terms of their structural and chemical properties and/or biological activity.

2.4. Representative Cell-Based Partitioning Schemes

The currently perhaps most popular approach to cell-based partitioning in low-dimensional chemical spaces focuses on the so-called the BCUT metric *(10,11)* and has successfully been applied in library and diversity analysis *(12)* or classification of active compounds *(13)*. In essence, BCUTs are uncorrelated complex descriptors that combine information about molecular connectivity, interatomic distances, and molecular properties such as hydrogen-bonding potential or charge. Calculation of these complex descriptors permits the generation of low-dimensional partitioning spaces that capture many chemical properties and that are typically formed by six orthogonal axes. If compounds are partitioned according to specific biological activity, the dimensionality of six-dimensional BCUT spaces can often be further reduced to three-dimensional representation by applying the concept of receptor-relevant subspaces *(11)*, thus permitting visualization of compound distributions. In this case, dimension reduction is facilitated by application of an algorithm that selects those BCUT axes around which most compounds having similar activity are located (areas considered as receptor-relevant subspace). The algorithm eliminates those axes that are not important for concentrating compounds having similar activity.

Another approach to cell-based partitioning makes use of principal component analysis *(14)* of descriptor spaces and has been intensely studied in our laboratory *(15,16)*. Principal component analysis (PCA) is a mathematical procedure that determines the variance within a dataset relative to selected variables and transforms these variables into a smaller number of uncorrelated ones for data representation. Thus, PCA is one of the dimension reduction methods that attempt to derive a smaller set of new complex descriptors from the original ones. For each molecule in a dataset, descriptor values are calculated and the eigenvalues and corresponding eigenvectors of the resulting matrix are determined. Eigenvectors constitute the principal components. These components are linear combinations of the original descriptors and account differently for the variance in the dataset (i.e., the first principal component makes the greatest contribution, followed by the second, and so on). Owing to their cumulative contributions, a relatively small number of components is often sufficient to capture the variance of a dataset (*see also* **Note 3**). For example, the first six or seven principal components might be sufficient to account for all, or nearly all, of the data variance of a compound set in a 15-dimensional descriptor space. Importantly, PCA removes correlation of original variables and, in consequence, principal components form an uncorrelated and orthogonal reference space. This also provides a basis for data visualization. For example, the first three principal components alone might account for about 70% of variance in a specific molecular dataset. Thus, using them as a three-dimensional coordinate system makes it possible to generate an approximate view of a computed compound distribution. **Figure 2** illustrates the different stages of the PCA-based partitioning process, as discussed above.

2.5. Machine Learning

Important questions are how to identify descriptors that are suitable for a specific partitioning analysis and how to determine preferred calculation conditions. There are no generally preferred molecular descriptors for compound partitioning and, in many cases, it is impossible to guess most suitable descriptors and calculation parameters. Therefore, partitioning algorithms can be combined with machine learning techniques such as genetic algorithms *(17)* in order to optimize

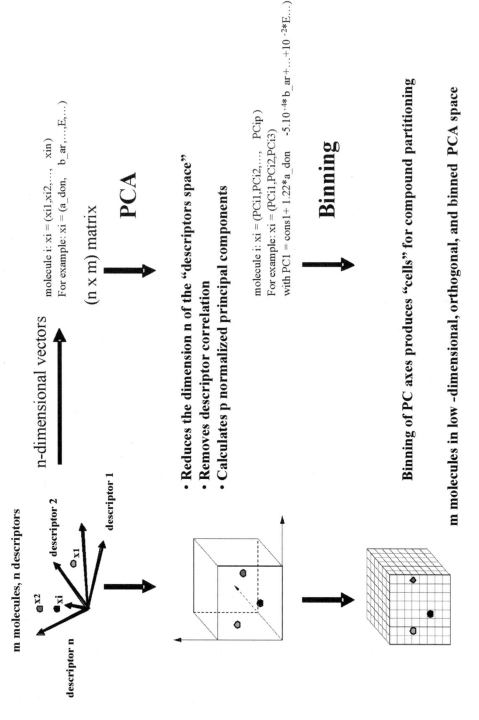

m molecules, n descriptors

descriptor 2

descriptor 1

descriptor n

x2

xi

x1

n-dimensional vectors

molecule i: xi = (xi1,xi2,..., xin)

For example: xi = (a_don, b_ar,...,E,...)

(n x m) matrix

PCA

• **Reduces the dimension n of the "descriptors space"**
• **Removes descriptor correlation**
• **Calculates p normalized principal components**

molecule i: xi = (PCi1,PCi2,..., PCip)

For example: xi = (PCi1,PCi2,PCi3)

with PC1 = cons1+ 1.22*a_don -5.10^{-4}*b_ar+...+10^{-2}*E...)

Binning

Binning of PC axes produces "cells" for compound partitioning

m molecules in low -dimensional, orthogonal, and binned PCA space

descriptor selection and partitioning calculations (*see* **Note 4**). For PCA-based partitioning, as described herein, a chromosome would represent, for example, a pool of possible molecular descriptors and, in addition, variable calculation parameters such as the maximum number of principal components and the number of bins per axis *(16)*. The combination of these two parameters determines the total number of cells that are generated. During these calculations, automatically selected descriptor combinations and calculation parameters are submitted to partitioning analysis, and the obtained results are evaluated using a predefined fitness or scoring function. For activity-oriented compound partitioning, a fitness function would typically monitor the prediction accuracy for classification of compounds having similar activity (taking into account both false-positives and false-negatives) and produce a corresponding score for each descriptor and parameter combination. Descriptor and parameter selections are modified through genetic algorithm calculations in order to improve the score of the fitness function during many cycles of selection and partitioning until a convergence criterion is reached. This automated process is usually much more effective than educated guesses and manual parameter adjustments.

2.6. Application Example

Table 2 summarizes the results of a study applying cell-based partitioning to classify molecules belonging to diverse biological activity classes *(16)*. Here, the PCA technique described above was coupled to a genetic algorithm and used to systematically partition a total of 317 active molecules belonging to 21 different biological activity classes (including various enzyme inhibitors, receptor agonists, and antagonists).

As can be seen, prediction accuracy of 70% or better could be achieved by PCA of various descriptor combinations followed by partitioning in lower-

---

Fig. 2. *(see opposite page)* Compound partitioning based on principal component analysis. As an example, a three-dimensional principal component space is generated. Dots represent molecules. As shown in this schematic illustration, *n* descriptors initially define an *n*-dimensional chemical space. Each of *m* test molecules is assigned an *n*-dimensional vector of descriptor coordinates. Thus, for all descriptors and test molecules, an *n*-by-*m* matrix is obtained. This matrix is then subjected to principal component analysis, which removes descriptor correlations and generates a set of *p* normalized principal components (linear combinations of the original descriptors, with coefficients reflecting their relative importance for capturing data variance). A limited set of principal components accounting for all, or almost all, of the variability constitute the newly derived orthogonal and lower-dimensional space. Application of a binning algorithm to the principal component axes produces cells for partitioning of the *m* test molecules, for which the new descriptor (component) values are calculated.

Table 2
PCA-Based Partitioning of Active Molecules[a]

D	PC	B	Sc	PA	P	Np	S	M
13	8	8	0.85	74.4	70	236	65	3
12	8	8	0.80	73.2	61	232	62	6
16	10	10	0.77	72.6	68	230	79	3
17	7	9	0.74	71.6	68	227	66	5
15	5	9	0.74	71.6	66	227	81	3
17	8	7	0.72	71.0	70	225	78	5
17	7	7	0.71	71.0	68	225	83	3
17	8	8	0.71	70.7	62	224	76	5

[a]"D" reports the number of original descriptors; "PC" the number of principal components; "B" the number of axis bins; "P" is the number of pure and "M" the number of mixed partitions; "S" the number of singletons; "Np" reports the total number of compounds in pure partitions; "PA" stands for prediction accuracy (%), defined as Np/N_{total} (with N_{total} being the total number of database compounds). "Sc" is the score of the fitness function (see text). Pure partitions contain only compounds having similar activity (desired result), whereas mixed partitions contain compounds belonging to different activity classes (classification failure). Singletons are compounds not recognized as similar to any others (classification failure). Data were taken from **ref. 16**.

dimensional space. The desired classification result was achieved when only compounds having similar activity occurred in the same cell (*see also* **Note 5**). For preferred chemical space representations listed in **Table 2**, the majority of compounds (>70%) were found in pure partitions.

These results were obtained by coupling a genetic algorithm for descriptor and calculation parameter (PC, bins) selection to PCA-based partitioning. In these calculations, descriptors were chosen from a pool of approx 150 different ones, and both the number of PCs and bins were allowed to vary from 1 to 15. An initial population of 300 chromosomes was randomly generated with initial bit occupancy of approx 15%. Rates for mutation and crossover operations were set to 5% and 25%, respectively. After PCA-based partitioning, scores were calculated for the following fitness function:

$$ S = 100 \times \frac{N_p}{N_m + C_s + (C/C_a)\, N_{total}} \frac{1}{} \tag{1} $$

In this formulation, N_p is the total number of the compounds in pure classes, N_m the number of compounds in mixed classes, and N_{total} the total number of active compounds. C is the total number of classes obtained by PCA analysis and C_a the number of different activity classes in the database. Thus, according to this scoring scheme, high scores were obtained if many compounds occurred in a small number of pure classes. A scale factor of 100 was arbitrarily applied to obtain top scores greater than 1.

Following partitioning calculations, the best scoring 150 chromosomes were saved and subjected to crossover and mutation operations. The resulting chromosomes represented the next generation. The process was repeated until scores remained unchanged for at least 1000 generations (convergence criterion).

3. Notes

1. Despite the conceptual elegance of partitioning in low-dimensional descriptor spaces, dimensional reduction is not essential for effective partitioning, as has been shown, for example, by application of statistical partitioning methods *(4)*.
2. Binning is also responsible for one of the potential drawbacks of cell-based partitioning, the occurrence of boundary effects. For example, modification of binning schemes can substantially change the relative occupancy of cells. Compounds occurring in the same cell in a partitioning analysis might shift into neighboring cells when calculation parameters are slightly modified and, consequently, would no longer be recognized as similar. In addition, some test molecules may map to boundaries between cells.
3. Because principal component analysis attempts to account for all of the variance within a molecular dataset, it can be negatively affected by "outliers," i.e., compounds having at least some descriptor values that are very different from others. Therefore, it is advisable to scale principal component axes or, alternatively, pre-process compound collections using statistical filters to identify and remove such outliers prior to the calculation of principal components.
4. In genetic algorithms, model parameters are encoded as "chromosomes" that yield possible (but not necessarily optimal) solutions to a given problem by optimization of a fitness function. Chromosomes are bit string representations where each bit—if set on—contributes a parameter to the calculation. Subpopulations of chromosomes yielding best intermediate solutions are subjected to operations that are analogous to genetic mutation and gene recombination in order to produce the next generation. This process continues until the solutions reach a convergence criterion of the fitness function.
5. In the context of compound partitioning, it should also be considered that relationships between structural and biological similarity can differ significantly. Much of the current molecular similarity research is based on the fundamental, and rather intuitive, "similar property principle" *(18)*, which states that compounds with similar structures should generally have similar biologically activity. On the other hand, it is well known that minute structural modifications of active com-

pounds can greatly alter or abolish their activity; a phenomenon that we—in light of the similar property principle—have called the "similarity paradox" *(19)*. These differences can represent major obstacles for molecular similarity analysis and virtual screening. In some ways, the similar property principle and similarity paradox mark opposite ends of a continuous spectrum of structure–activity relationships that are often difficult to explore and differentiate by computational analysis.

References

1. Willett, P., Wintermann, V., and Bawden, D. (1986) Implementation of non-hierarchic cluster analysis methods in chemical information systems: Selection of compounds for biological testing and clustering of substructure search output. *J. Chem. Inf. Comput. Sci.* **26,** 109–118.
2. Barnard, J. M. and Downs, G. M. (1992) Clustering of chemical structures on the basis of two-dimensional similarity measures. *J. Chem. Inf. Comput. Sci.* **32,** 644–649.
3. Mason, J. S. and Pickett, S. D. (1997) Partition-based selection. *Perspect. Drug Discov. Design* **7/8,** 85–114.
4. Stahura, F. L. and Bajorath, J. (2003) Partitioning methods for the identification of active molecules. Curr. Med. Chem. 10, 707–715.
5. Livingstone, D. J. (2000) The characterization of chemical structures using molecular properties. A survey. *J. Chem. Inf. Comput. Sci.* **40,** 195–209.
6. Bajorath, J. (2001) Selected concepts and investigations in compound classification, molecular descriptor analysis, and virtual screening. *J. Chem. Inf. Comput. Sci.* **41,** 233–245.
7. Chen, X., Rusinko, A. III, and Young, S. S. (1998) Recursive partitioning analysis of a large structure-activity data set using three-dimensional descriptors. *J. Chem. Inf. Comput. Sci.* **38,** 1054–1062.
8. Agrafiotis, D. K., Lobanov, V. S., and Salemme, R. F. (2002) Combinatorial informatics in the post-genomics era. *Nature Drug Discov. Rev.* **1,** 337–346.
9. Bayley, M. J. and Willett, P. (1999) Binning schemes for partition-based compound selection. *J. Mol. Graph. Model.* **17,** 10–18.
10. Pearlman, R. S. and Smith, K. M. (1998) Novel software tools for chemical diversity. *Perspect. Drug Discov. Design* **9,** 339–353.
11. Pearlman, R. S. and Smith, K. M. (1999) Metric validation and the receptor-relevant subspace concept. *J. Chem. Inf. Comput. Sci.* **39,** 28–35.
12. Schnur, D. (1999) Design and diversity analysis of large compound libraries using cell-based methods. *J. Chem. Inf. Comput. Sci.* **39,** 36–45.
13. Pirard, B. and Pickett, S. D. (2000) Classification of kinase inhibitors using BCUT descriptors. *J. Chem. Inf. Comput. Sci.* **40,** 1431–1440.
14. Glen, W. G., Dunn, W. J., and Scott, D. R. (1989) Principal component analysis and partial least squares regression. *Tetrahedron Comput. Methodol.* **2,** 349–376.
15. Xue, L. and Bajorath, J. (2000) Molecular descriptors for effective classification of biologically active compounds based on principal component analysis identified by a genetic algorithm. *J. Chem. Inf. Comput. Sci.* **40,** 801–809.

16. Xue, L. and Bajorath, J. (2002) Accurate partitioning of compounds belonging to diverse activity classes. *J. Chem. Inf. Comput. Sci.* **42,** 757–764.

17. Forrest, S. (1993) Genetic algorithms—principles of natural selection applied to computation. *Science* **261,** 872–878.

18. Johnson, M. A. and Maggiora, G. M. (eds.) (1990) *Concepts and applications of molecular similarity.* Wiley, New York, NY.

19. Bajorath, J. (2002) Integration of virtual and high-throughput screening. *Nature Drug Discov. Rev.* **1,** 337–346.

10

Partitioning in Binary-Transformed Chemical Descriptor Spaces

Jeffrey W. Godden and Jürgen Bajorath

Abstract

Here we describe a statistically based partitioning method called median partitioning (MP), which involves the transformation of value distributions of molecular property descriptors into a binary classification scheme. The MP approach fundamentally differs from other partitioning approaches that involve dimension reduction of chemical spaces such as cell-based partitioning, since MP directly operates in original, albeit simplified, chemical space. Modified versions of the MP algorithm have been implemented and successfully applied in diversity selection, compound classification, and virtual screening. These findings have demonstrated that dimension reduction techniques, although elegant in their design, are not necessarily required for effective partitioning of molecular datasets. An attractive feature of statistical partitioning approaches such as decision tree methods or MP is their computational efficiency, which is becoming an important criterion for the analysis of compound databases containing millions of molecules.

Key Words: Biological activity; chemical descriptors; chemical spaces; classification methods; compound databases; decision trees; diversity selection; partitioning algorithms; space transformation; statistics; statistical medians.

1. Introduction

In chemoinformatics research, partitioning algorithms are applied in diversity analysis of large compound libraries, subset selection, or the search for molecules with specific activity *(1–4)*. Widely used partitioning methods include cell-based partitioning in low-dimensional chemical spaces *(1,3)* and decision tree methods, in particular, recursive partitioning (RP) *(5–7)*. Partitioning in low-dimensional chemical spaces is based on various dimension reduction methods *(4,8)* and often permits simplified three-dimensional representation of

From: *Methods in Molecular Biology, vol. 275:*
Chemoinformatics: Concepts, Methods, and Tools for Drug Discovery
Edited by: J. Bajorath © Humana Press Inc., Totowa, NJ

computed compound distributions. The ability to visualize compound sets in chemical space invaluably aids in the analysis of partitioning results (and also other calculations), which may be one of the reasons for the popularity of cell-based partitioning techniques.

Whereas some of the mathematical operations involved in dimension reduction techniques are rather complex and often not easily applicable to very large compound sets, statistical partitioning approaches are generally not affected by such restrictions and are therefore computationally very efficient. Decision tree methods such as RP are typically not designed for diversity analysis or subset selection, but rather for the identification of active compounds or the separation of active from inactive molecules (in biological screening sets, for example). Recursive partitioning typically begins with a learning set consisting of known active and inactive compounds and divides this dataset in subsequent steps along a decision tree consisting of multiple test features or descriptors. At every branch of the tree, one or more descriptors are employed to subdivide the dataset into subsets that either have or do not have the tested features *(7,8)*. The primary goal is to obtain subsets of the smallest possible size that are highly enriched with active compounds and to associate these partitions with specific descriptor settings or pathways. Because these descriptor-based models are linked to a specific biological activity or class of compounds, they provide search tools for the identification of novel molecules with desired properties.

Median partitioning is another statistical method distinct from RP. The development of this methodology was driven by the need to select representative subsets from very large compound pools. Hierarchical clustering techniques *(4,9)* and dissimilarity-based methods *(10–12)* have typically been applied for such tasks but are computationally too complex to handle compound collections consisting of millions of molecules. Therefore, MP was originally designed as a computationally less demanding subset selection method *(13)* and later on was also adapted for the classification of active compounds *(14)* and for virtual screening of large databases *(15)*. This conceptually straightforward, yet very versatile, partitioning method is described in the following.

2. Methods

First, we introduce the underlying idea of MP and some of its basic requirements. Then automation and algorithmic details are discussed. Finally, we compare different partitioning approaches.

2.1. Concept of Median Partitioning

2.1.1. Statistical Medians of Descriptor Distributions

Like other partitioning or clustering techniques *(4)*, MP relies on the use of descriptors of molecular structure and properties *(16,17)* for the definition of

Table 1
Descriptor Medians[a]

Molecular descriptor	Median 1 (317)	Median 2 (2,317)
Number of aromatic atoms	12	10
Number of H-bond donors	2	1
Number of heavy atoms	26	21
Number of hydrophobic atoms	17	14
Number of aromatic bonds	12	11
Number of double non-aromatic bonds	1	1
Atomic connectivity index (chi 1)	19.1	15.3
VDW surface area of H-bond acceptors	27.9	19.3

[a]The table reports median values for a number of descriptors that were calculated for two overlapping compound datasets. Median 1 was calculated for 317 active compounds belonging to different biological activity classes. Median 2 was calculated after 2000 randomly collected molecules were added to this set of active compounds. Most median values differ for these two compound sets (*see* **Note 3**). VDW stands for van der Waals. Data were taken from **ref. 14**.

chemical reference spaces (*see also* **Note 1**). For each of m compounds in a database, values of n descriptors are initially calculated. In statistics, the median is defined as the value that separates a population of values into two equal subpopulations above and below the median *(18)*. Thus, for each descriptor a median can be calculated given the values of m molecules. It is important to point out that molecular descriptors suitable for calculation of medians must have continuous value ranges or, at least, a number of discrete values. For two-state descriptors such as, for example, structural fragments (that are either present or absent in a molecule), a meaningful calculation of medians is not possible (*see* **Note 2**). Furthermore, descriptors suitable for MP analysis usually benefit from having high information content *(13)*, which can be determined and quantified by descriptor entropy calculations in compound databases *(19,20)*. **Table 1** shows some examples of descriptors and calculated medians.

2.1.2. Partitioning Calculations

Once a basis set of descriptor medians is obtained, MP proceeds in a stepwise manner. In each of n subsequent steps, molecules with a value of the particular descriptor above (or equal to) the median are assigned 1 and molecules with value below the median are assigned 0. For n descriptors, a total of 2^n unique partitions are created, each of which is characterized by a unique n-digit partitioning code (for example, 10 descriptors produce 1024 partitions). Ultimately, each test molecule falls into a unique partition and is assigned its signature code

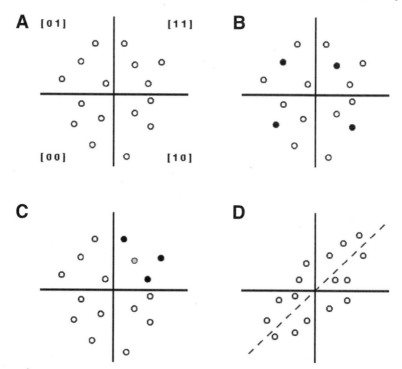

Fig. 1. Median partitioning and compound selection. In this schematic illustration, a two-dimensional chemical space is shown as an example. The axes represent the medians of two uncorrelated (and, therefore, orthogonal) descriptors and dots represent database compounds. In **A**, a compound database is divided in into equal subpopulations in two steps and each resulting partition is characterized by a unique binary code (shared by molecules occupying this partition). In **B**, diversity-based compound selection is illustrated. From the center of each partition, a compound is selected to obtain a representative subset. By contrast, **C** illustrates activity-based compound selection. Here, a known active molecule (gray dot) is added to the source database prior to MP and compounds that ultimately occur in the same partition as this bait molecule are selected as candidates for testing. Finally, **D** illustrates the effects of descriptor correlation. In this case, the two applied descriptors are significantly correlated and the dashed line represents a diagonal of correlation that affects the compound distribution. As can be seen, descriptor correlation leads to over- and underpopulated partitions.

(*see* **Note 4**). The MP process is illustrated in **Fig. 1**. A basic assumption of partitioning approaches including MP is that molecules falling into the same partition are similar and share similar properties (such as biological activity), which provides the basis for diversity- or activity-oriented compound selections, as illustrated in **Fig. 1**.

In contrast to partitioning methods that involve dimension reduction of chemical reference spaces, MP is best understood as a direct space method. However, n-dimensional descriptor space is simplified here by transforming property descriptors with continuous or discrete value ranges into a binary classification scheme. Essentially, this binary space transformation assigns less complex n-dimensional vectors to test molecules, with each dimension having unity length of either 0 or 1. Thus, although MP analysis proceeds in n-dimensional descriptor space, its dimensions are scaled and its complexity is reduced.

2.1.3. Descriptor Correlation

A major practical issue affecting MP calculations is caused by use of correlated molecular descriptors. During subsequent MP steps, exact halves of values (and molecules) are only generated if the chosen descriptors are uncorrelated (orthogonal), as shown in **Fig. 1A**. By contrast, the presence of descriptor correlations (and departure from orthogonal reference space) leads to overpopulated and underpopulated, or even empty, partitions (*see also* **Note 5**), as illustrated in **Fig. 1D**. For diversity analysis, compounds should be widely distributed over computed partitions and descriptor correlation effects should therefore be limited as much as possible. However, for other applications, the use of correlated descriptors that produce skewed compound distributions may not be problematic or even favorable (*see* **Note 5**).

2.2. Algorithmic Details

2.2.1. Automatic Descriptor Selection

For partitioning analysis, regardless of the methods applied, it is in general difficult to predict which descriptor combinations might perform best. Because there are no general rules, machine learning techniques such as genetic algorithms (GAs) *(21)* can conveniently be applied to select descriptors (*see also* **Note 1**). For GA calculations, descriptors can be encoded in chromosomes and automatically selected and subjected to MP. Obtained results are then evaluated using specific scoring functions that are optimized during subsequent rounds of GA calculations until predefined convergence criteria are reached. Thus, the basic MP process can be tuned for specific applications by use of different scoring schemes that optimize desired partitioning outcomes *(13–15)*.

2.2.2. Diversity Assessment

As mentioned above, the MP approach was originally designed to aid in diversity evaluation of large compound collections and selection of representative subsets (*see* **Note 6**). In this case, an MP grid with a predefined number of partitions is superposed on the compound dataset. In order to identify descriptor combinations that create as much diversity as possible during the MP process, the following scoring function was designed *(13)*:

$$S_1 = <IC>/<CC>$$

where <IC> is the average information content *(13,19)* and <CC> the average correlation coefficient of a descriptor combination. Thus, descriptor combinations are sought that have high information content and low correlation. In order to assess the effectiveness of selected descriptor combinations, the number of populated partitions is monitored during MP (as a measure of diversity).

2.2.3. Compound Classification

The MP method has also been adapted for classification of bioactive compounds, a task that substantially differs from diversity analysis. Here the key is to find descriptor combinations that place compounds with similar activity into the same partition, separate them from others, and avoid the creation of partitions containing molecules having diffcrent activity. Therefore, the following scoring function was optimized *(14)*:

$$S_2 = \frac{100}{N_{total}} \times \frac{1}{(N_{total} - N_p) + C / C_{act}}$$

Here N_{total} is the total number of active database compounds and N_p the number of compounds occurring in "pure" partitions that only contain molecules belonging to the same activity class. Both the number of compounds in "mixed" partitions (containing molecules having different activity) and singletons are considered classification failures. C is the total number of partitions containing active compounds (pure, mixed, or singletons) and C_{act} is the number of different activity classes in the database. A scaling factor of 100 is arbitrarily applied (to obtain top scores greater than 1). According to this scoring scheme, high scores are obtained if many compounds with similar activity occur in a small number of pure partitions (*see* **Note 5**).

2.2.4. Dispersive MP

A similar approach can also be applied to search databases for novel active molecules. In this case, several known active compounds are added to a source database as baits and descriptor combinations are identified that place these bait molecules into the same partition. Successful co-partitioning of known actives essentially serves as an internal control. If MP correctly recognizes the similarity of the baits, database compounds occurring in the same partition are thought to have a higher probability than others to exhibit activity similar to the bait molecules *(15)*. Algorithmically, this type of search for active compounds can be facilitated in different ways. Thus far, we have mainly focused on what we call dispersive MP. For this purpose, a fitness function was designed to balance two objectives:

- Find descriptor combinations that successfully co-partition known actives.
- Create greatest possible diversity among database compounds.

During diversity spreading, only database compounds with distinct similarity to co-partitioned bait molecules are expected to remain "close" to them. Among various scoring schemes we investigated for dispersive MP, the following simple function consistently produced best results *(15)*:

$$S_3 = A(cp) * P(pop)$$

Here $A(cp)$ is the number of successfully co-partitioned known actives (subsets of which may occur in different partitions) and $P(pop)$ the number of populated partitions. The total number of populated median partitions serves as a measure of the diversity spread among database compounds (just as in diversity analysis, as discussed above).

2.2.5. Recursive MP

When searching very large databases for active compounds, a single-step MP analysis often does not sufficiently reduce database compounds to a small enough number for testing (e.g., fewer than 100). Therefore, we have devised a recursive procedure for MP (called RMP) that proceeds as follows *(15)*:

- Find descriptor combinations that successfully co-partition known actives
- Pool database compounds from active partitions and discard others
- Add all bait molecules again to the pool
- Re-calculate medians, re-initialize descriptor selection, and re-partition
- Go through subsequent recursions
- Until a sufficiently small number of test compounds is obtained.

Following this algorithm, the size of the source database is reduced during each recursion until only a very small number of candidate compounds remains for testing. The methodology has two key aspects. First, descriptor medians are re-calculated each time after the source database is reduced in size to avoid statistical errors (*see* **Note 3**). Second, descriptor selection is initiated *de novo* at the beginning of each recursion (without transfer of information from previous steps). This is done in order to generate independent chemical space solutions and avoid database-dependent bias. Using our dispersive-recursive MP approach, it was possible for different biological activity classes (for example, tyrosine kinase inhibitors or serotonin receptor antagonists) to reduce approx 1.3 million database

Table 2
Classification of Active Compounds by Median and Cell-Based Partitioning[a]

Ds	D	%P	P	nP	S	M	nM
GA-PCA							
18	6	**55.2**	57	175	82	19	60
GA-MP							
19	19	**63.1**	69	200	86	22	31

[a]The test database consisted of 317 active compounds belonging to 21 biological activity classes and 2000 randomly selected background molecules. PCA stands for principal component analysis, the basis of the cell-based partitioning method used here *(23)*. Ds reports the number of original (GA-selected) descriptors and D the dimensionality of the partitioning space (PCA involves dimension reduction). %P is the percentage of active compounds in pure partitions as a measure of the prediction accuracy. P is the total number of pure partitions, nP the total number of active compounds in pure partitions, S the number of singletons (only one active compound; classification failure), M the number of mixed partitions (containing either molecules having different activity or active and background compounds), and nM the total number of active compounds in mixed partitions (classification failure). Data were taken from **ref.** *14*.

compounds to 20–100 candidate molecules in just two to five recursions. In these calculations, RMP produced hit rates of up to approx 20% *(15)*.

2.3. Median vs Cell-Based Partitioning

We have also compared MP to cell-based partitioning in a compound classification study focusing on a number of different activity classes. Both partitioning techniques were coupled to a GA and scoring function S2 (see above) was optimized. Results are summarized in **Table 2**.

In this study, both partitioning approaches produced promising results, with more than half of active compounds occurring in pure partitions. As a direct space method, MP compared favorably to cell-based partitioning. These findings encouraged us to apply RMP methodology for virtual screening of large compound databases *(15)*.

3. Notes

1. A brief overview of different types of molecular descriptors is given in Chapter 9 about cell-based partitioning by Xue et al.; this chapter also includes a description of genetic algorithm calculations.
2. Descriptor requirements present a significant difference between MP and decision tree methods such as RP. Whereas two-state descriptors are not suitable for MP, these types of descriptors are typically required for decision tree algorithms because at each branch the presence or absence of specific feature(s) must be detected in order to recursively divide a molecular dataset.

3. Descriptor median values naturally depend on the composition and size of compound databases. Whenever source databases are changed, reduced, or extended in size, descriptor medians need to be re-calculated to ensure accurate MP analysis. Relatively small changes in median values can significantly alter partitioning results.
4. Computationally, MP is a very efficient method. Median statistics and partitioning calculations (which are, in essence, a compound sorting process) are very fast. Generally, the major time-limiting step is the calculation of many potential descriptors for large numbers of compounds. Excluding descriptor calculations, median statistics, partitioning calculations, and partition code assignments for diversity analysis of approx 2.5 million molecules required only approx 2 h of CPU time on a 600 MHz PC processor *(13)*.
5. In practice, it is very difficult, if not impossible, to find sets of uncorrelated molecular property descriptors. Thus, although we try to limit descriptor correlation effects in diversity analysis, unevenly populated or empty partitions usually occur during MP. In fact, when generating high-dimensional reference spaces for MP analysis, propagating descriptor correlation effects can lead to large numbers of empty partitions (even if pairwise correlations are small). For example, when selecting a representative subset of approx 100,000 compounds from approx 2.5 million molecules in a 19-dimensional MP space, an overall partition occupancy rate of 21% was observed *(13)*. However, depending on the application, this does not necessarily mean that MP results are negatively affected by descriptor correlation. In compound classification, for example, descriptor correlation effects can even improve the accuracy of the predictions *(14)* (probably because sets of similar compounds are easier to "isolate" when distributions over partitions are skewed).
6. We needed to develop a classification technique that could efficiently select representative subsets from compound pools containing millions of molecules. Analysis of compound datasets of this size makes it necessary to avoid pairwise molecular comparisons (as involved in clustering) and complex mathematical transformations (as often involved dimension reduction of chemical spaces). The MP approach fulfills these requirements. Other algorithms have been designed to evaluate the diversity of very large compound collections that employ probability sampling of smaller subsets to estimate global diversity *(22)*.

References

1. Pearlman, R. S. and Smith, K. M. (1998) Novel software tools for chemical diversity. *Perspect. Drug Discov. Design* **9**, 339–353.
2. Mason, J. S. and Pickett, S. D. (1997) Partition-based selection. *Perspect. Drug Discov. Design* **7/8**, 85–114.
3. Bajorath, J. (2002) Integration of virtual and high-throughput screening. *Nature Drug Discov. Rev.* **1**, 337–346.
4. Stahura, F. L. and Bajorath, J. (2003) Partitioning methods for the identification of active molecules. *Curr. Med. Chem.* **10**, 707–715.
5. Friedman, J. A. (1977) Recursive partitioning decision rules for non-parametric classification. *IEEE Trans. Comput.* **26**, 404–408.

6. Chen, X., Rusinko, A. III, and Young, S. S. (1998) Recursive partitioning analysis of a large structure-activity data set using three-dimensional descriptors. *J. Chem. Inf. Comput. Sci.* **38,** 1054–1062.

7. Rusinko, A. III, Farmen, M. W., Lambert, C. G., Brown, P. L., and Young, S. S. (1999) Analysis of a large structure/biological activity data set using recursive partitioning. *J. Chem. Inf. Comput. Sci.* **39,** 1017–1026.

8. Agrafiotis, D. K., Lobanov, V. S., and Salemme, R. F. (2002) Combinatorial informatics in the post-genomics era. *Nature Drug Discov. Rev.* **1,** 337–346.

9. Ward, J. H. (1963) Hierarchical grouping to optimize an objective function. *J. Am. Stat. Assoc.* **58,** 236–244.

10. Snarey, M., Terrett, N. K., Willett, P., and Wilton, D. J. (1997) Comparison of algorithms for dissimilarity-based compound selection. *J. Mol. Graph. Model.* **15,** 372–285.

11. Higgs, R. E., Bemis, K. G., Watson, I. A., and Wikel, J. H. (1997) Experimental designs for selecting molecules from large chemical databases. *J. Chem. Inf. Comput. Sci.* **37,** 861–870.

12. Willett, P. (1999) Dissimilarity-based algorithms for selecting structurally diverse sets of compounds. *J. Comput. Biol.* **6,** 447–457.

13. Godden J. W., Xue, L., Kitchen, D. B., Stahura, F. L., Schermerhorn, E. J., and Bajorath, J. (2002) Median partitioning: A novel method for the selection of representative subsets from large compound pools. *J. Chem. Inf. Comput. Sci.* **42,** 885–893.

14. Godden, J. W., Xue, L., and Bajorath, J. (2002) Classification of biologically active compounds by median partitioning. *J. Chem. Inf. Comput. Sci.* **42,** 1263–1269.

15. Godden, J. W., Furr, J. R., and Bajorath, J. (2003) Recursive median partitioning for virtual screening of large databases. *J. Chem. Inf. Comput. Sci.* **43,** 182–188.

16. Livingstone, D. J. (2000) The characterization of chemical structures using molecular properties. A survey. *J. Chem. Inf. Comput. Sci.* **40,** 195–209.

17. Xue, L. and Bajorath, J. (2000) Molecular descriptors in chemoinformatics, computational combinatorial chemistry, and virtual screening. *Combin. Chem. High Throughput Screen.* **3,** 363–372.

18. Meier, P. C. and Zünd, R. E. (2000) *Statistical methods in analytical chemistry.* Wiley, New York, NY.

19. Godden, J. W. and Bajorath, J. (2002) Chemical descriptors with distinct levels of information content and varying sensitivity to differences between selected compound databases identified by SE-DSE analysis. *J. Chem. Inf. Comput. Sci.* **42,** 87–93.

20. Shannon, C. E. and Weaver, W. (1963) *The mathematical theory of communication.* University of Illinois Press, Urbana, IL.

21. Forrest, S. (1993) Genetic algorithms—principles of natural selection applied to computation. *Science* **261,** 872–878.

22. Agrafiotis, D. K. (2001) A constant time algorithm for estimating the diversity of large chemical libraries. *J. Chem. Inf. Comput. Sci.* **41,** 159–167.

23. Xue, L. and Bajorath, J. (2002) Accurate partitioning of compounds belonging to diverse activity classes. *J. Chem. Inf. Comput. Sci.* **42,** 757–764.

11

Comparison of Methods Based on Diversity and Similarity for Molecule Selection and the Analysis of Drug Discovery Data

Raymond L.H. Lam and William J. Welch

Abstract

The concepts of diversity and similarity of molecules are widely used in quantitative methods for designing (selecting) a representative set of molecules and for analyzing the relationship between chemical structure and biological activity. We review methods and algorithms for design of a diverse set of molecules in the chemical space using clustering, cell-based partitioning, or other distance-based approaches. Analogous cell-based and clustering methods are described for analyzing drug-discovery data to predict activity in virtual screening. Some performance comparisons are made. The choice of descriptor variables to characterize chemical structure is also included in the comparative study. We find that the diversity of a selected set is quite sensitive to both the statistical selection method and the choice of molecular descriptors and that, for the dataset used in this study, random selection works surprisingly well in providing a set of data for analysis.

Key Words: Biological activity; cell-based partitioning; chemical descriptors; classification; clustering; distance-based design; diversity selection; high-throughput screening; quantitative structure-activity relationship.

1. Introduction

Finding bioactive compounds is inherently a sequential process. Even a large screening program where 500,000 to 1,000,000 compounds are screened is a modest sampling of the many millions of compounds that are available commercially. Moreover, there are billions of possible compounds that could be made using standard reactions and reagents. An exhaustive search of the vastness of chemical space is not feasible, and drug discovery, like other optimizations, is necessarily a sequence of steps in hopefully the right direction.

From: *Methods in Molecular Biology, vol. 275:*
Chemoinformatics: Concepts, Methods, and Tools for Drug Discovery
Edited by: J. Bajorath © Humana Press Inc., Totowa, NJ

Almost always, drug discovery starts with an initial screen, with the screening results leading to screening further, possibly newly synthesized, compounds.

A number of researchers are pushing the sequential screening paradigm in the direction of smaller initial screening datasets and in the use of data mining methods for determining a structure–activity relationship. The initial screening sets of 10,000–15,000 compounds are very small by discovery standards. There have been extensive benchmarking studies using historical datasets *(1–5)*. All these investigators reached similar conclusions: for example, several cycles of sequential screening often identify about 80% of the hits by testing only about 20% of the entire compound collection *(2)*.

There are a number of possible objectives for sequential screening. Some screeners want to find all the active compounds in their collection. Some chemists would like to find all the active chemical classes in the collection. We think sequential screeners should adopt the more modest goal of finding several active chemical classes. The follow-up process of drug discovery is frightfully expensive, so even large companies cannot afford to follow up more than two or three chemical classes for a target. Sequential screening should attempt to match downstream capacity.

The purpose of this chapter is to benchmark various aspects of sequential screening. In **Subheading 2.** we look at several methods for defining and selecting a diverse initial screening set from a chemical database. **Subheading 3.** describes two similarity-based methods for analyzing structure-activity data and identifying active compounds. These methods of design and analysis are benchmarked in **Subheading 4.** Finally, **Subheading 5.** draws some conclusions.

2. Methods for Designing a Diverse Set of Compounds

2.1. Chemical Descriptors

The measure of chemical diversity of a set of compounds clearly depends on the descriptor variables chosen to characterize their chemical structures. Similarly, the utility of a structure–activity analysis will depend on how well the descriptor variables capture the important chemical features.

There is a vast array of possible descriptor sets. Todeschini and Consonni's catalog *(6)* is encyclopedic in scope; Leach and Gillet provide a useful summary *(7)*. There is relatively little literature benchmarking one set of descriptors against another, however. Brown and Martin found that 2D descriptors were more effective than computationally intensive 3D descriptors when used in conjunction with a clustering method to select active molecules *(8)*. Feng et al. compared several types of descriptors computed with Dragon software (www.disat.unimib.it/chm/Dragon.htm) using four datasets and three different statistical methods and found all the descriptors about equally effective *(9)*. Clearly, much more benchmarking needs to be done.

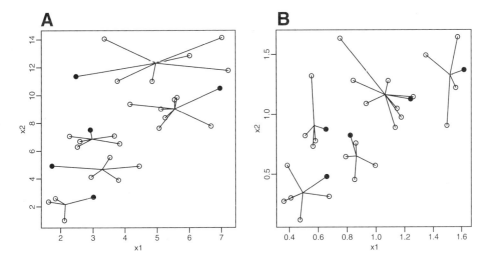

Fig. 1. Thirty molecules (open and solid circles) are grouped into five clusters in a two-dimensional chemical space. In **A**, the original, unscaled variables are used, whereas the variables are scaled to have unit sample standard deviations in **B**. The lines connect each molecule to its cluster center. Solid circles denote the compounds chosen at random; open circles are unselected compounds.

In **Subheading 4.** we compare two very different descriptor sets: six BCUTs, based on the work of Burden *(10)* and Pearlman and Smith *(11)*, and 46 constitutional descriptors from Dragon. BCUTs summarize whole-molecule properties based on graph-theoretic arguments. Constitutional descriptors are simple and describe general properties of the compound without resort to molecular geometry. They include such variables as number of bonds, numbers of specific atom types, number of rings, and molecular weight. In general, we denote the number of descriptors by k.

2.2. Clustering

One method of choosing a diverse set of compounds from a molecular database is to first cluster them (*see*, for example **ref.** *12*) and then select one molecule from each cluster. Clustering ideally groups the molecules into well-separated, compact groups with respect to the descriptor variables. If this is the case, then each cluster or group can be represented by one of its members. This method of choosing a diverse set of objects goes back at least to Zemroch *(13)* in the statistics literature and has been widely used for chemical databases *(14,15)*.

Figure 1 illustrates clustering with a simple example having just two descriptors, x_1 and x_2, and 30 compounds. The 30 compounds denoted by circles are clustered into five groups; the lines connect each compound to the center of its cluster. The *K*-means algorithm *(12)* is being used here and in **Subheading 4.** for a much larger database, as it is reasonably fast when dealing with hundreds of thousands of compounds. Its computational complexity is roughly linear with the number of compounds, much better than most clustering methods. One molecule is randomly selected from each group—the points denoted by solid circles. The *K*-means algorithm iterates by assigning each point to the nearest cluster center. The definition of "nearest" clearly depends on the scaling of the variables (as well as the choice of variables and the distance metric). In **Fig. 1A** the raw variables are used with the Euclidean distance metric, whereas in **Fig. 1B** the distance metric for clustering is computed after scaling so that both variables have unit sample standard deviation. A change of scale can lead to different clusters, as here, and hence different selected molecules.

2.3. Cell-Based Algorithms

2.3.1. Cell-Based Selection

In a standard cell-based method, the range of each of k numerical descriptors is subdivided into m bins, yielding m^k cells. To select a representative set of molecules from a database, one molecule is selected at random from each cell *(16)*. The method can also be used to assess the diversity of an existing molecular database by asking how many cells are represented *(17)*.

The method is straightforward, but runs into a major problem. For similar biological activity, two molecules must have fairly similar values of all critical descriptors *(18)*, so the number of bins per dimension, m, should be large. With a high-dimensional descriptor space (large k), there will be so many cells that most are empty in the database.

2.3.2. Uniform Cell Coverage

As it is essentially impossible to cover a high-dimensional space finely with a modest number of compounds, Lam and co-workers proposed a cell-based method that uniformly covers all low-dimensional subspaces formed by subsets of descriptors *(19,20)*. Typically, they would consider all one-dimensional (1D), 2D, and 3D subspaces. In addition to practical feasibility, this is consistent with Pearlman and Smith's notion of a relevant subspace *(21)*: a particular activity mechanism will likely involve only a few relevant descriptor variables.

With cells formed from only one, two, or three descriptors at a time, it is possible to divide each descriptor's range into fairly fine bins. Suppose, for example, we want 4096 cells. In one dimension, a descriptor can have 4096 bins. For two-dimensional cells, the two variables each have 64 bins, giving $64 \times 64 = 4096$ cells. Similarly, in three dimensions, 16 bins per variable lead to $16 \times 16 \times 16 = 4096$ cells. Lam and co-workers also formed larger bins at

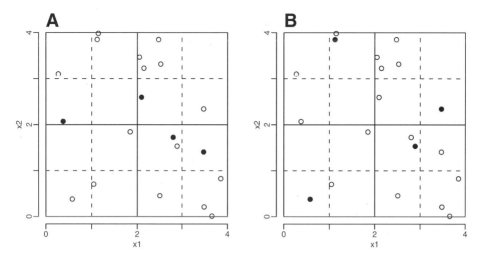

Fig. 2. Cells and selected molecules in a 2D descriptor space formed by variables x_1 and x_2. There are four bins for each 1D descriptor (solid or dashed lines) and four cells in a 2×2 arrangement in two dimensions (solid lines). Solid and open circles represent four molecules selected from 20 and the remaining unselected molecules, respectively. Panels **A** and **B** show poor and good selections, respectively, according to the UCC criterion.

the edges of each variable's range, where there are often extreme values, to keep the interior cells small *(19,20)*. Thus, all subspaces, whether 1D, 2D, or 3D, have the same number of cells. Some cells might be empty in some subspaces, but, because the number of cells is controlled (thousands instead of millions), the proportion empty tends to be much smaller than with traditional cell-based methods.

Choosing one molecule at random from each cell in a particular subspace will not necessarily give good coverage in other subspaces, and an optimization algorithm is necessary. Lam and co-workers introduced a uniform-cell-coverage (UCC) criterion *(19,20)* to measure the discrepancy between a particular choice of molecules and the ideal of one molecule per cell, accumulated over all subspaces. The UCC criterion forms the objective function for a fast exchange algorithm, yielding a UCC design.

Figure 2 illustrates the generation of cells and the UCC criterion with a very simple example involving the choice of four molecules from 20 in a two-dimensional descriptor space formed by variables x_1 and x_2. The space is divided into four bins for each 1D descriptor (solid or dashed lines) and into four cells in a 2×2 arrangement in two dimensions (solid lines). Solid circles represent the four selected molecules, while open circles are unselected.

Figure 2A shows a poor selection according to UCC: in 1D, the second x_1 bin and the first and last x_2 bins are empty. Similarly, in 2D, the lower left cell is empty. Correspondingly, there are overrepresented cells with more than one molecule selected. Mathematically, the UCC criterion averages penalty contributions of the form $(n - c)^2$ across all cells in all subspaces, where for a particular cell n is the number of molecules selected and c is the ideal for the cell (1 if the cell has at least one molecule in the database falling in that cell, 0 otherwise). The design in **Fig. 2A** generates penalties for the empty and over-populated 1D or 2D cells mentioned above. In contrast, the selection in **Fig. 2B** has a perfect UCC score of 0 as all cells in all subspaces are occupied once.

The adaptations introduced in the fast exchange algorithm to optimize the UCC criterion allow selection from databases of hundreds of thousands of compounds. Currently, the implementation is limited to tens of continuous descriptors, though discrete descriptors like fragment counts could be handled in principle. Further work is also needed for even larger databases with hundreds of descriptors.

2.4. Algorithms Based on Distance Metrics

Choosing a set of design points according to dissimilarity or distance measures underlies the algorithm of Kennard and Stone *(22)*. Johnson et al. *(23)* formalized two classes of distance-based designs: (1) "maximin" designs maximize the minimum distance between design points and spread the points maximally throughout the space of interest; and (2) "minimax" distance designs minimize the maximum distance between candidate points and the design points, making every candidate close to a design point and hence the design covers the candidate space. **Figure 3** illustrates these criteria. It is seen that a maximin design **(Fig. 3A)** tends to push many of the chosen points to the edge of the space, whereas a minimax design **(Fig. 3B)** can often get closer to all the points by drawing in from the edges. Similar ideas have been widely described in chemical contexts, e.g., **ref. *24*.** As in clustering (*see* **Subheading 2.2.**), scaling of the variables is an issue. The wider use of these methods is mainly limited by the prohibitive computational cost of optimizing distance-based criteria.

3. Methods for Predicting Activity via Similarity
3.1. Cluster Classification

The clustering method of choosing a diverse set of points (**Subheading 2.2.**) leads directly to a method of analysis of the resulting activity data. It is assumed that molecules in the same cluster have similar chemical structure and hence are likely to have similar activity. If a selected molecule shows activity,

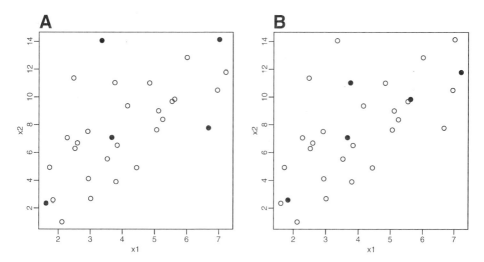

Fig. 3. Five points (solid circles) are selected from 30 (open and solid circles) using distance-based design criteria: **(A)** maximize the minimum distance between design points; **(B)** minimize the maximum distance from any point to its nearest design point.

then all the members of its cluster are considered to be promising candidates and assayed. Conversely, if a selected molecule turns out to be inactive, all members of its cluster are thought to be inactive and discarded.

3.2. Cell-Based Analysis

Cell-based analysis *(19,25)* is related to cell-based design *(see* **Subheading 2.3.**). When the compounds in the initial set are assayed, the cells in the various subspaces are scored according to the proportion of active compounds. A new and not assayed compound can then be rated by combining the scores of the cells to which it belongs. Cells for analysis are typically made a little larger than those used for design, so that each cell has about 10 assayed compounds and the proportion that are active is a reasonably reliable measure. This leads to reliable scores for new compounds.

The logic of cell-based analysis parallels that of classification based on clusters. Just as molecules in the same cluster should share similar chemical structures and may have similar activities, molecules falling in highly scored cells are likely to share the chemical structures crucial for activity. Unlike clustering, however, cell-based scoring can assign more weight to important subsets of variables. The method is capable of finding multiple, highly localized active regions in chemical space. Yi et al. conducted a fractional factorial experiment aiming at tuning the efficiency of cell-based analysis *(26)*.

4. Results

4.1. Experimental Plan

In our study we compare two diversity-driven design methods (uniform cell coverage and clustering), two analysis methods motivated by similarity (cell-based analysis and cluster-classification), and two descriptor sets (BCUT and constitutional). Thus, our study addresses some of the many questions arising in a sequential screen: how to choose the initial screen, how to analyze the structure–activity data, and what molecular descriptor set to use. The study is limited to one assay and thus cannot be definitive, but it at least provides preliminary insights and reveals some trends.

For example, we address the following questions. Does diversity generated by one method and descriptor set correspond to diversity according to another? How do various designs compare with random selections? In structure–activity analysis, does one method outperform another in the identification of active compounds?

We use assay data from a National Cancer Institute HIV/AIDS database in our study (http://dtp.nci.nih.gov/docs/aids/aids_data.html). As descriptors, we apply a set of six BCUT descriptors and a set of 46 constitutional descriptors computed by the Dragon software. These descriptors could be computed for 29,374 of the compounds in the database. The assay classifies each compound as confirmed inactive (CI), moderately active (CM), or confirmed active (CA). We treat the data as a binary classification problem with two classes: inactive (CI) and active (CM or CA). According to this classification, 542 (about 1.8%) of the compounds are active.

For consistent assessment of the design and analysis methods, the database is divided randomly into two halves: training and test data. However, the two halves are balanced to have roughly equal numbers of active compounds. All design methods choose 4096 compounds from the 14,688 compounds in the training data; the remaining training compounds are discarded. All analysis methods are compared on the same set of 14,686 test compounds. Thus, the comparisons of the analysis method use consistent test data. Therefore, design comparisons and analysis comparisons are independent from each other.

4.2. Diversity Design

Two designs of 4096 compounds are selected from the training data by each of the following methods:

- At random, to serve as a benchmark.
- Using the uniform-cell-coverage (UCC) criterion in **Subheading 2.3.**, with 4096 cells in every 1D, 2D, and 3D subspace of a descriptor set.
- Using the clustering method in **Subheading 2.2.**, with 4096 clusters formed.

Table 1
**Uniform-Cell-Coverage (UCC) Criterion Evaluated
for Three Descriptor Sets and Various Designs**[a]

		UCC criterion		
Design method	Descriptor set used for design	BCUT	Constitutional — 6 PCs	Constitutional — 20 PCs
Random	NA	21,659	13,729	37,852
UCC	BCUT	7,058	13,105	31,575
	Constitutional — 6 PCs	21,316	4,512	18,675
	Constitutional — 20 PCs	19,603	7,295	10,704
Clustering	BCUT	18,906	13,477	37,030
	Constitutional — 6 PCs	20,017	12,778	33,470
	Constitutional — 20 PCs	19,362	13,083	32,664
	Constitutional	20,674	13,016	32,306

[a]Only the first of two replicates is reported for each design. The UCC criterion measures the discrepancy from the ideal of one compound per cell in all 1D, 2D, and 3D subspaces; small values of UCC are desirable. No descriptors are required for a random design, hence the "NA" for "not applicable" in the table.

Generating two replicate designs provides a measure of variability within a method due to chance.

The UCC and clustering methods require a descriptor set—BCUT or constitutional descriptors. As our implementation of UCC requires continuous descriptors, the 46 constitutional descriptors, which include discrete counts, were also reduced to either the first 6 or the first 20 principal components (PCs). Thus, the UCC algorithm was applied to the BCUT descriptors and either 6 or 20 PCs from the constitutional descriptors. In addition to these three sets, clustering was also applied to the 46 raw constitutional descriptors. The random design requires no descriptors.

Thus, there are eight design-method/descriptor-set combinations to compare, as shown in the first two columns of **Table 1**. We use UCC to measure diversity, as it provides a comprehensive assessment of coverage in all low-dimensional subsets of variables. Recall that a small value of UCC is better. Furthermore, no matter how the design is generated, UCC can be measured according to the BCUT or constitutional descriptors (6 or 20 PCs). The results are very similar for the two replicates, hence only the first replicate is reported.

If the BCUT descriptors are used for evaluating a design according to UCC, the UCC design based on BCUTs is of course optimal. Surprisingly, at least to us, however, the third column of **Table 1** shows that all the remaining designs

Table 2
Cell Coverage in 1D, 2D, and 3D Subspaces
for Various Descriptor Sets and Designs[a]

Design method	Descriptor set used for design	Percentage of covered cells		
		BCUT	Constitutional — 6 PCs	Constitutional — 20 PCs
Random	NA	65.0	63.8	61.6
UCC	BCUT	85.3	67.1	66.3
	Constitutional — 6 PCs	67.2	84.2	75.2
	Constitutional — 20 PCs	68.2	77.3	81.8
Clustering	BCUT	69.9	65.3	63.6
	Constitutional — 6 PCs	67.3	67.6	65.9
	Constitutional — 20 PCs	68.0	67.5	67.0
	Constitutional	66.5	67.3	66.1

[a]Only the first replication is reported for each design. Large percentages are desirable.

have much larger UCC/BCUT values. In other words, a design chosen for diversity via clustering with any descriptor set (including BCUTs) or via UCC with a different descriptor set performs about the same as a random design in terms of UCC/BCUT. Similar results pertain in the last two columns of **Table 1** when UCC is evaluated using the constitutional descriptors. The conclusion is that a "diverse" design turns out to be not much more diverse than a random choice when evaluated according to a different method or descriptor set, which we find surprising.

Table 2 gives analogous results for the percentage of 1D, 2D, and 3D cells covered by the various designs. This measure is somewhat easier to interpret than UCC. For example, if UCC and BCUTs are used for design, approx 85% of the cells in BCUT space are covered. For any other design, the coverage in BCUT space drops substantially.

Table 3 reports the number of active compounds found in the initial screen by each design. None of the methods deviates substantially from the 76 hits expected under random sampling. The UCC designs are highly optimized; hence, the two replicates have many common compounds, as shown in the last column of **Table 3**. The cluster-based designs choose one compound at random from each cluster; there is much chance occurrence in this process and the two replicates share only about the same number of compounds as random sampling. Therefore, the random and cluster-based designs vary substantially and at least two runs are required for evaluation purposes.

Table 3
**Number of Active Compounds in the Initial Design
of 4096 Compounds Found by Various Methods[a]**

Design method	Descriptor set used for design	No. active compounds		No. common compounds
		Rep 1	Rep 2	
Random	NA	73	66	1,358
UCC	BCUT	81	78	3,708
	Constitutional — 6 PCs	86	87	3,511
	Constitutional — 20 PCs	74	73	3,935
Clustering	BCUT	59	81	1,343
	Constitutional — 6 PCs	69	89	1,309
	Constitutional — 20 PCs	77	71	1,399
	Constitutional	59	69	1,302

[a]Both replicates are reported and the number of compounds they share. Under random sampling conditions, the expected number of active compounds is 76.

Table 4
Number of Active Compounds Found by Cell-Based Analysis

Design method	Descriptor set used for design	No. active compounds	
		100 selected	200 selected
Random	NA	52, 42	62, 53
UCC	BCUT	40, 35	47, 44
	Constitutional — 6 PCs	31, 37	46, 58
	Constitutional — 20 PCs	30, 31	40, 40

[a]Reported is the number of active compounds found by CBA when 100 or 200 top scoring compounds are selected from various designs, each replicated twice. In all cases, CBA uses the six BCUT descriptors for analysis.

4.3. Structure–Activity Analysis

Here we compare cluster classification (**Subheading 3.1.**) and cell-based analysis (CBA, **Subheading 3.2.**) in terms of the number of hits found in the test data.

Table 4 presents the results for CBA. Four designs from the training data are considered, but only the BCUT descriptors are used here for analysis. CBA prioritizes the test compounds, and those with the highest scores are selected;

Table 5
Number of Active Compounds Found
by Cluster Classification[a]

Descriptor set	No. active compounds/ No. compounds selected
BCUT	44/274, 58/293
Constitutional — 6 PCs	31/218, 33/259
Constitutional — 20 PCs	54/240, 46/203
Constitutional	45/220, 45/243

[a]Reported is the number of active compounds found versus number of compounds selected by the cluster classification for four descriptor sets (two replicates).

we report the number of hits found when the 100 or 200 compounds with the highest scores in the test data are selected.

The most surprising finding in **Table 4** is that random designs outperform the diverse UCC designs, even when the BCUT descriptors are also used at the design stage. This contradicts previous results *(19,25)*, where it was found that a cell-based analysis using BCUT descriptors was improved if a matching UCC/BCUT design was used.

Table 5 provides analogous performance results for cluster-classification. Each test compound is assigned to the nearest cluster. If the cluster is active, i.e., the compound randomly chosen from the cluster in the training data was active, the test compound is selected for testing. Results from clustering according to the four possible descriptor sets are reported. With cluster classification, the number of test compounds selected is random and not easily controlled; 31–58 active compounds are found in 218–293 selected. CBA finds 40–62 active compounds among 200 (*see* **Table 4**), suggesting that CBA performs somewhat better in this case than cluster classification.

Young and Hawkins have analyzed the same dataset using recursive partitioning and the same designs from the training data. Comparison with their results reported in Chapter 12 suggests that both cluster classification and CBA are competitive with recursive partitioning as predictors of active compounds.

5. Conclusions

To our surprise, the comparisons in **Subheading 4.2.** of diversity design strongly suggest that a design constructed to be diverse according to one method and descriptor set is not much more diverse than random when assessed by a different diversity criterion. In the absence of compelling reasons for a particular descriptor set and diversity measure, these results suggest that random sampling is about equally effective.

The results in **Subheading 4.3.** on performance of classification methods in identifying active compounds do not clearly favor either the BCUT or constitutional descriptors. Again, these results are surprising, given that the two descriptor sets are qualitatively different. Cell-based analysis performs slightly better than cluster classification. Probably the most surprising result of all is that random initial compound sets were as good as diverse sets for cell-based analysis. Similar findings have indeed been obtained for recursive partitioning *(27)*. We would expect CBA to be advantaged by a matching cell-based uniform-coverage design, however, as the design would tend to ensure that every cell is well-populated, leading to reliable scores, during analysis.

The above findings relate to one assay and one data set built up over time, possibly with many analogs of active compounds, and the findings might be different for commercial molecular databases. More benchmarking along these lines is needed.

Acknowledgments

This work was funded by MITACS and NSERC of Canada. We thank Hugh Chipman, Geoffrey Salloum, and Xu Wang for their help with the cluster-classification method and Stan Young for valuable discussions and contributions to this work.

References

1. Abt, M., Lim, Y.-B., Sacks, J., Xie, M., and Young, S. S. (2001) A sequential approach for identifying lead compounds in large chemical databases. *Stat. Sci.* **16,** 154–168.
2. Engels, M. F. M. and Venkatarangan, P. (2001) Smart screening: approaches to efficient HTS. *Curr. Opin. Drug Disc. Dev.* **4,** 275–283.
3. Jones-Hertzog, D. K., Mukhopadhyay, P., Keefer, C. E., and Young, S. S. (1999) Use of recursive partitioning in the sequential screening of G-protein-coupled receptors. *J. Pharmacol. Toxicol.* **42,** 207–215.
4. van Rhee, A. M., Stocker, J., Printzenhoff, D., Creech, C., Wagoner, P. K., and Spear, K. L. (2001) Retrospective analysis of an experimental high-throughput screening data set by recursive partitioning. *J. Comb. Chem.* **3,** 267–277.
5. Warmuth, M. K., Liao, J., Rätsch, G., Mathieson, M., Putta, S., and Lemmen, C. (2003) Active learning with support vector machines in the drug discovery process. *J. Chem. Inf. Comput. Sci.* **43,** 667–673.
6. Todeschini, R. and Consonni, V. (2000) *Handbook of molecular descriptors.* Wiley-VCH, Weinheim, Germany.
7. Leach, A. R. and Gillet, V. J. (2003) *An introduction to chemoinformatics.* Kluwer Academic Publishers, London, UK.

8. Brown, R. D. and Martin, Y. C. (1996) Use of structure-activity data to compare structure-based clustering methods and descriptors for use in compound selection. *J. Chem. Inf. Comput. Sci.* **36,** 572–584.

9. Feng, J., Lurati, L., Ouyang, H., et al. (2003) Predictive toxicology: benchmarking molecular descriptors and statistical methods. *J. Chem. Inf. Comput. Sci.* **43,** 1463–1470.

10. Burden, F. R. (1989) Molecular identification number for substructure searches. *J. Chem. Inf. Comput. Sci.* **29,** 225–227.

11. Pearlman, R. S. and Smith, K. M. (1998) Novel software tools for chemical diversity. *Persp. Drug Disc. Des.* **09/10/11,** 339–353.

12. Hastie, T., Tibshirani, R., and Friedman, J. (2001) *The elements of statistical learning: data mining, inference, and prediction.* Springer, New York, NY.

13. Zemroch, P. J. (1986) Cluster analysis as an experimental design generator, with application to gasoline blending experiments. *Technometrics* **28,** 39–49.

14. Hansch, C., Unger, S. H., and Forsythe, A. B. (1973) Strategy in drug design. Cluster analysis as an aid in the selection of substituents. *J. Med. Chem.* **16,** 1217–1222.

15. Hodes, L. (1989) Clustering a large number of compounds. 1. Establishing the method on an initial sample. *J. Chem. Inf. Comput. Sci.* **29,** 66–71.

16. Cummins D. J., Andrews C. W., Bentley J. A., and Cory, M. (1996) Molecular diversity in chemical databases: Comparison of medicinal chemistry knowledge bases and databases of commercially available compounds. *J. Chem. Inf. Comput. Sci.* **36,** 750–763.

17. Menard, P. R., Mason, J. S., Morize, I., and Bauerschmidt, S. (1998) Chemistry space metrics in diversity analysis, library design, and compound selection. *J. Chem. Inf. Comput. Sci.* **38,** 1204–1213.

18. McFarland, J. W. and Gans, D.J. (1986) On the significance of clusters in the graphical display of structure-activity data. *J. Med. Chem.* **29,** 505–514.

19. Lam, R. L. H. (2001) *Design and analysis of large chemical databases for drug discovery*, Ph.D. Dissertation, University of Waterloo.

20. Lam, R. L. H., Welch, W. J., and Young, S. S. (2002) Uniform coverage designs for molecule selection. *Technometrics* **44,** 99–109.

21. Pearlman, R. S. and Smith, K. M. (1999) Metric validation and the receptor-relevant subspace concept. *J. Chem. Inf. Comput. Sci.* **39,** 28–35.

22. Kennard, R. W., and Stone, L. A. (1969) Computer aided design of experiments. *Technometrics* **11,** 137–148.

23. Johnson, M. E., Moore, L. M., and Ylvisaker, D. (1990) Minimax and maximin distance designs. *J. Statist. Plan. Infer.* **26,** 131–148.

24. Higgs, R. E., Bemis, K. G., Watson, I. A., and Wikel, J. H. (1997) Experimental designs for selecting molecules from large chemical databases. *J. Chem. Inf. Comput. Sci.* **37,** 861–870.

25. Lam, R. L. H., Welch, W. J., and Young, S. S. (2002) *Cell-based analysis of high throughput screening data for drug discovery.* Research Report RR-02-02, Institute for Improvement in Quality and Productivity, University of Waterloo.

26. Yi, B., Hughes-Oliver, J. M., Zhu, L., and Young, S. S. (2002) A factorial design to optimize cell-based drug discovery analysis. *J. Chem. Inf. Comput. Sci.* **42,** 1221–1229.

27. Young, S. S., Farmen, M., and Rusinko, Λ. III (1996) Random versus rational: Which is better for general compound screening? Network Science online publication, available at URL: www.netsci.org/Science/Screening/feature09.html.

12

Using Recursive Partitioning Analysis to Evaluate Compound Selection Methods

S. Stanley Young and Douglas M. Hawkins

Abstract

The design and analysis of a screening set for high throughput screening is complex. We examine three statistical strategies for compound selection, random, clustering, and space-filling. We examine two types of chemical descriptors, BCUTs and principal components of Dragon Constitutional descriptors. Based on the predictive power of multiple tree recursive partitioning, we reached the following tentative conclusions. Random designs appear to be as good as clustering and space-filling designs. For analysis, BCUTs appear to be better than principal components scores based upon Constitutional Descriptors. We confirm previous results that model-based selection of compounds can lead to improved screening hit rates.

Key Words: Decision trees,; high throughput screening; initial screening sets; random recursive partitioning; recursive partitioning; sequential screening.

1. Introduction

Many of the initial leads for drug development originate from high-throughput screening (HTS); there, many hundreds of thousands of compounds are typically tested for biological activity. Both the number of compounds available for screening and the number of targets for screening are increasing, so there is a need to consider methods for making this process much more time and cost efficient.

We give a cause-and-effect, fishbone, or Ishikawa (1) diagram in **Fig. 1** to organize our conception of the early drug discovery process. The diagram is organized in time sequence from left to right. There are a number of distinct steps in finding lead compounds. The first two steps are the identification of a suitable biological target and development of an assay to assess that target. We

From: *Methods in Molecular Biology, vol. 275:*
Chemoinformatics: Concepts, Methods, and Tools for Drug Discovery
Edited by: J. Bajorath © Humana Press Inc., Totowa, NJ

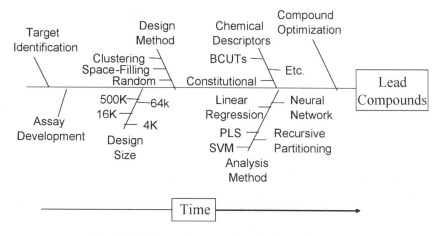

Fig. 1. Fishbone diagram of early drug discovery.

merely list those steps here and in **Fig. 1** to put our current efforts in context. We also list compound optimization as the next step in the process without going into any detail on that step.

We are most interested in how to design a set of compounds for initial screening: the *design method*, the *design size*, and the *method of statistical analysis*, and concentrate on factors that might influence the success of this operation. We would like to find a sample size that is large enough to provide useful information, but not so large as to increase discovery costs unreasonably. There are various methods for selecting representative compounds from a collection; three of these are random, clustering, and space-filling (*2*, hereafter LWY). Various methods have been used to analyze HTS data; we use recursive partitioning (RP), which has been very successful (*3–5*), so we will concentrate on RP and use the results of statistical analysis and prediction of holdout compounds to assess the selection method.

One approach to drug discovery is to screen sequentially, whereby a relatively small set of compounds is selected and assayed and the results are analyzed statistically to produce a mathematical model (*6,7*). The model is used to predict activity and also to identify additional compounds for screening— *see* **Fig. 2**. The new compound bioassay results are added to the results for the initial set and a new model is fitted. The process iterates, with new interesting candidate compounds being added. The focus of this chapter is to evaluate how the selection of a training set of compounds influences model building, and how the success of model building points to a good method for selecting training compounds. It is presumed, but not known, that the size and quality of the initial screening set will affect the subsequent model building and,

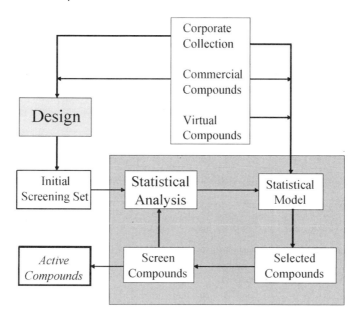

Fig. 2. Drug discovery paradigm. [Reproduced with permission from *Current Drugs* and Young, S. S., Lam, R. L. H., and Welch, W. J. (2002) Initial compound selection for sequential screening. *Current Opinion in Drug Discovery Development* **5,** 422–427. © 2002 PharmaPress Ltd.]

hence, the efficiency of finding active compounds. A good review of computational methods for early drug discovery is given by Xu and Hager *(8)*.

2. Single Tree

RP *(9–11)* is a family of data analysis techniques that works by dividing (partitioning) a dataset into smaller, disjoint sets. These groups are then analyzed as if they were an original dataset and are, in turn, divided in subgroups **(Fig. 3)**. There are three issues involved in performing RP: how to form groups, how to decide which grouping to use for splitting, and how to stop. As a division takes place, there is a grouping or segmentation step. Each predictor variable is converted into a small number of groups or classes. If the predictor is nominal, then groups are amalgamated by grouping classes with similar response. If the predictor is continuous, then it is cut into segments such that the within-segment variances are minimized subject to the constraint of the number of groups under consideration. It is instructive to consider an example tree **(Fig. 4)**. The compounds are rated active (coded 1) or inactive (coded 0), and the mean hit rate is low, 0.020, or 2%, a rate quite typical in drug discovery. The algorithm examines six continuous BCUT variables

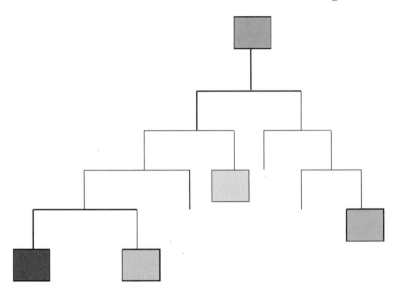

Fig. 3. Recursive partitioning. Recursive partitioning divides compounds into progressively smaller groups using specific features. The splitting features are selected using the potency of the compounds.

(12,13), and splits using BCUT4 into four segments. Most of the compounds, 3191, are in the first segment. Only 1.2% of these compounds are active. The next two segments contain more active compounds. They can be split and will be discussed in turn. The rightmost segment also contains mostly inactive compounds; 2% are active. Node names are given in the lower left hand corner of each node. The topmost node is the parent node and the nodes without daughter nodes are called terminal leaves or terminal nodes. The mean, u=, and standard deviation, s=, of the objects in a node are given.

The dendrogram lists a number of *p*-values for each node that is split. These *p*-values can be used to judge the veracity of a split. Keep in mind that the algorithm is examining a very large number of potential splits. Because there is such a thorough search over so many possibilities, there needs to be adjustment in the statistics used for splitting. The first *p*-value given, P=, is the "raw" *p*-value. This is the *p*-value for the *t*-test, *F*-test, or chi-square test for the split, computed as if this split was the only preplanned comparison. The chi-squared value of the four-way split of this "root" node is 973 with three degrees of

Fig. 4. *(see facing page)* Example tree. An RP tree was built using compounds selected by a space-filling design; BCUT descriptors were used for the analysis.

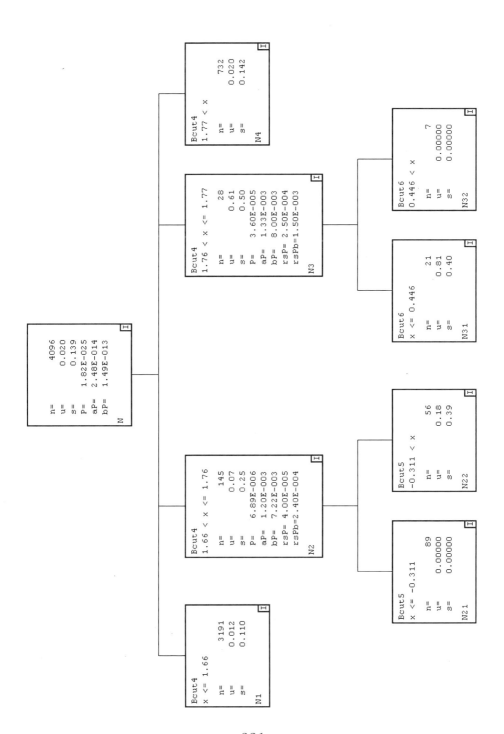

321

freedom. If we knew before we collected the dataset that we would split the variable BCUT4 into these four groups and got this chi-squared, the p value would be 1.82×10^{-25}. However, this split was actually arrived at by combing through BCUT4 to pick the most significant cutpoints. Adjusting the p value to reflect this multiple testing brings it down to $ap = 2.48 \times 10^{-14}$. We see that ap, although 10^{11} times larger than p, is still highly statistically significant. There is one more adjustment to the p-value given in this node. After segmentation, we still need to take into account the number of variables, in this case six. Here we do a simple Bonferroni adjustment, we multiply ap by six to get bp. It is the bp that is used to select the split variable and segmentation, where we select the split with the smallest bp.

We now turn our attention to node N2 with 145 compounds and 7% active. Here the p-value, $bp = 7 \times 10^{-3}$, looks good for making a split. Illustrating an additional option for split evaluation, we report two additional p-values obtained by resampling. Resampling gives an independent method of computing p-values *(14)*. In this case the observations in node N are placed at random into the four daughter nodes while maintaining the sample sizes of the daughter nodes. This is done many times and each time the test statistic is computed. By looking at the placement of the original statistic in the distribution of the resampling-based statistics, we can judge the veracity of the p-value computed from theory. The agreement in p-values is good. That the resampling p value is appreciably lower than the Bonferroni is an expected reflection of the fact that the Bonferroni p value is conservative whereas the resampling value is not. Both p-values, 7×10^{-3} and 2×10^{-4}, are statistically highly significant, supporting making the indicated split. Looking at N22, we see that 18% of the 56 compounds are active. Node N31 also looks good with 81% of the 21 compounds active.

It is useful to examine the predictions from a RP analysis. The original NCI HIV dataset was divided into two groups with the first used for modeling. We now cascade the second group down the tree constructed from the 4096 compounds selected by the space-filling algorithm. Compounds are sent down the tree following the values of their BCUTs and the dictates of the original tree. For example, a compound with BCUT4=1.77 and BCUT6=0.43 will go into node N31. These predictions for the holdout compounds are given in **Fig. 5**; the predictions are in good qualitative agreement with the results of the original calibration dataset in that the nodes predicted to have activity well above or well below average do so, although the actual size of the enhancement or

---

Fig. 5. *(see facing page)* Holdout set in SF/BCUT design tree.

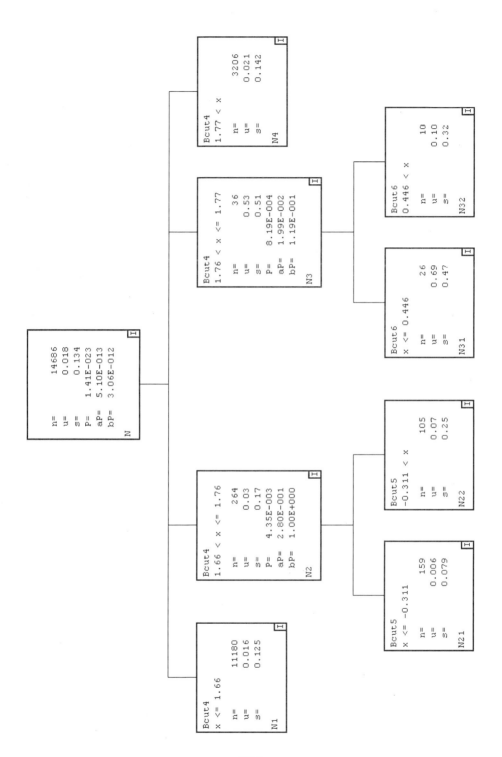

reduction is generally smaller in the holdout data. This is a "regression to the mean" effect, and is also expected.

The primary result of a recursive partitioning analysis is a tree-like model or *dendrogram*. All the data are in the top or parent node and the terminal nodes are a disjoint partitioning of the data. The rules that trace along the arms of a tree are important predictor variables. Recursive partitioning has many attractive qualities. One of the most useful features of a tree is the ability to convey complex relationships easily. From a statistical point of view, first and foremost, the technique is free of many of the restrictive assumptions associated with standard linear regression models. In a standard linear model, it is assumed a single model fits the data. In RP analyses, in stark contrast, each node (subgroup) is analyzed independently of the other nodes; thus, no single model is fit to the entire dataset. If there are multiple mechanisms, then they may be separated out in the different arms of the tree. This flexibility allows models that would be difficult to construct in a standard linear model. Second, in a standard linear model we often make strong distributional assumptions about the nature of the error, and these assumptions must be checked to ensure the validity of our inference. In recursive partitioning, it is possible to use robust methods, freeing us of strong distributional assumptions. We repeat, the result of a recursive partitioning analysis is the dendrogram, which is easily read and understood by non-statisticians. Thus, recursive partitioning is gaining ascendancy in the analysis of large, complex datasets.

3. A Forest of Trees

Recursive partitioning is a feature selection method. As such it shares the deficiencies of other feature selection methods such as stepwise or subset regression. The major deficiencies are as follows:

1. It provides just a single answer, whereas there may be several substantively different models giving roughly equally good results.
2. The tree selected is not necessarily the best tree, even among trees of the same "complexity," the same number of terminal nodes.
3. It can be confounded by highly interactive variables, variables that are useless on their own, but show synergy when used together.

The solution to these problems lies in creating, not a single tree, but a forest of trees (*see* **Fig. 6**); the reasoning is if one tree is good, then a forest should be even better. Random recursive partitioning (RRP) incorporates some randomness into the splitting procedure in place of the conventional method's deterministic approach so that running the analysis many times will generate a number of different trees.

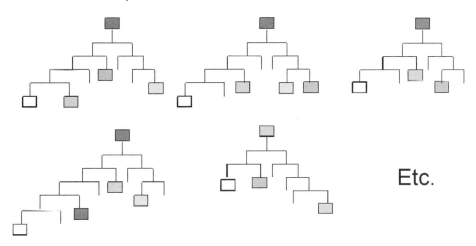

Fig. 6. Multiple trees.

There are two basic ways of introducing randomness into the tree generation—you can put a random element into the data and leave the split selection step fixed; or you can put a random element into the split selection step and leave the data fixed. Bootstrapping uses the first of these approaches. You create many new datasets by randomly sampling the original data set with replacement. So, for example, if a dataset had 10 cases numbered 1 through 10, a bootstrap sample might consist of 3 copies of case 4, 2 each of cases 3 and 10, and 1 each of cases 1, 7, 8. Putting many such randomly sampled datasets through the "greedy, pick-the-best-split" algorithm will usually give a variety of trees.

The second approach leaves the data fixed, and introduces a random element into the selection of the splitting variable. So if, for example, predictors x29, x47, and x82 were the only significant splitters and had multiplicity-adjusted p values of say 2×10^{-7}, 5×10^{-8}, and 3×10^{-3}, the conventional greedy algorithm would pick x47 as the splitting variable as it was the most significant. The RRP procedure would pick one of these three at random. Repeating the analysis with fresh random choices would then lead to a forest of trees; different random choices will create different trees.

Once we have generated the forest of trees, the next question is what to do with the information it contains. To explore this, recall that the analysis has two possible purposes—*prediction* and *feature selection*. Prediction is the problem that arises if we have a new compound whose activity is unknown and wish to predict its activity on the basis of the relationships seen in the calibration sample. A good way to use the forest to make such a prediction is "bagging."

You run the unknown compound through each of the trees in the forest and average the predictions that the different trees make for it. The term "bagging" is a contraction of "bootstrap aggregating," and so it would seem to apply only to forests created by bootstrapping, but in fact bagging is effective also with RRP forests.

The second potential purpose of an RP analysis is feature selection—trying to identify which predictors are strongly associated with high activity. This is a standard use of RP in sequential screening, where you will use the apparently important features as a guide to locate or synthesize new compounds that contain the features associated with high activity and avoid those associated with low. Feature selection is not done by averaging across the forest. Rather it consists of looking at the structure of the different trees. Each different tree morphology gives an indicator of a different set of features that are associated with differences in activity. Common findings among the different trees are the following:

- Alternative models. In complex high-dimensional data sets there will commonly be a number of very different-looking models all of which describe the data about equally well. Scanning the forest uncovers these alternative models. The alternative models can look different but be relatively trivial, based on correlated variables. Or they can point to multiple mechanisms.
- Substitutability—if two predictors are seen often, but never in the same tree, then this is an indication that they are mutually substitutable. "Substitutable" here is not meant to imply anything about structural chemistry, but is a purely descriptive term. If all the compounds in a library contain both feature A and feature B, or neither feature A nor feature B, and if feature A causes biological activity, then analysis of the data could wrongly suggest that feature B was important. The error in this will be discovered when the random forest shows that A and B are substitutable. This situation would suggest finding or synthesizing compounds with A alone or B alone to decouple the features.
- Synergy is the converse of this, where all trees contain either feature A and feature B; or neither feature A nor feature B. This implies that there is a synergistic interaction between the two features. Some more detail of how to read the forest to find synergies and variables that substitute is given in Hawkins and Musser *(15)*, who give some formal approaches for measuring the similarity of trees in the forest and analyzing the dependencies between pairs of features.
- In any recursive partitioning technique, power drops dramatically as we split our data into smaller and smaller groups so that, except in huge samples, the final model selected understates the actual number of useful predictors. By giving all significant predictors the opportunity to be used for splitting, RRP makes it easy to find a more complete set of relevant variables.

We use FIRMplus® for this analysis *(16)*.

Standard RP uses a greedy algorithm to build its trees and, as such, it is not guaranteed to find a globally "optimal" tree. RRP, if run long enough, should be able to find the optimal tree. Clearly, there is ample justification for considering RRP. Having multiple trees does present a problem: how to *interpret* the multitude of trees. Comparing two trees is relatively easy; we can view two trees or dendrograms at the same time and make simple visual comparisons to answer basic questions: Do the trees use the same number of predictors? Do the trees have the same number of terminal nodes? However, comparing more trees is much harder: even answering basic questions, such as how many terminal nodes each tree has, becomes cumbersome to do by hand; answering complex questions that require pairwise comparisons between trees requires tools beyond paper and pencil. Thus, creating multiple trees is easy, but interpreting them is not.

There is extensive literature showing that multiple trees generally give better predictions than single trees *(17)*.

4. NCI Data

The NCI maintains databases for research on the treatment of HIV/AIDS. We use a NCI database in this paper: dtp.nci.nih.gov/docs/aids/aids_data

5. Experimental Plan

We are interested in the question of how the selection of compounds, the design, might affect the predictive power of the analysis. Compounds can be selected at random or they can be selected based on some statistical algorithm, space-filling or clustering. The statistical selection method operates on numerical descriptions of the compounds and here we use four sets of descriptors for the design selection process. BCUT descriptors *(12,13)* are becoming popular and have been shown to effectively capture chemical information *(18–20)*. We use six BCUT descriptors. We also use either 6 or 20 principal components scores, PC6 or PC20, based upon the so-called Constitutional Descriptors computed by the Dragon software *(21)*. We have a total of eight experimental designs and these are given in the margin of **Table 1**. Lam and Welch computed these designs and they are described in Chapter 11. For each design, 4096 compounds are selected from the 14,688 compounds in the training set.

We decided to examine only one sample size for the design, 4096. Abt et al. *(6)* examined sample size, among other factors, when studying sequential screening. Yi et al. *(20)* also used a sample size of 4096 when studying the optimization of a statistical analysis method for this dataset. Both studies indicated that relatively small sample sizes of 5000 to 10,000 compounds could be used to produce useful trees. Clearly, large sample sizes should lead to better

Table 1
Statistical Analysis[a]

Design selection	Design descriptors		Analysis descriptors					
			BCUT		C6		C20	
Random	NA	Rep1	0.395	86	0.111	99	0.282	85
		Rep2	0.186	97	0.270	89	0.274	95
Clustering	Const		0.176	148	0.155	187	0.049	486
	BCUT		0.183	109	0.042	1707	0.042	1707
	C6		0.234	94	0.018	112	0.084	687
	C20		0.398	93	0.085	686	0.085	686
Space-filling	BCUT		0.183	109	0.008	245	0.030	198
	C6		0.245	98	0.245	94	0.235	98
	C20		0.208	96	0.230	100	0.128	94

[a]Three statistical methods were used for design selection—random, clustering and space-filling. For space-filling and clustering there were three sets of chemical descriptors used, BCUTs, and either 6 or 20 principal component scores computed from Constitutional Descriptors. For clustering we also used 46 individual Constitutional Descriptors. The random selection was replicated twice. We give the fraction active for multiple trees using three different types of descriptors for the N compounds predicted to be most active.

models, but as we are interested in reducing the cost of drug discovery, we chose a number of compounds for the training set near the lower bound that should be effective in producing usable models.

There is a subtle point. The original dataset is divided into training and testing sets. The designs are selected from the training set and the tree model is based on the compounds in the design from the training set. We are going to test the design quality by the quality of the model predictions in the testing set. We are not actually using the training compounds that are not in the design. There is a potential problem in selecting the design from the whole dataset and using the remaining compounds as the test set (as is often done in this type of study). The space-filling and clustering design methods are constructed to cover the space as uniformly as possible so they may select most of the thinly populated areas. In these sparse regions, there may be actives. When the analysis and prediction is done, there may be no unusual compounds remaining in the testing set. We have chosen to attempt to remove this potential bias by dividing the compounds from the beginning into the training and testing sets.

We give a two-way plot of randomly selected and space-filling selected compounds, BCUT4 vs BCUT3, in **Fig. 7**. It is clear that the space-filling algorithm of LWY selects compounds more uniformly from the collection. The compound density is spread out more.

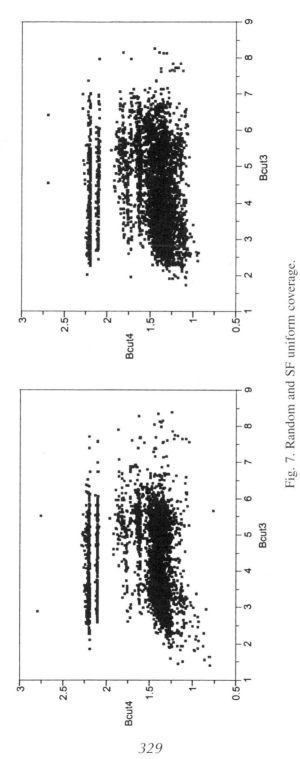

Fig. 7. Random and SF uniform coverage.

329

6. Analysis Results

The basic results of these analyses are presented in **Table 1**. On the left margin are the design methods and the descriptors used in the design phase. Note that it is not necessary to use descriptors with a random design so the design descriptors are given as not applicable (NA). For the space-filling design of LWY we used BCUTs, and 6 and 20 principal components from the Dragon Constitutional Descriptors. For clustering we added a clustering design using 46 individual Constitutional Descriptors. Computational considerations limit our space-filling code to 10 dimensions, so we did not attempt a space-filling design with the Constitutional Descriptors. At the top of the table we give the descriptors used in the RRP analysis. BCUTs have been used successfully in QSAR analysis *(18–20)*, so we expected BCUTs to be effective. We know less about the effectiveness of the Constitutional Descriptors. Simple descriptors, like the Constitutional Descriptors, have been used successfully *(22)*. We did not know if 20 principal component scores would be necessary, or if 6 would be sufficient. This question is more complex than many principal component users suppose it to be. The principal components are pure linear functions of the predictors. While it is true that by using all components you should be able to duplicate any model accuracy got using the original variables, it is not necessarily the case that the predictive principal components will be those that explain a high proportion of the variance of the original predictors. In other words, even if a few principal components explain a high proportion of variance, they will not necessarily capture any of the information important for predicting biological activity. In the context of our immediate problem, this means that we should decide between using 6 and using 20 principal components on the basis of the quality of the models fitted using these components, and not on the basis of their proportion of variance explained.

Given a design set of compounds, an analysis can be run based upon any descriptors. We use three sets of descriptors, BCUT, PC6, or PC20. Consider the body of **Table 1** where we tabulate the results for the analysis of each design for each of the three sets of descriptors; this table summarizes the results for 24 different multiple tree statistical analyses. For each design/descriptor combination we give two numbers: the fraction of the compounds that are active and the number of compounds for which this fraction is computed. Note that each statistical model will make a prediction for each compound in the testing dataset. The predicted compounds are ranked by their predicted values. Because trees make predictions based on the average of the compounds in a terminal node, these predictions are a step function. We selected at the step that made predictions for approx 100 compounds. To give a sense of the variability of this process, we ran two replications of the random selection, Rep1 and Rep2.

We computed an analysis of variance over **Table 1**, followed by tests of specific effects. Two results were statistically significant. Random selection of compounds was better than cluster or space-filling selection. BCUT descriptors were better for analysis than either of the principal component descriptor sets.

7. Discussion

By and large, the trees were valid in that the predicted activities from trees agreed with the actual mean activities of the corresponding nodes in the holdout samples. There is, and is expected to be, some "regression to the mean," in that where the calibration tree had a node predicting extremely high or extremely low activity, the observed means of the holdout samples will tend toward the average. This is not a problem, but is a reminder that the dendrogram can identify very active or very inactive groups of compounds, but tends to overstate their unusualness. Even so, the promising nodes uncovered in the calibration have a hit rate for the hold out sample that is about 12 times the background hit rate of 2%. This improved hit rate is in line with previous results *(20,23)* and others.

There were however some cases where the tree on the hold out set did not confirm the original tree; compounds in nodes predicted to be active were not. As the holdout set was bigger, approx 14K vs approx 4K in the training set, these discrepancies are not likely to be the result of random variability in the holdout data, and they need some further investigation.

It is worth making some general comments on chemical databases. Chemicals are not typically made for random reasons; chemicals are made for some purpose. In particular, once a good chemical is identified, it is common practice to make many variants of that chemical, making slight changes in an attempt to make a better molecule. When screeners assemble chemical databases, they will often augment their collection with compounds similar to active compounds in their current collection, "analog by catalog," as it is much cheaper to buy a ready-made compound than to make one from scratch. All of this maneuvering with compounds and databases improves the chances of useful discovery, but means that most chemical databases cannot be viewed as "a random collection of molecules." Most chemical collections will have many subsets of compounds that are very similar to one another, for example, numerous steroids are in corporate collections. So, if you select a random set of compounds as an initial screening set, there is a good chance that there will be groups of similar compounds in the set. There is a tension between diversity and redundancy; to cover more chemical space, you want diversity, but to statistically analyze screening data you need feature redundancy in the screened set to give the statistical algorithms replication. One basic test that is used is the *t*-test and that compares compounds that are grouped by the presence and absence of a specific chemical feature. If all the compounds are completely unique, then all the comparisons will be one compound against the rest and we will not be using the power inherent in averaging. The space-filling statistical algorithm used for selecting the initial screening set has the effect of spreading the selected compounds uniformly through the chemical space and there is no specific attention to building redundancy into the set. Only if enough compounds are selected, will they be close enough to one another to provide this redundancy. It is an open question as to how densely the chemical space needs to be covered.

The nature of the chemical collections also makes it difficult to measure the performance of specific screening strategies. We would like to say that a successful screening strategy validates the entire process—the molecular descriptors, the initial screening set selection method, and the statistical algorithm used for model building. In particular, we would like the features associated with activity to have chemical meaning and be useful in finding other active compounds that have those specific features. As chemical databases are filled with close analogs, what we may be doing is very fancy analog finding. Analog finding can be done with other methods. There is some evidence that statistical model building is doing something beyond analog finding in that the hit rates for statistical models are typically better than gestalt analog finding. Usually statistical model–based selection is better than gestalt analog finding, approx 10 times random selection versus approx 5 times, but this would need to be established for each situation of descriptor type and analysis method.

Building predictive models when the hit rate is low is a challenge; there is relatively little information in the data to guide the model building process. Using a continuous response measure should be better than a binomial response. We examined the quality of the model building process in the following way. We defined a good node as one with a hit rate of 10% or greater, approx 5 times the hit rate in the dataset. For each of the eight design methods (nine designs as we have two designs for the random selection), we computed the average number of good nodes over the three types of analysis descriptors. We note a trend toward more good nodes if the hit rate in the training set is higher; *see* **Fig. 8**.

The hope was that having a good design would make for a better model. We expected that the design quality would be in the order random, clustering, space-filling. Basically none of the designs beat a random design. We suspect two factors contribute to the success of random designs: The random design has better redundancy, and the number of compounds selected, 4096, may not be large enough to densely cover chemical space. The NCI dataset probably has redundancy of actives in that it was augmented over time with analogs to active

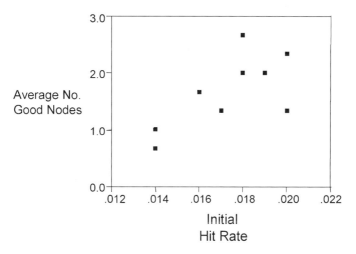

Fig. 8. Number of good notes versus the initial hit rate.

compounds so the random design has a better chance of dense coverage in these active regions. Random versus rational selection of compounds has been discussed *(24)*.

References

1. Ishikawa, K. (1986) *Guide to quality control*, Productivity, Inc., Shelton, CT. *See also*, www.hci.com.au/hcisite2/toolkit/causeand/htm.
2. Lam, R. L. H., Welch, W. J., and Young, S. S. (2002) Uniform coverage designs for molecule selection. *Technometrics* **44**, 99–109.
3. Hawkins, D. M., Young, S. S., and Rusinko, A. (1997) Analysis of a large structure–activity data set using recursive partitioning. *Quantitaive Structure-Activity Relationship* **16**, 296–302.
4. Rusinko, A. III, Farmen, M. W., Lambert, C. G., Brown, P. L., and Young, S. S. (1999) Analysis of a large structure/biological activity data set using recursive partitioning. *J. Chem. Inf. Comput. Sci.* **39**, 1017–1026.
5. van Rhee, A. M., Stocker, J., Printzenhoff, D., Creeh, C., Wagoner, P. K., and Spear, K. L. (2001) Retrospective analysis of an experimental high-throughput screening data set by recursive partitioning. *J. Comb. Chem.* **3**, 267–277.
6. Abt, M., Lim, Y-B., Sacks, J., Xie, M., and Young, S. S. (2001) A sequential approach for identifying lead compounds in large chemical databases. *Stat. Sci.* **16**, 154–168.
7. Engels, M. F., and Venkatarangan, P. (2001) Smart screening: approaches to efficient HTS. *Current Opinion Drug Discovery & Development* **4**, 275–283.
8. Xu, J. and Hagler, A. (2002) Review: chemoinformatics and drug discovery. *Molecules* **7**, 566–600.

9. Hawkins, D. M. and Kass, G. V. (1982) Automatic interaction detection. In *Topics in applied multivariate analysis*, Hawkins, D. M. (ed.), Cambridge Univ. Press, pp. 269–302.

10. Breiman, L., Friedman, J., Olshen, R. A., and Stone, C. J. (1984) *Classification and regression trees.* Wadsworth, New York, NY.

11. Quinlan, J. R. (1992) *C4.5 programs for machine learning.* Morgan Kaufmann Publishers, San Mateo, CA.

12. Burden, F. R. (1989) Molecular identification number for substructure searches. *J. Chem. Inf. Comput. Sci.* **29,** 225–227.

13. Pearlman, R. S. and Smith, K. M. (1999) Metric validation and the receptor-relevant subspace concept. *J. Chem. Inf. Comput. Sci.* **39,** 28–35.

14. Westfall, P. H. and Young, S. S. (1993) *Resampling-based multiple testing.* Wiley, New York, NY.

15. Hawkins, D. M. and Musser, B. J. (1999) One tree or a forest? Alternative dendro-graphic models. *Computing Science and Statistics* **30,** 534–542

16. FIRMPlus® www.goldenhelix.com.

17. Breiman, L. (2001) Statistical modeling: the two cultures. *Stat. Sci.* **16,** 199–231.

18. Stanton, D. T. (1999) Evaluation and use of BCUT descriptors in QSAR and QSPR studies. *Chem. Inf. Comput. Sci.* **39,** 11–20.

19. Lam, R. L. H. (2001) *Design and analysis of large chemical databases for drug discovery.* Ph.D. Dissertation, University of Waterloo.

20. Yi, B., Hughes-Oliver, J. M., Zhu, L., and Young, S. S. (2002) A factorial design to optimize cell-based drug discovery analysis. *J. Chem. Inf. Comput. Sci.* **42,** 1221–1229.

21. Dragon, www.disat.unimib.it/chm/Dragon.

22. Burden, F. R., and Winkler, D. A. (2000) A quantitative structure-activity relation-ships model for the acute toxicity of substituted benzenes to *Tetrahymena pyriformis* using Bayesian-regularized neural networks. *Chem. Res. Toxicol.* **13,** 436–440.

23. Jones-Hertzog, D. K., Mukhopadhyay, P., Keefer, C. E., and Young, S. S. (1999) Use of recursive partitioning in the sequential screening of G-protein-coupled receptors. *J. Pharmacol. Toxicol.* **42,** 207–215.

24. Young, S. S., Farmen, M., and Rusinko, A. III. Random versus rational: Which is better for general compound screening? www.netsci.org/Science/Screening/feature09.

13

Designing Combinatorial Libraries Optimized on Multiple Objectives

Valerie J. Gillet

Abstract

The recent emphasis in combinatorial library design has shifted from the design of very large diverse libraries to the design of smaller more focused libraries. Typically the aim is to incorporate as much knowledge into the design as possible. This knowledge may relate to the target protein itself or may be derived from known active and inactive compounds. Other factors should also be taken into account, such as the cost of the library and the physicochemical properties of the compounds that are contained within the library. Thus, library design is a multi-objective optimization problem. Most approaches to optimizing multiple objectives are based on aggregation methods whereby the objectives are assigned relative weights and are combined into a single fitness function. A more recent approach involves the use of a Multiobjective Genetic Algorithm in which the individual objectives are handled independently without the need to assign weights. The result is a family of solutions each of which represents a different compromise in the objectives. Thus, the library designer is able to make an informed choice on an appropriate compromise solution.

Key Words: Combinatorial libraries; combinatorial synthesis; computational filtering; drug-like; library enumeration; genetic algorithms; MOGA; molecular descriptors; Multiobjective Genetic Algorithm; multiobjective optimization; simulated annealing.

1. Introduction

The last decade has seen a shift from the traditional approach to chemical synthesis, based on one compound at a time, to the use of robotics allowing the synthesis of large numbers of compounds in parallel, in what are known as combinatorial libraries. The related technique of high-throughput screening (HTS) allows tens to hundreds of thousands of compounds to be tested for biological activity in a single day *(1)*. Thus, the throughput of the synthesis and

From: *Methods in Molecular Biology, vol. 275:*
Chemoinformatics: Concepts, Methods, and Tools for Drug Discovery
Edited by: J. Bajorath © Humana Press Inc., Totowa, NJ

test cycle has increased enormously. However, despite the increase in the number of compounds that can be handled, they still represent a very small fraction of the number of drug-like compounds that could potentially be made; for example, it has been estimated that as many as 10^{40} such compounds could exist *(2)*. Thus, it is clear that there is a need to be selective about the compounds that are made in combinatorial libraries *(3)*.

In the early days of combinatorial synthesis the emphasis was on synthesizing as many diverse compounds as possible on the assumption that maximizing diversity would maximize the coverage of different types of biological activity. However, these early libraries gave disappointing results: they had lower hit rates than expected and the hits that were found tended to have unfavorable physico-chemical properties to provide good starting points for lead discovery *(4)*.

It is now clear that if the new technologies are to be effective for drug discovery, the libraries need to be designed very carefully. Consequently, the emphasis has shifted away from large diverse libraries to the design of smaller libraries that incorporate as much knowledge about the target as is available. At one extreme, the three-dimensional (3D) structure of the biological target may be known, in which case structure-based methods such as docking or *de novo* design can be used in an attempt to design compounds that will fit into the binding site *(5,6)*. It is still the case, however, that in most drug-discovery programs the 3D structure of the target is unknown. When several actives and inactives are known, it may be possible to generate a model of activity in the form of a quantitative-structure activity relationship (QSAR), the model could then be used to design libraries consisting of compounds with high predicted activities *(7)*. Other approaches are based on similarity methods *(8)* where compounds are selected based on their 2D or 3D similarity to one or more known active compounds. Diverse libraries are appropriate when they are to be screened against a range of biological targets or when little is known about the target of interest. As a general rule, the amount of diversity required is inversely related to the amount of information that is available about the target.

Whether the primary aim is to design diverse or focused libraries, or indeed to provide a balance between the two, many other criteria should also be taken into account. For example, the compounds should possess appropriate physico-chemical properties to enable them to be progressed through the drug-discovery pipeline *(9)*. In addition, the reactants should be readily available, for example, already present in in-house collections or cheap to purchase with acceptable delivery times. Thus, library design is increasingly being treated as a multi-objective optimization problem that requires the simultaneous optimization of several criteria. In common with most real world optimization problems, the criteria are often in conflict, for example, optimizing diversity simultaneously with drug-like properties, and thus a compromise in the objectives is usually

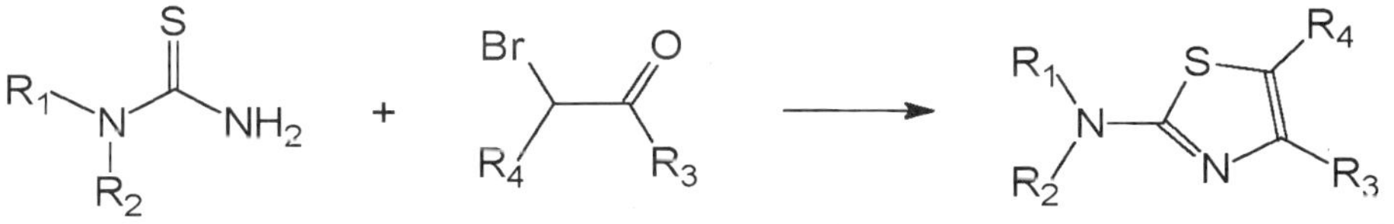

Fig. 1. A 2-aminothiazole library synthesized from α-bromoketones and thioureas.

sought. This chapter discusses approaches for the optimization of combinatorial libraries based on multiple objectives.

2. Methods

2.1. Reactant- versus Product-Based Designs

A simple two component combinatorial synthesis is shown in **Fig. 1**. The reaction involves the coupling of α-bromoketones and thioureas. Multiple products (2-aminothiazoles) can be synthesized in parallel by selecting different examples of each of the components, or reactants. The positions of variability in the reactants are indicated by the R groups.

In general, there are many more examples of the reactants available than can be handled in practice and thus selection methods must be used. For example, when designing peptides: there are 20 amino acids and hence 20 × 20 or 400 dipeptides; 8000 tripeptides; 32K tetrapeptides, and so on. When designing libraries of small drug-like compounds, in general there could be tens or even hundreds of possible reactants available for each position of variability. Thus, even when libraries are limited to a single reaction scheme, the numbers of compounds that could potentially be made can be very large.

Library design methods can be divided into reactant-based or product-based design. In reactant-based design, reactants are chosen without consideration of the products that will result. For example, diverse subsets of reactants are selected in the hope they will give rise to a diverse library of products. In product-based design, the selection of reactants is determined by analyzing the products that will be produced.

Reactant-based design is computationally less demanding than product-based design, since there are fewer molecules to consider. Consider a two-component reaction where there are 100 examples of each type of reactant. Now assume that the aim is to design a library of 100 products with configuration 10 × 10, i.e., 10 examples of each reactant. There are approx 10^{13} different possible subsets of size 10 contained within 100 compounds, as determined by the equation below:

$$\frac{N!}{n!(N-n)!}$$

Examining this number of subsets is clearly not feasible. Hence, a number of computationally efficient, albeit approximate, methods have been devised for performing reactant-based selection *(10)*. Product-based design, however, is much more computationally demanding and would require the analysis of 100×100 potential products (i.e., 10^4 molecules). Despite the increased computational cost of product-based design, it has been shown that it can result in better optimized libraries especially when the aim is to optimize library-based properties such as diversity *(11,12)*. Product-based design is even more appropriate for targeted or focused designs where it is the properties of the product molecules themselves that are to be optimized, for example, similarity to a known active compound.

Product-based approaches can be divided into those that take the combinatorial constraint into account such that each reactant in one pool appears in a product with every reactant from every other reactant pool, and those that merely pick product molecules without consideration of the synthetic constraint. The latter approach is often referred to as cherry-picking and is synthetically inefficient as far as combinatorial synthesis is concerned. In this chapter the emphasis is on product-based library design methods that take the combinatorial constraint into account.

2.2. Filtering

The first step in library design is to identify potential lists of reactants. This can be done by searching databases of available compounds, for example, in-house databases or databases of compounds that are available for purchase such as the Available Chemicals Directory *(13)*. The next step is to filter the reactant lists. This is a very important step because it can vastly reduce the computational complexity of the subsequent library design step. The aim is to remove reactants that could not possibly lead to "good" products. A variety of filtering techniques can be used. For example, removal of compounds that contain functionality that will interfere with the synthesis or that contain functional groups known to be toxic. In addition, thresholds on various physicochemical properties could also be applied, for example, removal of compounds with more than eight rotatable bonds or molecular weights greater than 300, because compounds with these properties are not generally considered as drug-like.

2.3. Library Enumeration

Enumeration is the computational equivalent of carrying out a combinatorial synthesis. The result is a virtual library of product molecules that can then be analyzed using a library design program to select compounds of interest. Two different approaches to library enumeration have been developed: fragment marking and the reaction-transform approach *(14)*.

Fragment marking involves representing a library by a central core (for example, a benzodiazepine ring) that is common to all compounds in the virtual library with one or more R groups to indicate the positions of variability. The library is enumerated by creating bonds between the core template and the reactants. The reactant lists must first be "clipped," for example, the hydoxyl group must be removed from a carboxylic acid selected to be combined with an amine group in the formation of an amide bond. Fragment-marking approaches usually require that there is a central core template that can be defined and that fragment clipping can be automated; however, this may not always possible, for example, for a Diels–Alder reaction.

The reaction-transform approach is based on a computer-readable representation of the reaction mechanism that describes the transformation of the atoms in the reactants to the product. The transform is applied to the input reactants themselves to generate the products. The reaction-transform approach thus more closely mimics the actual synthetic process; however, it can be difficult to construct efficient transforms. This is the approach used in the ADEPT software (*14*).

2.4. Design Criteria

As discussed in **Subheading 1.**, the primary design criterion is often based on either similarity or diversity. Quantifying these measures requires that the compounds are represented by numerical descriptors that enable pairwise molecular similarities or distances to be calculated or that allow the definition of a multidimensional property space in which the molecules can be placed.

A variety of different descriptors have been used in library design (*15,16*). They can be divided into descriptors that represent whole molecule properties; descriptors that can be calculated from the 2D graph representations of molecules including topological indices and 2D fingerprints; and descriptors calculated from 3D representations of molecules. Whole molecule properties include physicochemical properties such as molecular weight, molar refractivity, and calculated log$P$. Topological indices are single-valued descriptors that characterize structures according to their size, degree of branching, and overall shape. Many different topological indices have been devised and they are often used together with a molecule being represented by a vector of real numbers. 2D fingerprints are binary vectors and can be divided into fragment-based methods and path-based methods. In the fragment-based methods, each bit in the vector corresponds to a particular substructural fragment and is set to "on" or "off" to indicate the presence or absence of the substructure within a molecule. In the path-based methods, all paths up to a given length in the molecule are determined and each path is hashed to a small number of bits that are then set to "on."

The most commonly used 3D descriptors are pharmacophore keys, which are usually represented as binary vectors (*17*). The starting point when generating a pharmacophore key is a 3D conformation of a molecule that is represented by its pharmacophoric features, that is, its atoms or groups of atoms that can form interactions with a receptor such as hydrogen bond donors, acceptors, aromatic centres, anions, and cations. In three-point pharmacophore keys, each bit in the vector represents three pharmacophoric features together with a set of distance ranges that define how the features are positioned in 3D space. As with 2D fragment-based fingerprints, a bit is set to "on" to indicate the presence of a pharmacophore triplet within a molecule, otherwise it is set to "off."

When molecules are represented by high-dimensional descriptors such as 2D fingerprints or several hundred topological indices, then the diversity of a library of compounds is usually calculated using a function based on the pairwise (dis)similarities of the molecules. Pairwise similarity can be quantified using a similarity or distance coefficient. The Tanimoto coefficient is most often used with binary fingerprints and is given by the formula below:

$$S_{AB} = \frac{c}{a + b - c}$$

where there are a bits set to "on" in molecule A, b bits set to "on" in molecule B, and c "on" bits common to both A and B. When molecules are represented by real-numbered vectors, then the comparison is usually based on Euclidean distance. Various diversity functions have been suggested for library design including the average nearest-neighbor distance and the sum of pairwise dissimilarities *(18)*.

When molecules are represented by low-dimensional descriptors, then the descriptors can be used to define the axes of a chemistry space. Typical descriptors are a small number of physicochemical properties or the principal components generated by the application of principal components analysis to high-dimensional descriptors. Each descriptor then defines one axis and is divided into a series of bins. The combination of all bins over all descriptors defines a set of cells over a chemistry space. Molecules can be mapped onto the cells according to their physicochemical properties. A diverse library is one that occupies a large number of cells in the space, whereas a focused library is one where the molecules occupy a small localized region of the space.

The optimization of physicochemical properties can be dealt with by applying simple thresholds such as Lipinski's rule-of-five *(19)*. The rule states that if a compound violates any two of the following rules it is predicted to have poor oral absorption:

- Molecular weight > 500
- log$P$ > 5

- More than five hydrogen bond donors (defined as the sum of OH and NH groups)
- More than ten hydrogen bond acceptors (defined as the number of N and O atoms)

Alternatively, they can be optimized by matching the profile of properties in the library to some collection of known drug-like molecules. The latter method will typically allow some compounds to be present in the library that violate the more stringent rules. Several groups have developed more sophisticated methods for predicting drug-likeness *(20)* and, more recently, lead-likeness (because it has been recognized that lead compounds tend to be less complex than drugs) *(21,22)*.

2.5. Optimization Methods

The computational complexity of product-based library design has led to the development of programs that are based on optimization techniques such as genetic algorithms and simulated annealing. The methods require the definition of a function that is able to measure the degree to which a potential solution meets the library design criteria. The optimization technique then attempts to maximize (or minimize) the given function. Typically, many potential solutions are explored during the operation of the algorithm and thus the function must be relatively rapid to calculate.

Several groups have approached multiobjective library design by combining individual objectives into a single combined fitness function. This is a widely used approach to multiojective optimization and effectively reduces a multiobjective optimization problem to one of optimizing a single objective.

This approach has been adopted in the SELECT library design program *(23)*. SELECT is based on a GA and aims to identify a combinatorial subset of predetermined size and configuration, from within a virtual, fully enumerated library. The chromosome representation in SELECT encodes potential subsets as the lists of reactants from which the library will be synthesized. Thus, the chromosome is an integer string that is partitioned according to the number of positions of variability in the library. The size of a partition is determined by the number of reactants to be selected. Thus, when configured to select an $n_A \times n_B$ subset from a virtual library of size $N_A \times N_B$, the chromosome consist of $n_A + n_B$ integers. Each integer corresponds to one of the possible reactants available. The standard genetic operators of crossover and mutation are used with the special condition that the same reactant must not appear more than once in a partition.

SELECT has been designed to allow optimization of a variety of different objectives. Diversity (and similarity) is optimized using functions either based on pairwise dissimilarities and fingerprints or using cell-based measures. The physicochemical properties of libraries are optimized by minimizing the difference in the distribution of the library being designed and some reference distribution, such as that seen in the World Drug Index (WDI) *(24)*. Cost is optimized simply by minimizing the sum of the cost of the reactants. Each objective is usually standardized to be in the range 0 to 1 and user-defined weights are applied prior to summing the contributions into a weighted-sum fitness function as show below:

$$f(n) = w_1.diversity + w_2.cost + w_3.property1 + w_4.property2 + \dots$$

The HARPick program also tackles multiobjective library design by combining individual objectives, via weights, into a single function. HARPick uses Monte Carlo simulated annealing as the optimization technique *(25)* with library design being based on pharmacophore keys. A library is represented by an ensemble pharmacophore key, which is the union of the individual molecule keys. In HARPick the pharmacophore keys are integer vectors that indicate the frequency of occurrence of each three-point pharmacophore. The fitness function is composed of several individual functions: diversity is based on the number of unique pharmacophore triplets covered by the library and is tuned to force molecules to occupy relative voids (underrepresented three-point pharmacophores) as well as absolute voids; libraries can be optimized to fill voids underrepresented in an existing library; a function based on the number of conformations per molecule is used to control molecular flexibility; various properties are calculated that are crude measures of molecular shape with the aim of producing an even distribution of shapes in the library; and finally a count of the total number of pharmacophores present is used to limit the inclusion of promiscuous molecules (that is, molecules that contain a large number of pharmacophore triplets). As in the SELECT program, the individual functions are combined into a single fitness function via user-defined weights.

The method has subsequently been extended to include four-point pharmacophores and to allow pharmacophoric measures to be combined with 3D BCUT descriptors *(26)*. BCUT descriptors were designed to encode atomic properties relevant to intermolecular interactions. They are calculated from a matrix representation of a molecule's connection table where the diagonals of the matrix represent various atomic properties such as atomic charge, atomic polarizability, and atomic hydrogen bonding ability, and the off-diagonals are assigned the interatomic distances. The eigenvalues of the matrix are then extracted for use as descriptors. Five such descriptors were calculated: two based on charge, two on atomic polarizability, and one on hydrogen bond acceptors. These descriptors then define a 3D BCUT chemistry space, as for the cell-based methods described previously, with BCUT diversity being measured as the ratio of occupied cells to the total possible occupied cells. Pharmacophore diversity is based on the number of unique pharmacophores and the total number of pharmacophores in the product subset. An overall score for a library is then calculated by summing the two diversity measures. The method has been tested on a virtual library of 86,140 amide products in which pharmacophores were calculated on-the-fly, i.e., during the optimization process itself, with pharmacophore keys being stored for reuse as they are calculated.

Other similar aggregation approaches to multiobjective library design include the methods described by Agrafiotis *(27)*, Zheng et al. *(28)*, and Brown et al. *(29)*.

2.6. Multiobjective Optimization Using a MOGA

The aggregation approach to multiobjective optimization in which multiple objectives are combined into a single fitness function is limited for a number of reasons, some of which are identified here. First, the selection of weights for the individual components is non-intuitive especially when comparing different properties, for example, diversity and calculated log*P*. Second, the use of weights limits the search space that is explored. Third, in general, the methods are restricted to finding a single solution that represents one particular compromise in the objectives; assigning a different set of weights will typically result in a different solution, one that may be equally valid but that represents a different compromise in the objectives. Thus, in practice, it is usual to perform a number of trial-and-error runs using different weights in order to identify a "good" solution.

Multiobjective evolutionary algorithms (MOEAs) belong to a class of algorithms that is based on optimizing each objective independently and thus avoids the need to assign weights to individual objectives *(30)*. They exploit the population nature of evolutionary algorithms in order to explore multiple solutions in parallel. The MOGA is one example of a MOEA and is based on a GA *(31)*. In MOGA, the fitness ranking in a traditional GA is replaced by Pareto ranking. Pareto ranking is based on the concept of dominance, where, in a given population, one solution dominates another if it is better in all objectives and a non-dominated solution is one for which no other solution is better in all the objectives. In MOGA, an individual is assigned fitness according to the number of individuals by which it is dominated. Parent selection is then biased toward the least dominated individuals so that all non-dominated solutions have equal chance of being selected and they have a higher chance of being selected than solutions that are dominated. The non-dominated individuals form what is known as the Pareto surface. In the absence of further information, all solutions on the Pareto surface are equally valid with each one representing a different compromise in the objectives.

The MOGA algorithm has been adopted in the MoSELECT library design program *(32–34)*. MoSELECT derives from the earlier SELECT program with the original GA being replaced by a MOGA. Thus, in MoSELECT different objectives such as diversity, similarity, physicochemical property profiles, and cost are treated independently to generate a family of different compromise solutions as will be shown in **Subheading 3.**

2.7. Varying Library Size and Configuration

Many library design methods require that the size (number of products) and configuration (numbers of reactants selected for each component) of the library are specified upfront. However, it is often difficult to determine optimum values *a priori* and usually there is a trade-off between these criteria and the other criteria to be optimized. Consider the design of a library where the aim is to maximize coverage of some cell-based chemistry space. It is clear that as more products are included in the library the chance of occupying more cells increases. Thus, an optimal library is likely to be one that represents a compromise in size and diversity.

MoSELECT has been adapted so that size and configuration can be optimized simultaneously with other library design criteria. Size is allowed to vary by using a binary chromosome representation. The chromosome is partitioned, as before, with one partition for each position of variability. However, now each partition is of length equal to the number of reactants available with each reactant represented by a binary value. The value "1" indicates that a reactant has been selected and the value "0" indicates that it has not been selected for the final library. Thus the chromosome is now of length $N_A + N_B$ (as opposed to $n_A + n_B$ as described earlier). The application of the genetic operators results in different reactants being selected and deselected, and library size (and configuration) is thus varied by altering the number of bits set to "1."

As described previously, diversity and library size are usually in conflict with larger libraries resulting in greater cell coverage. Thus, when optimizing on diversity alone there will be a tendency to select very large libraries. Thus, in MoSELECT size is included as an objective alongside diversity with each objective being handled independently. This allows the trade-off between size and diversity to be explored in a single run.

2.8 Multiobjective Design Under Constraints

The MOGA approach allows the mapping of the entire Pareto surface with solutions at the extremes being identified as well as a range of solutions in between the extremes. When optimizing size and diversity, this means that a wide range of solutions is possible, from libraries consisting of a single product up to the library size that achieves maximum cell coverage. While having the ability to map the entire Pareto surface can provide useful insights into the shape of the search space of a particular library design problem, in practice there are often external constraints that must be taken into account. For example, constraints on library size may arise from the equipment available or simply on the basis of cost.

Library configuration can be a factor in cost as well as library size. Typically it is desirable to minimize the total number of reactants required. Thus, if the aim is to synthesize a library of 400 products from two positions of variability, then the most efficient use of reactants is achieved for the configuration 20×20. Other configurations (40×10, 25×16, etc.) would require access to a greater number of unique reactants.

Constraints can be implemented within the MOGA to direct the search toward restricted regions of the search space. Constraints are handled by penalizing solutions that violate the constraints. Such infeasible solutions are allowed to exist within the population (rather than being removed entirely) because their presence may lead to feasible solutions later in the search through the use of crossover. They are penalized so that they have a lower chance of being selected for reproduction and so that they do not appear in the final solution set. In the example described in the next section, constraints are applied on library size and configuration; however, they could equally be applied to any of the objectives incorporated within the library design.

3. Results: Designing 2-Aminothiazole Libraries

The two-component 2-aminothiazole library shown in **Fig. 1** is used to illustrate different library design scenarios using the SELECT and MoSELECT programs.

As discussed, the starting point for library design is to identify available reactants, for example, by searching in-house databases and/or by identifying reactants that can be purchased. In this case, substructure searches were performed on the ACD. When constructing a query, it is often necessary to place constraints on the compounds to be returned as hits. Thus, the α-bromoketone substructure was constrained so that it should not be embedded within a ring and explicit hydrogens were attached to one of the nitrogen atoms in the thiourea query with the additional constraint that substitution on the sulfur atom was prohibited.

Once initial sets of reactants were found computational filters were applied to remove reactants that are known to be undesirable. This was done using the ADEPT software (*14*) with the following compounds being removed: reactants having molecular weight greater than 300; reactants having more than eight rotatable bonds; and a series of substructure searches were performed to remove reactants containing undesirable substructural fragments. After filtering there were 74 α-bromoketones and 170 thioureas remaining, which represents a virtual library of 12,850 product molecules. The next step in the design

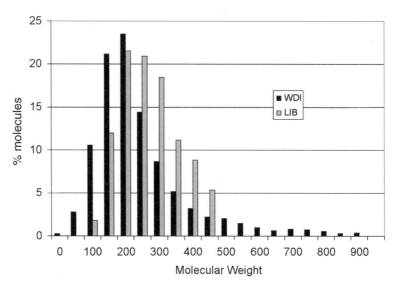

Fig. 2. The molecular weight profile of the library designed using SELECT (LIB) is shown together with the profile of molecular weights in WDI.

process was to enumerate the full virtual library, which was done using the transform method in ADEPT.

The virtual library was then characterized using the Cerius^2 default topological descriptors and physicochemical properties *(35)*. The 50 default descriptors were reduced to three principal components using principal components analysis, and this defined a 3D chemistry space into which the virtual library could be plotted. The chemistry space consisted of 1134 cells and, when the virtual library was mapped into the space, it was found to occupy 364 of the cells; thus, this represents the maximum cell coverage that is achievable.

The SELECT program was then used to design a 15 × 30 library that was simultaneously optimized on diversity (measured by the number of occupied cells) and to have a drug-like molecular weight profile (measure by the RMSD between the profile of the library and the profile of molecular weights found in the WDI). The resulting library was found to occupy a total of 234 cells and its molecular weight profile is shown in **Fig. 2** together with the profile of molecular weight found in WDI. When optimizing a library on diversity alone, the best library found occupies 282 cells and, when optimizing on molecular weight profile alone, the best library was found to occupy 169 cells. Thus, when optimizing both objectives simultaneously using the weighted-sum approach in SELECT, the resulting library represents a compromise in the two objectives.

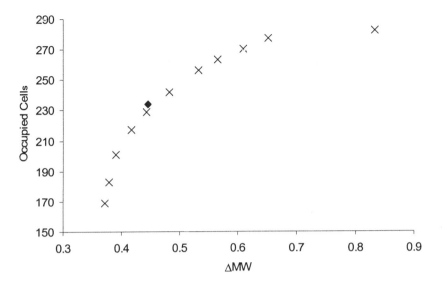

Fig. 3. A family of libraries (shown by the crosses) is found when optimizing molecular weight profile simultaneously with cell-based diversity when using the MoSELECT program. The single SELECT solution is shown by the solid diamond.

Performing a single run of SELECT with one set of weights does not allow the library designer to explore the relationship between the two objectives and a single somewhat arbitrary solution was produced.

The relationship between molecular weight profile and diversity was then explored using the MOGA approach implemented in MoSELECT. The result was a total of 11 different libraries with each library representing a different trade-off between the objectives, as shown by the crosses in **Fig. 3**. The most drug-like library (the library with the best molecular weight profile) is the least diverse (169 cells occupied), whereas the most diverse library (282 cells occupied) has the least drug-like profile. The SELECT solution found previously is shown by the solid diamond.

Thus far, the size and configuration of the libraries were fixed. The relationship between library size and diversity was investigated by performing multiple runs of the SELECT program with each run configured to find a library of increasing size. The results of performing this exercise are shown in **Fig. 4**, where it can be seen that diversity (cell coverage) increases as library size increases.

MoSELECT allows the trade-off in library size and diversity to be investigated in a single run. The libraries found are shown by the solid squares

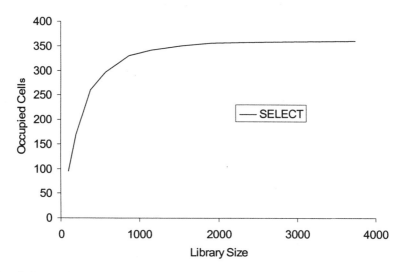

Fig. 4. Exploring library size and diversity with the SELECT program requires multiple runs with different input values.

(superimposed on the SELECT results) in **Fig. 5**. Thus, the full range of library sizes is explored, from very small libraries with low diversity up to a library size of 1392, which has the maximum diversity that is possible: it occupies all 364 cells that are occupied by the full virtual library.

The remaining library designs are based on applying the MOGA under various constraints. In **Fig. 6**, the libraries are constrained to contain between 250 and 500 products. Finally, the libraries are constrained to contain between 15 and 20 reactants in each component. The libraries found when no constraint is placed on configuration are shown by the crosses in **Fig. 7A**, and the libraries found when the constraints are applied are shown by the solid squares. **Figure 7B** illustrates that the constrained (more efficient) libraries were found without any loss in diversity.

4. Discussion and Notes

Combinatorial library design is a complex procedure that can be divided into several steps as indicated above. A wide variety of different computational tools are available that can be applied to the different steps; however, effective use of the tools can require considerable user interaction in order to maximize the chances of finding useful compounds. Thus, the tools should not be considered as black boxes.

For a given reaction scheme, the first step is usually to identify available reactants. Care should be taken when constructing substructural queries to

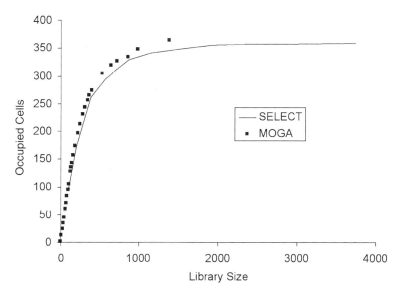

Fig. 5. Library size and diversity can be explored in a single run using the MoSELECT program. The family of solutions found is shown by the solid squares and is superimposed on the SELECT curve repeated from **Fig. 4**.

ensure that the compounds retrieved are indeed capable of undergoing the reaction; for example, when searching for primary amines, it may be desirable that hits are restricted to those that contain a single amine group. Visual inspection of the results can be used to ensure that the substructural query was correctly specified and it can also be useful in determining which computational filters to apply. For example, the presence of highly flexible molecules in the answer set may suggest the use of a filter to remove reactants where the number of rotatable bonds is above some threshold value. Filters are extremely important because the early removal of undesirable compounds can simplify the later stages of library design.

Once the reactant pools have been filtered, the next step in product-based designs is usually to enumerate the full virtual library. This can be a very time-consuming step and hence a useful precursor can be to enumerate carefully chosen subsets that will give an indication of the success or otherwise of the full virtual experiment. Thus, in a two component reaction it can be useful to take the first reactant in the first pool and combine it with all the reactants in the second pool (to generate $1 \times n_B$ products). This should then be followed by the enumeration of one reactant in the second pool with all reactants in the first pool to give $n_A \times 1$ products. If either of these two partial enumeration steps fail, then the full enumeration will also fail. Thus, troublesome reactants can be identified early.

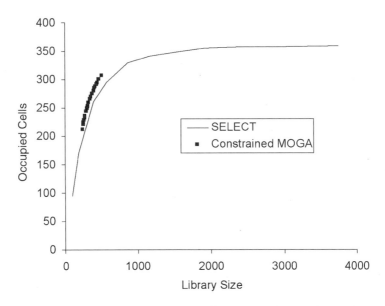

Fig. 6. Library sized is constrained to between 250 and 500 products.

The next step is to determine the descriptors to use for the library optimization. It is important that descriptors are chosen that are relevant to the type of compounds that the library is being designed for. The descriptors should result in a high degree of similarity between compounds that are known to have the desired properties. Thus, if some active compounds are known, then, ideally, these should cluster together within the descriptor space. Another criterion to take into account when choosing descriptors is the number of compounds in the virtual library. Some descriptors can be costly to compute, especially 3D descriptors when the conformational flexibility of the compounds is taken into account. Thus, it is important to be aware of the computational resources that will be required for a given library design strategy.

Finally, the optimization step itself usually involves human intervention. With the traditional aggregation approaches to library design, the user must decide on appropriate weights for the various objectives being optimized. This can involve several trial-and-error experiments where different combinations of weights are applied. In the novel library design method based on a MOGA, the user no longer needs to determine relative weights; however, a family of different compromise solutions is found and hence the user must apply his or her own knowledge to decide which library represents the best compromise in the objectives.

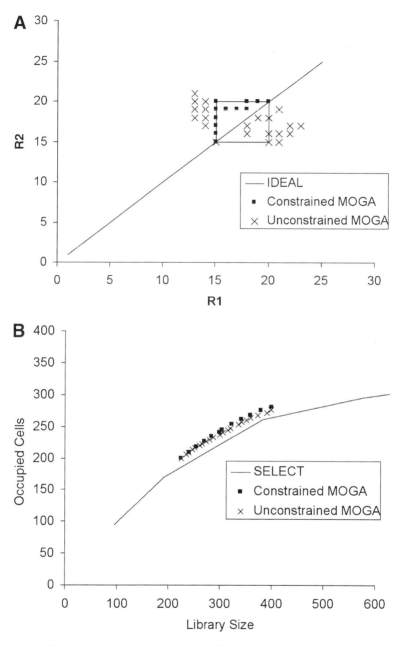

Fig. 7. **(A)** The crosses show a run where library size is constrained, but no constraints are placed on library configuration. The solid squares show the effect of also constraining configuration so that between 15 and 20 reactants are used from each pool. The solid line shows the ideal solution in terms of efficiency, that is, equal numbers of reactants are selected from each reactant pool. **(B)** No loss of diversity is seen in the configuration-constrained library relative to the less efficient unconstrained solutions.

Acknowledgments

The author wishes to thank the following for their contribution to the work described here: Peter Fleming, Darren Green, Illy Khatib, Stephen Pickett, Peter Willett, and Trudi Wright.

References

1. Wolcke, J. and Ullmann, D. (2001) Miniaturized HTS technologies—HTS. *Drug Discov. Today* **6,** 637–646.
2. Valler, M. J. and Green, D. (2000) Diversity screening versus focussed screening in drug discovery. *Drug Discov. Today* **5,** 286–293.
3. Rose, S. and Stevens, A. (2003) Computational design strategies for combinatorial libraries. *Current Opin. Chem. Biol.* **7,** 331–339.
4. Martin, E. J. and Critchlow, R. E. (1999) Beyond mere diversity: tailoring combinatorial libraries for drug discovery. *J. Comb. Chem.* **1,** 32–45.
5. Beavers, M. B. and Chen, X. (2002) Structure-based combinatorial library design: methodologies and applications. *J. Mol. Graph. Model.* **20,** 463–468.
6. Leach, A. R., Bryce, R. A. and Robinson, A. J. (2000) Synergy between combinatorial chemistry and *de novo* design. *J. Mol. Graphics Model.* **18,** 358–367.
7. Kubinyi, H. (2002) From narcosis to hyperspace: the history of QSAR. *Quantit. Struct.-Act. Relat.* **21,** 348–356.
8. Barnard, J. M., Downs, G. M., and Willett, P. (1998) Chemical similarity searching. *J. Chem. Inf. Comput. Sci.* **38,** 983–996.
9. van de Waterbeemd, H. and Gifford, E. (2002) ADMET in silico modelling: towards prediction paradise? *Nat. Rev. Drug Discov.* **2,** 192–204.
10. Gillet, V. J. and Willett, P. (2001) Dissimilarity-based compound selection for library design. In *Combinatorial library design and evaluation. Principles, software tools and applications in drug discovery*, Ghose, A. K. and Viswanadhan, A. N. (eds.), Marcel Dekker, New York, pp. 379–398.
11. Gillet, V. J., Willett, P., and Bradshaw, J. (1997) The effectiveness of reactant pools for generating structurally diverse combinatorial libraries. *J. Chem. Inf. Comput. Sci.* **37,** 731–740.
12. Jamois, E. A., Hassan, M., and Waldman, M. (2000) Evaluation of reactant-based and product-based strategies in the design of combinatorial library subsets. *J. Chem. Inf. Comput. Sci.* **40,** 63–70.
13. ACD. Available Chemicals Directory, MDL Information Systems, Inc. 14600 Catalina Street, San Leandro, CA 94577. http://www.mdli.com.
14. Leach, A. R., Bradshaw, J., Green, D. V. S., Hann, M. M., and Delany III, J. J. (1999) Implementation of a system for reagent selection and library enumeration, profiling and design. *J. Chem. Inf. Comput. Sci.* **39,** 1161–1172.
15. Brown, R. D. (1997) Descriptors for diversity analysis. *Perspect. Drug Discov. Design* **7/8,** 31–49.

16. Bajorath, J. (2001) Selected concepts and investigations in compound classification, molecular descriptor analysis, and virtual screening. *J. Chem. Inf. Comput. Sci.* **41**, 233–245.

17. Pickett, S. D., Mason, J. S., and McLay, I. M. (1996) Diversity profiling and design using 3D pharmacophores: Pharmacophore-derived queries (PDQ). *J. Chem. Inf. Comput. Sci.* **36**, 1214–1223.

18. Waldman, M., Li, H., and Hassan, M. (2000) Novel algorithms for the optimization of molecular diversity of combinatorial libraries. *J. Mol. Graphics Model* **18**, 412–426.

19. Lipinski, C. A., Lombardo, F., Dominy, B. W., and Feeney, P. J. (1997) Experimental and computational approaches to estimate solubility and permeability in drug discovery and development settings. *Adv. Drug Delivery Rev.* **23**, 3–25.

20. Clark, D. E. and Pickett, S. D. (2000) Computational methods for the prediction of "drug-likeness." *Drug Discov. Today* **5**, 49–58.

21. Hann, M. M., Leach, A. R., and Harper, G. (2001) Molecular complexity and its impact on the probability of finding leads for drug discovery. *J. Chem. Inf. Comput. Sci.* **41**, 856–864

22. Oprea, T. I. (2000) Property distributions of drug-related chemical databases. *J. Comput-Aided Mol. Des.* **14**, 251–264.

23. Gillet, V. J., Willett, P., and Bradshaw, J. (1999) Selecting combinatorial libraries to optimise diversity and physical properties. *J. Chem. Inf. Comput. Sci.* **39**, 167–177.

24. WDI: The World Drug Index is available from Derwent Information, 14 Great Queen St., London W2 5DF, UK.

25. Lewis, R. A., Pickett, S. D., and Clark, D. E. (2000) Computer-aided molecular diversity analysis and combinatorial library design. In *Reviews in computational chemistry*, Lipkowitz, K. B. and Boyd, D.B. (eds.), VCH Publishers, New York, Vol. 16, pp. 1–51.

26. Mason, J. S. and Beno, B. R. (2000) Library design using BCUT chemistry-space descriptors and multiple four-point pharmacophore fingerprints: simultaneous optimisation and structure-based diversity. *J. Mol. Graph. Model.* **18**, 438–451.

27. Agrafiotis, D. K. (2002) Multiobjective optimisation of combinatorial libraries. *J. Comput.-Aid. Mol. Design* **5/6**, 335–356.

28. Zheng, W., Hung, S. T., Saunders, J. T., and Seibel, G. L. (2000) PICCOLO: a tool for combinatorial library design via multicriterion optimization. In *Pacific Symposium on Biocomputing 2000*, Atlman, R. B., Dunkar, A. K., Hunter, L., Lauderdale, K., and Klein, T. E. (eds.), World Scientific, Singapore, pp. 588–599.

29. Brown, J. D., Hassan, M., and Waldman, M. (2000) Combinatorial library design for diversity, cost efficiency, and drug-like character. *J. Mol Graph. Model.* **18**, 427–437.

30. Coello, C. A., van Veldhuizen, D. A., and Lamont, G.B. (2002) *Evolutionary algorithms for solving multi-objective problems.* Kluwer Academic Publishers, New York.

31. Fonseca, C. M. and Fleming, P. J. (1995) An overview of evolutionary algorithms in multiobjective optimization. In *Evolutionary computation*, De Jong, K. (ed.), The Massachusetts Institute of Technology, Cambridge, MA, Vol. 3, No. 1, pp. 1–16.
32. Gillet, V. J., Khatib, W., Willett, P., Fleming, P., and Green, D. V. S. (2002) Combinatorial library design using a multiobjective genetic algorithm. *J. Chem. Inf. Comput. Sci.* **42,** 375–385.
33. Gillet, V. J., Willett, P., Fleming P., and Green, D. V. S. (2002) Designing focused libraries using MoSELECT. *J. Mol Graph. Model.* **20,** 491–498.
34. Wright, T., Gillet, V. J., Green, D. V. S., and Pickett, S. D. (2003) Optimising the size and configuration of combinatorial libraries. *J. Chem. Inf. Comput. Sci.* **43,** 381–390.
35. Cerius^2 is available from Accelrys Inc., 9685 Scranton Road, San Diego, CA 92121.

14

Approaches to Target Class Combinatorial Library Design

Dora Schnur, Brett R. Beno, Andrew Good, and Andrew Tebben

Abstract

The wealth of information available from the solution of the human genome has dramatically altered the nature of combinatorial library design. While single-target-focused library design remains an important objective, creation of libraries directed toward families of receptors such as GPCRs, kinases, nuclear hormone receptors, and proteases, has replaced the generation of libraries based primarily on diversity. Although diversity-based design still plays a role for receptors with no known ligands, more knowledge-based approaches are required for target class design. This chapter discusses some of the possible design methods and presents examples where they are available.

Key Words: 3D pharmacophores; library design; combinatorial library; structure-based design; target class library; gene family; target class knowledge database; cell-based library design methods; BCUTs; privileged substructure; DiverseSolutions; ClassPharmer™.

1. Introduction

With the onslaught of data that has arisen from the mapping of the human genome, there has been a distinct shift in the nature of combinatorial library design. Initially, library design efforts focused on the production of large numbers of diverse products to augment high-throughput screening (HTS) decks *(1–8)*. Improvements to the pure diversity approach included the design of drug-like diverse libraries that utilized Lipinski's rule of 5 *(9)*, polar surface area *(10)*, and other metrics to produce compounds having desirable ADME properties *(11)*. More recently, the focus has moved from diversity in favor of combinatorial libraries designed to target specific receptors or enzymes *(12)*. While these single-target-focused libraries remain a key component of many drug-discovery programs, and are useful in both "hit to lead" and "lead optimization" contexts,

From: *Methods in Molecular Biology, vol. 275:*
Chemoinformatics: Concepts, Methods, and Tools for Drug Discovery
Edited by: J. Bajorath © Humana Press Inc., Totowa, NJ

creation of target class libraries has largely replaced generation of purely diversity-based libraries.

These target class libraries fall between the two extremes of diverse and target-focused libraries *(13)*. These are combinatorial libraries in which the products are biased toward multiple members of families of related receptors or enzymes, rather than individual targets *(14)*. The basis for the design and synthesis of target class combinatorial libraries is the observation that receptors and enzymes that belong to the same functional family (e.g., kinases, Class I GPCRs) often share similar steric and electronic features in their binding/active sites. Kinases, which have been shown to have highly similar active sites, provide one example of this *(15)*. Another example is provided by the Family A GPCR receptors, of which several require aromatic rings and basic moieties in their ligands *(16)*. Identification and exploitation of these intrafamily similarities affords the opportunity to design and synthesize target class combinatorial libraries in which the products contain features that are complementary to the common motifs found in the binding/active sites of the receptors or enzymes comprising the target family.

Target class libraries are well suited to augment large HTS decks with drug-like compounds designed to include key receptor/enzyme binding features. In addition, they are likely to prove even more valuable in focused screening campaigns where compounds are assayed against multiple targets from the same family (presumably the family for which the library was designed). Another potential application of target class libraries is the de-orphaning of biological targets of unknown function.

There are two basic paradigms for the design of target class combinatorial libraries. These are applicable for target class libraries composed of compounds "cherry-picked" from a larger screening set, as well as combinatorially synthesized libraries. The following descriptions assume an ultimate library design goal of a combinatorially synthesized, target class library of 10,000 compounds for a target class composed of 10 members.

In the first design approach, the common features required for ligand binding to all (or many) of the target family members are identified, then used to derive a model for selecting library products for a 10,000 compound library based on one or more combinatorial templates. In the second approach, ten 1000 compound combinatorial libraries are designed, where each library is directed at a single member of the target class using target-specific computational models. These 10 focused libraries are then combined to form the large 10,000 compound target class library. The amount of effort required (both computational and synthetic) for the first method is much less than that required for the second approach. However, intuitively, a library of this type would be expected to provide weak, non-selective hits against members of the target class because the model used to design the library emphasizes their similarities, rather than the differences that are responsible for ligand specificity.

The second approach, although requiring more effort, has the potential to provide some combinatorial products that are potent against the individual targets, and other products that bind to members of the target family which were not explicitly considered in the design effort. Potency against the individual targets depends on the quality of the individual focused designs that make up the target class library. However, even the most successful focused library designs provide product sets in which only a fraction of the products bind to their intended targets. Combinatorial products, which, as a result of some unfavorable interaction, do not bind to the target for which they were designed, may bind to a related target where the unfavorable interaction is absent. This latter approach for target class library design has the added benefit of providing "more shots on goal."

There are no published examples directly comparing these two paradigms for target class combinatorial library design. However, in practical experience, it is often the case that compounds which were designed during lead optimization phases of projects focused on particular biological targets are identified as hits in HTS assays run for other targets within the same family. By extension, it is reasonable to expect that compounds from combinatorial libraries designed against one member of a target family, may also bind to other enzymes/receptors within that same family.

Regardless of which target class library design paradigm is employed, computational methods that can identify the interactions responsible for ligand–receptor binding and/or the molecular features needed to form these interactions are required for the library design process. The preferred method is direct examination of high-resolution crystal structures of the enzymes or receptors co-crystallized with ligands. This provides information regarding the explicit interactions relevant to ligand binding, and also allows the shapes of the binding/active sites to be compared. Given this type of data, docking is an extremely powerful computational tool that can be utilized for target class library design.

Unfortunately, it is often the case that crystal structures are not available for targets of interest. This limitation is especially acute for GPCRs, which are the biological targets of as many as 50% of recently launched drugs *(16)*. The paucity of structural data for GPCR targets is offset, at least partially, by the large amount of data available for classes of ligands that bind to these targets.

Computational models relating molecular structure and/or properties to biological activity are required for the design of both target-focused and target class combinatorial libraries based on known active ligands. These models are developed from descriptors, which encode information about molecular properties and structure. Many different descriptor types ranging from simple physico-chemical properties [e.g., molecular weight, cLog*P (17)*, rotatable bond count] to 2D descriptors based on molecular connection tables [e.g., atom pairs *(18)*, Daylight Fingerprints *(17)*] to 3-D pharmacophores *(19–21)* and 3D property-derived BCUTs *(22)* have been utilized for library design purposes.

An essential starting point for ligand-based designs is the development of a target class knowledge database. Known drugs, analogs, and other active compounds along with their biological response information have to be collected from the literature, commercial drug databases, and proprietary sources. The importance of these databases has been sufficiently recognized in the pharmaceutical industry that numerous companies such as Aureus Pharmaceuticals, Jubilant Biosystems, Sertanty, and Biowisdom have developed products to address the need.

2. Methods

Most of the available computational methods for library design can be applied to target class libraries. In this chapter, rather than striving for a complete review of all possible methods, we will focus on several significant applications. Among them are 3D pharmacophore descriptor based design applications, privileged substructure methods, cell-based design methods, and structure-based methods. Where target class design examples exist, they will be discussed.

2.1. Three-Dimensional (3D) Pharmacophore Descriptors

Three-dimensional (3D) pharmacophore descriptors essentially quantify what the medicinal chemist envisions when considering biological pharmacophores relevant to ligand–receptor binding: several key molecular features/functional groups in a specific relative orientation. The molecular features encoded in 3D pharmacophore descriptors include hydrogen-bond donors and acceptors, lipophiles, aromatic rings, and acidic and basic moieties. Each of these can play a role in ligand–receptor binding interactions. The relative positioning of combinations of these features within a molecule is determined from 3D conformational models represented by a single low-energy conformation or multiple conformations (**Fig. 1**). Typically, 3D pharmacophores composed of three or four features (three-point and four-point 3D pharmacophores) separated by three or six distances, respectively, are utilized for CADD and combinatorial library design purposes. In order to limit the number of possible 3D pharmacophore descriptors to a manageable quantity, distances are generally binned. Detailed discussions of methods for calculating 3D pharmacophores are found in the literature *(19,20,23)*.

If the bioactive conformation of a ligand for a particular receptor is known, then a single three- or four-point 3D pharmacophore that is crucial for the

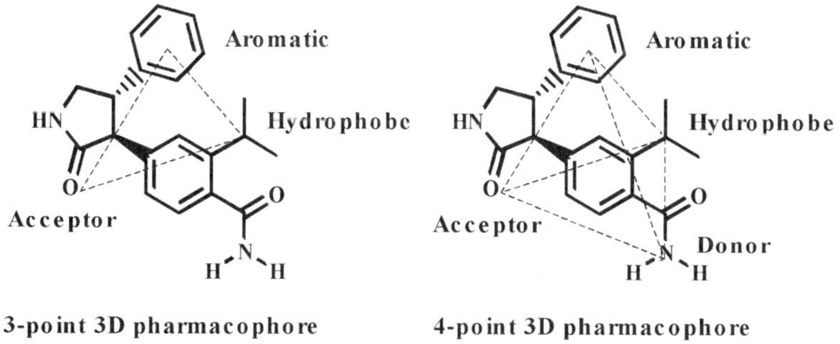

3-point 3D pharmacophore   4-point 3D pharmacophore

Fig. 1. Schematic illustrating three- and four-point 3D pharmacophores. Three-point 3D pharmacophores encode three functional group types and the three distances separating them, and four-point 3D pharmacophores encode four functional group types and the six distances separating them. Functional group types commonly included are acids, bases, hydrophobes, H-bond acceptors, H-bond donors, and aromatic systems. Distances are assigned to bins (e.g., 2.5–4.0 Å) to limit the individual 3D pharmacophore descriptors to a tractable number, and to aid in comparing the individual 3D pharmacophores.

binding of that ligand to its receptor may be identified. Other compounds, which contain the 3D pharmacophore of interest, can then be identified via virtual screening or specifically designed.

Alternatively, bitstrings in which the state of each bit (0 or 1) represents the presence or absence of a single three- or four-point 3D pharmacophore can be utilized. These 3D pharmacophore "fingerprints" encode all of the three- or four-point 3D pharmacophores that can be attributed to a particular molecule (within the limits of conformational sampling resolution). Pharmacophore fingerprints can also be generated for sets of compounds by performing a logical OR operation on the fingerprints for the individual molecules. The similarity of one molecule to another can be assessed by calculating the Tanimoto coefficient *(24)* of the 3D pharmacophore fingerprints for the two molecules.

Mason and coworkers reported one of the first examples of a target class library design utilizing 3D pharmacophore descriptors *(20)*. In this example, the authors designed a set of GPCR-targeted libraries based on Ugi chemistry *(25)*. A key feature of the design is the incorporation of a GPCR privileged substructure in each of the combinatorial products. GPCR-privileged substructures are chemical moieties that occur with high frequency in the ligands of multiple GPCRs *(16)*. Examples include biphenyl tetrazole, indole, and biphenyl-methyl groups. Methods to derive them will be discussed below.

In the published example, 502 compounds from the MDL Drug Data Report (MDDR) *(26)* that were active against a GPCR target and also contained a biphenyl tetrazole moiety were used to generated a "privileged" four-point 3D pharmacophore fingerprint. A privileged four-point 3D pharmacophore is a four-point 3D pharmacophore in which one of the four molecular features is a privileged moiety, and the other three are members of the standard set of feature types (H-bond donors, acids, etc.) In this case, the privileged feature was represented by the centroid of the biphenyl tetrazole moiety in each compound. The four-point 3D pharmacophore fingerprint for the set of 502 GPCR ligands was the union of the fingerprints of the individual molecules, and represented approx 161,000 privileged four-point 3D pharmacophores.

Utilizing a simple greedy algorithm, a set of 22 acid reagents (along with 12 aldehydes and 8 isonitriles to yield 2112 products) was selected to maximize the intersection of the privileged four-point 3D pharmacophore fingerprint of the combined combinatorial products with the GPCR-privileged 3D pharmacophore fingerprint derived from the MDDR compounds. Approximately 49% of the GPCR-privileged 3D pharmacophores found in the GPCR-privileged fingerprint were covered by the products of the optimized reagents. Subsequent libraries were designed to cover the four-point 3D pharmacophores present in the GPCR reference fingerprint that were not covered by the original library.

The GPCR target class bias in this first example was achieved using two key design elements. The first is the incorporation of a GPCR-privileged substructure, and the second is maximal coverage of GPCR-privileged four-point 3D pharmacophores found in known GPCR ligands. This approach weights all of the four-point 3D pharmacophores found in the set of known GPCR ligands equally in terms of their importance for receptor–ligand binding.

In a similar target class design effort utilizing a set of 3321 GPCR ligands with reported in vivo activity, Lamb and coworkers identified a set of 1.8 million two-, three-, and four-point pharmacophores predicted to be important for GPCR binding *(27)*. However, in this case, rather than treating all of the 3D pharmacophores found in the known actives as equally important, only those 3D pharmacophores that occurred in at least 10 active compounds were included in the GPCR-reference 3D pharmacophore key. Utilizing this reference key, the Dupont Pharmaceuticals group designed a library of 7865 products that covered 66% of the 1.8 million GPCR-relevant 3D pharmacophores that were identified. The use of a 3D pharmacophore "frequency count" in the analysis of known active ligands improves the odds of identifying 3D pharmacophores that are actually relevant to ligand–receptor binding *(28)*.

The previous two examples both utilized the 3D pharmacophores found in known GPCR-active ligands to design GPCR target class combinatorial libraries. The following example illustrates an extension of the pharmacophore methodology in which 3D pharmacophore fingerprints from known *inactives* are also utilized to help further focus in on those 3D pharmacophores that are important for ligand–receptor binding. Although the designed combinatorial library is more accurately termed a focused library, rather than a target class library, the techniques employed are directly extensible to target class library design.

Utilizing a set of 43 known α_1-adrenergic receptor ligands with K_i values <5 nM (actives), and a set of 62 compounds with K_i values >5 μM against α_1 receptor subtypes (inactives), Bradley and coworkers derived a 3D pharmacophore ensemble model that correctly identified 80% of the actives and only 10% of the inactives as active compounds in validation studies *(29)*. This ensemble model was composed of a set of 500 two-, three-, and four-point 3D pharmacophores with the highest "information content" found in the analysis of the active and inactive compounds in the model training set. The information content for each 3D pharmacophore was calculated using an equation derived from information theory. Essentially, those 3D pharmacophores that occur with high frequency in known actives, but are absent or occur with low frequency in known inactives for a particular target are high in "information content" and may be used in combination to discriminate actives from inactives.

Bradley and coworkers used the 3D pharmacophore ensemble model to filter a virtual combinatorial library of 3924 N-substituted glycine peptoids *(30)* containing three known α_1 actives down to a set of 639 products. Using a "cut-down" technique, a 160 compound combinatorial library was designed in which the number of compounds that passed the ensemble model filter was maximized. This library contained two of the three known actives present in the original 3924 compound virtual library. This represents a substantial enrichment [(2 actives/160 products) × 100 = 1.25% vs (3 actives/3924 products) × 100 = 0.076%].

Beno and Mason reported an alternative design approach based on 3D pharmacophore frequency counts that used the same set of 43 known α_1 ligands, and a virtual library of 10,648 N-substituted glycine peptoids *(30,31)*. The virtual library contained at least three products known to be active at α_1. In this case a library of 343 products (7 R1 × 7 R2 × 7 R3) was selected with a simulated annealing procedure that maximized the similarity of the normalized four-point 3D pharmacophore frequency distributions of the active α_1 ligands and the products comprising the selected virtual library subset. In this case, one of the three known α_1 actives was found in the final library. Comparison of these results to those of Bradley et al. *(29)* suggests the importance of including inactive compounds when deriving 3D pharmacophore based computational models. The inclusion of two- and three- as well as four-point 3D pharmacophores may also lead to models with improved discriminating power.

Other approaches that could be extended to target class library design include work by McGregor and Muskal *(13,19)*. These utilized PharmPrint™ 3D pharmacophore descriptors (three-point pharmacophores) and partial least squares and principal component analysis to develop models for focused and drug-like libraries, respectively.

The examples provided above all use (or could use) multiple-point 3D pharmacophores from sets of known active ligands, and in some cases, inactive ligands as well, to generate models for library design. These models discern to varying degrees the 3D pharmacophores that are relevant to binding of ligands to their receptors, and may be derived from large numbers of diverse compounds covering many different chemotypes. These models represent the common ligand features that may be recognized by different members of a biological target class. Thus, they are well suited to the design of target class libraries, which emphasize the commonalties between related targets.

Multiple-point 3D pharmacophore fingerprints can also be used to calculate the similarity between pairs of molecules using the Tanimoto coefficient, or similar metrics. Individual target-focused libraries may be designed by maximizing the 3D pharmacophore similarity of product compounds to ligands known to be active against the target of interest *(32)*. Target class combinatorial libraries may then be created by combining smaller libraries focused to individual, related targets.

Multiple-point 3D pharmacophore descriptors are also useful for designing libraries when crystal structures are available for the target(s) of interest. Fingerprints consisting of 3D pharmacophores that are complementary to binding site features can be created and used in conjunction with docking studies to select products with optimal shape and pharmacophoric features from virtual combinatorial libraries *(20,33,34)*. This technique has been used to design Factor Xa *(20)* and cyclin-dependent kinase (CDK-2) *(35)* focused libraries. This approach could be extended to multiple targets within a target class by calculating multiple-point 3D pharmacophore fingerprints that are complementary to the binding/active site for each target, and then performing a logical AND operation on all of the fingerprints to determine their intersection. The resultant fingerprint of receptor-complementary, common 3D pharmacophores could then be used in conjunction with a docking algorithm to select products from a virtual combinatorial library.

Target class combinatorial libraries are intended to contain products that are active against multiple members of a family of biological targets. However, activity/potency is not the only concern. Optimally, the combinatorial products should be as drug-like as possible, with minimal ADMET liabilities. This is a difficult goal to achieve. However, computational models utilizing multiple-point 3D pharmacophore descriptors may be used to address some of these issues as well. A 3D pharmacophore model for PGP substrates has been published *(36)*, and key pharmacophores common to many CYP3A4 inhibitors *(37,38)* have been identified as well. These may be utilized for target class library design.

For example, one might design a GPCR target class library in which the coverage of GPCR-relevant 3D pharmacophores is maximized, while the coverage of PGP substrate pharmacophores is minimized in the selected products.

At present, there are relatively few reported examples of target class library design efforts that utilize multiple-point 3D pharmacophore descriptors. However, multiple-point 3D pharmacophores are well suited for target class library design efforts owing to their ability to encode common features recognized by receptors/enzymes and displayed by small molecules. They can be utilized with protein structures, collections of ligands, or single ligands. Models that predict desirable biological activity or potential ADMET liabilities can be developed with 3D pharmacophore descriptors. As interest in target class libraries increases, multiple-point 3D pharmacophore descriptors should see extensive use in combinatorial library design.

2.2. Privileged Substructures for Target Class Library Design

One of the early and effective approaches to target class library design was the analysis of a set of ligands for frequently occurring chemical moieties or substructures. Various methods including both pharmacophores *(20)* and frameworks analysis *(39)* have been employed to find these substructures. To use the latter method to find privileged substructures, one first selects a set of literature structures such as "Family A" or "Family B" GPCR non-peptide ligands in the MDDR and performs frameworks analysis. One then performs maximum common substructure (MCS) analysis on all the frameworks and removes the ligands with that substructure from the superset of ligands. The frameworks analysis, MCS analysis, and ligand removal are iterated until 90% of the ligands have been accounted for. For a ligand set from the 1999 version of the MDDR, 15 SLNs (SYBYL line notation structures) *(40)* accounted for 90% of the Family A and B GPCR ligands *(41)*.

A more recent variation on privileged substructure analysis involved the use of ClassPharmer™ *(42,43)*. This software tool uses graph-based analysis to derive keys that capture substructure common features in the ligand training set. The resultant classes or clusters of compounds represented by common substructures can be further analyzed using the R-table generation module and through importation of activity/selectivity data as property attributes of the classes. The substructures, which are displayed by the viewer module with attached R-group attachment positions indicated, potentially provide a rich source of scaffolds for combinatorial library elaboration. Because a redundancy setting controls the number of classes in which a compound may appear, ligands can be broken into a variety of substructure fragments that may not be identified with methods that allow a compound to be assigned only to one cluster. Additionally, compounds that are singletons appear as separate classes.

Because test lists of compounds may be filtered through the classes, retention of singletons is an important feature for subsequent virtual screening of compound sets or libraries.

In a preliminary application of this methodology to target class or gene family ligand analysis, Schnur and Hermsmeier *(43)* looked at the ClassPharmer™ analyses of sets of GPCR, ion channel, and NHR ligands from the MDDR. For the NHR's, 88 thyroid hormone-like ligands yielded 15 classes and 4 singletons, while the 564 estrogenic ligands yielded 48 classes with 3 singletons. For the ion channels, the glutamate cationic family set of 145 compounds yielded 17 classes and 4 singletons while the nicotinicoid anionic set of 550 compounds yielded 57 classes with 4 singletons. A set of 65 Family B GPCR ligands yielded only four classes but gave 39 singletons. This is not surprising because most of the ligands were peptidic and ClassPharmer™ is not optimized for peptides. A set of 6230 Family A GPCR ligands yielded 503 classes and 333 singletons.

This last set was utilized for a proof of principle for target selectivity analysis. The 96 activity keys associated with the compounds in the MDDR were assigned a number from 1 to 96 and imported as an attribute for each compound into ClassPharmer™. Visualization as a distribution histogram for the compounds of each class allowed a crude gauge of the specificity of the classes with regard to GPCR targets. As expected, some classes were more selective than others. The utility of this result was confirmed by filtering a 10K combinatorial library and a 10K random compound set (from the corporate inventory) through the GPCR classes. Because the library was designed using frameworks/MCS-derived privileged structures to filter starting reagents into GPCR-like and diversity-based, it was not surprising that 90% of the compounds fell into 32 ClassPharmer™ classes. The remaining 10% of the compounds did not fall into any of the classes. This was an expected result because a focused/diverse library design had been employed. A number of the classes represented in the library were relatively non-selective; in accord with this, the library was active in a number of GPCR target screens. In contrast, only a third of the 10K random set of compounds occupied 220 of the GPCR ClassPharmer™ classes. The much greater number of occupied classes reflects the diversity of the compound set relative to the combinatorial library that was derived from a relatively small number of starting reagents. The low compound occupation for this set needs to be viewed with caution however. Not all GPCR targets were represented by the initial MDDR compound set and proprietary compound classes that might be intended for GPCR targets were not represented in the MDDR set used for the analysis. Nonetheless, ClassPharmer™ seems to be a promising tool for finding privileged substructures and designing either selective or promiscuous libraries by filtering virtual libraries through classes defined by a gene family ligand test set.

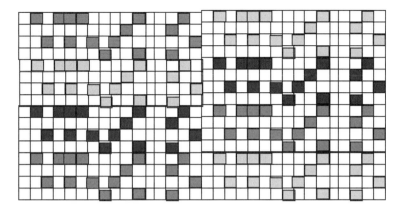

Fig. 2. 2D representation of two compound sets in a cell based chemistry space. Cells occupied by set one in black, by set two in light gray, and by both sets in dark gray. Empty cells are white.

2.3. Cell-Based Library Design Methods

Cell-based methods for combinatorial library design have been discussed at length in the literature *(44)*. The method divides each axis of a multidimensional property space into bins and, thereby divides the space into hypercubes or cells. The known ligands of individual targets or an entire target class can be associated with the cells they occupy. Unlike clustering methods that define clusters based on the compounds in the set, cell-based analyses allow comparison of molecules not originally in the definition set without alteration of the chemistry space (**Fig. 2**). A basic assumption of this method is that compounds that are near neighbors of known ligands are more likely to be active for a particular target or class of targets. Clearly, the validity of this assumption is related to the validity of the descriptors used as axes of the chemistry space. This method easily lends itself to ligand-based target class design if a knowledge database of the target ligands is available to define a target class space that contains regions where ligands for specific targets cluster.

The most commonly used software tool for the purpose, DiverseSolutions *(45)*, employs a unique set of descriptors, BCUTs *(22)*, that are based on both connectivity-related and atomic properties such as charge, polarizability, and hydrogen bonding abilities which appear to correlate with ligand receptor binding and activity *(46,47)*. An example *(48)* is shown (**Fig. 3**) for an ion channel target. Channel openers and blockers are differentiated in the cell-based space derived from an optimally derived diversity space for the entire combinatorial library that contained them. Because the diversity space in this case has four dimensions and the plots are 3D, it is possible to observe that some subsets of the

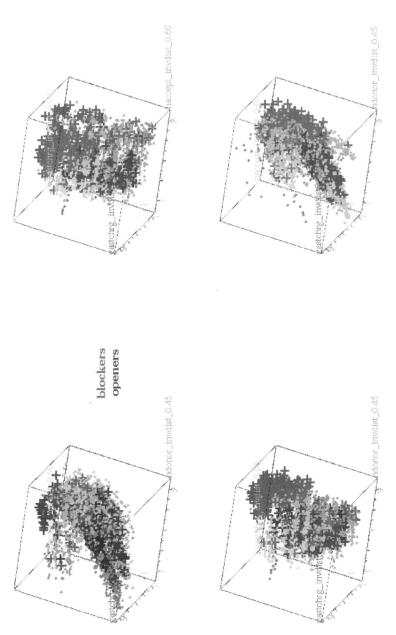

blockers
openers

Fig. 3. An ion-channel-based combinatorial library in 3D subspaces of a 4D Diverse Solutions chemistry space. Channel openers are shown in black, blockers in dark gray and the rest of the combinatorial library is shown in light gray. Axes are 3D H-hydrogen suppressed BCUTs based on hydrogen bond donor (A) and acceptor properties (B) and Gasteiger-Huckel charges (C and D). The off-diagonals of the matrices for A, B, C were inverse distance (1/d). For D the off-diagonal was $1/d^6$. For A, B and D the BCUT was the highest eigenvalue. For C, the BCUT corresponds to the lowest Eigenvalue. Clockwise from the upper left the XYZ axes, respectively, are ABC, BCD, ABD and ACD.

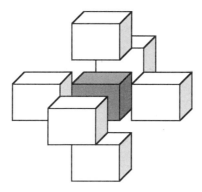

Fig. 4. Representation of "interesting" or "promising" cells. The list of promising cells was chosen to include the cell containing the active ligand plus one layer of the adjacent cells. Additional layers of cells could be added to cover a larger region around the known active to decrease the possibility of missing a hit in the designed library.

descriptors (chemistry space axes) seem to cluster and separate the blockers and openers better than others. Observations of this type *(46)* led to the development and implementation of the concept of receptor-relevant subspaces *(47)* in the DiverseSolutions software package. Stewart et al. have used DiverseSolutions to find a receptor-family-relevant chemistry space for nuclear hormone receptors that distinguished 907 known NHR ligands from other inactive compounds *(49)*.

Distance-based similarity searching around a known active is a well-known approach that yields lists of nearest-neighbor compounds, which are presumed to have an increased likelihood of activity against the same target. Pearlman and Smith implemented a list-based nearest-neighbor-searching algorithm within Diverse Solutions *(45)*, which can also be used for target-directed combinatorial library design. Recent versions of DiverseSolutions and of Pearlman's Windows-based LibraryDesigner application *(50)* also offer several novel library design options of varying appropriateness for target class libraries. Ideally suited for target class library design is a unique cell-based "fill-in" library design option. A set of known active ligands from the target class knowledge database is used to identify "promising cells" in chemistry space (**Fig. 4**). The space used may have been derived either from the entire target class knowledge database of ligands, the virtual library from which the combinatorial library will be designed, or from a standard corporate chemistry space. The reactant-biased, product-based library design algorithm is then used to design a library, of whatever desired size, which best fills these "promising cells." The degree of target focus is controlled by the number of bins per axis and the number of cell radii from the known ligand used to define the size of the "promising cell." The "focused" design approach in DiverseSolutions and LibraryDesigner uses a set of target ligands to score all the compounds in the virtual library based on their distance to the actives and then selects a designed library that optimizes the average virtual activity. An example of using this method to select GPCR compounds for screening to validate the library design approach has been reported by Wang and Saunders *(51)*. The algorithm also permits use of externally determined activity scores such as those from docking, QSAR models, pharmacophore models, or other sources. Recent versions of DiverseSolutions and of Pearlman's Windows-based LibraryDesigner application *(50)* also offer a novel "focused/diverse" library design option, which yields products that are focused with respect to receptor-relevant axes of the chemistry space and are diverse with regard to the receptor-irrelevant axes. Because it is unlikely that an entire target class of receptors will have the same sets of relevant and irrelevant axes, use of this algorithm should be limited to individual targets or at best closely related targets.

The "receptor relevance" of BCUT descriptors has inspired several groups to apply them in conjunction with other methods. Beno and Mason reported the use of simulated annealing to optimize library design using BCUT chemistry space and four-point pharmacophores concurrently *(33)* and the use of chemistry spaces in conjunction with property profiles *(52)*. The application of such composite methods to target class library design is readily apparent. Pirard and Pickett reported the application of the chemometric method, partial least squares discriminant analysis, with BCUT descriptors to successfully classify ATP-site-directed kinase inhibitors active against five different protein kinases *(53)*. Manallack et al. used BCUTs as input parameters to neural networks that selected compounds that targeted specific gene families *(54)*. Their training sets were derived from the MDDR and included three classes: protein kinase inhibitors, GPCR Class A biogenic amines, and Class A peptide-binding-type GPCRs. Clearly, the literature involving DiverseSolutions and/or BCUT descriptions for target class library design is currently limited, but will continue to grow.

2.4. Structure-Based Methods

The advantages inherent in a structure-based approach to computational chemistry manifest themselves equally clearly in target class design strategies. The concept of target class forms a mainstay of the structure-based drug-design process. A fundamental example of this is the common structural motif principle comprising the heart of homology modeling methodology *(55–57)*. The tools of structure-based target class library design share a large degree of overlap with those applied to library design in general [reviewed extensively elsewhere *(58–60)*]. The primary differences in approach are exhibited in the methods used

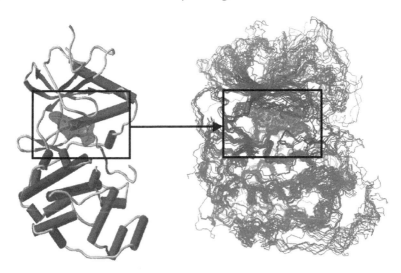

Fig. 5. Superposition of 26 kinase structures via their conserved structural elements, with ATP binding site highlighted. Adapted from **ref. *61***.

to define design constraints. Rather than delineating library space using a single active site, constraints are created based on the similarities and differences that become apparent upon class structural motif superposition. As a consequence, a number of new target class strategies are possible when compared with ligand-based design, both from the perspective of ligand and protein. Ligand super-positions can be directly constrained by their binding modes. Key interactions with conserved active site regions can also be determined, allowing the abstraction and design of novel ligand binding motifs. Furthermore, regions of structural variation can be pinpointed to permit the design of selective inhibitors.

Structure-based target-class-design approaches have been applied over a number of protein classes *(15,61–66)*. It is for the ATP competitive binding site of the kinase gene family, however, that most work has been published, and it is this class that will serve as our primary example. Target class structural conservation, selectivity analyses, and the transferability of structural constraints between class members is elegantly highlighted in the work of Naumann and Matter *(15)*. In these studies 26 different crystal structures were superimposed by their ATP binding pockets based on conserved tertiary structure **(Fig. 5)**. The authors exploited such superpositions to both map out the active sites for various kinase targets using GRID *(67)* and to superpose a CDK1 purine inhibitor set within the confines of the cyclin dependent kinase 2 (CDK 2) binding site. Principal component analysis of the GRID maps nicely separated the class by target subtype (CDK/MAP/PKA/SRC), while QSAR

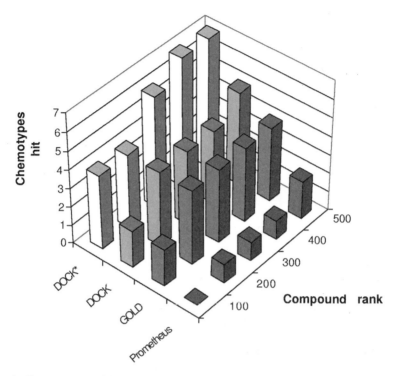

Fig. 6. Chemotype enrichment rates using a variety of structure-based virtual screening algorithms and constraint settings for CDK2. DOCK search incorporating target class critical pharmacophore constraints denoted by the * mark. Adapted from **ref. 70**.

field analysis using CoMFA *(68)* and CoMSIA *(69)* yielded models with robust statistical parameters.

The potential power of structure-based class constraints is exemplified by work undertaken in the field of kinase screening library selection *(70)*. Kinase structures pose significant problems for VS calculations because of the inherent flexibility of the ATP binding site, and the structural differences inherent between inactivated versus activated enzyme *(71)*. Good et al. undertook a series of searches based on CDK2 using three different tools: GOLD *(72)*, DOCK *(73)*, and PROMETHEUS *(74)*. A 10,000 compound dataset seeded with 85 active molecules spanning 14 different chemotypes was used as the search deck. Screens were undertaken using the generic methodology search protocols of each method. In addition, a DOCK search was created including pharmacophore search constraints based on generic target class interactions of ATP and its inhibitors, as observed in various kinase crystal structures. Search results are shown in **Fig. 6** with chemotype enrichment employed as the primary measure

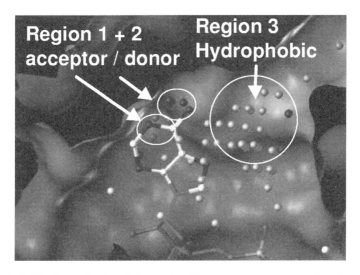

Fig. 7. DOCK site point breakdown for the kinase receptor study. Three primary critical regions were defined: (1) adenine acceptor zone, (2) adenine donor zone, (3) kinase ATP inhibitor rear hydrophobic pocket binding region. Adapted from **ref. 70**.

of success. The target class constraints used are highlighted in **Fig. 7**. The poor performance of the complex scoring function used in PROMETHEUS is a testament to the difficulties inherent to kinase structure-based virtual screening. The enhanced performance of the constrained search provides a practical example of the utility of target class information in library selection. Others have had success applying variants of this approach. A pertinent example is derived from the work of Furet et al. *(75)*, who undertook *de novo* scaffold design based on the ability of a novel molecular core to map out the key binding requirements of the CDK 1/2 ATP active sites. The resulting 5-aryl-1H-pyrazole substructure was used to search the corporate collection and a number of novel low micromolar inhibitors of both CDK 1 and 2 were discovered.

A final example illustrating the unique power of a structure-based approach to target class design comes from the work of Honma et al. *(63,64)*. Starting from a novel class of CDK4 inhibitors derived from *de novo* structure-based design *(63)*, the authors undertook an extensive sequence analysis of approx 400 kinases. The least conserved regions were determined particularly with respect to other CDK targets. Targeting these difference residues through modification of their initial lead (which exhibited essentially no selectivity), libraries were designed that produced molecules with up to 180-fold selectivity with respect to CDK2 **(Fig. 8)**.

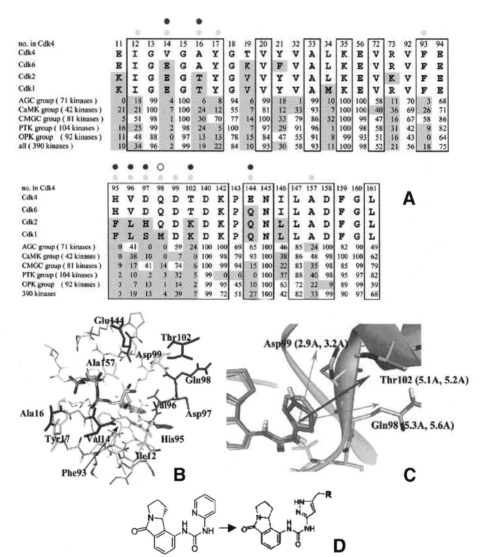

Fig. 8. CDK4 selective library design process of Honma et al. *(64)*. **(A)** Align sequences of 390 kinases. Dark circles denote residues with <40% conservation or subject to replacement in CDK1/2/6. **(B)** Darker residues in ATP binding site pinpoint the least conserved residues highlighted in **(A)**. **(C)** Map lead structure onto difference residues. Arrows denote direction and distance to said amino acids. **(D)** Design library according to these constraints. Resulting compounds show up to 180-fold selectivity for CDK4 with respect to CDK2. Adapted from **ref. *64*.**

3. Conclusions

Many of the methodologies for diversity based and for focused library design are applicable to target class libraries. Those presented in this chapter—3D pharmacophores, privileged substructures, cell-based designs, and structure-based designs—are a representative sampling. Whatever design tools are employed, from 2D property-based profiles and scoring methods *(76)* to those described above, the resultant design quality is highly dependent on the knowledge database of ligands or structural data used to develop the design. As these knowledge databases grow, target class library design examples will undoubtedly become more prevalent in the literature. The ultimate contribution of target class combinatorial library design to drug discovery will be determined.

Acknowledgments

The authors wish to thank Robert Pearlman and Mark Hermsmeier for helpful comments during the preparation of this chapter.

References

1. Bures, M. G. and Martin, Y. C. (1998) Computational methods in molecular diversity and combinatorial chemistry. *Curr. Opin. Chem. Biol.* **2,** 376–380.
2. Van Drie, J. H. and Lajiness, M. S. (1998) Approaches to virtual library design. *Drug Discovery Today* **3,** 274–283.
3. Spellmeyer, D. C. and Grootenhuis, P. D. J. (1999) Recent developments in molecular diversity: Computational approaches to combinatorial chemistry. *Annu. Rep. Med. Chem.* **34,** 287–296.
4. Drewry, D. H. and Young, S. S. (1999) Approaches to the design of combinatorial libraries. *Chemom. Intell. Lab. Syst.* **48,** 1–20.
5. Agrafiotis, D. K., Myslik, J. C., and Salemme, F. R. (1999) Advances in diversity profiling and combinatorial series design. *Annu. Rep. Comp. Chem. Mol. Diversity* **2,** 71–92.
6. Leach, A. R. and Hann, M. M. (2000) The *in silico* world of virtual libraries. *Drug Discovery Today* **5,** 326–336.
7. Lewis, R. A., Pickett, S. D., and Clark, D. E. (2000) Computer-aided molecular diversity analysis and combinatorial library design. In *Reviews in Computational Chemistry*, Lipkowitz, K. B. and Boyd, D. B. (eds.), Wiley-VCH, New York, Vol. 16, pp. 1–51.
8. Willett, P. (2000) Chemoinformatics—similarity and diversity in chemical libraries. *Curr. Opin. Biotechnol.* **11,** 85–88.
9. Lipinski, C. A., Lombardo F., Dominy, B. W., and Feeney, P. J. (1997) Experimental and computational approaches to estimate solubility and permeability in drug discovery and development settings. *Adv. Drug Deliv. Rev.* **23,** 3–25.
10. Palm, K., Stenberg, P., Luthman, K., and Artursson, P. (1997) Polar molecular surface properties predict the intestinal absorption of drugs in humans. *Pharm. Res.* **14,** 568–571.

11. van de Waterbeemd, H., Smith, D. A., Beaumont, K., and Walker, D. K. (2001) Property-based design: optimization of drug absorption and pharmacokinetics. *J. Med. Chem.* **44,** 1313–1333.

12. Schneider, G. and Nettekoven, M. (2003) Ligand-based combinatorial design of selective purinergic receptor (A2A) antagonists using self-organizing maps. *J. Comb. Chem.* **5,** 233–237.

13. McGregor, M. J. and Muskal, S. M. (2000) Pharmacophore fingerprinting. 2. Application to primary library design. *J. Chem. Inf. Comput. Sci.* **40,** 11–125.

14. Schuffenhauer, A., Zimmermann, J., Stoop, R., van der Vyver, J.-J., Lecchini, S., and Jacoby, E. (2002) An ontology for pharmaceutical ligands and its application for in silico screening and library design. *J. Chem. Inf. Comput. Sci.* **42,** 947–955.

15. Naumann, T. and Matter, H. (2002) Structural classification of protein kinases using 3d molecular interaction field analysis of their ligand binding sites: Target family landscapes. *J. Med. Chem.* **45,** 2366–2378.

16. Klabunde, T. and Hessler, G. (2002) Drug design strategies for targeting G-protein coupled receptors. *Chembiochem* **3,** 929–944.

17. Daylight Chemical Information Systems, Inc., 27401 Los Altos, Suite 360, Mission Viejo, CA 92691.

18. Carhart, R. E., Smith, D. H., and Venkataraghavan, R. (1985) Atom pairs as molecular features in structure-activity studies: definition and applications. *J. Chem. Inf. Comput. Sci.* **25,** 64–73.

19. McGregor, M. J. and Muskal, S. M. (1999) Pharmacophore fingerprinting. 1. Application to QSAR and focused library design. *J. Chem. Inf. Comput. Sci.* **39,** 569–574.

20. Mason, J. S., Morize, I., Menard, P. R. Cheney, D. L., Hulme, C., and Labaudiniere, R. F. (1999) New 4-point pharmacophore method for molecular similarity and diversity applications: overview of the method and applications, including a novel approach to the design of combinatorial libraries containing privileged substructures. *J. Med. Chem.* **42,** 3251–3264.

21. Beno, B. R. and Mason, J. S. (2001) The design of combinatorial libraries using properties and 3D pharmacophore fingerprints. *Drug Disc. Today* **6,** 251–258.

22. Pearlman, R. S. (1996) Novel software tools for addressing chemical diversity, *Network Science,* http://www.awod.com/netsci/Science/combichem/feature08.html.

23. Mason, J. S., Good, A. C., and Martin, E.J. (2001) 3-D pharmacophores in drug discovery. *Curr. Pharm. Design* **7,** 567–597.

24. Willett, P., Barnard, J. M., and Downs, G. M. (1998) Chemical similarity searching. *J. Chem. Inf. Comput. Sci.* **38,** 983–996.

25. Ugi, I. and Steinbruckner, C. (1961) Isonitriles. II. Reaction of isonitriles with carbonyl compounds, amines, and hydrazoic acid. *Chem. Ber.* **94,** 734–742.

26. MDL Drug Data Report, MDL Information Systems, San Leandro, CA, USA.

27. Lamb, M. L., Bradley E. K., Spellmeyer, D. C., Suto, M. J., and Grootenhuis, P. D. J. Iterative design of gene-family directed screening libraries. Book of Abstracts, 222nd ACS National Meeting, Chicago, Aug 26–30, 2001.

28. Good, A. C. and Lewis, R. A. (1997) New methodology for profiling combinatorial libraries and screening sets: cleaning up the design process with HARPick. *J. Med. Chem.* **40,** 3926–3936.

29. Bradley, E. K., Beroza, P., Penzotti, J. E, Grootenhuis, P. D. J., Spellmeyer, D. C., and Miller, J. L. (2000) A rapid computational method for lead evolution: description and application to α_1-adrenergic antagonists. *J. Med. Chem.* **43,** 2770–2774.

30. Zuckerman, R. N., Martin, E. J., Spellmeyer, D. C., et al. (1994) Discovery of nanomolar ligands for 7-transmembrane G-protein-coupled receptors from a diverse *N*-(substituted)glycine peptoid library. *J. Med. Chem.* **37,** 2678–2685.

31. Beno, B. R. and Mason, J. S. Combinatorial library design using both properties and 3D pharmacophore fingerprints. Book of Abstracts, 221st ACS National Meeting, San Diego, 2001.

32. Pickett, S. D., McLay, I. M., abd Clark, D. E. (2000) Enhancing the hit-to-lead properties of lead optimization libraries. *J. Chem. Inf. Comput. Sci.* **40,** 263–272.

33. Mason, J. S. and Beno, B. R. (2000) Library design using BCUT chemistry-space descriptors and multiple four-point pharmacophore fingerprints: Simultaneous optimization and structure-based diversity. *J. Mol. Graphics Model.* **18,** 438–451.

34. Murray, C. M. and Cato, S. J. (1999) Design of libraries to explore receptor sites. *J. Chem. Inf. Comput. Sci.* **39,** 46–50.

35. Eksterowicz, J. E., Evensen, E., Lemmen, C., et al. (2002) Coupling structure-based design with combinatorial chemistry: application of active site derived pharmacophores with informative library design. *J. Mol. Graph. Model.* **20,** 469–477.

36. Penzotti, J. E., Lamb, M. L, Evensen, E., and Grootenhuis, P. D. J. (2002) A computational ensemble model for identifying substrates of P-glycoprotein. *J. Med. Chem.* **45,** 1737–1740.

37. Ekins, S., Bravi, G., Binkley, S., et al. (1999) Three- and four-dimensional quantitative structure activity relationship analyses of cytochrome P-450 3A4 inhibitors. *J. Pharm. Exp. Ther.* **290,** 429–438.

38. Ekins, S., Bravi, G., Wikel, J. H., and Wrighton, S.A. (1999) Three-dimensional-quantitative structure activity relationship analysis of cytochrome P-450 3A4 substrates. *J. Pharm. Exp. Ther.* **291,** 424–433.

39. Bemis, G. W. and Murcko, M. A. (1996) The properties of known drugs. 1. Molecular frameworks. *J. Med. Chem.* **39,** 2887–2893.

40. The SYBYL modeling package is available from Tripos Associates, St Louis, MO.

41. Vaz, R., private communication, 1999.

42. ClassPharmer™ is available from Bioreason, Inc., Santa Fe, NM.

43. Schnur, D. M. and Hermsmeier, M., Recent approaches to target class design, 36th MARM of the ACS, 2003.

44. Schnur, D. and Venkatarangan, P. (2001) Applications of cell-based diversity methods to combinatorial library design. In *Combinatorial library design and evaluation,* Ghose, A. K. and Viswadhan, V. N. (eds.), Marcel Dekker, Inc., New York, NY.

45. DiverseSolutions was developed by R. S. Pearlman and K. M. Smith at the University of Texas at Austin and is distributed by Optive Research, Inc. http://www.optive.com, and Tripos Inc., http://www.tripos.com.

46. Schnur, D. (1999) Design and diversity analysis of large combinatorial libraries using cell-based methods. *J. Chem. Inf. Comput. Sci.* **39,** 36–45.
47. Pearlman, R. S. and Smith, K. M. (1999) Metric validation and the receptor-relevant subspace concept. *J. Chem. Inf. Comput. Sci.* **39,** 28–35.
48. Schnur, D. M. (2001) Approaches to target class library design, CHI Conference on Molecular Diversity, San Diego, CA.
49. Stewart, E. L., Brown, P. J., Bentley, J. A., and Wilson, T. M. (2001) Abstracts of Papers, 222nd ACS National Meeting, Chicago, IL, August 26–30.
50. LibraryMaker and LibraryDesigner are distributed by Optive Research, Austin, TX; http://www.optiveresearch.com.
51. Wang, X. and Saunders, J. (2001) Abstracts of Papers, 222nd ACS National Meeting, Chicago, IL, August 26–30.
52. Beno, B. R. and Mason, J. S., unpublished.
53. Pirard, B. and Pickett, S. D. (2000) Classification of kinase inhibitors using BCUT descriptors. *J. Chem. Inf. Comput. Sci.* **40,** 1431–1440.
54. Manallack, D. T., Pitt, W. R., Gancia, E., et al. (2002) Selecting screening candidates for kinase and G-protein-coupled receptor targets using neural networks. *J. Chem. Inf. Comput. Sci.* **42,** 1256–1262.
55. Sitkoff, D. F., Krystek, S. R., Bassolino, D. A., et al. (2001) Protein family clustering as an aid to drug design. *Abstr. Pap. Am. Chem. Soc. 221st*, COMP-161.
56. Montelione, G. T. (2001) Structural genomics: an approach to the protein folding problem. *Proc. Natl. Acad. Sci. USA* **98,** 13,488–13,489.
57. Peitsch, M. C., Schwede, T., Diemand, A., and Guex, N. (2002) Protein structure prediction by comparison: homology-based modeling. *Current Topics in Computational Molecular Biology*, 449–466.
58. Bohm, H.-J. (2001) Progress in structure-based library design. In *Rational approaches to drug design: Proceedings of the 13th European Symposium on QSAR*, Höltje, H.-D. and Sippl, W. (eds.), Prous Science, Barcelona, pp. 367–371.
59. Stahl, M. (2000) Structure-based library design. *Meth. Prin. Med. Chem.* **10,** 229–264.
60. Leach, A. R., Bryce, R. A., and Robinson, A. J. (2000) Synergy between combinatorial chemistry and de novo design. *J. Mol. Graph. Model.* **18,** 358–367.
61. Gray, N. S., Wodicka, L., Thunnissen, A.-M. W. H., et al. (1998) Exploiting chemical libraries, structure, and genomics in the search for kinase inhibitors. *Science* **281,** 533–538.
62. Gehlhaar, D. K., Bouzida, D., and Rejto, P. A. (1999) Reduced dimensionality in ligand-protein structure prediction: covalent inhibitors of serine proteases and design of site-directed combinatorial libraries. *ACS Symposium Series* **719,** 292–311.
63. Honma, T. Hayashi, K., Aoyama, T., et al. (2001) Structure-based generation of a new class of potent cdk4 inhibitors: new de novo design strategy and library design. *J. Med. Chem.* **44,** 4615–4627.
64. Honma, T., Yoshizumi, T., Hashimoto, N., et al. (2001) A novel approach for the development of selective Cdk4 inhibitors: library design based on locations of Cdk4 specific amino acid residues. *J. Med. Chem.* **44,** 4628–4640.

65. Diller, D. J. (2001) Homology models, high throughput docking, and drug design. Molecular modeling. *Abstr. Pap. Am. Chem. Soc. 222nd*, COMP-050.

66. Sippl, W. (2002) GPCR Dopamine D3 antagonist design, in *Proceedings of the 14th European symposium on QSAR*, Livingstone, D. and Ford, M. (eds.), Wiley-VCH, Basel. http://www.iainm.demon.co.uk/euroqsarws2.htm.

67. GRID version 18, Molecular Discovery Ltd., West Way House, Elms Parade, Oxford UK.

68. Clark, M., Cramer, R. D., Jones, D. M., Patterson, D. E., and Simeroth, P. E. (1990) Comparative molecular field analysis (CoMFA). 2. Towards its use with 3D-structural databases. *Tetrahedron Comput. Methodol.* **3,** 47–59.

69. Klebe, G., Abraham, U., and Mietzner, T. (1994) Molecular similarity indices in a comparative analysis (CoMSIA) of drug molecules to correlate and predict their biological activity. *J. Med. Chem.* **37,** 4130–4146.

70. Good, A. C., Cheney, D. L., Sitkoff, D. F., et al. (2003) Analysis and optimization of structure-based virtual screening protocols (2). Examination of docked ligand orientation sampling methodology; mapping a pharmacophore for success. *J. Mol. Graph. Mod.* **22,** 31–40.

71. Engh, Richard A. and Bossemeyer, D. (2002) Structural aspects of protein kinase control—role of conformational flexibility. *Pharmacol. Therapeut.* **93,** 99–111.

72. GOLD version 1.2, developed and distributed by the CCDC, 12 Union Road, Cambridge, CB2 1EZ, UK. URL: http://www.ccdc.cam.ac.uk/prods/gold/index.html.

73. DOCK, developed and distributed by the Kuntz group, Dept. of Pharmaceutical Chemistry, 512 Parnassus, University of California, San Francisco, CA, USA. URL: http://www.cmpharm.ucsf.edu/kuntz.

74. Baxter, C. A., Murray, C. W., Waszkowycz, B., et al. (2000) New approach to molecular docking and its application to virtual screening of chemical databases. *J. Chem. Inf. Comput. Sci.* **40,** 254–262.

75. Furet, P., Meyer, T., Strauss, A., Raccuglia, S., and Rondeau, J-M. (2002) Structure-based design and protein X-ray analysis of a protein kinase inhibitor. *Bioorg. Med. Chem. Lett.* **12,** 221–224.

76. Balakin, K. V., Tkachenko S. E., Lang, S. A., Okun, I., Ivashchenko, A. A., and Savchuk, N. P. (2002) Property-based design of GPCR-targeted library. *J. Chem. Inf. Comput. Sci.* **42,** 1332–1342.

15

Simulated Annealing

*An Effective Stochastic Optimization Approach
to Computational Library Design*

Weifan Zheng

Abstract

We describe here a stochastic optimization protocol for computational library design based on the principle of simulated annealing (SA). We also demonstrate via computer simulation studies that the SA-guided diversity sampling affords higher information content than random sampling in terms of cluster hit rates. Using a tripeptoid library, we show that the SA guided similarity focusing provides important information about reagent selection for combinatorial synthesis. Finally, we report a system that employs the SA protocol for the simultaneous optimization of multiple properties during library design. We propose that the SA technique is an effective optimization method for computational library design.

Key Words: Combinatorial chemistry; library design; simulated annealing; diversity analysis; targeted library design; drug-likeness; multicriterion optimization.

1. Introduction

Combinatorial chemistry for drug discovery has evolved from what was initially described as a shotgun approach to a technology that often employs rational computational design. The goal of rational design is to ensure that a maximum amount of information can be obtained from designed libraries while a minimum number of compounds are synthesized and tested, and ultimately to discover novel active compounds in a highly efficient fashion. From a practical standpoint, computational library design is a process in which subsets of available reagents are selected for a given scaffold in an experimental synthesis based on a set of computational criteria in order to achieve the aforementioned goal. These

From: *Methods in Molecular Biology, vol. 275:*
Chemoinformatics: Concepts, Methods, and Tools for Drug Discovery
Edited by: J. Bajorath © Humana Press Inc., Totowa, NJ

criteria are often different for libraries that are designed for different purposes, which include diverse libraries for general screening, target-focused libraries, drug-like libraries, and, more recently, gene-family-targeted libraries.

In the context of general screening, computational library design involves the selection of a subset of compounds that are optimally diverse and representative of available classes of compounds, leading to a non-redundant chemical library for biological testing. Methods reported in the literature include (a) cluster analysis, which first identifies a set of compound clusters followed by the selection of one or more representative compounds from each cluster *(1–4)*; (b) partitioning methods, which either place all the compounds into a low-dimensional space divided into cells or partition all compounds through median partitioning, and then choose compounds from each partition as representatives *(5,6)*; (c) direct sampling, which tries to obtain a subset of optimally diverse compounds by optimizing a diversity function *(7–10)*. Even though the general trend in the pharmaceutical industry is moving away from general screening of pure diverse libraries, the design principle of diversity analysis remains valid and can be employed in conjunction with other criteria.

In a targeted screening project, however, computational library design involves the selection of subsets of reagents from an available pool of chemical structures that afford a focused library with high percentage of compounds that are predicted to be active against the underlying target. The activity prediction can be based on library similarity to known leads, pharmacophore models, QSAR models and/or molecular docking in cases where the biological target structure is known. Many applications in this category have appeared in the literature in the past several years *(11–15)*.

Owing to drug developability requirements, design criteria such as Lipinski's rules of 5 *(16)*, Veber's "rotatable bond rule" *(17)*, and drug-likeness concept *(18)* are increasingly being incorporated into the design process as additional factors. These factors and ultimately compound solubility, membrane permeability, and cytochrome P450 liabilities have to be considered in a comprehensive library design practice. Selected literature methods that address these issues include HarPick *(19)*, SELECT *(20)*, PICCOLO *(21)*, MoSELECT *(22)*, and others *(23)*.

With the advances in genomics, families of novel targets have emerged as potential drug targets and gene-family-based research has become a central theme of discovery research in many pharmaceutical companies *(24)*. Thus, computational library design has to address the issue of how to optimally select compounds for related targets in a given gene family. These issues and proposed solutions have been discussed in recent meetings *(25)*.

Although the above-mentioned aspects of computational library design are multifaceted and complex, they can be tackled systematically using a comprehensive library design tool that employs the principle of multicriterion optimization. These methods include simulated annealing (SA) *(26)*, and genetic algorithms (GA) *(27)*. This chapter summarizes one of these methods— a simple yet effective approach from our own work that employs the simulated annealing as the optimization technique. Also highlighted in this chapter are the applications of this technique in diverse library design *(28)*, target-focused library design *(12)*, and drug-like library design *(21)*.

2. Methods

2.1. The Simulated Annealing (SA) Optimization Protocol

The methods of simulated annealing *(26)*, genetic algorithms *(27)*, and taboo search *(29)* are three of the most popular stochastic optimization techniques, inspired by ideas from statistical mechanics, theory of evolutionary biology, and operations research, respectively. They are applicable to our current problem and have been used by researchers for computational library design. Because SA is employed in this chapter, a more-detailed description of the (generalized) SA is given below.

The idea of SA is to simulate the physical process called annealing, in which a system is heated to a high temperature, and then is gradually lowered to a preset temperature value (e.g., room temperature). During this process, the system samples possible configurations according to Boltzmann distribution. At equilibrium, low energy states will be mostly populated. The first implementation of the SA procedure was described by Metropolis et al. *(30)*, followed by the development of a generalized mathematical optimization protocol. The implementation of SA in our project is as follows:

1. Generate a trial solution to the underlying problem. For combinatorial library design, a random selection of a subset of building blocks is generated.
2. Calculate the value of a fitness function (F_{curr}) that characterizes the quality of the trial solution to the underlying problem (e.g., the diversity or predicted activity of the combinatorial library built upon the selection of building blocks from **step 1**).
3. Perturb (i.e., slightly modify) the trial solution to obtain a new solution (e.g., a part of the selected building blocks are changed to other building blocks in order to build a new combinatorial library).
4. Calculate the value of the fitness function (F_{new}) for the new solution generated in **step 3**.
5. For the purpose of minimization, if $F_{new} \leq F_{curr}$, the new solution is accepted and used to replace the old solution. If $F_{new} > F_{curr}$, the new solution is accepted only if the following Metropolis criterion is satisfied, i.e.,

$$rnd < e^{-(F_{new}-F_{curr})/T} \qquad (1)$$

where *rnd* is a random number uniformly distributed between 0 and 1, and T is a parameter analogous to the temperature in Boltzmann distribution law.

6. **Steps 3–5** are repeated until the termination condition is satisfied. The temperature scheme and the termination condition used in this work have been adopted from Sun et al. *(31)*. Every time when a new solution is accepted or when a preset number of successive trial solutions do not lead to a better result, the temperature is lowered e.g., by 10%. The calculations are terminated when either the current temperature of simulations is lowered to the value of $T = 10^{-6}$ or the ratio between the current temperature and the temperature corresponding to the best solution found is equal to 10^{-6}.

2.2. The SA Guided Diversity Sampling

The above-described principle of simulated annealing optimization can be applied to diverse sampling *(28)*, which is to select a subset of molecules from an available pool such that the selected subset represents as many classes of compounds as possible. In the practice of database mining or combinatorial library design, compounds are first represented by molecular descriptors, such as molecular connectivity indices *(32)*, and atom pair descriptors *(33)*. Then, a subset of M molecules is selected from a pool of N molecules. A special diversity function (see below) can be designed to measure the diversity of selected compounds. Comparison of the diversity values of different subsets of M compounds using the above-described SA technique leads to the most diverse subset that will be suggested for use in combinatorial synthesis or for biological testing as in database mining projects.

In order to apply the SA protocol, one of the keys is to design a mathematical function that adequately measures the diversity of a subset of selected molecules. Because each molecule is represented by molecular descriptors, geometrically it is mapped to a point in a multidimensional space. The distance between two points, such as Euclidean distance, Tanimoto distance, and Mahalanobis distance, then measures the *dissimilarity* between any two molecules. Thus, the diversity function to be designed should be based on all pairwise distances between molecules in the subset. One of the functions is as follows:

$$D = \frac{1}{\sum\limits_{i}^{m-1} \sum\limits_{j>i}^{m} \dfrac{1}{d_{ij}^{a}}} \tag{2}$$

The summation is over all pairwise distances between the M selected points (molecules). Power a was set to 1 in all of the experiments reported below; however, it could be set to any value between 1 and 6 empirically.

2.3. The SA Guided Focusing of Libraries

The goal of targeted library design is to select building blocks that can be used to construct libraries with a high content of compounds predicted to be active against a target. The activity prediction can be based on similarity analysis with respect to lead molecules, pharmacophore matching scores, activities predicted by QSAR models, or molecular docking scores. The example described here is based on the similarity principle that is widely employed in medicinal chemistry. The virtual library compounds (trial solutions) are generated by a random combination of available building blocks based on the underlying chemical reaction. Once a trial solution has been generated, the enumerated compounds are then characterized by molecular descriptors, and the similarity between a library molecule and the probe (lead) molecule is measured by the Euclidean distance between them in the descriptor space. With the similarity measure as the fitness function, the SA protocol is then employed to maximize the similarity between enumerated virtual molecules and the lead molecule. Finally, frequency distribution analysis of building blocks found in the molecules with the highest similarity to the lead molecule is performed, and the building blocks found more frequently than random expectation are suggested as candidates for combinatorial synthesis *(12)*.

2.3.1. Building Block Frequency Analysis

The SA-guided sampling of the virtual chemical library produces a set of compounds with the highest similarities to the lead molecule. The resulting set is then analyzed in terms of relative frequency of each building block, f_i, which is calculated as:

$$f_i = \frac{N_i}{N_t} \tag{3}$$

where N_i and N_t are the number of occurrences for a building block i and the total number of building blocks in the top scoring compounds, respectively. The value of f_i is compared with the expected frequency (i.e., if the selection were random) which is calculated as $1/N$ (N is the total number of available building blocks). The building blocks with frequency of occurrence higher than random expectations are considered as candidates for combinatorial synthesis of the targeted library.

2.4. The SA Guided Simultaneous Optimization of Multiple Properties

The SA protocol has also been successfully applied to optimize drug-like properties or ADME parameters while maximizing diversity and/or predicted

activity of library compounds *(21)*. Two important aspects of this implementation are the formulation of a fitness function and the perturbation scheme used
to effectively generate the trial solutions during simulated annealing. These are
explained in detail as follows.

2.4.1. Perturbation Method

We consider three aspects of perturbation. (1) The choice of which substitution group (R) on a scaffold to be sampled on a given iteration; (2) the choice
of reagents to be picked from the selected reagent pool from **step 1**; (3) the
choice of reagents to be ejected from the current trial solution (i.e., the current
reagent selection). The first question is addressed by considering the relative
number of reagents being selected for each R group, as well as the size of the
reagent pool for each R group. The R groups are sampled randomly with probability determined by the average ratios of the size of a pool N_i to the total
number of reagents in all pools and the number of selected reagents K_i to the
total number of selected reagents. This empirical rule biases the sampling
toward the R groups that need more sampling, while still ensuring that each
R group is sampled reasonably well. The second sampling decision is handled
by a uniform random sampling approach. The reagent pool is randomized at the
start of the optimization, with reagents selected in order. After the pool has
been fully sampled, the sampling begins again from the start of the list. This
sampling method is more efficient than a purely random approach, and
converges faster. Finally, the reagent that is ejected from the chosen R group of
the library is selected purely at random.

2.4.2. Fitness Function

The fitness function can contain terms related to diversity, similarity, developability, activity, and practicality. Two diversity terms can be encoded: the
first, *reagent diversity*, describes the degree of self-similarity among the
reagents at each substitution position. The second term, *product novelty*,
depends on the similarity between the products of the library and an existing
collection of compounds. Developability terms include molecular weight,
lipophilicity, and hydrogen bond donor/acceptor counts. Other terms related primarily to practical issues may include reagent price and product flexibility. The
overall fitness function *E(S)* of a solution *(S)* is defined as the weighted sum of
individual penalty scores $E_i(S)$ for all the terms under consideration. That is,

$$E(S) = \sum Wi * Ei(S) \tag{4}$$

where W_i is the weight given to the *i*th term. Each term is described below.

2.4.3. Reagent Diversity

A simple method is employed to penalize the selected library for excessive self-similarity. An *S*-optimality criterion or a measure described in **Eq. 2** is computed for the reagents of each R group based on the Daylight fingerprint Tanimoto (*34*) distances among members of that R group. This has the effect of minimizing the maximum similarity between members of an R group.

2.4.4. Product Novelty

An important goal of many library designs is to augment a screening collection with compounds that populate previously unexplored regions of chemical space. In order to avoid the time-consuming pairwise comparison of library products with hundreds of thousands of compounds at each iteration of the optimization, we chose to implement a low-dimensional cell-based method. In this implementation, compounds from the screening collection are represented in a six-dimensional feature space, mapped onto a grid with 20 divisions on each axis. The cell occupancies are stored in memory. During each iteration, molecular descriptors are calculated for each new library member, its location on the grid is determined in an extremely rapid lookup. The average cell count for the library is used as the penalty score for this term.

2.4.5. Developability Penalties

Lipinski's "Rule of 5" (*16*) states that compounds associated with good developability properties have MW less than 500, log*P* less than 5, and no more than 5 donors or 10 acceptors. We took these four terms as our initial set of developability parameters, in each case taking the term to be minimized as the fraction of the total number of molecules in the library that fall outside of the limit for each term. Lipinski's values for each term are used as defaults, but all are variables under the control of the user.

2.4.6. Focusing Term

One or more lead molecules may be used as a focusing target. Similarity metrics include Daylight fingerprint Tanimoto similarity. The penalty score for each compound in the library is defined as the distance between it and the most similar lead molecule. The penalty score for the library is the average of the individual compound penalty scores. QSAR predictions and docking scores can also be used in this term.

3. Applications

3.1. The SA-Guided Diversity Sampling—
Hit-Rate-Simulation Experiments

The major goal of this example is to demonstrate the behavior of the SA-guided diversity sampling protocol, which could be approached in two different ways. One of them is through retrospective analysis of a chemical database with known structures and activities, and the other is through analysis of simulated datasets of known distribution. To better separate the issues of descriptor validation and computational protocol characterization, the latter approach has been adopted here in the hope that one can obtain a basic understanding of the sampling strategy itself without noises introduced by molecular descriptors when dealing with real datasets. Because simulated datasets are used to replace real chemical databases, compound selection becomes choosing a subset of points from a total collection of points. Three aspects of experiments were performed in the original report *(10)*: (a) visualization of the sampled points in two-dimensional space; (b) quantification of the information content obtained from the SA-guided sampling in terms of percentage coverage of data clusters; and (c) computer simulation of hit rates obtained by both the SA-guided sampling and random sampling. Included here are the results from hit-rate-simulation experiments obtained by the SA-guided sampling and random samplings. Details of the dataset and experimental design are explained as follows.

3.1.1. Dataset

This simulated dataset is generated as follows. First, nine cluster centers are defined at different locations in a 2D space with coordinate values within [–3.0, 3.0]. Second, a random number (between 1 and 100) of points is generated around each cluster center within a distance of 0.5. Finally, additional points are generated, which are randomly distributed in the 2D space so that a total of 1000 points is obtained. This dataset simulates the situation where clusters of molecules exist in their descriptor space, and the number of members for each cluster is different, i.e., some regions are more densely populated than other regions.

3.1.2. Definition of Active Clusters

C active clusters with size R are defined by randomly placing C non-overlapping circles of radius R into the 2D space of the simulated dataset. Points that happened to be within each of the C circles are defined as active points, which simulate C clusters of active molecules while points outside the circles are defined inactive. Each cluster with active points is referred to as an active cluster.

3.1.3. Definition of an Individual Hit and a Cluster Hit

If a point sampled happened to be an active point, it is counted as an individual hit. Thus, the number of active points sampled by a particular method is defined as the *individual hit rate* obtained by that method. On the other hand, in order to characterize the representativeness of a sampling, we define the concept of a *cluster hit* as follows. If one or more points are sampled from an active cluster, we define that this active cluster is sampled and counted as a cluster hit. Therefore, the number of active clusters sampled by a particular method is defined as the *cluster hit rate* obtained by that method.

3.1.4. Simulation Experimental Design

In order to simulate different scenarios in real chemical database mining and library design, several important factors, which could influence hit rates, are examined. The variable factors include (1) the geometrical size of each active cluster *(R)*, (2) the number of active clusters (C) in a dataset, (3) locations of active clusters in the descriptor space. Thus, the experimental design is as follows. For each of three geometrical sizes (i.e., $R = 0.1$, 0.2, and 0.3), C active clusters are defined for the simulated dataset (where $C = 5$, 10, 15, ..., 30), and their locations in the 2D space are randomly defined. For instance, when $R = 0.1$, we first define $C = 5$ active clusters, then $C = 10$, 15 active clusters, and so on. For each case of C, the locations of the active clusters in the space can be different. To simulate this effect, the process of defining C active clusters is repeated for L (=100) times using different random seeds, leading to L (=100) different distributions of active clusters in the 2D space. Then, for each of the L cases, both the SA-guided sampling and random samplings are applied to sample M points (e.g., $M = 40$), and the individual hit rate and cluster hit rate (see above definition) are determined for both methods. Therefore, for both the SA-guided sampling and the random sampling, an average individual hit rate as well as an average cluster hit rate are obtained from the L (100) individual hit rates and L (100) cluster hit rates, respectively. The same procedure is repeated when $M = 80$, 100, and so on. Finally, the average individual hit rates for both methods are reported at different M's when $C = 5$, 10, 15, ..., 30 as in **Figs. 1A, 2A** for $R = 0.1$ and 0.3, respectively. Similarly, the average cluster hit rates for both methods are also given as in **Figs. 1B, 2B** for $R = 0.1$ and 0.3, respectively.

Each figure displays the average hit rates obtained by the SA-guided sampling and random sampling in cases of different C's (number of active clusters present in the dataset). For instance, **Fig. 1A** compares the average individual hit rates obtained by the SA-guided sampling and random sampling when $C = 5$, 10, 15, 20, 25, and 30. For each case of C, both the SA sampling and the random sampling are applied at different M's (number of

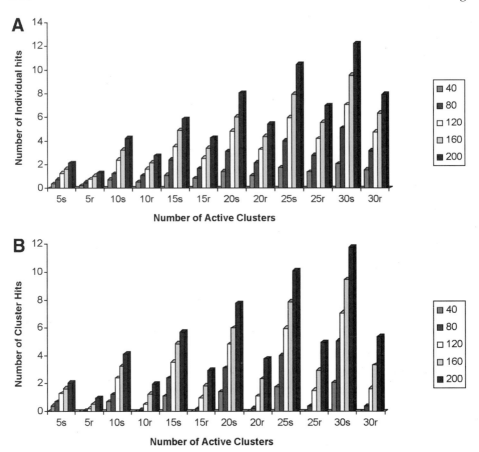

Fig. 1. (**A**) Comparison of individual hits obtained by the SA sampling and random sampling (cluster size $R = 0.1$). The comparison was performed when different numbers of active clusters exist in the data set. (**B**) Comparison of cluster hits obtained by the SA sampling and random sampling (cluster size $R = 0.1$). The comparison was performed when different numbers of active clusters exist in the data set.

points sampled, where $M = 40, 80$, etc.). Thus, the bars corresponding to 5s and 5r compare the hit rates obtained by the SA sampling and the random sampling at different M's when $C = 5$. Similarly, the bars corresponding to 10s vs 10r compare the hit rates obtained by the SA sampling and the random sampling at different M's when $C = 10$.

When $R = 0.1$, the percentage of active points (active compounds) in the dataset was from 0.65% to 3.96%. In all cases of different C's, the individual hit rates obtained by the SA-guided sampling are higher than that obtained by corresponding random sampling. An even better performance of the SA sampling over random sampling is observed when cluster hit rates are considered, which better characterizes the information content obtained by a sampling method. For all different *C*'s, the cluster hit rates given by the SA sampling are no less than 100% higher than that obtained by corresponding random sampling (**Fig. 1B**).

When $R = 0.2$, the percentage of active points (i.e., active compounds) in the dataset is from 2.56% to 12.6%. When individual hit rates are considered, the SA sampling performs about the same as or slightly better than random sampling in all cases of different *C*'s (data not shown). However, when cluster hit rates are considered, the SA sampling performs clearly better than corresponding random sampling, especially when the number of active clusters (*C*) increased (data not shown).

When *R* continues to increase to 0.3, the percentage of active points (i.e., active compounds) in the dataset increased to 5–16.8%. In this case, the SA sampling performs about the same or even slightly worse than the corresponding random sampling in terms of the individual hit rates (**Fig. 2A**). Nevertheless, when cluster hit rates are considered, the SA sampling still performs the same as or slightly better than random sampling, especially when the number of active clusters increases (**Fig. 2B**).

The above observation implies that when the percentage of active compounds in the library or database is low (in the range of 0.65–4%), the SA sampling performs much better than random sampling. This is encouraging, because in most of the combinatorial chemical synthesis projects the percentage of active compounds is as small as that in this simulated case. However, if the percentage of active compounds increases, the number of active compounds obtained by random sampling increases proportionally. This suggests that when the percentage of active compounds in the library is very high, the SA sampling (or any other cluster sampling) performs no better than random sampling in terms of the *individual hit rate*. There is a common view that the worse performance of cluster sampling strategies is due to non-ideal descriptors. On the contrary, our simulation indicates that this in fact is the nature of this kind of strategy regardless of what descriptors are used, because we have used simulated data sets, in which descriptors are *ideal*. Nevertheless, when *cluster hit rate* is considered as the criterion, the SA sampling performs better than or the same as random sampling in all tested cases, which indicates that information content obtained by the SA sampling is always better than random sampling.

3.2. The SA Guided Focusing—Designing a Tripeptoid Library

The SA protocol has been applied to the design of a tripeptoid library based on similarity to lead compounds (*12*). The experimental work on this library was described by Zuckermann et al. (*35*) who have shown that a few members

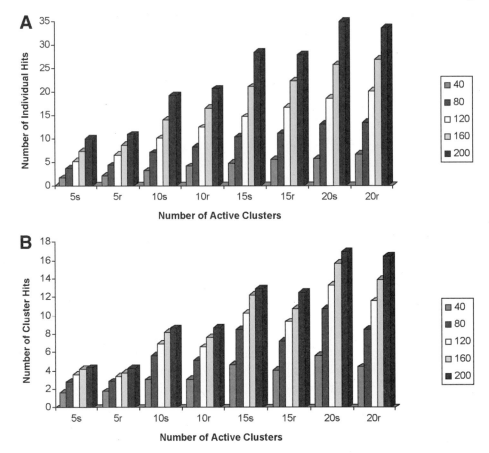

Fig. 2. **(A)** Comparison of individual hits obtained by the SA sampling and random sampling (cluster size $R = 0.3$). The comparison was performed when different numbers of active clusters exist in the data set. **(B)** Comparison of cluster hits obtained by the SA sampling and random sampling (cluster size $R = 0.3$). The comparison was performed when different numbers of active clusters exist in the data set.

of the library had high affinities for α_1-adrenergic or μ-opiate receptors. The results of that work are used as a test case to evaluate the effectiveness of the SA protocol. When met-enkephalin is used as a lead, the SA protocol suggested almost all building blocks found in peptoids with opioid activity. When morphine is used as a lead, the SA protocol also suggested several building blocks that were found in active opioid peptides. Standard hypothesis testing indicates that the results of the SA-guided similarity focusing are statistically significant.

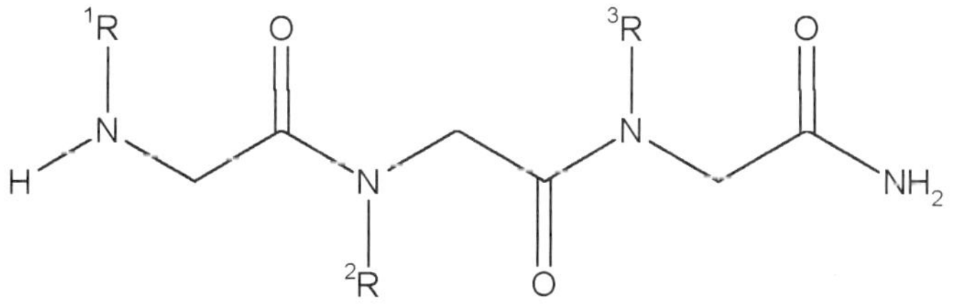

Fig. 3. Markush structure of tripeptoids. ^{1}R, ^{2}R, and ^{3}R are positions where various side chains (building blocks) are attached.

3.2.1. Building Blocks

Computational methods described in this work are tested using a tripeptoid combinatorial library described by Zuckermann et al. *(35)*. These authors described chemical structures of 24 amines used as building blocks for the peptoid synthesis. The common Markush structure of tripeptoids is shown in **Fig. 3** where R1, R2, and R3 are the alkyl portions of primary amines used as building blocks. The structures of the building blocks are shown in **Fig. 4** and we followed the abbreviations used in the original publication.

3.2.2. Active Peptoids

The structures of several active peptoids found by these authors are shown in **Table 1**. CHIR2279, CHIR2283, and CHIR2276 are high-affinity ligands for the α_1-adrenergic receptor, whereas CHIR4531, CHIR4534, and CHIR4537 were found to have high affinity for μ-opiate receptor.

3.2.3. Peptide as a Lead Compound

The main objective of this experiment was to demonstrate that a peptide lead compound could be used in rational design of a non-peptide library. One of the natural opiates, met-enkephalin, is used as a hypothetical lead compound. The averaged frequency distribution based on four SA runs is obtained (data not shown). Based on this result, O3 had the highest frequency, and the frequencies of A4, D11, D13, D14, D16, D2, D3, D5, and D9 are also above random expectation. Apparently, O3 appeared in all the reported active peptoids with opioid activity (cf. **Table 1**). Comparison of the structure of met-enkephalin **(Fig. 5)** with O3 indicated that O3 is similar to the side chain of tyrosine, which is the N-terminal residue of met-enkephalin. Among other building blocks found more frequently than random expectation, A4, D3, and D13 are present in the reported opioid peptoids (cf. **Table 1**). Thus, the SA sampling correctly identified four

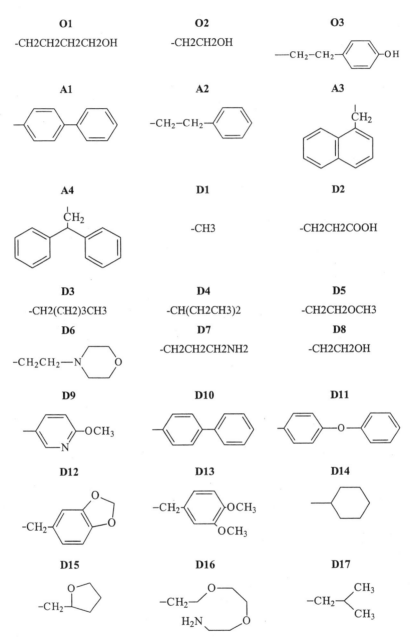

Fig. 4. The building blocks and their abbreviations as described by Zuckermann et al. *(36)*.

Table 1
Structures of Peptoids with α_1-Adrenergic
and μ-Opiate Activity (as Reported in ref. *36*)

Compound ID	Structure	K_i (nM)
CHIR2279	O3-D10-A2	5^a
CHIR2283	O3-D11-A2	140^a
CHIR2276	O3-D10-A1	310^a
CHIR4531	A4-D12-O3	6^b
CHIR4534	A4-D3-O3	46^b
CHIR4537	A4-D13-O3	31^b

[a]Data for α_1-adrenergic receptor binding.
[b]Data for μ-opiate receptor binding.

out of five building blocks found in the active peptoids. In addition to these building blocks, the SA protocol also selected D2, D3, D5, D9, D11, D14, and D16, which could be tested experimentally.

3.2.4. Morphine as a Lead Compound

This experiment represents a scenario when an organic lead compound is available. We chose morphine, a known opiate receptor ligand of non-peptide chemical nature, as a hypothetical lead compound. The averaged frequency distribution based on all four SA runs is obtained (data not shown). The most frequent building block was D11. Building blocks D10, D12, D14, and O3 were less frequent, but all above random expectation.

Comparison between the structures of D11 and morphine makes it obvious that D11 is similar to a substructure of morphine. Among other building blocks found more frequently than random expectation, D12 appears in CHIR4531, and O3 is found in all reported active peptoids (**Table 1**). Thus, in this test, we correctly identified two out of five building blocks found in the active opioid peptoids. It is interesting that with morphine as a lead, we identified D12 (found in CHIR4531) that we missed when met-enkephalin was used as a probe. Thus, with two lead molecules of non-peptoid nature, we could identify all five building blocks found experimentally in active opioid peptoids. The statistical significance of all these results has been demonstrated (*12*).

3.2.5. The SA Guided Similarity Focusing vs Exhaustive Experimental Evaluation

The design of a peptoid library using non-peptoid leads such as met-enkephalin and morphine represents an important practical instance of a rational

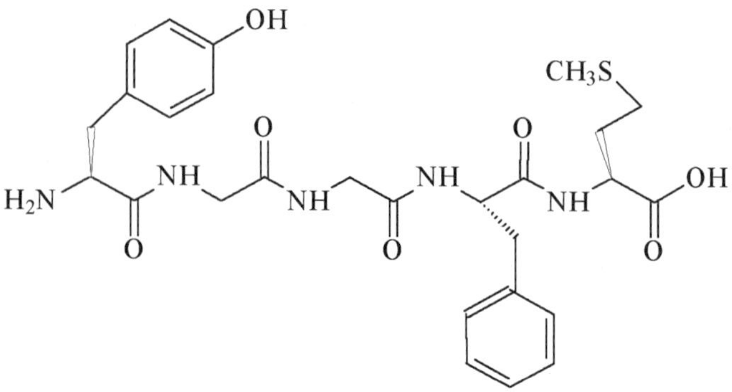

Fig. 5. Chemical structure of met-enkephalin.

library design. The use of met-enkephalin and morphine as leads could have been attempted, in principle, prior to the experimental synthesis and biological testing of the peptoid library developed by Zuckermann et al. Our results indicate that the SA-guided similarity focusing proposed 12 building blocks on a rational basis (when a composite probe was used), which included all five building blocks found in the three reported active opioid peptoids. Simple evaluation shows that if all combinations of building blocks were explored in a true sense of combinatorial chemical synthesis, as many as $24^3 = 13,824$ compounds would have to be synthesized and tested. On the other hand, if the experiments were limited to using only 12 building blocks suggested by the SA similarity focusing, only $12^3 = 1728$ compounds would have to be synthesized. Our results show that the same active compounds would be a part of this smaller library and therefore they would be identified. Thus, if the suggestions made by the SA-guided similarity focusing, using non-peptoid leads, were accepted prior to the synthesis and testing, the total number of compounds subjected to experimental screening would be reduced by almost an order of magnitude.

3.3. The SA Guided Simultaneous Optimization of ADME Properties

A published synthetic scheme *(36)* of a four component Ugi reaction (**Fig. 6**) has been used as an example to demonstrate the use of the SA optimization protocol for the simultaneous optimization of multiple properties. Because two of the four components are fixed in the scheme, only two diversity sites remain for optimization. These two sites come from primary amines (R1NH2) and aldehydes (R2CHO), respectively. We have collected from the ACD (Available Chemical Directory) structures of primary amines and aldehydes available from ALDRICH and LANCASTER. Compounds with reactive or unstable structural patterns are removed. As a result, 779 primary amines and 246 aldehydes are considered.

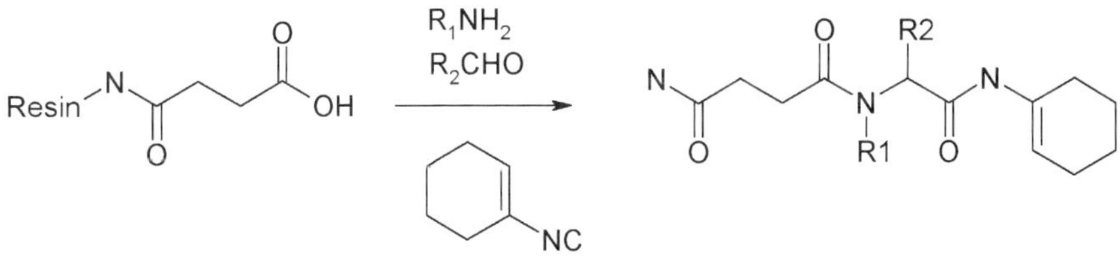

Fig. 6. A four-component Ugi reaction.

Table 2
Spreadsheet Showing the Best Three Solutions and the Initial Random Solution

Solutions	SDiv	Novelty	MW	HBD	HBA	clogP	MS
Best	2.1	334	1.9	0.0	10.0	0.9	0.34
2nd best	2.1	353	1.85	0.0	10.0	0.9	0.34
3rd Best	2.1	359	1.85	0.0	10.0	0.9	0.34
. . .							
Initial	73.0	126	70	0.4	28	39	0.08

3.3.1. Design of An 864-member Ugi Library

An 864-member library is being designed with 24 primary amines (R1) and 36 aldehydes (R2). The default ranges for developability parameters are set according to Lipinski. The weights have been selected based on the ranges of values observed in most cases. The program records all the accepted solutions during the SA process. These solutions and their associated penalty scores are presented in a spreadsheet. For the 864-member Ugi library, a spreadsheet showing the best three solutions and the initial random solution are given in **Table 2**. One can see that molecular weight and clogP penalties went from 70% and 39% for the initial solution down to 1.9% and 0.9% for the best solution. Hydrogen bond donor and acceptor counts penalties went from 0.4% and 28% down to 0.0% and 10.0%, respectively. Reagent diversity (SDiv) penalty also went down from 73 to 2.1. Because we gave a very small weight to hole-filling (Hfil) and zero weight to mass spectral redundancy (MS) in this experiment, their penalty scores actually went up. This indicates that we can emphasize those terms that we care about most by giving larger weights to them and sacrifice those that we do not care by giving smaller weights. This example also indicates that we can reduce the penalty for multiple terms simultaneously.

One can use this program to compare two different library "shapes" and find out which design may be better. For instance, a second 864-member Ugi library was designed using

36 primary amines and 24 aldehydes. Compared with the 24-by-36 library, it has a better diversity (1.9 for 36-by-24 vs 2.1 for 24-by-36), a better hole-filling (254 vs 334), a similar clog$P$ score (0.69 vs 0.93) and a better H-bond acceptor score (8.0 vs 10.0). It is, however, worse on MW (8.3 vs 1.9).

One can bias the library toward a developability criterion. For instance, when a larger weight was given to clog$P$ when designing a 36-by-24 Ugi library, a solution with 0.0% penalty on clog$P$ was obtained, as opposed to 0.69 in the previous case. This is not a dramatic change due to the nature of this particular library, but it can make a huge difference in other situations. This solution is also better on MW (2.6 vs 8.3), better on H-bond acceptor penalty (3.8 vs 8.0). As expected, the diversity of the library (2.28 vs 1.92) was sacrificed to achieve the above goals.

4. Conclusions

In this chapter, we have presented a stochastic optimization protocol for computational library design based on the principle of simulated annealing *(26)*. We demonstrated via computer simulation studies that the SA-guided diversity sampling affords higher information content than random sampling in terms of cluster hit rates. Using a tripeptoid library, we have shown that the SA guided similarity focusing could provide important information about reagent selection for combinatorial synthesis. Our analysis indicates that a much smaller library could be synthesized while still yielding the same set of active compounds if our design were adopted prior to the synthesis. Finally, we have reported a system that employs the SA protocol for the simultaneous optimization of multiple properties during library design. We conclude that the SA technique is an effective optimization method for computational library design.

References

1. Willett, P., Winterman, V., and Bawden, D. (1986) Implementation of nonhierarchic cluster analysis methods in chemical information systems: selection of compounds for bilogical testing and clustering of substructures search output. *J. Chem. Inf. Comput. Sci.* **26,** 109–118.
2. Lawson, R. G. and Jurs, P. C. (1990) Cluster analysis of acrylates to guide sampling for toxicity testing. *J. Chem. Inf. Comput. Sci.* **30,** 137–144.
3. Shemetulskis, N. E., Dunbar, J. B., Dunbar, B. W., Moreland, D. W., and Humblet, C. (1995) Enhancing the diversity of a corporate database using chemical database clustering and analysis. *J. Comp.-Aid Molec. Design* *9(5), 407–416.*
4. Barnard, J. M. and Downs, G. M. (1992) Clustering of chemical structures on the basis of two-dimensional similarity measures. *J. Chem. Inf. Comput. Sci.* **32(6),** 644.
5. Godden, J. W., Xue, L., Kitchen, D. B., Stahura, F. L., Schermerhorn, E. J., and Bajorath, J. (2002) Median partitioning: a novel method for the selection of

representative subsets from large compound pools. *J. Chem. Inf. Comput. Sci.* **42,** 885–893.

6. Pearlman, R. S. and Smith, K. M. (1998) Novel software tools for chemical diversity. *Perspect. Drug Discov. Design* **9,** 339–353.

7. Martin, E. J., Blaney, J. M., Siani, M. A., Spellmeyer, D. C., Wong, A. K., and Moos, W. H. (1995) Measuring diversity: experimental design of combinatorial libraries for drug discovery. *J. Med. Chem.* **38(9),** 1431–1436.

8. Agrafiotis, D. K. (1997) Stochastic algorithms for maximizing molecular diversity. *J. Chem. Info. Comput. Sci.* **37(5),** 841.

9. Hassan, M., Bielawski, J. P., Hempel, J. C., and Waldman, M. (1996) Optimization and visualization of molecular diversity and combinatorial libraries. *Mol. Div.* **2,** 64–74.

10. Zheng, W., Cho, S. J., Waller, C. L., and Tropsha, A. (1997) Simulated annealing guided evaluation (sage) of diversity: a novel computational tool for diverse chemical library design and database mining. *Books Abstracts*, 213th ACS National Meeting, San Fracisco, CA, CINF-015.

11. Sheridan, R. P. and Kearsley, S. K. (1995) Using a genetic algorithm to suggest combinatorial libraries. *J. Chem. Inf. Comput. Sci.* **35,** 310–320.

12. Zheng, W., Cho, S. J., and Tropsha, A. (1998) Rational combinatorial library design 1. focus-2d: a new approach to the design of targeted combinatorial chemical libraries. *J. Chem. Inf. Comput. Sci.* **38(2),** 251–258.

13. Zheng, Q. and Kyle, D. J. (1996) Computational screening of combinatorial libraries. *Bioorg. Med. Chem.* **4(5),** 631–638.

14. Kick, E. K., Roe, D. C., Skillman, A. G., et al. (1997) Structure-based design and combinatorial chemistry yield low nanomolar inhibitors of cathepsin D. *Chem. Biol.* **4(4),** 297–307.

15. Sun, Y., Ewing, T. J., Skillman, A. G., and Kuntz, I. D. (1998) CombiDOCK: structure-based combinatorial docking and library design. *J. Comput. Aided Mol. Des.* **12(6),** 597–604.

16. Lipinski, C. A., Lombardo, F., Dominy, B. W., and Feeney, P. (1997) Experimental and computational approaches to estimate solubility and permeability in drug discovery and development settings. *Adv. Drug Delivery Rev.* **23,** 3–25.

17. Veber, D. F., Johnson, S. R., Cheng, H. Y., Smith, B. R., Ward, K. W., and Kopple, K. D. (2002) Molecular properties that influence the oral bioavailability of drug candidates. *J. Med. Chem.* **45(12),** 2615–2623.

18. Ajay, A., Walters, W. P., and Murcko, M. A. (1998) Can we learn to distinguish between "drug-like" and "nondrug-like" molecules? *J. Med. Chem.* **41(18),** 3314–3324. Sadowski, J. and Kubinyi, H. A. (1998) A scoring scheme for discriminating between drugs and nondrugs. *J. Med. Chem.* **41(18),** 3325–3329.

19. Good, A. C. and Lewis, R. A. (1997) New methodology for profiling combinatorial libraries and screening sets: cleaning up the design process with HARPick. *J. Med. Chem.* **40(24),** 3926–3936.

20. Gillet, V. J., Willett, P., Bradshaw, J., and Green, D. V. S. (1999) Selecting combinatorial libraries to optimize diversity and physical properties. *J. Chem. Inf. Comput. Sci.* **39,** 169–177.

21. Zheng, W., Hung, S. T., Saunders, J. T., and Seibel, G. L. (2000) PICCOLO: a tool for combinatorial library design via multicriterion optimization. *Pac. Symp. Biocomput.* 588–599.

22. Gillet, V. J., Khatib, W., Willett, P., Fleming, P. J., Green, and D. V. (2002) Combinatorial library design using a multiobjective genetic algorithm. *J. Chem. Inf. Comput. Sci.* **42(2),** 375–385.

23. Agrafiotis, D. K. (2002) Multiobjective optimization of combinatorial libraries. *J. Comput. Aid. Mol. Des.* **16,** 335–356.

24. Frye, S. (1999) Structure-activity relationship homology (SARAH): a conceptual framework for drug discovery in the genomic era. *Chem. Biol.* **6(1),** R3–R7.

25. Zheng, W. and Lampe, J. (2002) Combinatorial optimization approaches to the design of focused, diverse, and target class oriented libraries. *Cambridge Healthtech Institute's Sixth Annual Cheminformatics,* Philadelphia, PA.

26. Kirkpatrick, S., Gelatt, C. D. Jr., and Vecchi, M. P. (1983) Optimization by simulated annealing. *Science* **220,** 671–680.

27. Forrest, S. (1993) Genetic algorithms: principles of adaptation applied to computation. *Science* **261,** 872–878.

28. Zheng, W., Cho, S. J., Waller, C. L., and Tropsha, A. (1999) Rational combinatorial library design. 3. Simulated annealing guided evaluation (SAGE) of molecular diversity: a novel computational tool for universal library design and database mining. *J. Chem. Inf. Comput. Sci.* **39(4),** 738–746.

29. Cvijovic, D. and Klinowski, J. (1995) Taboo search—an approach to the multiple minima problem. *Science* **267,** 664–666.

30. Metropolis, N., Rosenbluth, A. W., Rosenbluth, M. N., and Teller, A. H. (1953) Equation of state calculations by fast computing machines. *J. Chem. Phys.* **21,** 1087–1092.

31. Sun, L., Xie, Y., Song, X., Wang, J., and Yu, R. (1994) Cluster analysis by simulated annealing. *Comput. Chem.* **18,** 103–108.

32. Kier, L. B. and Hall, L. H. (1976) *Molecular connectivity in chemistry and drug research.* Academic Press, New York.

33. Carhart, R. E., Smith, D. H., and Venkataraghavan, R. (1985) Atom pairs as molecular features in structure-activity studies: definition and applications. *J. Chem. Inf. Comput. Sci.* **25,** 64–73.

34. Daylight Chemical Information Software, version 4.51, Daylight Chemical Information Systems, Inc., 27401 Los Altos, Mission Viejo, CA 92691.

35. Zuckermann, R. N., Martin, E. J., Spellmeyer, D. C., et al. (1994) Discovery of nanomolar ligands for 7-transmembrane g-protein-coupled receptors from a diverse n-(substituted)glycine peptoid library. *J. Med. Chem.* **37,** 2678–2685.

36. 4-component Ugi reaction. *Advanced ChemTech handbook of combinatorial and solid phase organic chemistry.* Advanced ChemTech, p. 65.

16

Genetic Algorithms for Classification of Olfactory Stimulants

Barry K. Lavine, Charles E. Davidson, Curt Breneman, and William Kaat

Abstract

We have developed and tested a genetic algorithm (GA) for pattern recognition, which identifies molecular descriptors that optimize the separation of the activity classes of olfactory stimulants in a plot of the two or three largest principal components of the data. Because principal components maximize variance, the bulk of the information encoded by these descriptors is about differences between olfactory classes in the dataset. In addition, the GA focuses on those classes and or samples that are difficult to classify as it trains using a form of boosting to modify the fitness landscape. Boosting minimizes the problem of convergence to a local optimum, because the fitness function of the GA is changing as the population is evolving toward a solution. Over time, compounds that consistently classify correctly are not as heavily weighted in the analysis as compounds that are difficult to classify. The pattern recognition GA learns its optimal parameters in a manner similar to a neural network. The algorithm integrates aspects of both strong and weak learning to yield a "smart" one-pass procedure for feature selection and classification.

Key Words: Structure–activity relationship studies; genetic algorithms; pattern recognition; olfaction; musks; classification; molecular descriptors.

1. Introduction

There is an enormous demand within the fragrance industry for methodology that will allow for the development of new compounds with specialized olfactory properties. In a traditional framework, the introduction of a new odorant is a lengthy, laborious, and costly discovery and development process. We propose to streamline this process by taking advantage of existing olfactory databases available through the open scientific literature as input for a new structure/activity correlation methodology in order to develop fundamental relationships between

From: *Methods in Molecular Biology, vol. 275:*
Chemoinformatics: Concepts, Methods, and Tools for Drug Discovery
Edited by: J. Bajorath © Humana Press Inc., Totowa, NJ

chemical structure and the olfactory properties of molecules. The first step in this so-called rational approach to odorant design is to characterize each molecule in a training set by using an appropriate set of descriptors capable of representing key intermolecular interaction mechanisms. To accomplish this task, we will use an enhanced version of Breneman's Transferable Atom Equivalent (TAE) descriptor methodology to create a large set of electron-density-derived shape/property-encoded surface translator (PEST), wavelet coefficient (WCD), and TAE histogram descriptors *(1)*. These descriptors will then be used to create improved qualitative structure activity relationship models that characterize and predict the behavior of olfactory stimulants.

Existing QSAR methodologies have met with mixed success. Numerous groups have demonstrated the effectiveness of QSAR within homogeneous sets of molecules *(2)*, but traditional QSAR methodologies are much less effective when applied to datasets containing a great deal of structural variation. Much of this difficulty can be traced to the type of molecular property descriptors used to represent the problem. Commonly used fragment-based descriptors relying on 2D topology of molecules are not highly correlated with most biological responses. In contrast to previous attempts at SAR, our use *(3)* of shape-aware electron-density-based molecular property descriptors has removed many of the limitations brought about by the use of descriptors based on substructure fragments, molecular connectivity indices, or other whole molecule descriptors.

Another reason for the mixed success of past QSAR efforts can be traced to the nature of the underlying modeling problem, which is often quite complex. To meet these challenges, a genetic algorithm for pattern-recognition analysis has been developed *(4,5)* that selects descriptors that create class separation in a plot of the two largest principal components *(6)* of the data while simultaneously searching for features that increase the clustering of the data. The efficacy of this methodology has been evaluated using a structurally diverse database consisting of 331 macrocyclic and nitroaromatic compounds (192 musks and 139 nonmusks).

2. Materials

Compounds used in the database were obtained from literature reports of chemical structure and odor quality *(7–11)*. In **Table 1**, a list of the compounds comprising the database is given. The macrocyclic and nitroaromatic musks are of strong, medium, weak, or unspecified odor intensity; the nonmusks are odorless or have an odor other than musk. Information about odor quality and intensity is contained in the activity label associated with each compound. It should be emphasized that a musk compound labeled as weak, medium, or strong refers only to the change in its odor threshold, not to any change in its odor quality. Structural classes present in the dataset are shown in **Fig. 1**. Natural musks, whose sources include both rare animal and plant species, are

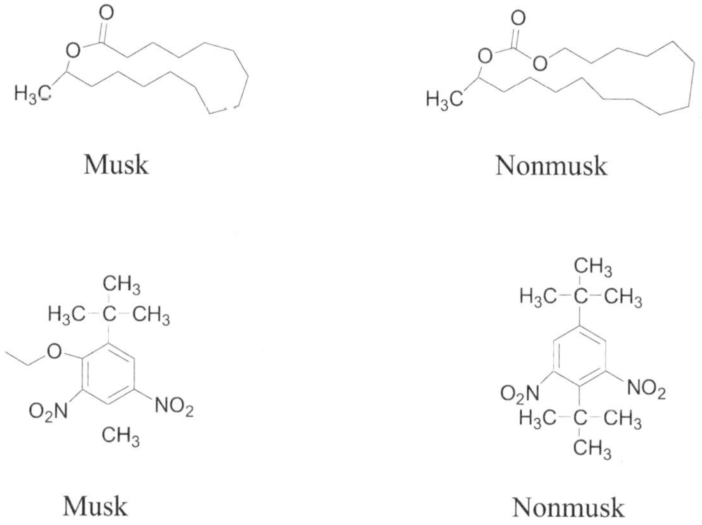

Fig. 1. Two very strong musks and two nonmusks representing the two major structural classes of compounds found in the data set. Reproduced with permission from the American Chemical Society (B. K. Lavine et al. (2003), *Journal of Chemical Information and Computer Sciences* **43,** 1890–1905.)

macrocycles, whereas the first synthetic musks prepared were nitrated derivatives of benzene.

Two-dimensional representations of the compounds were generated by drawing each compound on a graphics terminal using Chembase (Molecular Design Limited), which converted the graphical representation of the structures into molecular connection tables. A three-dimensional molecular model was also generated for each compound in the database using a molecular mechanics model building routine that employed the CHARMM force field contained in the modeling program Quanta (Molecular Simulations). The PEST algorithm *(12)* was then used to generate wavelet, histogram, and hybrid shape/property descriptors from the connection tables and the three-dimensional models. Molecular descriptors were computed individually for each structural group of musks, allowing for easy separation and modeling of the structural classes.

3. Methods

3.1. Electron-Density-Derived Descriptors

To effectively characterize the potential olfactory properties of any molecule, it is necessary to use an appropriate set of molecular descriptors. While

(text continues on page 411)

Table 1
Compounds Comprising the Musk Database[a]

Index	Label	Compound Name
1	MSTR	8-Cyclohexadecanone
2	MSTR	2(1H) Benzocyclododecenone,3,4,5,6,7,8,9,10,11,12,13,14-dodecahydro
3	MSTR	Cyclotetradecone, 4 methyl
4	MWEA	2(1H) Benzocyclododecenone, tetradecahydro-
5	MMED	Cyclopentadecanol
6	MSTR	Cyclopentadecanone, 5-methyl
7	MSTR	4-Cyclopentadecen-1-one
8	MSTR	2-Cyclopentadecen-1-one, 3-methyl
9	MSTR	4-Cyclopentadecen-1-one, (Z)-
10	MMED	17-oxabicyclo [14.1.0] heptadecane
11	MSTR	5-Cyclohexadecen-1-one
12	MMED	Thiacyclopentadecane
13	MMED	Oxacyclotridecan-2-one
14	MMED	Oxacyclotridecan-2-one, 14-methyl-
15	MSTR	Oxacyclotridecan-2-one, 15-methyl-
16	MSTR	Oxacyclotridec-6-en-2-one, (Z)-
17	MSTR	Oxacyclotridecan-2-one, 16-methyl-
18	MSTR	1,5-Dioxacyclopentadecan-2-one
19	MMED	Oxacyclopentadecane-2, 15-Dione
20	MSTR	Cyclopentadecanone, 2-hydroxy-
21	MMED	1,5-Dioxacyclopentadecane-6, 15-Dione
22	MSTR	Oxacyclohexadec-11-en-2-one
23	MSTR	1,3-Dioxacycloheptadec-10-en-2-one
24	MSTR	1,4-Dioxacyclohexadecane-5, 16-dione
25	MOTH	2-Cyclotetradecen-1-one
26	MMUS	3-Cyclotetradecen-1-one
27	MOTH	1-(1-cyclododecen-1-yl)-1-acetyl-1-cyclododecene
28	MOTH	1-Butanone, 1-(1-cyclododecen-1-yl)-1-butyryl-1-cyclododecene
29	MMUS	1-Cyclododecene-1-methanol, .alpha. -methyl-
30	MMUS	Cyclododecanemethanol, alpha. -methyl-
31	MSTR	Cycloheptadecanone
32	MMUS	9-Cycloheptadecen-1-one, (Z)
33	MSTR	Cyclopentadecanone
34	MWEA	Cyclooctadecanone
35	MSTR	Cyclohexadecanone
36	MSTR	Cyclotetradecanone
37	MMUS	1,5-Dioxacyclopentadecan-2,4-dione
38	MMUS	1,4-Dioxacyclotetradecan-2, 3-dione

Table 1 *(continued)*

Index	Label	Compound Name
39	MMUS	1,3-Dioxacyclopentadecan-2-one
40	MMUS	Oxacyclotridecan-2, 13-dione
41	MMUS	Azacycloheptadecane
42	MSTR	Oxacycloheptadecan-2-one
43	MMUS	Oxacycloheptadec-8-en-2-one
44	MSTR	Cyclcopentadecanone, 3-methyl-
45	MWEA	Cyclopentadecanone, 2-methyl-
46	MMUS	Cyclopentadecanone, 4-methyl-
47	MSTR	Oxacyclohexadecan-2-one
48	MMUS	1,3-Dioxacycloheptadecan-2-one
49	MSTR	Oxacyclopentadecan-2-one
50	MMUS	1,3-Dioxacyclohexadecan-2-one
51	MMUS	Oxacyclotetradecan-2-one
52	MMUS	1,4-Dioxacyclopentadecan-2, 3-dione
53	MMUS	1H-Cyclopentacyclododecan-1-one, tetradecahydro
54	MMUS	2(1H) Benzocyclododecenone 4,5,6,7,8,9,10,11,12-dihydro
55	MOTH	Cyclododecapyrimidine, 5, 6, 7, 8, 9,10, 11, 12,13, 14-Decahdyro-N
56	MOTH	Cyclododecan
57	MOTH	Bicyclo [10.1.0] tridecane, 1-methoxy
58	MMUS	Oxacycloletadec-9-en-2-one
59	MMUS	Cyclohexadecanolid
60	MMUS	Ethanone, 1-(2, 5, 5-trimethylcycloheptyl)-
61	MMUS	Oxacyclohexadecane-2, 13, dione
62	MMUS	Oxacyclohexadecane-2, 13, dione, 16, 16, dimethyl
63	MMUS	5-Cyclopentadecen-1-one (Z) and (E)
64	MMUS	Cyclotetradecanon
65	MWEA	Oxacyclopentadecane
66	MWEA	Oxacyclohexadecane
67	MMUS	Thiacyclotetradecane
68	MMUS	Thiacycloheptadecane
69	MMUS	Azacyclotetradecane
70	MMUS	Azacyclotetradecane, 1-methyl-
71	MMUS	Azacyclopentadecane
72	MMUS	Azacyclopentadecane, 1-methyl-
73	MMUS	Azacyclohexadecane
74	MMUS	Azacyclohexadecane, 1-methyl-
75	MMUS	Azacycloheptadecane, 1-methyl-
76	MMUS	Azacyclooctadecane
77	MMUS	Azacyclooctadecane, 1-methyl-

(continued)

Table 1 *(continued)*

Index	Label	Compound Name
78	MMUS	Cyclotridecanone
79	MSTR	Cyclohexadecanone, 3-methyl
80	MMUS	Oxacyclohexadecan-6-one
81	MMUS	1, 3 Dioxacyclotetradecan-2-one
82	MMUS	1, 3 Dioxacycloheptadecane
83	MWEA	Oxacyclooctadecan-2-one
84	MMUS	Cyclopentadecom-1, 2, 3-trione
85	MMED	1,4-Dioxacycloheptadecan-5-one
86	MMED	1,5-Dioxacycloheptadecan-6-one
87	MMUS	1,4-Dioxacyclohexadecane-2, 3-dione
88	MMUS	1,4-Dioxacyclotetradecane-5, 14-dione
89	MMUS	1,4-Dioxacyclopentadecane-5, 15-dione
90	MMUS	1,5-Cyclopentadecanedione
91	MWEA	2H-Benzocyclotridecen-2-one, hexadecahydro
92	MWEA	Cyclononadecanone
93	MMED	1,7-Dioxacycloheptadecan-2-one
94	MWEA	1-Oxa-5-thiacyclohexadecan-2-one
95	MMUS	5-Cyclotetradecen-1-one, (Z)-
96	MMUS	1,4-Dioxacycloheptadecane-5, 17-dione
97	MMUS	Pyridin
98	MMUS	16-Azabicyclo [10.3.1] hexadeca- 1(16),12, 14, triene, 3-methyl-,(.+-.)-
99	MSTR	1,8-Dioxacylcycloheptadecan-9-one
100	MSTR	1,7-Dioxacycloheptadecan-8-one
101	MMED	1,6-Dioxacycloheptadecan-7-one
102	MWEA	1-Oxa-6-thiacycloheptadecan-17-one
103	MWEA	1-Oxa-7-thiacycloheptadecan-18-one
104	MWEA	1-Oxa-5-thiacycloheptadecan-16-one
105	MMUS	1,5-Dioxacyclohexadecan-6-one
106	NOTH	Cyclododecanone
107	NOTH	Bicyclo [7.2.0] undec-s-en-2-ol, 2,6,10,10-tetramethyl
108	NOTH	Bicyclo [7.2.0] undec-5-ene-2-Acetaldehyde, 6,10,10-trimethyl
109	NOTH	Cyclododecan-1, 3,dioxole, 3a alpha, 4,5,6,7,8,9,10,11,12,13,13a beta-dodecahydro-2-methyl
110	NOTH	Cyclododeca-1,2 dioxane, 5, 6, 7, 8, 9, 10, 11,12,13,14-decahydro
111	NOTH	Cyclododeca [b] furan, tetradecahydro
112	NOTH	Cyclododecane, 1-methoxy-2 methyl
113	NOTH	5-cyclododecene-1-methoxy methoxy
114	NOTH	Ketone, methyl, 2,6,10-trimethyl-1 cyclododecen-1yl

Table 1 *(continued)*

Index	Label	Compound Name
115	NOTH	Cyclododecan[c] Furan, 1,3,3a, 4,5,6,7,8,9,10,11,13a-dodecahydro
116	NOTH	Cyclododecyl-1, 5, 9-trimethy, 10-acetyl, 1,8-diene
117	NOTH	Cyclodocecyl-1-ene-1,5,9-trimethyl-5,6-epoxide
118	NOTH	3-Cyclooctene-1-methanol, 7-hydroxy, diformate
119	NOTH	Cyclooctane (methoxy methoxy)
120	NOTH	Cyclooct [e] isobenzofuran, tetradecahydro-3a-methyl
121	NOTH	6-Azulenol, 2, 3, 3A, 4,5,6,7,8-octahydro-1 methyl-4 methylene-7-(1-methylethyl)
122	NOTH	6(1H)-Azulenone, 2,3,3A, 7,8,8A,hexahydro-3A-methyl-1-(1methylethyl)-
123	NOTH	4-Azulenemethanol, decahydro-8-methyl-2-(1-methylethenyl)-acetate
124	NOTH	Cyclononanone
125	NFAI	1,3-Dioxolan-2-one
126	NFAI	1,3-Dioxan-2-one
127	NOTH	1,3-Dioxonan-2-one
128	NOTH	1,3-Dioxecan-2-one
129	NOTH	1,3-Dioxacyloundecan-2-one
130	NOTH	1,3-Dioxacyclotridecan-2-one
131	NOTH	1,3-Dioxepane
132	NOTH	1,3-Dioxocane
133	NOTH	1,3-Dioxonane
134	NOTH	1,3-Dioxacyclododecane
135	NOTH	1,3-Dioxacyclotridecane
136	NOTH	Oxacycloundecan-2-one
137	OLES	2,5-Furandione, dihydro
138	OLES	2H-Pyran-2, 6 (3H)-dione, dihydro
139	NFAI	2, 7-Oxepandedione
140	NOTH	2, 10-Oxecanedione
141	NOTH	Oxacycloundecan-2, 11-dione
142	NOTH	Oxacyclododecane-2, 12-dione
143	OLES	Cyclopentadecan-1, 7-dione
144	OLES	Cyclopentadecan-1, 8-dione
145	NOTH	Cyclodecanone
146	NOTH	Cycloundecanone
147	NOTH	Cyclododeane (1,1-dimethylethoxy)
148	NOTH	Cyclododecane, (methoxy methyl)-
149	NOTH	Cyclododecane, (ethoxymethyl)-

(continued)

Table 1 *(continued)*

Index	Label	Compound Name
150	NOTH	Cyclododecane, [(1-methylethoxy) methyl]-
151	NOTH	Cyclododecane, [2-propenyoxy) methyl]-
152	NOTH	Cyclopentanone
153	NOTH	Cyclohexanone
154	NOTH	Cycloheptanone
155	NOTH	Cyclooctanone
156	OLES	Cycloeicosanone
157	OLES	Cycloheneicosanone
158	NONM	2-cyclopentadecen-1-one
159	NONM	Oxacyclotridecan-2-one, 13-methyl
160	NONM	1,3 dioxacyclooctadec-2-one
161	NONM	Oxacyclotetradecane-2, 14-dione
162	NONM	1,4-Cyclopentadecanedione
163	NONM	1,6-Cyclopentadecanedione
164	NONM	1H-Indene, 2,3-dihydro-1, 1, 2,4,6-pentamethyl-5, 7-dintro
165	NONM	Benzene, 1,3,5-trinitro
166	NONM	Benzene, 2-methyl-1, 3,5-trinitro
167	NONM	Benzene, 1,3,5-trimethyl-2, 4,6-trinitro
168	NONM	Benzene, 2,4,dimethyl, 1,3,5-trinitro
169	NONM	Benzene, 1,3-Bis (1,1-dimethylethyl)-2,4-dinitro
170	NONM	Benzene, 2-methoxy-1, 3-Bis (1-methylethyl)-5-nitro
171	NONM	Benzene, 2-(1,1-dimethylethyl)-1,3,5-trinitro
172	NONM	Benzene, 1,5-Bis (1,1-dimethylethyl)-3, methyl-2, 4-dinitro
173	NONM	Benzene, 2-Methoxy-4-methyl-1-(4-methylpentyl)-3,5-dinitro
174	NONM	Benzene, 1-(1,1-dimethylethyl)-2-methoxy-4 methyl-3-nitro
175	NONM	Benzene, 1,4-Bis (1,1-dimethylethyl)-2-methoxy-3-nitro
176	NONM	Benzene, 1,3-Bis (1,1-dimethylethyl)-2-methoxy-4-methyl-5-nitro
177	NONM	Benzaldehyde, 6-(1,1-dimethylethyl)-2-methoxy-3-nitro
178	NONM	Benzene, 1-(1,1-dimethylethyl)-2methoxy-3, 4,dimethyl-5-nitro
179	NONM	Benzene, 1-(1,1-dimethylethyl)-2,3-dimethoxy-4-nitro
180	NONM	Benzoic acid, 2-(1,1-dimethylethyl)-4,6-dimethyl-3, 5-dinitro
181	NONM	Benzene, 2 butyl-4-methyl-1, 3,5-trinitro
182	NONM	Benzene, 2 methyl-4 (3-methylbutyl)-1,3,5-trinitro
183	NONM	Benzaldehyde, 2, 6 - Bis (1,1-dimethylethyl)-3-methoxy-5-nitro
184	NONM	Benzene, 1-bromo-4 butyl-2-methyl-3, 5-dinitro
185	NONM	Benzamine, 4-(1,1-dimethylethyl)-2,6-dimethyl, 3-5, dinitro
186	NONM	Benzene, 1-(1,1-dimethylethyl)-4-methoxy-3-methyl-2, 5,6-trinitro
187	NONM	Benzene, 1,3-dibromo-4- (1,1-dimethylethyl)-2,6-dimethyl, 5-nitro

Table 1 *(continued)*

Index	Label	Compound Name
188	NONM	Benzaldehyde, 4-(1,1-dimethylethyl)-3-nitro
189	NONM	Benzaldehyde, 4-(1,1-dimethylethyl)-3,5-dinitro
190	NONM	Benzene, 2-(1,1-dimethylethyl)-4,5 dimethyl-1, 3-dinitro
191	NONM	Benzoic acid, 4-(1,1-dimethylethyl)-2methyl 3,5-dinitro
192	NONM	Benzene, 1(1,1-dimethylethyl)-3,4-dimethyl-6- (1methylethyl)-2,5 dinitro
193	NONM	Benzene, 1(1,1-dimethylethyl)-4 methoxy-3, 5-dimethyl-2-nitro
194	NONM	Benzene, 2 methoxy-1, 3 dimethyl-4, 5 dinitro
195	NONM	Benzene, 1(1,1-dimethylethyl)-3,5-dimethyl-2, 4-dinitro-6[Phenylmethyl]sulfonyl
196	NONM	Benzamine, 2(1,1-dimethylethyl)-4,6-dimethyl-3, 5-dinitro
197	NONM	Benzene, 1(1,1-dimethylethyl)-3 methoxy-2, 4-dinitro
198	NONM	Methanone, [2-(1,1-dimethylethyl)-4,6-dimethyl-3, 5-dinitrophenyl] Phenyl-
199	NONM	Benzene, 1-(1,1-dimethylethyl)-3,5-dimethyl-2, 6-dinitro-4 [Phenylmethyl] sulfonyl
200	NONM	Benzene, 2-ethyl-5-isooctyl-4-methoxy-1, 3-dinitro
201	NONM	Benzene, 1-isoheptyl-2-methoxy-4-methyl-3, 5-dinitro
202	NONM	Benzene, 1-isooctyl-2-methoxy-4-methyl-3, 5-dinitro
203	NONM	Ethanone, 1- [3-(1,1-dimethylethyl)-2-methoxy-5-nitrophenyl
204	NOTH	Benzene, 1,3-dibromo-2-isopropyl-5-methoxy-4-nitro
205	OLES	Benzene, 1, 3-BIS- (1,1-dimethylethyl)-5-nitro
206	OLES	Benzaldehyde, 5 (1,1-dimethylethyl)-2-methoxy-3-nitro
207	OLES	Benzene, 1, 5-BIS- (1,1-dimethylethyl)-2 methoxy-4 methyl 3-nitro
208	OLES	Ethanone, 1- [3-(1,1-dimethylethyl)-4-methoxy-5-nitrophenyl
209	OLES	Benzaldehyde, 2 (1,1-dimethylethyl)-4-methoxy-5-nitro
210	OLES	Benzene, 1, 4-BIS- (1,1-dimethylethyl)-2 methoxy-5-nitro
211	OLES	Benzene, 1-(1, 1-dimethylethyl)-2, 5-dimethoxy-4-nitro
212	OLES	Benzene, 1-(1, 1-dimethylethyl)-2-methoxy-4 methyl-5-nitro
213	NOTH	Benzaldehyde, 5- (1,1-dimethylethyl)-2-methyl-3-nitro
214	OLES	Benzaldehyde, 2- (1,1-dimethylethyl)-4,5,6-trimethyl-3-nitro
215	OLES	Benzene, 5-(1, 1-dimethylethyl)-2-methoxy-1, 3-dinitro
216	OLES	Benzene, 1-(1, 1-dimethylethyl)-4-methoxy-2-methyl 3-5-dinitro
217	OLES	Benzene, 2-bromo-5- (1, 1-dimethylethyl)-4-methoxy-1, 3-dinitro
218	OLES	Benzene, 2-butoxy-1- (1, 1-dimethylethyl)-4-methyl-3, 5-dinitro
219	OLES	Benzene, 2-methoxy-4 methyl-1- (1-methylpropyl)-3,5-dinitro
220	OLES	Benzene, 2-methoxy-4 methyl-1- (2-methylpropyl)-3,5-dinitro
221	OLES	Benzene, 2-(1,1-dimethylethyl)-4-methoxy-5-methyl-1, 3-dinitro

(continued)

Lavine et al.

Table 1 *(continued)*

Index	Label	Compound Name
222	OLES	Benzene, 1-(1,1-dimethylethyl)-5-methoxy-2, 4-dintro
223	OLES	Benzaldehyde, 2-(1,1-dimethylethyl)-4-methoxy-3, 5-dinitro
224	OLES	Phenol, 4-(1,1dimethylethyl)-2,6-diethyl-3, 5-dinitro
225	OLES	Benzene, 1-(1,1-dimethylethyl)-4-methoxy-3, 5-dimethyl-2, 6-dinitro
226	OLES	Benzene, 5-(1,1-dimethylethyl)-2-methyl-1, 3-dintro
227	OLES	Benzene, 2,5-Bis- (1,1-dimethylethyl)-1,3-dinitro
228	OLES	Benzene, 5-(1,1-dimethylpropyl)-2-methyl-1, 3-dintro
229	OLES	Benzene, 1-(1,1-dimethylethyl)-3,5-diethyl-2, 4,6-trinitro
230	OLES	Benzofuran, 2, 3, -dihydro-3, 3,6-trimethyl-5, 7-dinitro
231	OLES	Benzene, 1, 4-Bis- (1,1-dimethylethyl)-2-methoxy-3, 5-dinitro
232	OLES	Benzenemethanol, 4 - (1,1-dimethylethyl)-2, 6-dimethyl -3, 5-dinitro
233	OLES	1H-Indene, 6-(1,1-dimethylethyl)-2, 3 dihydro-4, 5,7-trinitro
234	OLES	Benzaldehyde, 2, 4-Bis- (1,1-dimethylethyl)-5-methoxy-3-nitro
235	NONM	Benzene, 2-(1,1-dimcthylethyl)-4-methoxy-1, 3, 5-trinitro
236	NONM	Benzene, 2-methoxy-1- (2-methylpropyl)-3,5 dinitro-4-(trifluoromethyl)
237	NONM	Benzene, 1-(1,1-dimethylbutyl)-2-methoxy-4-methyl-3-5-dinitro
238	NONM	Benzene, 1-(1,1-dimethylpentyl)-2-methoxy-4-methyl-3-5-dinitro
239	NONM	Benzene, 2-methoxy-1, 5-Bis (1methylethyl)-3-nitro
240	NONM	Benzene, 1-(1,1-dimethylpentyl)-2-methoxy-4, 5-dimethyl-3-nitro
241	NONM	Benzenemethanol, 4 - (1,1-dimethylethyl)-2, 6-dimethyl -3, 5-dinitro-, acetate (ester)
242	NONM	Benzene, 1-(1,1-dimethylethyl)-3, 4, 5-trimethyl-2-nitro
243	NONM	Benzene, 1-(1,1-dimethylethyl)-2, 3, 4, 5-tetramethyl-6-nitro
244	NONM	1H-Indene, 2, 3 -dihydro-1, 1,4,6-tetramethyl 5,7-dinitro
245	NONM	1H-Indene, 6-ethyl-2, 3 dihydro-1, 1-dimethyl 5,7-dinitro
246	MMUS	Benzene, 1-bromo-4 (1,1-dimethylethyl)-2,6-dimethyl-3, 5-dinitro
247	MSTR	Benzene, 1-azido-4 (1,1-dimethylethyl)-2,6-dimethyl-3, 5-dinitro
248	MSTR	Ethanone, 1-[2(1,1-dimethylethyl)-4,6-dimethyl-3, 5-dinitrophenyl]
249	MMUS	Benzaldehyde, 2-(1,1-dimethylethyl)-4,6-dimethyl-3, 5-dinitro
250	MMUS	Benzonitrile, 4-(1,1-dimethylethyl)-2, 6-dimethyl-3, 5-dinitro
251	MMUS	Benzene, 1-(1, 1-dimethylethyl)-2-fluoro-3, 5-dimethyl-2, 6-dinitro
252	MMUS	Benzene, 1-(1, 1-dimethylethyl)-4-fluoro-3, 5-dimethyl-2, 6-dinitro

Table 1 *(continued)*

Index	Label	Compound Name
253	MMUS	Ethanone, 1-(4-methoxy-2-methyl -3, 5-dinitrophenyl)
254	MMUS	Ethanone, 1-[4(1,1-dimethylethyl)-2,3,6-trimethyl-5-nitrophenyl]
255	MSTR	Benzene, 1-(1,1-dimethylethyl)-3,5-dimethyl-2, 4,6-trinitro
256	MMUS	Benzene, 1-bromo-3- (1,1-dimethylethyl)-5-methyl-2, 4, 6-trinitro
257	MMUS	Benzene, 2-(1,1-dimethylethyl)-4-methyl-1, 3,5-trinitro
258	MMUS	Benzene, 1-chloro-3- (1,1-dimethylethyl)-5-methyl-2, 4, 6-trinitro
259	MWEA	Benzene, 1, 3-Bis (1,1-dimethylethyl)-5-methyl-2, 4, 6-trinitro
260	MMUS	Benzene, 3-(1,1-dimethylethyl)-1-fluoro-5-methyl-2, 4, 6-trinitro
261	MWEA	Benzene, 2-hexyl-4-methyl-1, 3, 5- trinitro
262	MMUS	Benzene, 2-methyl-4- (1-methylethyl)-1, 3, 5-trinitro
263	MSTR	Benzene, 1-(1,1-dimethylethyl)-2-ethoxy-3, 5-dinitro
264	MSTR	Benzene, 1-(1,1-dimethylethyl)-2-ethoxy-4 ethyl 3, 5-dinitro
265	MSTR	Benzene, 1-(1,1-dimethylpropyl)-4 ethyl-2-methoxy- 3, 5-dinitro
266	MSTR	Benzene, 1, 3-Bis (1,1-dimethylethyl)-4-methoxy-6-methyl-2, 5-dinitro
267	MSTR	1H-Indene, 2-ethyl, 2, 3 -dihydro-1, 1,3, 3, 5-pentamethyl 4, 6-dinitro
268	MSTR	Silane, (3, 5-dimethyl-2, 4, 6-trinitrophenyl) trimethyl-
269	MMUS	Benzene, 1, 3-Bis (1,1-dimethylethyl)-2-methoxy-5-nitro
270	MMUS	Benzene, 1-(1,1-dimethylethyl)-2-methoxy-3-nitro
271	MMUS	Benzene, 2-methoxy-4-methyl-1, 3,5-trinitro
272	MMUS	Benzaldehyde, 3-(1,1-dimethylethyl)-2-methoxy-5-nitro
273	MMUS	Benzene, 2-bromo-4- (1,1-dimethylethyl)-1,3, 5-trinitro
274	MMUS	Benzene, 1-(1,1-dimethylethyl)-2, 4-dimethoxy-5, 6-dimethyl-3-nitro
275	MMUS	Benzene, 2-methyl-4- (2-methylpropyl)-1,3,5-trinitro
276	MMUS	Benzene, 5-(1,1-dimethylethyl)-2-ethyl-1, 3-dinitro-
277	MMUS	Ethanone, 1-(2-butyl-3-methyl-4, 6-dinitrophenyl)-
278	MMUS	Benzene, 1-(1,1-dimethylethyl)-2-methoxy-3, 5-dimethyl-4, 6-dinitro
279	MMUS	Benzene, 2-(1,1-dimethylpropyl)-4-methyl-3- (1-methylethyl)-1,5-dinitro
280	MMUS	Benzene, 1 (1,1-dimethylethyl)-3-methyl-2, 4-dinitro
281	MMUS	Benzoyl chloride, 6-(1,1-dimethylethyl)-3-methyl-2, 4-dinitro-
282	MMUS	Benzene, 1, 3-dibromo-2- (1,1-dimethylethyl)-5-methoxy-4-nitro
283	MMUS	Benzonitrile, 2-(1,1-dimethylethyl)-4, 5-dimethyl-3-nitro-
284	MMUS	Benzene, 1-(1,1-dimethylethyl)-3-methoxy-5-methyl-2, 4, 6-trinitro

(continued)

Table 1 *(continued)*

Index	Label	Compound Name
285	MMUS	Benzene, 2-(1,1-dimethylethyl)-4-methyl-3- (1-methylethyl) 1, 5-dinitro
286	MMUS	Benzene, 1-(1, 1-dimethylpropyl)-2, 4-dimethoxy-3, 5-dinitro-
287	MWEA	Benzene, 2, 4-Bis- (1,1-dimethylethyl)-1-nitro
288	MSTR	Ethanone, 1-[4-(1,1-dimethylpropyl)-2,6-dimethyl-3, 5-dinitrophenyl]
289	MSTR	Benzene, 1-(1,1-dimethylpropyl)-3, 4, 5-trimethyl-2,6-dinitro-
290	MMUS	Benzene, 1-(1,1-dimethylethyl)-2-methoxy-3,5-dinitro-
291	MMUS	Benzene, 4-(1, 1-dimethylethyl)-6-methyl-1, 3-dinitro
292	MSTR	Benzene, 6-(1,1-dimethylethyl)-3-ethyl-1-methoxy-2, 4-dinitro
293	MWEA	Benzene, 6-(1,1-dimethylethyl)-1-methoxy-3- (1-methylethyl)-2-4-dinitro-
294	MSTR	Benzene, 6-(1,1-dimethylethyl)-1-ethoxy-3-methyl-2, 4-dinitro-
295	MWEA	Benzene, 6-(1,1-dimethylethyl)-3-methyl-1- (1-methyl ethoxy)-2, 4-dinitro-
296	MMUS	Benzaldehyde, 4-(1,1-dimethylethyl)-2,6-dimethyl-3, 5-dinitro-
297	MMED	Benzoic acid, 2-(1,1-dimethylethyl)-4,6-dimethyl-3, 5-dinitro-methyl ester
298	MWEA	Benzene, 5-(1,1-dimethylpropyl)-2-ethyl-1, 3-dinitro-
299	MWEA	Benzene, 2-ethyl-1, 3-dinitro-
300	MSTR	Benzene, 2-(1,1-dimethylpropyl)-4,6-dimethyl-1, 3, 5-trinitro-
301	MSTR	1H-Indene, 3-ethyl, 2, 3 -dihydro-1, 1,3, 5-tetramethyl 4, 6-dinitro .
302	MMUS	Naphthalene, 1,2,3,4- tetrahydro-1,1,4,4-tetramethyl-6-(1methylethyl)-5,7-dinitro
303	MMUS	Naphthalene, 6-tert-butyl-1,2,3,4- tetrahydro-1,1,4, 4-tetramethyl-5,7-dinitro
304	MMUS	Naphthalene,1,2,3,4-tetrahydro-7-isopropyl-1,1,2,4, 4-pentamethyl-6,8-dinitro
305	MMUS	Naphthalene,1,2,3,4-tetrahydro 1,1,4-trimethyl-6, 8-dinitro
306	MWEA	1-propanone,1-[2-(1,1-dimethylethyl)-4,6-dimethyl-3, 5-dinitrophenyl]-
307	MMUS	Benzene,1,3-dibromo-5-(1,1-dimethylethyl)-2-methoxy-6-methyl-2-nitro
308	MSTR	1H-Indene, 2, 3 -dihydro-1, 1,3, 3, 5-pentamethyl 4,6-dinitro
309	MSTR	Benzene,2-(1,1-dimethylethyl)-4,5,6-trimethyl-1,3-dinitro-
310	MSTR	Ethanone, 1-[4-(1,1-dimethylethyl)-2,6-dimethyl-3, 5-dinitrophenyl]-
311	MMUS	Benzene, 1-(1,1-dimethylethyl)-2-methoxy-4-methyl-3,5-dinitro-
312	MMUS	Ethanone, 1-[6-(1,1-dimethylethyl)-3-ethyl-2,4-dinitrophenyl]-

Table 1 *(continued)*

Index	Label	Compound Name
313	MMUS	Benzene, 1-bromo-6-(1,1-dimethylethyl)-3-methoxy-2,4-dinitro-
314	MMUS	Benzaldehyde, 5-(1,1-dimethylethyl)-4-methoxy-3-nitro-
315	MMUS	Benzaldehyde, 5-(1,1-dimethylethyl)-4-ethoxy-3-nitro-
316	MWEA	Benzene,4,6-Bis- (1,1-dimethylethyl)-1-methoxy-2-nitro
317	MSTR	Benzene,6-(1,1-dimethylethyl)-1,3-dimethoxy-2,4-dinitro
318	MSTR	Benzene,6-(1,1-dimethylpropyl)-1-methoxy-3-methyl-2,4-dinitro-
319	MMUS	Benzonitrile,2-(1,1-dimethylethyl)-4,6-dimethyl-3,5-dinitro-
320	MMUS	Benzene,1-bromo-2-(1,1-dimethylethyl)-4,6-dimethyl-3,5-dinitro
321	MWEA	Benzoyl chloride, 2-(1,1-dimethylethyl)-4,6-dimethyl-3,5-dinitro-
322	MWEA	Benzoyl chloride, 4-(1,1-dimethylethyl)-2,6-dimethyl-3,5-dinitro-
323	MWEA	Benzoic acid, 4-(1,1-dimethylethyl)-2,6-dimethyl-3,5-dinitro,-methylester
324	MSTR	Benzene,2-(1,1-dimethylethyl)-4-ethyl-6-methyl-1,3,5-trinitro
325	MMUS	1H-Indene, 2, 3 -dihydro-1, 1,2, 3, 3, 5-hexamethyl 4,6-dinitro
326	MMUS	1H-Indene, 5-ethyl- 2, 3-dihydro-1, 1, 3, 3 -tetramethyl 4,6-dinitro
327	MMUS	1H-Inden-5-ol, 2-ethyl- 2, 3-dihydro-1, 1, 3, 3 -tetramethyl 4,6-dinitro
328	MMUS	1H-Indene, 5-ethyl- 2, 3-dihydro-1, 1, 2, 3, 3 -pentamethyl 4,6-dinitro
329	MMUS	1H-Indene, 3-ethyl- 2, 3-dihydro-1, 1, 2, 3, 3 -pentamethyl 4,6-dinitro
330	MWEA	Benzene, 1, 5-Bis- (1,1-dimethylethyl)-3-methyl-2-nitro-
331	NONM	Benzenesulfonic acid, 4-butyl-2-methyl-3, 5-dinitro

[a]MSTR, strong musk; MMED, medium musk; MWEA, weak musk; MMUS, musk of unspecified odor strength; MOTH, musk that has a secondary odor note that is not musk; OLES, odorless; NOTH, specified odor other than musk; NONM, nonmusk. Table 1 is reproduced with permission from the American Chemical Society (B. K. Lavine et al. (2003), *Journal of Chemical Information and Computer Sciences*, **43**, 1890–1905.)

many types of descriptors exist in the literature, the present work emphasizes the use of electron-density-derived descriptors. The underlying methodology relies on the hypothesis that a causative relationship exists between observed odor properties and the distribution of certain molecular electronic properties as sampled on molecular van der Waals surfaces. An additional hypothesis of PEST shape/property hybrid descriptor validation is that the spatial arrangement of surface electronic properties contains pertinent chemical information. Both of these hypotheses have been previously validated *(13)* in studies involving biological and nonbiological molecular behavior.

A library of integrated atomic basins as defined by AIM theory *(14)* is used to rapidly construct representations of molecular electron density distributions and van der Waals electronic surface properties. Ten electronic surface properties obtained from these reconstructions have been identified as containing useful information. The distribution of these electronic properties on molecular surfaces may be characterized in several ways. One way involves the recording of the distribution of these properties as surface histograms that quantify the molecular surface area with specific ranges of each property value. In addition to these histogram descriptors, extrema, average values, and standard deviations of the property distributions (in some cases with separate σ values for positive and negative portions of the range) were included in the descriptor set. Surface property distributions may also be characterized by the use of discrete wavelet transforms. Wavelet coefficient descriptors (WCDs) produced through these reconstructions are also additive at the atomic level and convey more chemical property information as a result of the data compression methods used to generate them. Only eight scale and eight detail coefficients are able to represent each molecular surface property distribution with a high degree of fidelity. The lower set of scalar coefficients approximate the shape of the property distribution, whereas values for from the detail set may be associated with deviations from the scalar shape.

The surface property distributions can also be subjected to Zauhar "Shape Signature" ray tracing approach *(15)* to generate shape descriptors. A ray is initialized with a random location and direction within the molecular surface and reflected throughout inside the electron density isosurface until the molecular surface is adequately sampled. Molecular shape information is obtained by recording the ray path information including segment lengths, reflection angles, and property values at each point of incidence. Path information (segment length and point of incidence values) can be summarized into 2D histograms to obtain a surface shape profile. For a single electronic property, a 2D histogram having the distribution of distance (x axis) versus the associated property value (y axis) can give a characteristic distribution (z axis) based on the overall shape and property value of the molecule. Such a 2D-histogram can be created for every surface property. Each bin of the two-dimensional histogram becomes a hybrid/shape property descriptor.

3.2. Pattern-Recognition Analysis

For pattern-recognition analysis, each compound was initially represented by 896 computer-generated molecular descriptors. Before a descriptor could

Table 2
Musk Dataset

Training Set (Index Numbers/Table 1): 1–12, 14–30, 32–61, 63–74, 77, 78, 80-88, 90–149, 151–162, 164, 166–175, 178–193, 195–220, 222–232, 234–256, 258 287, 289–307, 309–322, 324–331
Prediction Set (Index Numbers/Table 1): 13, 31, 62, 75, 76, 79, 89, 150, 163, 165, 176, 177, 194, 221, 233, 257, 288, 308, 323

---

be entered into the study, it was checked to see if it had the same value for every compound in the dataset. Descriptors were eliminated from the study if they were invariant. Prior to pattern-recognition analysis, the descriptors were autoscaled to zero mean and unit standard deviation to alleviate any problems arising from differences in scaling.

The musk database was divided into a training set of 312 compounds and a prediction set of 19 compounds (*see* **Table 2**). Compounds in the prediction set were randomly chosen. Discriminating relationships uncovered in the training set could be validated using the compounds from the prediction set.

A genetic algorithm (GA) for pattern-recognition analysis was used to identify molecular descriptors from which discriminating relationships could be found. The pattern-recognition GA selected descriptors that increase clustering while simultaneously searching for descriptors that optimize the separation of the classes (musk versus nonmusk) in a plot of the two or three largest principal components of the data. Because principal components maximize variance, the bulk of the information encoded by these features will be about differences between classes in the dataset. The idea is demonstrated in **Fig. 2**, which shows a plot of the two largest principal components of a dataset prior to feature selection. The dataset consisted of 30 compounds distributed between three classes (weak, medium, and strong odor activity). Each compound is characterized by 10 molecular descriptors. However, only four of these measurements contain information about the QSAR. When a principal component map of the data is developed using only these four measurements, sample clustering on the basis of class is evident.

There are many advantages in using this approach to feature selection. First, chance classification is not a serious problem because the bulk of the variance or information content of the feature subset selected is about the classification problem of interest. Second, features that contain discriminatory information about a particular classification problem are usually correlated, which is why feature selection methods using principal component analysis or other variance-based methods are generally preferred. Third, the principal component plot

Before Feature Selection

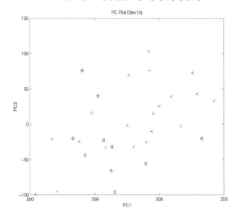

Feature Selection

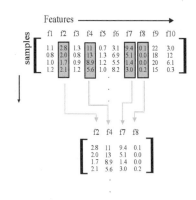

After Feature Selection

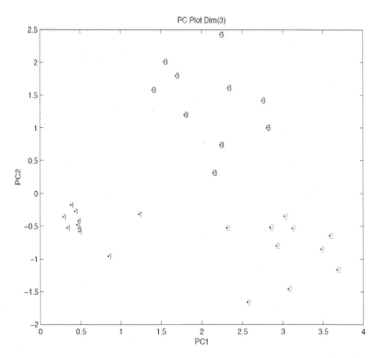

Fig. 2. A plot of the two largest principal components developed from all of the features in the dataset does not show class separation. When principal components are developed from the features that contain information about the classes, sample clustering on the basis of class is evident in a principal component plot of the data.

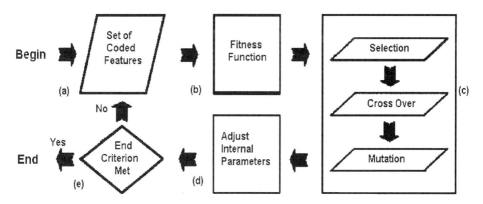

Fig. 3. Block diagram of the pattern-recognition GA.

functions as an embedded information filter. Feature sets are selected based on their principal component plots. A good principal component plot can only be generated using features that maximize group differences. Hence, principal component analysis limits our search to these types of feature subsets, significantly reducing the size of the search space.

To perform this search, it was necessary to use a genetic algorithm *(16–18)*, which employs a survival of the fittest approach. Genetic algorithms exploit knowledge contained in a population of solutions to generate new and better solutions while simultaneously using random choice as a tool to guide a highly exploitive search of the data. Genetic algorithms do not make any assumptions about the geometry of the response surface beyond the fitness of a potential solution to the optimization problem. Discontinuities or singularities, which often rule out the use of derivative-based methods, do not pose a problem for genetic algorithms because many points in different regions of the search space are simultaneously investigated while searching for the best solution. Therefore, results are more robust in terms of the starting location than so-called hill-climbing techniques. The genetic algorithm's search of the solution space is efficient, and the computational environment offered by a genetic algorithm can be readily adjusted to match a particular application. Genetic algorithms are best suited to problems whose underlying optimization function is unknown, poorly understood, exceedingly complex, or error prone, or some combination thereof such as feature selection.

A block diagram of our pattern recognition GA is shown in **Fig. 3**. Selected feature subsets are coded as binary strings called chromosomes. Each chromosome describes a unique set of features. A particular feature is present in a chromosome or binary string if the corresponding bit in the string is set to 1. The length of each chromosome is equal to the number of features in the data set. The number of chromosomes in the initial population is ϕ, which is usually set at 50 or 100. The chromosomes or binary strings comprising the initial population (the population at generation 0) are generated at random to minimize potential bias.

The fitness function of the pattern recognition GA scores the principal component plots and thereby identifies a set of features that optimize the separation of the classes in a plot of the two or three largest principal components of the data. To facilitate the tracking and scoring of the principal component plots, class and sample weights, which are an integral part of the fitness function, are computed:

$$CW(c) = 100 \frac{CW(c)}{\sum_{c} CW(c)} \tag{1}$$

$$SW(s) = CW(c) \frac{SW(s)}{\sum_{s \in c} SW(s)} \tag{2}$$

$CW(c)$ is the weight of class c (with c varying from 1 to the total number of classes in the data set). $SWc(s)$ is the weight of sample s in class c. The class weights sum to 100, and the sample weights for the objects comprising a particular class sum to a value equal to the weight of the class in question.

Each principal component plot generated for each feature subset after it has been extracted from its chromosome is scored using the K-nearest-neighbor classification algorithm *(19)*. For a given data point, Euclidean distances are computed between it and every other point in the principal component plot. These distances are arranged from smallest to largest. A poll is taken of the point's K_c nearest neighbors. For the most rigorous classification, K_c equals the number of samples in the class to which the point belongs. Thus, K_c usually has a different value for each class. The number of K_c nearest neighbors with the same class label as the sample point in question, the so-called sample hit count, $SHC(s)$, is computed as $[0 \leq SHC(s) \leq K_c]$ for each sample. It is then a simple matter to score a principal component plot (*see* **Eq. 3**). First, the contribution to the overall fitness by each sample in class 1 is computed, with the scores of the samples comprising the class summed to yield the contribution by this class to the overall fitness. This same calculation is repeated for classes 2, 3, etc., with the scores from each class summed to yield the overall fitness, $F(d)$.

$$F(d) = \sum_{c} \sum_{s \in c} \frac{1}{K_c} \times SHC(s) \times SW(s) \tag{3}$$

To understand scoring, consider a dataset with two classes, which have been assigned equal weights. Class 1 has 10 samples, and class 2 has 20 samples. For uniformly distributed sample weights, class 1 samples will have a weight of 5 and class 2 samples will have a weight of 2.5, since each class has a weight of 50 and the sample weights in each class are uniformly distributed. Suppose a sample in class 1 has, as its nearest neighbors, seven class 1 samples in a principal component plot developed from a particular feature subset. Hence, $SHC(s)/K_c = 7/10$, and the contribution of the sample to the fitness function for the particular feature subset equals 0.7×5 or 3.5. Multiplying SHC/K_c by $SW(s)$ for each sample and summing up the corresponding product for the 30 samples in the dataset yields the value of the fitness function for this particular feature subset.

Selection, crossover, and mutation operators are applied to the chromosomes. Fit strings are retained and selected for breeding, a process called selection, which is the first step toward population reorganization. The fit feature subsets are then broken up, swapped, and recombined, thus creating new feature subsets, which are introduced into the population of potential solutions. This process is called crossover. In this study, the selection and crossover operators are implemented by ordering the population of strings, i.e., potential solutions, from best to worst, while simultaneously generating a copy of the same population and randomizing the order of the strings in this copy with respect to their fitness. A fraction of the population is then selected as per the selection pressure, which is set at 0.5. The top half of the ordered population is mated with strings from the top half of the random population, guaranteeing the best 50% are selected for reproduction, while every string in the randomized copy has a uniform chance of being selected. This is due to the randomized selection criterion imposed on strings from this population. If a purely biased selection criterion were used to select strings, only a small region of the search space would be explored. Within a few generations, the population would consist of only copies of the best strings in the initial population.

For each pair of strings selected for mating, two new strings are generated using three-point crossover. A mutation operator is then applied to the new strings. The mutation probability of the operator is usually set at 0.01, so 1% of the feature subsets are selected at random for mutation. A chromosome marked for mutation has a single random bit flipped, which allows the GA to explore other regions of the parameter space. The resulting population of strings, both the parents and children, are sorted by fitness, with the top ϕ strings retained for the next generation. Because the selection criterion used for reproduction exhibits bias for the higher-ranking strings, the new population is expected to perform better on average than its predecessor. The reproductive operators used, however, also ensure a significant degree of diversity in the population, because the crossover points of each chromosome pair are selected at random.

The fitness function of the GA is able to focus on those samples and classes that are difficult to classify by boosting their weights over successive generations. Boosting the weights is referred to as adjusting the internal parameters in the block diagram of the genetic algorithm shown in the previous section. In order to boost, it is necessary to compute both the sample-hit rate (SHR), which is the mean value of SHC/K_c over all feature subsets produced in a particular generation (*see* **Eq. 4**), and the class-hit rate (CHR), which is the mean sample hit rate of all samples in a class (*see* **Eq. 5**):

$$SHR(s) = \frac{1}{\phi} \sum_{i=1}^{\phi} \frac{SHC_i(s)}{K_c} \tag{4}$$

$$CHR_g(c) = AVG(SHR_g(s) : \forall_{sec}) \tag{5}$$

In **Eq. 4**, ϕ is the number of chromosomes in the population, and AVG in **Eq. 5** refers to the average or mean value. During each generation, class and sample weights are adjusted by a perceptron (*see* **Eqs. 6** and **7**) with the momentum, P, set by the user ($g + 1$ refers to the current generation, whereas g is the previous generation). Classes with a lower class hit rate and samples with a lower sample hit rate are boosted more heavily than those classes or samples that score well:

$$CW_{g+1}(s) = CW_g(s) + P(1 - CHR_g(s)) \tag{6}$$

$$SW_{g+1}(s) = SW_g(s) + P(1 - SHR_g(s)) \tag{7}$$

The changes in the class weights are monitored throughout the run. If the average change in the class weights is greater than some tolerance, the genetic algorithm is said to be learning its optimal class weights. Once this tolerance has been reached, the class weights become fixed, and the sample weights in each class become uniformly distributed according to their class weight. This initiates the second stage. The momentum, which controls the rate at which the sample weights are changed, is initially assigned a value of 0.8 while the genetic algorithm is learning the class weights, but the momentum is adjusted to 0.4 once the class weights become fixed. These values have been chosen in part because they facilitate learning by the genetic algorithm but do not cause a particular sample or class to dominate the calculation, which would result in the other samples or classes not contributing to the scoring by the fitness function.

Boosting is crucial for the successful operation of the pattern-recognition GA because it modifies the fitness landscape by adjusting the values of the class and sample weights. This helps to minimize the problem of convergence to a local optimum. Hence, the fitness function of the GA is changing as the population is evolving toward a solution using information from the population to guide these changes.

During each generation, class and sample weights are updated using the class and sample hit rates from the previous generation. Evaluation, reproduction, and boosting of potential solutions are repeated until a specified number of generations are executed or a feasible solution is found.

4. Joint Study—Nitroaromatic and Macrocyclic Musks

The first step in this study was to apply principal component analysis to the data. Each principal component is a linear combination of the original molecular descriptors. Using this procedure is analogous to finding a new coordinate system that is better at conveying information present in the data than axes defined by the original measurement variables. The coordinate system is linked to variance. Often, only two or three principal components are necessary to explain all the information present in a dataset if there are a large number of interrelated measurement variables. Using principal component analysis, dimensionality reduction, classification of samples, and identification of clusters in high-dimensional data are possible.

Figure 4 shows a principal component plot of the 871 molecular descriptors and 312 compounds. The 1's are the macrocyclic nonmusks, 2's are the aromatic nitro nonmusks, 3's are the macrocyclic musks, and the 4's are aromatic nitro musks. It is evident from this plot that most of the information captured by the two largest principal components is about chemical structure, not odor quality because the macrocycles are well separated from the nitroaromatics in the first principal component. To identify molecular descriptors correlated with musk odor quality, it was necessary to use the pattern-recognition GA, which identified features by sampling key feature subsets, scoring their principal component plots, and tracking classes and/or samples that were most difficult to classify. The boosting routine used this information to steer the population to an optimal solution. After 100 generations, the pattern-recognition GA identified 15 molecular descriptors whose principal component plot (*see* **Fig. 5**) showed clustering of the compounds on the basis of odor quality.

A prediction set of 19 compounds (*see* **Table 2**) was used to assess the predictive ability of the 15 molecular descriptors identified by the pattern recognition GA. We chose to map the 19 compounds directly onto the principal component plot defined by the 312 compounds and 15 descriptors. **Figure 5** shows the prediction set samples projected onto the principal component map. Each projected compound lies in a region of the map with compounds that bare the same class label. Evidently, the pattern-recognition GA can identify molecular descriptors that are correlated to musk odor quality.

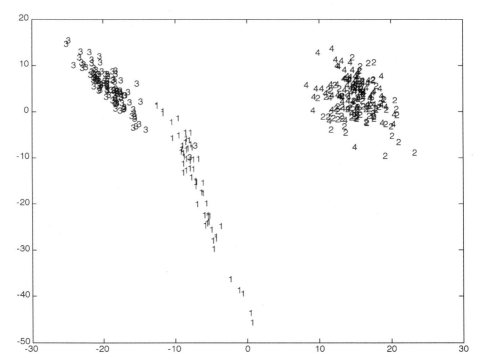

Fig. 4. A plot of the two largest principal components of the 312 compounds and the 871 molecular descriptors comprising the training set. 1 = macrocyclic nonmusk, 2 = aromatic nitro nonmusks, 3 = macrocyclic musks, and 4 = aromatic nitro musks. The plane defined by the two largest principal components accounts for 39% of the total cumulative variance.

Molecular descriptors that were identified by the pattern-recognition GA are listed in **Table 3**. Most of the descriptors identified by the pattern-recognition GA convey information about intermolecular interactions, which suggests their importance in defining musk odor quality. DGNH6 represents the rate of change of the G kinetic energy density normal to and away from the surface of the molecule. DKNW6, DKNW7, and DKNW16 are wavelet descriptors that describe the same basic values. All three descriptors are correlated to weak bonding interactions and probably describe some facet of the interaction between the musk and the receptor. PIPAVGP, PIPW15, and PIPB04 are descriptors that convey information about the local ionization potential of the molecule. BNPW18 and BNPB31 are so-called bare nuclear potential descriptors that probably describe interactions involving polar and hydrogen bonding. EPB03 and EPB43 are shape descriptors derived from ray traces of the molecule's electrostatic surface potential. GW15 and KW15, which are wavelet descriptors derived from the G and K

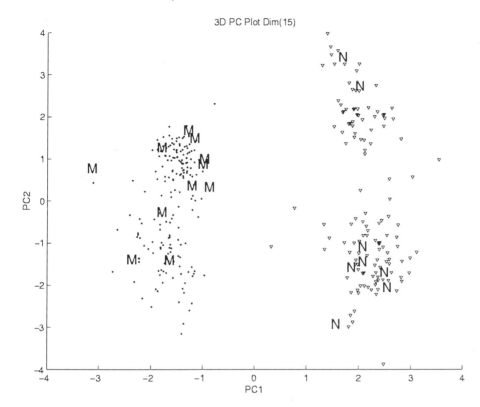

Fig. 5. A plot of the two largest principal components of the training set developed from the 312 compounds and 15 molecular descriptors identified by the pattern-recognition GA. The plane defined by the two largest principal components accounts for 35% of the total cumulative variance. Circles are the musks; inverted triangles are the nonmusks; M = musks from the prediction set projected onto the principal component plot; N = nonmusks from the prediction set projected onto the principal component plot.

kinetic energy reconstructions normal to and away from the surface of the molecule, describe hydrogen-bonding interactions. LAPLB24 is a shape descriptor derived from the second derivative of the electronic energy distribution with 2 meaning the shorter length rays are represented and 4 meaning that intermediate property values are represented. FUKB11 is also a shape descriptor derived from the Fukai radical reactivity index.

Figure 5 suggests that nitrated and nitro-free musks have common structural features that can be used to differentiate them from nonmusks. We consider this to be a significant result. Fragrance chemists have long sought to find the overlap between nitrated and nitro-free musks in terms of the structural features that a compound must possess in order to evoke a musk odor. Further-

Table 3
Final Set of Descriptors for the Musks

DGNH6	Descriptor describes the rate of change of the G kinetic energy density normal to and away from the surface of the molecule.
DKNW6	Wavelet descriptors that describe the same basic value as DGNH6.
DKNW7	Wavelet descriptors that describe the same basic value as DGNH6.
DKNW16	Wavelet descriptors that describe the same basic value as DGNH6.
PIPAVGP	Descriptor that conveys information about the local ionization potential of the molecule.
PIPW15	Descriptor that conveys information about the local ionization potential of the molecule.
PIPB04	Descriptor that conveys information about the local ionization potential of the molecule.
BNPW18	A so-called bare nuclear potential descriptors that probably describe interactions involving polar and hydrogen bonding.
BNPB31	A so-called bare nuclear potential descriptor that probably describe interactions involving polar and hydrogen bonding.
EPB03	Shape descriptor derived from ray traces of the molecule's electrostatic surface potential.
EPB43	Shape descriptor derived from ray traces of the molecule's electrostatic surface potential.
GW15	Wavelet descriptors derived from G kinetic energy reconstructions normal to and away from the surface of the molecule, describe hydrogen-bonding interactions.
KW15	Wavelet descriptor derived from K kinetic energy reconstructions normal to and away from the surface of the molecule, describe hydrogen-bonding interactions.
LAPLB24	Shape descriptor derived from the second derivative of the electronic energy distribution with 2 meaning the shorter length rays are represented and 4 meaning that intermediate property values are represented.
FUKB11	Shape descriptor derived from the Fukai radical reactivity index.

more, we were able to separate aromatic nitro musks from nonmusks. This is also a significant result since the SAR of aromatic nitro musks is not well understood because of the complex substitution pattern and the varied poly-functional character of the nitro group. One can therefore conclude that musk odor activity of aromatic nitro musks can be accurately modeled by the electron density derived descriptors used in this study.

5. Notes

1. Descriptors based on experimental data were not used in this study. It would be very difficult to obtain these types of data from the literature for a large set of compounds. Furthermore, it would not be possible to use the SAR developed in this study as a screening tool to identify new musks because the compounds would have to be synthesized in order to obtain the necessary experimental data.

2. There are a number of parameters that affect the performance of the pattern-recognition GA including the choice of crossover and mutation rate and the configuration of the initial population. Our experience with the pattern-recognition GA has shown that three-point crossover works. However, the number of features in each feature subset of the initial population is a critical parameter. If the feature sets are initially sparse, the probability of including features, which are neither good nor bad, is low since the principal component based fitness function does not provide additional points for adding them. Conversely, the probability of removing these features from less sparse feature subsets is also low because there is no advantage in deleting them. For datasets with a large number of good features, it is probably best not to employ sparse feature subsets in the initial population. Otherwise, it may take thousands of generations to ensure the inclusion of all good features in the solution.

3. To ensure removal of features, which are neither good nor bad, the corresponding loading plot that is generated with each principal component plot can be examined by the pattern-recognition GA. If the loadings for a particular feature are near zero for both principal components, the feature is a likely candidate for removal since its contribution to the principal component plot is negligible. This culling can be implemented every 10 generations to check for features, which are neither good nor bad. During the generation when culling is implemented, crossover would not be performed on the strings. Our experience with this culling algorithm, which allows the user to specify the critical threshold value for the loadings and the generations where culling occurs, indicates that correctly configuring the initial population is a better course of action to ensure that uninformative features are not present in chromosomes that are retained for crossover.

4. Varying the composition of the initial population or the mutation rate can prove beneficial in optimizing a solution but this fact should not be viewed negatively as suggested by some researchers because it allows the user to vary the search of the solution space ensuring a more careful analysis of the data. Given the small number of iterations required for a solution (usually less than 100), the advantages of using these two GA parameters as search variables outweighs any disadvantage that might be incurred due to increased complexity.

5. A drawback of any genetic algorithm is that one cannot control the rate of convergence, but convergence is not what we are seeking. A genetic algorithm can evade local optima, but this does not mean that convergence necessitates an optimal solution. Convergence as a benchmark for the success of a GA would suggest

that any genetic algorithm provides a deficient solution. However, the quality of the best solution found—and how quickly and reproducibly it is found—is the guide being used to determine the success of our method. The ease, speed, and reproducibility of our pattern-recognition GA have been demonstrated on a variety of datasets. We attribute the success of the pattern-recognition GA to the large number of preferred solutions that exist in the data as a result of the high degree of collinearity among the measurement variables.

References

1. Breneman, C. M., Thompson, T. R., Rhem, M., and Dung, M. (1995) Electron density modeling of large systems using the transferable atom equivalent method. *Comp. Chem.* **19,** 161–179.
2. Hansch, C. and Leo, A. (1995) Exploring QSAR, fundamentals and applications in chemistry and biology. ACS National Meeting, Washington, DC.
3. Whitehead, C. E., Breneman, C. M., Sukumar, N., and Ryan, M. D. (2003) Transferable atom equivalent multi-centered expansion method. *J. Comput. Chem.* **24,** 512–529.
4. Lavine, B. K., Davidson, C. E., Vander Meer, R. K., Lahav, S., Soroker, V., and Hefetz, A. (2003) Genetic algorithms for deciphering the complex chemosensory code of social insects. *Chemometrics Intell. Lab. Instrument.* **66,** 51–62.
5. Lavine, B. K., Davidson, C. E., and Moores, A. J. (2002) Genetic algorithms for spectral pattern recognition. *Vib. Spectros.* **28,** 83–95.
6. Jolliffe, I. T. (1986) *Principal component analysis*, Springer Verlag, New York.
7. Beats, M. G. J. (1978) *Structure activity relationships in human chemoreception*, Applied Science Publishers, London, UK.
8. Wood, T. F. (1970) *Chemistry of the aromatic musks*, Givaudanian, Clifton, NJ, pp. 1–37.
9. Bersuker, I. B., Dimoglo, A. S., Gorbachov, M., Yu, Vlad, P. F., and Pesaro, M. (1991) Origin of musk fragrance activity: the Electron-opological approach. *New J. Chem.* **15,** 307–320.
10. Ham, C. L. and Jurs, P. C. (1985) Structure activity studies of musk odorants using pattern recognition: monocyclic nitrobenzenes. *Chem. Senses* **10,** 491–502.
11. Theimer, E. T. (1982) *Fragrance chemistry, the science of the sense of smell.* Academic Press, New York.
12. Breneman, C., Bennett, Bi, J., Song, M., and Embrechts, M. (2002) New electron density-derived descriptors and machine learning techniques for computational ADME and molecular design. MidAtlantic Computational Chemistry Meeting, Princeton University, Princeton, NJ.
13. Breneman, C. M. and Rhem, M. (1997) QSPR Analysis of HPLC column capacity factors for a set of high-energy materials using electronic van der Waals surface property descriptors computed by transferable atom equivalent method. *J. Comput. Chem.* **18,** 182–197.
14. Bader, R. F. W. (1990) *Atoms in molecules: a quantum theory.* Oxford Univ. Press, Oxford, UK.

15. Zauhar, R. J. and Welsh, W. J. (2000) Application of the shape signatures approach to ligand-and-receptor based drug design. Abstracts of Papers of the American Chemical Society 220, 70-COMP, Part 1.
16. Michalewicz, Z. (1995) *Genetic Algorithms + Data Structures = Evolution Programs.* Springer Verlag, New York.
17. Mitchell, M. (1998) *An Introduction to Genetic Algorithms.* The MIT Press, Cambridge, MA.
18. Goldberg, D. E. (1989) *Genetic Algorithms in Search, Optimization, and Machine Learning.* Addison Wesley Publishing Company, Reading, MA.
19. James, M. (1992) *Classification.* John Wiley & Sons, New York.

17

How to Describe Chirality and Conformational Flexibility

Gordon M. Crippen

Abstract

Given atomic coordinates for a particular conformation of a molecule and some property value assigned to each atom, one can easily calculate a chirality function that distinguishes enantiomers, is zero for an achiral molecule, and is a continuous function of the coordinates and properties. This is useful as a quantitative measure of chirality for molecular modeling and structure–activity relations.

Key Words: Principal axes; symmetry; asymmetry; enantiomers; chirality; QSAR.

1. Introduction

Very loosely speaking, a chiral object is something that is not identical to its mirror image. Many different treatments *(1,2)* over many years has produced an enormous literature on the subject. Depending on the design criteria, different approaches for detecting, measuring, enumerating, or classifying chirality are better suited than others to particular applications.

Suppose several compounds inhibit a given enzyme to varying degrees, as determined by experiment. It is not uncommon for such effects to be stereo-specific, making it important to differentiate between enantiomers for simple chiral molecules. In the case of conformationally flexible molecules, at least part of the ligand will be fixed upon binding to a specific conformation that depends on interactions between the ligand and the enzyme, as well as the intra-ligand and ligand–solvent energetics. Thus, in order to correlate molecular structure with binding affinity, as in a quantitative structure–activity study (QSAR), one must describe the chirality of the ligand for the particular enzyme-bound conformation *(3)*. On the other hand, this chirality description

From: *Methods in Molecular Biology, vol. 275:*
Chemoinformatics: Concepts, Methods, and Tools for Drug Discovery
Edited by: J. Bajorath © Humana Press Inc., Totowa, NJ

may need to view molecular structure in terms of broader similarity than are commonly used in standard treatments of chirality. As an example of such bioisosterism *(5)*, a ring nitrogen can sometimes be replaced by a carbon with no loss of activity, whereas the standard Cahn–Ingold–Prelog (CIP) rules *(4)* treat the two atoms as always distinct. It may well be that binding affinity correlates with a particular arrangement in space of ligand hydrogen bond donor groups, and this arrangement must have a particular chirality in the enzyme-bound conformation. In such a case, all hydrogen bond donating groups would be treated as equivalent, and all other atoms would be ignored. For QSAR applications, it is preferable to have a quantitative measure of chirality, rather than discrete *R* vs *S* vs achiral. For example, a slightly left-handed arrangement of some atomic property may be preferred by the enzyme, but an achiral or slightly right-handed arrangement may be moderately acceptable, while a decidedly right-handed distribution is rejected.

For our purposes, a well-suited chirality measure must have four features:

1. It must be independent of rigid translation and (proper) rotation of the given atomic coordinates, although it may depend on conformation.
2. The values for two mirror images should have opposite sign but equal magnitude. This implies that the value for achiral molecules should be zero.
3. The value should depend not only on coordinates but also on some sort of atomic properties that may represent a relevant way to distinguish atoms or groups of atoms. The intent is to avoid arbitrary rules about which atoms are equivalent to which ones, when are two atoms adequately distinguishable, and, if so, which has the higher priority.
4. Otherwise the measure should be a continuous function of the given atomic coordinates and atomic property values, and it need not be independent of them.

As already mentioned, there are several other treatments of chirality, each with its proponents ready to defend it "to the death." These are not wrong or bad in some absolute sense, but rather they are not well suited to the sort of applications outlined above. For instance, the CIP rules are used to assign an absolute chirality designation to every asymmetric center in a molecule or to determine the center is in fact not asymmetric. This is well suited to enumerating stereoisomers that occur in biological molecules and may be synthesized and separated in the laboratory. The assignments are discrete and do not depend on conformational changes that may readily occur under normal experimental conditions. Hence, pseudorotations of cyclohexyl rings are disregarded, but it is assumed that there is no active racemase enzyme present. The rules clearly distinguish between *(R)*-CHDFCl and CH_2FCl, even though their properties may be essentially equivalent for most applications. In other words, the CIP approach does not satisfy properties 3 and 4 above. More recent methods may produce a continuous range of values with variation in conformation *(6)*, but they still depend on rules to order the four substituents of an asymmetric carbon.

Another long line of investigations is said to have started from Kitaigorodskii's suggestion that the normalized maximal overlap volume between a molecule and its mirror image could serve as a measure of chirality *(7)*. The general principle employed is that some molecular similarity measure is applied between a particular conformation of a molecule and its mirror image. The similarity measure D may be a continuous function of conformation and atomic properties, and it may even be a metric in the geometric sense, but at least for any two molecules A and B, $D(A, B) = D(B, A) \geq 0$, and $D(A, B) = 0$ if and only if $A = B$. This distinguishes chiral from achiral, but it fails to discriminate between a chiral molecule and its enantiomer, property 2 above. The molecular similarity measure used in some such approaches is simply the maximal overlap volume of the electron clouds of the two molecules *(8–11)*, which may not reflect important variations in atomic or group properties, such as hydrogen bond donor capacity, pK_a of a group, or atomic polarizability (property 3). Even so, molecular similarity measures of chirality in terms of steric volume overlap or electrostatic potential agreement have been shown to be useful in QSAR *(12)*.

As part of a general scheme for measuring symmetry properties of molecules represented as point atoms, Avnir and coworkers define a quantitative measure of chirality as the mean squared spatial distance between the original points and the closest achiral configuration of these same points *(13,14)*. This distinguishes chiral from achiral molecules, but once again does not differentiate between two enantiomers (property 2). While the idea of the nearest achiral configuration is certainly interesting, their algorithm for computing it is rather complicated. This chirality measure is quantitative with respect to geometry of the molecule, but it is qualitative in its treatment of atom labels. Thus, one of the complications in their algorithm is deciding which is the best one-to-one correspondence between several identically labeled atoms in the two different configurations.

The approach of Kuz'min et al. *(15)* is similar in that the molecule is treated as point atoms having qualitatively distinguishable or indistinguishable labels, and the quantitative degree of chirality is measured as the weighted sum of squared distances between corresponding points in the molecule and its optimally superimposed mirror image. The geometric part of the problem is neatly handled by exploiting the symmetry properties of the inertial tensor, but there remains the combinatorial optimization of the atom correspondence in the case of some indistinguishable labels such that the value of the chirality measure is minimized. Their level of dissymmetry measure is zero for achiral molecules and positive for chiral ones, so once again, enantiomers are not distinguished (property 2). While atom labels are used qualitatively to set up the optimal correspondence between a molecule and its mirror image, they are used quantitatively as positive weights in their measure, so the same chiral molecule might have different values when different atom properties are used as the weights, thus satisfying property 4 in part.

Starting with the semiempirical approach of Kauzmann et al. *(16)*, Ruch and Schönhofer developed a theory of chirality functions *(17,18)*. These amount to polynomials over a set of variables that correspond to the identity of substituents at various substitution positions on a particular achiral parent molecule. The values of the variables can be adjusted so that the polynomial evaluates to a good fit to the experimentally measured molar rotations of a homologous series of compounds *(2)*. Thus, properties 1 and 2 are satisfied, but the variables are qualitatively distinct for the "same" substituent at different positions or "different" substituents at the same positions, violating property 3. Furthermore, there is a different polynomial for each symmetry class of base molecule. Thus, chirality functions are not continuous functions of atom properties and conformation (property 4).

2. Methods

Kuz'min et al. *(15)* pointed out a standard result of classical mechanics: If a configuration of particles has a plane of symmetry, then this plane is perpendicular to a principal axis *(19)*. A principal axis is defined to be an eigenvector of the inertial tensor. Furthermore, if the configuration of particles possesses any axis of symmetry, then this axis is also a principal axis, and the plane perpendicular to this axis is a principal plane corresponding to a degenerate principal moment of inertia *(19)*.

Suppose we are given Cartesian coordinates a_i and mass m_i for each atom i. To convert the coordinates to principal axes frame of reference, first translate to center-of-mass coordinates

$$c_i = (c_{xi}, c_{yi}, c_{zi})^T = a_i - \left(\sum_j m_j a_j\right) \bigg/ \left(\sum m_j\right) \qquad (1)$$

where the superscript T indicates matrix transpose. Then

$$I = \begin{bmatrix} \sum m_i(c_{yi}^2 + c_{zi}^2) & -\sum m_i c_{xi} c_{yi} & -\sum m_i c_{xi} c_{zi} \\ -\sum m_i c_{xi} c_{yi} & \sum m_i(c_{xi}^2 + c_{zi}^2) & -\sum m_i c_{yi} c_{zi} \\ -\sum m_i c_{xi} c_{zi} & -\sum m_i c_{yi} c_{zi} & \sum m_i(c_{xi}^2 + c_{yi}^2) \end{bmatrix} \qquad (2)$$

is the inertial tensor. This matrix has three positive eigenvalues that are not necessarily all distinct, and corresponding to each is an eigenvector, but these are not uniquely determined in the degenerate case. However, the eigenvectors can always be ordered by eigenvalue, chosen to be orthonormal and forming a right-handed coordinate system. Let R be the 3×3 matrix whose columns are these ordered eigenvectors. Then the principal axis coordinates of each atom are just $(x_i, y_i, z_i)^T = Rc_i$.

Our chirality measure is defined in terms of the principal axes coordinates by

$$\chi = \begin{cases} 0 & \text{for degenerate eigenvalues} \\ \sum m_i x_i y_i z_i & \text{nondegenerate} \end{cases} \tag{3}$$

in accord with the desired properties. If the eigenvalues are degenerate, $\chi = 0$ straight away (property 2) regardless of initial coordinates (property 1), and properties 3 and 4 are trivial. In the nondegenerate case the principal axes coordinates are uniquely defined up to 180° flips about the three axes, and these have no effect on the value (property 1). A reflection through the xy, xz, or yz planes will reverse the sign of one of the coordinates of all atoms, thus reversing the sign of χ (property 2). A nonplanar but achiral molecule may have some atoms located on such planes, producing zero terms; otherwise, there will be pairs of corresponding atoms across one or more of these planes such that the pair of terms in **Eq. 3** cancels. The measure relies on coordinates and the m_is, rather than on distinguishability and priority rules (property 3), and it depends continuously on them via **Eqs. 1** and **2** (property 4). This is philosophically in line with the idea that the degree of chirality of a molecule is not an absolute concept, but depends on the atomic property of interest *(20)*.

The essence of the matter is **Eq. 3**, but a convenient scaled version is

$$\chi_{scaled} = 10^5 \frac{(\lambda_2 - \lambda_1)(\lambda_3 - \lambda_1)(\lambda_3 - \lambda_1)}{\lambda_1 \lambda_2 \lambda_3 \sum_i m_i} \sum_i \frac{m_i x_i y_i z_i}{(x_i^2 + y_i^2 + z_i^2)^{3/2}} \tag{4}$$

where the eigenvalues have been ordered $0 < \lambda_1 \leq \lambda_2 \leq \lambda_3$. If any two eigenvalues are nearly equal, then automatically $\chi_{scaled} \approx 0$; uniformly scaling the coordinates and/or the masses by some constant has no effect on χ_{scaled}; and otherwise the magnitudes are on the order of 1–100 for chiral molecules. Moreau *(21)* used the same basic idea as **Eq. 3** but came to a variant on **Eq. 4** that corresponds more closely to the standard idea of chiral centers by weighting the atoms according to how close they are to a chosen central atom. In that way, one can compare the chirality in the neighborhoods of two different asymmetric carbon atoms in one molecule, for example.

The calculations in the next section were performed using the above methods implemented in MOE molecular modeling software *(22)*.

3. Results

Let us first examine a few special cases that cover most common point groups. A linear molecule, such as HCN (point group $C_{\infty v}$) or acetylene ($D_{\infty h}$), will lie along one principal axis, say the z axis, so that the first eigenvalue of the inertial tensor vanishes and the other is doubly degenerate; alternatively, by the second case in **Eq. 3** $x_i = y_i = 0$ for all i, and thus $\chi = 0$.

Consider planar molecules, such as 1,2-dichlorobenzene (C_{2v}), glyoxal (**Fig. 1**, structure **6**; point group C_{2h}), orthoboric acid [$B(OH)_3$; structure **7**; point group C_{3h}), naphthalene (D_{2h}), or benzene (D_{6h}). Such a molecule will have all its atoms in one principal axes plane, say the yz plane, so that $x_i = 0$ for all i.

Nonplanar but highly symmetric molecules, such as CH_4 and adamantane (T_d) or the octahedral SF_6 (O_h), produce one triply degenerate eigenvalue and hence $\chi = 0$. Trigonal pyramidal NH_3 (C_{3v}) has one doubly degenerate eigenvalue corresponding to eigenvectors orthogonal to the C_3 symmetry axis, and hence $\chi = 0$.

Consider allene isomers (**Fig. 1**, structure **1**). Allene itself ($R_1=R_2=R_3=R_4=H$) belongs to the D_{2d} point group, and the S_4 axis is indicated by an arrow in the figure. Weighting the atom positions by their atomic masses, the eigenvalues of I are 3.5, 55.9, and 55.9 Dalton-$Å^2$. The first eigenvector coincides with the S_4 axis, and the two eigenvectors associated with the doubly degenerate eigenvalue span the plane of the two orthogonal C_2 axes of symmetry. Any linear combination of eigenvectors of a degenerate eigenvalue is still an eigenvector, so the two C_2 axes of symmetry are also eigenvectors, but they may not happen to be exactly the eigenvectors found when diagonalizing the inertial tensor. In any case, **Eq. 3** results in $\chi = 0$. For fluoroallene ($R_1=F$; point group C_s), the center of mass shifts somewhat from the central carbon toward the fluorine atom, the eigenvalues are no longer degenerate, and the first principal axis is no longer along the three carbon atoms, but lies slightly tilted in the F–C=C plane. Nonetheless, the mass distribution has a reflection symmetry plane (the plane of F–C–R_2) perpendicular to one of the other principal axes, and $\chi = 0$. The simplest chiral derivative, $R_1=R_3=F$ and $R_2=R_4=H$, has $\chi = -11.2$; its enantiomer, $R_1=R_4=F$ and $R_2=R_3=H$, has $\chi = +11.2$.

As an example of the C_{2v} point group, basketane (**Fig. 1**, structure **2**) results in nondegenerate eigenvalues, but the indicated C_2 symmetry axis is an eigenvector, and $\chi = 0$. For the D_{3h} point group, consider cyclopropane, structure **3**, all R=H. The indicated C_3 axis is the eigenvector corresponding to the largest eigenvalue, and the other eigenvalue is twofold degenerate, so $\chi = 0$. When $R_2=Cl$, there is no degeneracy, but still $\chi = 0$. Of course $R_1=R_2=Cl$ also has

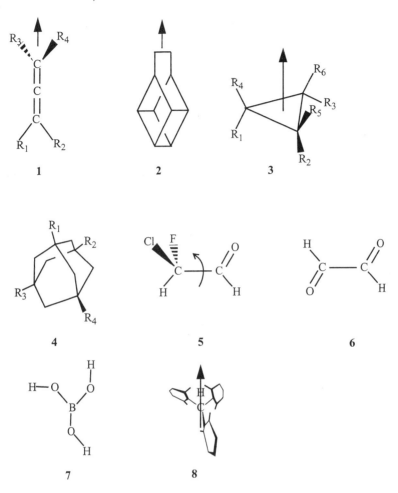

Fig. 1. Example molecular structures. Symmetry axes discussed in the text are indicated by arrows.

$\chi = 0$, but R_1=F and R_2=Cl yields $\chi = 1.67$. The more interesting enantiomeric pair of dichlorocyclopropanes, R_1=R_5=Cl vs R_4=R_2=Cl, have $\chi = \pm0.15$, respectively. Cyclobutane (D_{4h}) behaves like cyclopropane, producing $\chi = 0$ due to a doubly degenerate eigenvalue.

The T_d point group behaves as expected and offers no special problems. Of course, $\chi = 0$ for CH_4, CH_3Cl, and CH_2ClBr. For an asymmetric center (point group C_1), χ is a *quantitative* measure of *how* chiral is the distribution of the property in question, taken to be simply atomic mass in all these examples. Thus, χ is -0.0052 for *(R)*-CHDClBr, $+0.0052$ for *(S)*-CHDClBr, $+0.041$ for *(R)*-CHFClBr, and -0.041 for *(S)*-CHFClBr. In terms of other chirality approaches, this is equivalent to saying that D is nearly the same as H, but (the masses of) F and H are more clearly distinguishable (relative to the total mass of the molecule). In general, the sign of χ is not the same for all R or S configuration molecules, because CIP rules have their own precedent ordering, and this has no special relation to the calculated value of χ, using whatever atomic property values. Adamantane, structure **4**, behaves just like methane and has one triply degenerate eigenvalue, yielding $\chi = 0$. Substituting R_1=F results in one nondegenerate eigenvalue with its corresponding eigenvector being the C_3 symmetry axis through R_1, and a doubly degenerate eigenvalue, so $\chi = 0$. When R_1=F and R_2=Cl, $\chi = 0$, even though the symmetry has been disrupted both by the mass changes and by the longer halogen–carbon bond lengths. The enantiomers R_1=F, R_2=Cl, R_3=Br, R_4=H vs R_1=F, R_2=Cl, R_3=H, R_4=Br have $\chi = \pm 3.7$, respectively.

Ethane in its low-energy, precisely staggered conformation *(D_{3d})* has a doubly degenerate eigenvalue and therefore $\chi = 0$. In a higher-energy conformation between staggered and eclipsed *(D_3)*, the degeneracy remains, correctly giving $\chi = 0$. A high-energy D_2 conformation of ethene twisted somewhat out of plane, but not 90°, has nondegenerate eigenvalues and $\chi \neq 0$. The ethane derivative CHFClCHFCl in a staggered conformation with corresponding substituents on the two carbons *trans* to each other *(C_i)* has three nondegenerate eigenvalues, and the origin of the principal axes is at the inversion center between the two carbon atoms. The sum in **Eq. 3** evaluates to zero, in accord with C_i being achiral. Hydrogen peroxide, one of the few C_2 molecules, has nondegenerate eigenvalues and correctly gives $\chi \neq 0$.

On the other hand, a minimal energy structure of tris-(2,6-dichlorophenyl) methane (structure **8**) belongs to the chiral point group C_3 because the aromatic rings are skewed relative to the C_3 axis, like the blades of a fan. One principal axis coincides with the C_3 symmetry axis, and we can call it the z axis. Then the x and y axes correspond to a doubly degenerate eigenvalue, so $\chi = 0$. Because of the symmetry, the atoms and the terms of **Eq. 3** are grouped into triples having the same values of m_i, z_i, and $r = (x_i^2 + y_i^2)^{1/2}$. Converting to cylindrical coordinates, each term $m_i x_i y_i z_i$ has the form $m_i r^2 \cos\theta \sin\theta$. Each threefold symmetrical triple sums to zero because

$$\cos(\theta)\sin(\theta) + \cos(\theta + 2\pi/3)\sin(\theta + 2\pi/3) + \cos(\theta + 4\pi/3)\sin(\theta + 4\pi/3) = 0 \quad (5)$$

for any arbitrary phase angle θ between the first atom and the degenerate xy axes. In general, chiral molecules having C_n symmetry erroneously gives $\chi = 0$ when $n > 2$ because **Eq. 3** mistakes such symmetry for σ. Such molecules are so rare that they are unlikely to cause problems in practical QSAR applications.

As a very simple example of a conformationally flexible chiral molecule, consider structure **5**, *(R)*-fluorochloroacetaldehyde. Because χ clearly has a

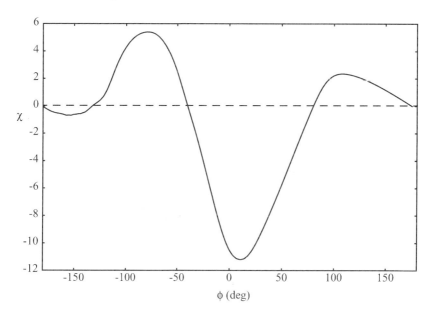

Fig. 2. Variation in χ for *(R)*-fluorochloroacetaldehyde (structure **5**) as a function of ϕ, the O=C–C–Cl dihedral angle.

geometric component, it comes as no surprise that it varies as a function of conformation (**Fig. 2**). This is the behavior of the whole molecule, but, of course, if we calculated χ only using the CHFCl–C atoms, χ would be constant and nonzero. Thus, at about dihedral angle $\phi=80°$, corresponding to nearly eclipsed hydrogens, the mass distribution is momentarily achiral, and $\chi = 0$. The most chiral distribution occurs when the O and Cl atoms are eclipsed at $\phi=0°$. The *(S)* isomer gives exactly the same trace with reversed sign, of course, so one might say that the *(R)* isomer has predominantly or an averaged $\chi < 0$, while the *(S)* has predominantly $\chi > 0$. This sort of behavior is generally seen in conformationally flexible but chiral molecules. For example, certain energetically reasonable conformations of *(R)*-glyceraldehyde have values of +5.5 and –9.5, and there are conformations between where $\chi = 0$. This is unsettling for people schooled in the idea that molecular chirality in every sense must be independent of conformation, yet it is a perfectly natural consequence of this particular approach. The given atomic property can be distributed in space over the molecule as a whole as sometimes a right-handed distribution, sometimes left-handed, and even symmetrically in a lower-dimensional subspace of all conformations. One can imagine a situation where a binding site on some protein recognizes a certain right-handed distribution of charge, say, and rejects the mirror image distribution. Then an important factor for binding would be the ability of a flexible molecule to assume some conformation with a right-handed charge distribution, regardless of whether the flexible molecule as a whole would be assigned R or S absolute configuration. On the other hand, χ remains constant and nonzero, independent of conformation, when only the asymmetric carbon and its immediate neighbors are included in the calculation. This is, after all, the equivalent of applying the CIP rules to this simple example.

In the example of structure **5**, we get $\chi = 0$ when the hydrogens are approximately eclipsed. The aldehyde oxygen atom is tipped slightly toward the fluorine so that *overall* there is a mirror symmetric mass distribution. The sum in **Eq. 3** adds up to zero, but there is not really a pairing of canceling terms corresponding to equivalent atoms related by one mirror reflection. We will call this a *balanced* but not achiral configuration. The algorithm for distinguishing between a truly achiral molecule and a balanced conformation of a chiral molecule is as follows. **Equation 3** judges atoms to be equivalent or nonequivalent by their atomic masses, m_i. Other atomic properties could equally well be chosen, such as partial charge or polarizability. Consider using m_i^p for different powers p. If there are n different values of the atom property, then the n equations $\chi(p) = 0$ for $p = 1, \ldots, n$ are linearly independent and can be satisfied only for a truly symmetric molecule where atoms are either on the plane of symmetry or are paired with equivalent, mirror symmetrically related atoms. Thus, in the *(R)*-fluorochloroacetaldehyde (nearly) balanced conformation, $\chi(1) = -003$, but $\chi(2) = -31.8$ and $\chi(3) = -535$. Likewise in the *(R)*-glyceraldehyde example, one conformation having $\chi(1) = 0$ has $\chi(2) = -11.25$ and $\chi(3) = -188.13$, thus demonstrating that the conformation is balanced but chiral. On the other hand, consider the achiral molecule difluoroacetaldehyde in the hydrogen eclipsed conformation, so that H–C–CHO are all coplanar, and the two fluorine atoms are above and below the mirror symmetry plane. Calculating χ in a computer program is always subject to numerical roundoff errors, but $\chi(1) = -0.00035$, $\chi(2) = -0.0024$, and $\chi(3) = -0.029$ can be taken to be essentially zero, showing that this is not a balanced conformation, but a genuinely achiral one. Incidentally, the CPU time required for these calculations is negligible by today's standards, even if carried out for two or three different property sets. The inertial tensor to be diagonalized is always a 3×3 matrix, and the rest of the calculations scale linearly with the number of atoms.

4. Conclusions

Equations 1–4 constitute an algorithm for determining from atomic coordinates and some property assigned to the atoms whether the molecule is achiral, and, if not, quantitatively how chiral. Compared to other methods, it is fast and simple because it avoids finding the globally optimal superposition of two enantiomers and assigning the optimal pairwise atom correspondence between them. In the case of relatively rare point groups, chiral molecules are incorrectly assigned $\chi = 0$, but otherwise even balanced configurations are correctly recognized as genuinely chiral. Achiral molecules always produce $\chi = 0$. It corresponds to conventional standards of chirality in that enantiomers have χ values of equal magnitude but opposite sign. It could be used on fragments of a molecule including an individual asymmetric center and its substituents, but, when applied to a whole molecule, it does not capture ideas like diastereomers. Instead, it contributes a new viewpoint to the general issue of chirality that is particularly well suited to certain modeling applications where the spatial distribution of some atomic property must be quantitatively described. In particular, we have been using it in QSAR applications *(23)*. Conceptually, it quantitates the equivalence of atoms, instead of relying on arbitrary rules about what atoms or groups are deemed equivalent.

The general idea of a standard positioning and distinguishing atoms by some assigned property has some interesting applications beyond chirality. Consider a conformational search that generates many conformations in local energy minima. If two of these differ by a 180° flip of an unsubstituted phenyl ring, then most search programs would consider them different because the atoms are all viewed as uniquely labelled in the computer's internal representation. However, both would map to equivalent principal axes positions where atoms of one structure are superimposed on atoms of the other having identical properties, such as mass or partial charge. This can really simplify the detection of equivalent conformations in an elegant way.

Acknowledgments

This work was supported by NSF (DBI-9614074), the Vahlteich Research Award Fund, and NIH (GM59097-01).

References

1. Barron, L. D. (1991) Fundamental symmetry aspects of molecular chirality. In *New developments in molecular chirality*, Mezey, P. G. (ed.), Kluwer Academic Publishers, Dordrecht, Understanding Chemical Reactivity, Vol. 5, pp. 1–55.
2. Derflinger, G. (1991) Chirality and group theory. In *Chirality. From weak bosons to the α-helix*, Janoschek, R. (ed.), Springer-Verlag, pp. 34–58.
3. Crippen, G. M. (1999) VRI: 3D QSAR at variable resolution. *J. Comput. Chem.* **20,** 1577–1585.
4. Cahn, R. S., Ingold, C. K., and Prelog, V. (1966) Specification of molecular chirality. *Angew. Chem., Internat. Ed. Engl.* **5,** 385–415.
5. Burger, A. (1991) Isosterism and bioisosterism in drug design. *Prog. Drug Res.* **37,** 287–371.

6. Aires-de-Sousa, J. and Gasteiger, J. (2002) Prediction of enantiomeric selectivity in chromatography. Application of conformation-dependent and conformation-independent descriptors of molecular chirality. *J. Mol. Graphics Mod.* **20,** 373–388.

7. Kitaigorodskii, A. (1961) *Organic chemical crystallography.* Consultant Bureau, New York, p. 230.

8. Mezey, P. G. (1997) A proof of the metric properties of the symmetric scaling-nesting dissimilarity measure and related symmetry deficiency measures. *Int. J. Quantum Chem.* **63,** 105–109.

9. Mezey, P. G. (1997) Chirality measures and graph representations. *Computers Math. Applic.* **34,** 105–112.

10. Mezey, P. G. (1998) The proof of the metric properties of a fuzzy chirality measure of molecular electron density clouds. *J. Molec. Struct. (Theochem.)* **455,** 183–190.

11. Mezey, P. G. (1998) Mislow's label paradox, chirality-preserving conformational changes, and related chirality measures. *Chirality* **10,** 173–179.

12. Seri-Levy, A., West, S., and Richards, W. G. (1994) Molecular similarity, quantitative chirality, and QSAR for chiral drugs. *J. Med. Chem.* **37,** 1727–1732.

13. Zabrodsky, H. and Avnir, D. (1995) Continuous symmetry Measures. 4. Chirality. *J. Am. Chem. Soc.* **117,** 462–473.

14. Salomon, Y. and Avnir, D. (1999) Continuous symmetry measures: Finding the closest C_2-symmetric object or closest reflection-symmetric object using unit quaternions. *J. Comput. Chem.* **20,** 772–780.

15. Kuz'min, V. E., Stel'makh, I. B., Bekker, M. B., and Pozigun, D. V. (1992) Quantitative aspects of chirality. I. Method of dissymmetry function. *J. Phys. Org. Chem.* **5,** 295–298.

16. Kauzmann, W., Clough, F. B., and Tobias, I. (1961) The principle of pairwise interactions as a basis for an empirical theory of optical rotatory power. *Tetrahedron* **13,** 57–105.

17. Ruch, E. and Schönhofer, A. (1968) Näherungsformeln für spiegelungsantimetrische Moleküleigenschaften. *Theoret. Chim. Acta* **10,** 91–110.

18. Ruch, E. and Schönhofer, A. (1970) Theorie der Chiralitätsfunktionen. *Theoret. Chim. Acta* **19,** 225–287.

19. Symon, K. R. (1960) *Mechanics,* 2nd ed., Addison-Wesley, Reading, MA, p. 432.

20. Harris, A. B., Kamien, R. D., and Lubensky, T. C. (1999) Molecular chirality and chiral parameters. *Rev. Mod. Phys.* **71,** 1745–1757.

21. Moreau, G. (1997) Atomic chirality, a quantitative measure of the chirality of the environment of an atom. *J. Chem. Inf. Comput. Sci.* **37,** 929–938.

22. Chemical Computing Group Inc., 1010 Sherbrooke Street West, Suite 910, Montreal, Quebec, Canada, H3A 2R7. http://www.chemcomp.com.

23. Wildman, S. A. and Crippen, G. M. (2002) Three-dimensional molecular descriptors and a novel QSAR method. *J. Mol. Graph Mod.* **21,** 161–170.

18

Novel Scoring Methods in Virtual Ligand Screening

Daniel Pick

Abstract

Several different approaches have been proposed in the last decade to assess the binding affinity of a virtual small molecule ligand to a target protein, particularly with respect to screening large compound databases. Here we review the methods that have been proposed, and discuss techniques for optimizing scoring functions that have been applied in industrial settings.

Key Words: Scoring functions; virtual ligand screening; computational drug discovery.

1. Introduction

In the last decade advances in computational chemistry have made it possible to virtually screen millions of small molecule compounds against high resolution protein structures in three dimensions (3D). This technique, known as "docking," achieved an early success in identifying haloperidol as a ligand conforming to the active binding site of HIV protease *(1)*. In early docking algorithms, both the receptor and the ligand were treated as rigid bodies; as the science developed, ligand conformational flexibility was taken into account so that both a large number of ligands and a large number of conformations of each ligand could be examined.

The sequencing of the human genome, together with advances in combinatorial chemistry, have led to explosive growth in both the number of potential protein targets and the size of corporate small molecule databases. Pharmaceutical and biotech companies, eager to fill drug development pipelines, have supported efforts to build improved docking software. The promise of virtual ligand screening has created a booming market for docking software development groups, both academic and commercial. At least

From: *Methods in Molecular Biology, vol. 275:*
Chemoinformatics: Concepts, Methods, and Tools for Drug Discovery
Edited by: J. Bajorath © Humana Press Inc., Totowa, NJ

10 different organizations offer docking packages today, all claiming superior accuracy and/or performance. A wide variety of techniques have been implemented in docking engines, including force-field computational grids, distance geometry techniques, internal coordinate mechanics solvers, Monte Carlo–based simulated annealing, and genetic algorithms. Most assume that a high-resolution structure of the protein target is available.

The output of all docking programs is a score that measures, in some sense, the complementarity between the receptor and a specific ligand conformation. The quest for a quickly computable, accurate scoring function has been an active area of research for much of the decade. The weakness of many scoring functions has been that, in many cases, they have performed no better than random selection in ranking the fit of ligand conformations to a particular target. This chapter reviews the considerations in designing a scoring function, the published efforts to engineer such functions, the accuracy and performance of the functions published in the literature, and efforts to develop better functions to improve the quality and accuracy of the small molecule hits obtained.

2. Scoring Function Design

The first question that scoring function designers must address is the quantities they are seeking to compute. Some scoring functions have been designed to approximate the change in the Gibbs free energy ΔG_{bind} between the bound and the unbound states of the receptor–ligand complex. Others have been designed to minimize the root-mean-square deviation (RMSD) of a virtual ligand pose, compared to the ligand pose found in crystallographic experiments on known crystal complexes.

All scoring functions have sought to address several issues:

- *Accuracy.* Accuracy has been measured in a number of ways, but an accurate scoring function attempts to minimize the difference between the calculated ΔG_{bind} and the experimentally determined figure, or the RMSD between the virtual and the experimental poses, or both.
- *Speed.* Given the growth in the size of corporate and research chemical databases, a scoring function must be computable in less than 2 min of CPU time to be useful.
- *Enrichment.* In some ways, enrichment is another form of accuracy. Given a database of a large number of decoy small molecules seeded with a few known binders to a specific target, a good scoring function should locate the known binders quickly, and rank them ahead of the decoys. Enrichment studies typically measure the percentage of the database scanned to retrieve a percentage of the known binders.
- *Predictive capacity.* Given that a scoring function that works well on a specific training set of complexes, a good scoring function should identify chemically interesting hits for novel receptors not included in the training set.

The most accurate method for predicting binding free energy for a wide variety of complexes has been the free energy perturbation (FEP) method, first developed by Zwanzig in 1954 *(2)*, and implemented in the AMBER and CHARMm software packages. Unfortunately, as Koehler et al. *(3)* note, its high computational expense limits its application in drug design. This expense is due to the lengthy sampling time needed to ensure that the conformational space is adequately sampled. For virtual ligand screening, the goal has been an automated procedure that would screen thousands of compounds efficiently. All VLS scoring functions, therefore, have sought to balance the tradeoff between calculating a physically meaningful quantity accurately, and calculating such a quantity in a reasonable amount of CPU time.

3. Force Field Approximations

The earliest designers of scoring functions recognized two fundamental contributions to receptor–ligand complementarity: shape and electrostatics. To account for 3D shape complementarity, they calculated some form of contact or van der Waals score, and to account for electrostatic interactions, they calculated some form of electrostatic potential score. In 1992 Kuntz and coworkers *(4)* combined these scores in DOCK 3.0 to compute a grid-based AMBER force-field approximation. They attempted to rank the ligand orientations by molecular mechanics interaction score, whose form was

$$E = \sum_{i=1}^{m}\sum_{j=1}^{n}\left[\frac{A_{ij}}{r_{ij}^{12}} - \frac{B_{ij}}{r_{ij}^{6}} + 332\frac{q_i q_j}{Dr_{ij}}\right]$$

In this formula, m and n are the number of ligand and receptor atoms, respectively; r is the interatomic distance between atoms i and j; the q's are the point charges on the atom, and A and B are adjustable van der Waals repulsion and attraction parameters, and D is the dielectric function. They assumed that this scoring function could account for hydrogen bond energies in the electrostatic term.

This score displays several features that define a model for future scoring functions:

1. It is computed pairwise over the receptor and ligand atoms. For the contact term the authors enabled the user to specify part or all of the receptor atoms; users could introduce a distance cutoff in the calculation.
2. A_{ij} and B_{ij} are introduced as adjustable repulsion and attraction parameters.
3. The score is computed as the sum of separable contact and electrostatic terms. This feature has been questioned by later authors such as Tame *(5)*, who point out that this additivity is assumed without comment or justification.

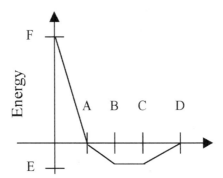

Fig. 1. The piecewise linear potential function, as described in **ref. 6**.

The success of DOCKscore was measured by its designers as its ability to minimize the RMSD of the virtual pose against the crystallographic orientation for four well-determined complexes, including dihydrofolate reductase (DHFR)/methotrexate. The test set was chosen to demonstrate different aspects of complementarity, including salt bridge formation, hydrogen bonding, and hydrophobic interactions.

In 1995 Gehlhaar et al. *(6)* published PLP score, a minimal scoring function, which included a steric term and a hydrogen bonding term, but no electrostatic term. Like the DOCKscore designers, their goal was to minimize the RMSD of the virtual ligand pose from the crystallographic orientation, but they were also interested in designing a scoring function that would be rapidly computable. PLPscore was also designed to enable flexible docking of ligands, that is, to perform a full conformational and positional search within a rigid binding site.

In PLPscore, both the steric and hydrogen bonding terms are calculated from a piecewise linear potential function (*see* **Fig. 1**), instead of a smooth 6-12 Lennard-Jones potential energy function. The difference between the two terms is simply in the parameter values chosen for each term.

In contrast to the two adjustable parameters in DOCKscore, the piecewise linear function contains six. In addition, PLPscore is calculated pairwise over all protein and ligand heavy atoms. Every protein–ligand pair of atoms is assigned an interaction type, either steric or hydrogen bond, according to whether each atom is a hydrogen bond donor, acceptor, donor–acceptor, or non-polar. Like DOCKscore, PLPscore was tested on DHFR/methotrexate. In 100 docking runs, 91 solutions were within 1.5 Å RMSD of the crystal structure. It was also tested on a complex of HIV-1 protease and AG-1343, an Agouron propietary potential drug against AIDS.

4. Empirical Functions

Beginning in the mid-1990s, a new class of scoring functions was published which sought to compute ΔG_{bind} from a sum of separable contributions, whose coefficients were determined by either multiple linear regression or partial least squares fitting on a large training set of receptor–ligand complexes. The designers of these scoring functions, including Böhm *(7)* and Eldridge and coworkers *(8)*, sought to predict ΔG_{bind}, instead of simply minimizing the RMSD of the ligand pose. They also sought to be less dependent on force field approximations, which would often be slow and unreliable when comparing ligands with different chemistries.

A typical empirical scoring function has the form

$$\Delta G_{bind} = \Delta G_{hbond} + \Delta G_{metal} + ... + \Delta G_0$$

where the number of terms on the right hand side of the equation, and the contributions calculated, vary from function to function. In Böhm's function, 4 terms are used; in ChemScore by Eldridge et al., 5 terms are used; in VALIDATE *(9)*, 12 terms are used. The terms attempt to quantify separable and distinct physical contributions to the binding affinity that are not significantly correlated, as the coefficients are calculated by regression techniques. Empirical scoring function designers measure the success of the scoring function by comparing the predicted to the experimentally found binding affinity.

The strength of empirical scoring function is that they are trained on a large number of receptor–ligand complexes taken from the PDB. For example, the training set of ChemScore included 17 aspartic proteases, 15 serine proteases, 15 metalloproteases, 16 sugar-binding proteins, and 19 other complexes. These classes were chosen to make the scoring function perform well on a variety of potential targets of interest to drug designers.

Because these scoring functions are constructed empirically, they are sensitive to the complexes represented in their training sets. To use them effectively, computational chemists must train them on complexes similar to those of their drug design projects, and continually update them as new complexes are solved. Although they are rapidly computable, empirical functions' sensitivity to the data in their training set makes them unsuitable for VLS projects, where the function is likely to encounter both novel ligands and novel ligand orientations.

5. Knowledge-Based Functions

By 1997 the weaknesses in the empirical approach had been noted in the CASP competition of docking methods *(10)*. At the end of the decade Muegge and Martin *(11)* in the US, Gohlke et al. *(12)* in Germany, and Mitchell and coworkers *(13)* in the UK independently introduced PMFScore, DrugScore, and BLEEP—three knowledge-based scoring functions. These functions returned to the concept of relying on an energy force potential to compute a score, which they compute from distance-dependent potentials of protein–ligand atom pairs. These potentials are built, following Sippl's derivation *(14)*, of an inverse Boltzmann relation between the energy of the complex and the relative frequencies of the atom pairs.

In these functions structural information from a large number of complexes was extracted from the PDB and used to construct pairwise atom potentials or preferences. These interaction potentials are constructed by typing both the protein and ligand atoms, and then constructing a potential for each type of interaction. In DrugScore 17 types are used for both protein and ligand atoms; in PMFScore, 16 protein atom types and 34 ligand atom types are defined. This gives rise to a large number of potential curves. The score for a specific protein–ligand complex is then computed by identifying the interactions that occur in the complex within a specified distance cutoff. The score is then computed by summing the interaction potentials for the complex.

Statistical potential designers assume each individual complex resides at the global minimum of its free energy, and that the distribution of complex molecules in solution obeys Boltzmann's law. They extend these assumptions to an entire database of complexes, each of which may or may not be in its own global energy minimum. The extension of these assumptions has been criticized by Thomas and Dill *(15)*, among others, as not reflecting the true underlying energies. Nevertheless, PMFScore achieved a standard deviation of 1.8 log K units from observed binding affinities on 77 complexes, and DrugScore ranked the best virtual pose less than 2 Å RMSD from the experimentally found pose in 73% of 91 complexes.

6. Consensus Approaches

By the beginning of the millennium, many different academic and commercial docking packages had appeared on the market, and each used a different method for scoring virtual ligand poses. Given so many different approaches, all claiming superior performance, how did a computational chemist select the appropriate method for screening virtual ligands against a particular target? Three different studies suggested that rather than selecting one individual method, a consensus approach reduced the number of false positives identified by individual scoring functions.

In the first study, Charifson and coworkers *(16)* performed virtual ligand screening on p38 MAP kinase, IMPDH, and HIV protease. For each of these targets, they chose 400 or more test compounds in three activity ranges, and seeded a database of 10,000 random commercial compounds that passed certain filters with these test compounds. They then docked and scored all the compounds with a dozen different scoring functions, both individually and in combinations of two or three. They found that ChemScore, DOCKScore, and PLPScore performed well across all three targets and activity ranges, but in addition found that when they took the intersection of the lists produced by each function, they obtained a significant reduction in the number of false positive compounds.

Subsequently, Bissantz et al. *(17)* performed virtual screening on thymidine kinase and estrogen receptor α with three different docking packages and seven different scoring functions. In their study they constructed a 1000 compound library containing 990 random compounds and 10 ligands known to bind. They found that while some scoring functions performed well in ranking ligands against thymidine kinase, they did poorly in ranking ligands against the estrogen receptor. However, they confirmed the Charifson group's results in that they found that consensus scoring outperformed single scoring regardless of the target or the docking tool. They also suggested a two-step protocol for virtual ligand screening: screening a reduced dataset with a few known ligands to find the optimal docking/scoring combination, and then applying the combination found to screening of the entire database.

In 2001 Stahl and Rarey *(18)* published a detailed analysis of four scoring functions for virtual ligand screening, including PLPScore, DrugScore, and PMFScore. They screened a database of more than 7500 compounds on a group of seven targets, including the estrogen receptor and p38 MAP kinase. Like the Bissantz group, they showed that each of the individual scoring functions performed well screening virtual ligands for some targets, but performed poorly on others. They also showed that consensus scoring was a more robust approach than single scoring.

7. Future Developments

As massively parallel distributed computing becomes more widely available, academic and corporate researchers will be able to perform large-scale virtual ligand screening experiments in a matter of hours. The requirements for such experiments are a parallel processing docking software package and sufficient computational resources. In such a computational environment, the balance between accuracy and speed in scoring function design will increasingly tilt toward accuracy, although experimenters are likely to enlarge the size of the chemical space they are willing to study through VLS experiments. Scoring functions that depend on adjustable parameters and that have given good results for specific classes of receptors will be tuned to those classes in accelerated drug discovery programs. Consensus scoring of large numbers of compounds assessed with several different scoring functions will likely produce a better pool of virtual drug leads faster.

Acknowledgments

The author wishes to thank Mike Tennant and Andy Jennings at Syrrx, Inc., Scott Dixon at Metaphorics, LLC, and G. Scott Weston at Scios, Inc. for their contributions to this work.

References

1. DesJarlais, R. L., Seibel G. L., Kuntz I. D., et al. (1990) Structure-based design of nonpeptide inhibitors specific for the human immunodeficiency virus 1 protease. *Proc. Natl. Acad. Sci. USA* **87,** 6644–6648.
2. Zwanzig, R. W. (1954) High-temperature equation of state by a perturbation method. I. Nonpolar gases. *J. Chem. Phys.* **22,** 1420–1426.
3. Koehler, K. F., Rao, S. N., and Snyder, J. P. (1996) Modeling drug-receptor interactions. In *Guidebook on molecular modeling in drug design*, Claude Cohen (ed.), Academic Press, New York, pp. 235–336.
4. Meng, E. C., Shoichet, B. K., and Kuntz, I. D. (1992) Automated docking with grid-based energy evaluation. *J. Comp. Chem.* **13,** 505–524.
5. Tame, J. R. H. (1999) Scoring functions: a view from the bench. *J. Comp.-Aid. Mol. Des.* **13,** 99–108.
6. Gehlhaar, D. K., Verkhivker, G. M., Rejto, P. A., et al. (1995) Molecular recognition of the inhibitor AG-1343 by HIV-1 protease: conformationally flexible docking by evolutionary programming. *Chem. Biol.* **2,** 317–324.
7. Böhm, H.-J. (1994) The development of a simple empirical scoring function to estimate the binding constant for a protein-ligand complex of known three-dimensional structure. *J. Comput. Mol. Design* **8,** 243.
8. Eldridge, M. D., Murray, C. W., Auton, T. R., Paolini, G. V., and Mee, R. P. (1997) Empirical scoring functions : I. The development of a fast empirical scoring function to estimate the binding affinity of ligands in receptor complexes. *J. Comput. Mol. Design* **11,** 425–445.
9. Head, R. D., Smythe, M. L., Oprea, T. I., Waller, C. L., Green, S. M., and Marshall, G. R. (1996). VALIDATE : a new method for the receptor-based prediction of binding affinities of novel ligands. *J. Am. Chem. Soc.* **118,** 3959–3969.
10. Dixon, J. S. (1997) Evaluation of the CASP2 docking section. *Proteins: Struct., Funct., Genet.* **Suppl. 1,** 198–204.
11. Muegge, I. and Martin, Y. C. (1999) A general and fast scoring function for protein-ligand interactions: a simplified potential approach. *J. Med. Chem.* **42,** 791–804.
12. Gohlke, H., Hendlich, M., and Klebe G. (2000) Knowledge-based scoring function to predict protein-ligand interactions. *J. Mol. Bio.* **295,** 337–356.

13. Mitchell, J. B. O., Laskowski, R. A., Alex, A., and Thornton, J. M. (1999) BLEEP-potential of mean force describing protein-ligand interactions: I. Generating potential. *J. Comp. Chem.* **20,** 1165–1176.

14. Sippl, M. J. (1993). Boltzmann's principle, knowledge-based mean fields and protein folding. An approach to the computational determination of protein structures. *J. Comp.-Aid. Mol. Des.* **7,** 473–501.

15. Thomas, P. D. and Dill, K. A. (1996) Statistical potentials extracted from protein structures : how accurate are they? *J. Mol. Bio.* **257,** 457–469.

16. Charifson, P. S., Corkery, J. S., Murcko, M. A., and Walters, W. P. (1999) Consensus scoring: a method for obtaining improved hit rates from docking databases of three-dimensional structures into proteins. *J. Med. Chem.* **42,** 5100–5109.

17. Bissantz, C., Folkers, G., and Rognan, D. (2000). Protein-based virtual screening of chemical databases. 1. Evaluation of different docking/scoring combinations. *J. Med. Chem.* **43,** 4759–4767.

18. Stahl, M. and Rarey, M. (2001) Detailed analysis of scoring functions for virtual screening. *J. Med. Chem.* **44,** 1035–1042.

19

Prediction of Drug-Like Molecular Properties

Modeling Cytochrome P450 Interactions

**Mehran Jalaie, Rieko Arimoto, Eric Gifford,
Sabine Schefzick, and Chris L. Waller**

Abstract

Preventing drug–drug interactions and reducing drug-related mortalities dictate cleaner and costlier medicines. The cost to bring a new drug to market has increased dramatically over the last 10 years, with post-discovery activities (preclinical and clinical) costs representing the majority of the spend. With the ever-increasing scrutiny that new drug candidates undergo in the post-discovery assessment phases, there is increasing pressure on discovery to deliver higher-quality drug candidates. Given that compound attrition in the early clinical stages can often be attributed to metabolic liabilities, it has been of great interest lately to implement predictive measures of metabolic stability/ liability in the drug design stage of discovery. The solution to this issue is wrapped in understanding the basic of the cytochrome P450 (CYP) enzymes functions and structures. Recently, experimental information on the structure of a variety of cytochrome P450 enzymes, major contributors to phase I metabolism, has become readily available. This, coupled with the availability of experimental information on substrate specificities, has lead to the development of numerous computational models (macromolecular, pharmacophore, and structure–activity) for the rationalization and prediction of CYP liabilities. A comprehensive review of these models is presented in this chapter.

Key Words: CYP P450; cytochrome P450; docking; structure-based drug discovery; pharmacophore; QSAR; homology models; databases; computational models; ADME/T.

1. Introduction

The pharmaceutical industry is currently faced with pressures heretofore unimagined. The driving forces for change in the industry may be attributed to increases in generic competition due to legislative changes (e.g., Waxman–Hatch Act of 1984) and changes in the healthcare industry, in general. With a majority of the population electing healthcare coverage through managed care

From: *Methods in Molecular Biology, vol. 275:*
Chemoinformatics: Concepts, Methods, and Tools for Drug Discovery
Edited by: J. Bajorath © Humana Press Inc., Totowa, NJ

rather than fee-for-service providers, and the mission of managed health care providers to provide quality healthcare on a managed budget, the number of individuals switching to generic forms of drugs post-patent coverage has increased dramatically *(1)*.

With an average time of 10–15 yr to discover and fully develop a new compound at an cost estimated to be in excess of 800 million dollars *(2)*, pharmaceutical companies are employing various strategies in order extract all of the possible revenues from their investments. Revenues yielded from a newly patented drug must recover the costs associated with research and development, marketing, previous failures, and the pursuit of new research and make a profit. The decreases in return on investment (ROI) on first in class new chemical entities (NCEs) is driving the industry, as a whole, to seek solutions to minimize the time compounds spend in discovery by expediting or anticipating failures in the preclinical or clinical stages.

In the post-discovery stages, investigational new drugs fail primarily due to deficiencies in absorption, metabolism, toxicity, or efficacy. As a result, pharmaceutical companies are aggressively pursuing strategies to increase the preclinical attrition rate. Primary among these strategies is the implementation of computational techniques (i.e., *in silico* screening) with a goal to incorporate "drug-like" features into molecules as early in the process as possible and to minimize the presence of those properties with potential to be liabilities in post-discovery in vitro and in vivo assessments *(3)*.

With respect to the identification of potential metabolic liabilities, the cytochrome P450 (hereafter referred to as CYP) enzyme superfamily is considered to be a major contributor to the high attrition rate in drug development process that exists in the pharmaceutical industry given that they play a major role in phase I metabolism of pharmaceutical, and other exogenous, chemical compounds. Therefore, a thorough understanding of CYPs from the structural points of view would enhance our appreciation of their functions, and ultimately would provide the opportunity for delivering better and more effective medicine sooner to the patients.

Table 1, taken from Lewis et al. *(4)*, gives a good overview about typical substrates, inhibitors, inducers, and the most significant properties or substrate classes for each isozyme.

2. Structure-Based Design

2.1. Homology Models of Cytochrome P450 Enzymes

2.1.1. Introduction

The ideal strategy in drug development from the ADME perspective is the design of medicine with desired metabolic profiles, such as enzyme specificity

Table 1
Overview of Different P450 Isozymes, Their Inhibitors and Inducers *(4)*

CYP	Substrate classes	Typical substrates	Inhibitors	Inducers	Carcinogens activated
1A1	Planar polyaromatic hydrocarbons (PAHs)	Benzo[*a*]pyrene	1-Ethynyl pyrene	TCDD, PAHs	Many PAHs
1A2	Planar poly (hetero)-aromatic amines and amides	Caffeine	Furafulline	TCDD, PAHs	Many heterocyclic amines
2A	Small to medium molecular weight ketones	Coumarin	Metyrapone	Poorly induced	Aflatoxin B_1, NNK, Coumarin
2B	Non-planar lipophilic molecules usually with V-shaped geometries	Phenobarbital	Secobarbital	Phenobarbital	Tienilic acid
2C	Non-planar molecules usually with hydrogen bond potential	Tolbutamide	Sulfaphenazole	Poorly induced	NNK
2E	Small molecular weight compounds of diverse structures	p-Nitrophenol	Disulfiram	Ethanol	Many haloalkenes and haloalkanes nitrosamines, benzenes
3A	Large molecular weight compounds of diverse structures	Erythromycin	Gestodene	Synthetic steroids	Aflatoxin B_1, senecionine
4A	Long-chain carboxylic acids	Lauric acid	10-Undecynoic acid	Clofibrate	Inducers are usually peroxisome proliferators

and half-life, and/or inhibitory potency. Cytochrome P450 plays a major role in phase I metabolism of drugs, therefore, understanding the structural basis of the enzyme-substrate/inhibitor interactions for CYPs is an essential part of the drug discovery process. While direct determination of the structure for the protein–ligand complex is ideal, crystallizing membrane-bound proteins is known to be difficult. Drug-metabolizing human CYPs are embedded in the membrane of the endoplasmic reticulum, thus are called microsomal CYPs. Bacterial CYPs are soluble cytosolic proteins and high-resolution crystal structures are available for a number of isoenzymes, CYP101, 102, 107, 108, 111, 119,

121, 152, and 175 *(5)*. There is only one crystal structure available for mammalian enzyme, rabbit CYP2C5, in the public domain to date *(6)*. To obtain crystals suitable for an X-ray diffraction study, it was necessary to cleave the N-terminal membrane-anchor region and mutate several residues in order to make the protein more soluble. When direct structural determination methods are not readily applicable, homology modeling is an alternative way to estimate protein structure. In addition to visually appreciating the protein–ligand interactions, structural models of the protein are also useful for rationalizing the shifts in substrate selectivity, substrate preference, and/or catalytic activity due to amino acid substitutions. For instance, metabolic deficiency associated with genetic polymorphism or selectivity/preference within a subfamily (e.g., CYP2C) can be best studied with homology-based approach.

Since the first bacterial enzyme, CYP101, was crystallized in 1985 *(7,8)*, structural models of human CYPs have continuously been developed and utilized to rationalize the enzyme-substrate/inhibitor interactions. **Table 2** summarizes the modeling studies for major drug-metabolizing CYPs. Instead of describing the details of each previously reported model, this section will discuss the strategies of homology modeling specifically applied to CYPs, following the standard steps, (1) template selection, (2) sequence alignment, (3) 3D coordinate assignment, (4) structural refinement, and (5) model validation.

2.1.2. Template Selection

Homologous proteins of the CYP superfamily with known structure serve as the templates for homology modeling. The sequence similarities and/or identities between the template and target proteins should be as high as possible. Several search methods such as FASTA *(40)* or BLAST *(41)* are available to retrieve template homologs from the PDB (Protein Data Bank) *(42)*.

Table 3 lists CYP isoenzymes that have been used as templates for modeling human CYPs, including CYP101, 102, 107A1, 108, 55A1, and 2C3/5, and the major human drug-metabolizing enzymes, namely, CYP1A2, 2B6, 2C9, 2D6, and 3A4. The sequence identities in the table were calculated by an automated multiple sequence alignment program *(43)*. When the sequence identity between the target (human CYP) and the template, except for the CYP2 family, is less than 30%, it is very difficult to align sequences. It is generally thought that the models are not accurate with sequence identity of less than 25% because the alignment is so poor *(44)*. Therefore, improving the sequence alignment is critical to the development of reliable models. Using multiple templates is the most appropriate approach when there are several crystal structures of homologues available.

The CYP superfamily is a typical example where the three-dimensional structure is conserved to a much greater extent than the sequence. **Figure 1**

Table 2
Summary of CYP Homology Models

Target		Template	Author (reference)	Year
CYP 3A4	CYP 101		Ferenczy and Morris (9)	1989
2D6	101		Koymans et al. (10)	1993
2B1	101		Szklarz et al. (11)	1994
2A1,4,5,6	102		Lewis and Lake (12)	1995
2D6	101,102,108		de Groot et al. (13)	1996
2D6	101,102,108		Modi et al. (14)	
2E1	102		Tan et al. (15)	1997
2B4	101,102,107A1,108		Chang et al. (16)	
1A2	102		Lozano et al. (17)	
3A4	101,102,107A1,108		Szklarz and Halpert (18)	
2B1	101,102,108		Dai et al. (19)	1998
1A2			Dai et al. (20)	
1A2,6, 2B6, 2C9,19, 2D6, 2E1, 3A4	102		Lewis (21)	1999
4A1,4,11	102		Lewis and Lake (22)	
2C9	101,102,107A1,108		Payne et al. (23)	
2C18,19	101,102,107A1,108		Payne et al. (24)	
1A2, 2D6, 3A4	101,102,107A1,108		De Rienzo et al. (25)	2000
2C9	2C5		Afzelius et al. (26)	2001
2C8,9,18,19	2C5		Ridderstrom et al. (27)	
2B6	2C5		Bathelt et al. (28)	2002
2D6	2C5		Bapiro et al. (29)	
2A6, 2B6, 2C8,9,19, 2D6, 2E1	2C5		Lewis (30)	
2B4	2C5		Sechenykh et al. (31)	
1A1	2C5		Szklarz and Paulsen (32)	
2B6	2C5		Wang and Halpert (33)	
2C5	101,102,107A1,108, 55A1		Kirton et al. (34)	
2D6	101,102,107A1,108, 2C5		Kirton et al. (35)	
2D2,6	2C5		Venhorst et al. (36)	2003
2E1	2C5		Lewis et al. (37)	
2A6			Lewis et al. (38)	
2B6, 2C8,9,19, 2D6			Lewis (39)	

shows three crystal structures—CYP102 (PDB code: 1JPZ) (45), CYP107A1 (1JIP) (46), and CYP2C5 (1DT6) (6)—structurally aligned (47). The 3D structure, particularly the core, is well conserved, whereas the sequence identity is not greater than 15% for any pair of the three structures. The overall fold of

Table 3
**Sequence Identity (%) Among Isoenzymes Commonly
Used as Template Structures for Homology Modeling
and Major Human CYPs Calculated by Clustal W *(43)***

CYP	101 (cam)	102 (BM-3)	107A (eryF)	108 (terp)	55A1 (Nor)	2C3/5
101	100%					
102	10	100				
107A1	17	**12**	100			
108	24	15	21	100		
55A1	19	8	29	25	100	
2C3/5	13	**15**	**15**	14	8	100
1A2	11	14	9	13	14	28
2B6	6	13	13	12	11	48
2C9	14	14	14	14	9	74
2D6	13	14	13	10	14	39
3A4	12	22	16	12	14	19

Pairs in Figure 1 are in bold.

CYP consists of 13 alpha helices (A, B, B′, and C–L) and five beta-sheets. The C-terminal half is alpha-helix-rich, and the N-terminal half is beta-sheet-rich. The heme group is placed between them. The region surrounding the heme group, helices I and L and heme-binding Cys, is highly conserved *(48,49)*. A number of sequence analyses and the structure of the mammalian enzyme (CYP2C5) support that these structural elements are present in human CYPs as well *(6,50–53)*. In addition, microsomal CYPs have the N-terminal membrane-anchor region and an insertion in the F-G loop, though the CYP2C5 structure is missing both regions. It has been suggested that the F-G loop is also inter-acting with the membrane *(48)*. With the overall fold being well defined, con-structing valid models is quite feasible, if the target sequence is correctly aligned to the template.

Template selections are certainly limited by the availability of the crystal structure. The first crystal structure was solved for CYP101 *(54)*, and the active site of CYP3A4 *(9)*, CYP2D6 *(10)*, and CYP2B1 *(11)* were modeled using the single template of CYP101. Until the structure of CYP2C5 was solved, selections had been among the cytosolic CYPs that are genetically very distant from the human-microsomal CYPs. The primary choice was CYP102, as it was the only class II enzyme (same functional class as microsomal CYPs) with known structure, and usually the one with highest sequence similarity to the

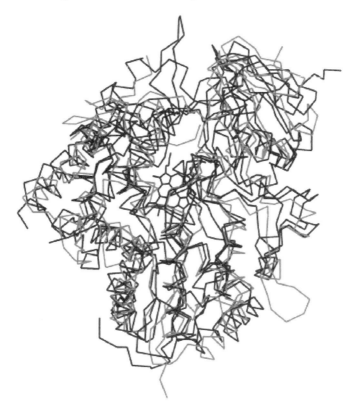

Fig. 1. Crystal structures of CYP2C5 (gray), CYP102, and CYP107A1 are overlapped. The PDB codes are 1dt6, 1jpz, and 1jip, respectively.

target. The CYP102 structure was used as the single template to model CYP1A *(17,21)*, CYP2A *(12)*, 2B *(21)*, 2C *(21)*, 2D *(21)*, 2E *(15,21)*, 3A *(21)*, and 4A *(22)*. Owing to the low confidence in the sequence alignment, using multiple templates was the most common strategy employed in these studies. The structures of CYP101, 102, and 108 *(13,14,20)*, and 107A1 were often included as well *(16,18,24,25)*. Kirton and coworkers experimentally constructed homology models of CYP2C5 using a single template of CYP102 and the multiple templates of CYP101, 102, 107A1, 108, and 55A1. The models were then compared with the crystal structure of CYP2C5. The results indicated that using a single template created a structure too similar to the template, whereas using multiple templates generated a more accurate structure *(34)*. The benefits of using multiple templates were evident when modeling had to rely on the homologs with low sequence identity. This study also demonstrated that a reasonable homology model could be built when sequence alignment was carefully optimized. The RMSD between all the Cα atoms in the best model and those in the 2C5 crystal structure was 4.7 Å. This was, in fact, "the best expected" homology model with such low sequence identity according to the statistics from CASP3 (Critical Assessment of Techniques for Protein Structure Prediction) meeting *(55)*. Since the structure of CYP2C5 was solved *(6)*, the modeling efforts have been mainly focused on the CYP2 family using a single template of CYP2C5 *(26–28,30,33,36,38,39)*. Although it is clear that CYP2C5 is the closest homolog to the human CYPs, using multiple templates can still be beneficial to modeling certain isoenzymes, particularly those with relatively low sequence identity with CYP2C5, e.g., CYP3A4. For modeling CYP2D6 (40% identity with 2C5), using a multiple templates (CYP101, 102, 107A1, 108, and 2C5) yielded a better structure in terms of mainchain stereochemistry and amino acid environment, compared to the model based only on CYP2C5 structure *(35)*. Interestingly, the 2C5-single-template model was better than the four-bacterial-template model with respect to the same structural criteria, thus indicating the limitation of homology modeling based on low sequence identities (approx 15% for CYP2D6/bacterial template). The model was improved by adding the bacterial sequences probably because that there were regions where using one of the bacterial CYPs as template was more appropriate.

2.1.3. Sequence Alignment

Before attempting to align the target sequence, the alignment among the template sequences must first be optimized. Because the sequence identities among the template homologs are most likely to be quite low, the sequences should be aligned based on structural elements. Automated sequence alignment methods that optimize sequence overlaps misplaced some of the structurally conserved regions when applied to CYP101, 102, and 108 sequences *(53)*. Structural alignment routines are available in various molecular modeling software packages, such as INSIGHT II and QUANTA (Accelrys, San Diego, CA). The web-based program Dali *(56)* performs multiple structural alignments of the submitted protein with its homologs found in PDB. The HOMSTRAD database *(47)* stores aligned homologs, including 12 crystal structures of CYPs. Once the alignment among the template sequences is optimized, the target sequence is aligned against the template. The alignment of the template should be fixed and treated as a profile. One can start with an automated alignment, but manual adjustment with additional information is absolutely necessary. The estimated secondary structure for the target sequence is most appropriate for the manual adjustment. Several methods such as PSIPRED *(57)* and PHD *(58)* are available for secondary structure prediction from the amino acid sequence. The sequence alignment is manually adjusted by placing the corresponding element (α-helices and β-sheets) with the template structures.

There are three highly conserved regions throughout the CYP superfamily that can be used to guide the sequence alignment: (1) (A/G)Gx(D/E)T in helix I; terminal Thr forms enzyme's oxygen binding pocket *(54)*; (2) a charge pair of ExxR in helix K (no substitution is tolerated); and (3) FxxGxxxCxG in helix L; forms the heme binding loop with Cys coordinating as the fifth ligand of the heme *(5)*. In addition, PGP in the N-terminal is highly conserved in mammalian CYPs, as well as W (H is often found in bacterial CYPs)xxxR in helix C. To further improve the alignment, multiple sequences of CYPs from the family or subfamily to which the target CYP belongs can be included into the multiple sequence alignment *(16)*. Highlighting the conserved regions becomes less ambiguous with multiple sequences as seen in the modeling study of CYP2 family *(12,27,30)*. Six substrate-recognition sites (SRS), referred as SRS1–SRS6, were proposed by sequence alignment of 10 CYP2 family enzymes with CYP101 *(50)*, and this definition is widely used to determine the active site.

Experimental data, such as site-directed mutation *(59,60)* and/or photolabeling *(61)*, can be incorporated into the sequence alignment process. Amino acid residues whose mutations significantly alter the enzyme activity are more likely to be within one of the substrate recognition sites. In a photolabeling experiment, the ligand is a photoaffinity probe that labels its nearby residue, thus identifying the amino acid residue located within the ligand-binding site. Mutation data have to be examined carefully because residues outside of the active site can still affect the enzyme's activity indirectly. In general, a mutagenesis study cannot differentiate direct and indirect interactions.

2.1.4. Assigning Coordinates

Once the sequence alignment is optimized, the 3D coordinates are assigned to the target sequence. The structure of the target can be constructed based on the weighted average of the templates *(11,18)*, regions from one of the homologs that are most similar to the target *(13,23,62)*, or based on spatial restraints *(63)* derived from the alignment *(14,25,34)*. The methods to be used vary among the modeling software packages. Dai and coworkers constructed homology models of CYP1A2 using QUANTA and LOOK (Molecular Application Group, Palo Alto, CA) and concluded that the difference was not critical *(20)*. The quality of the model relies most heavily on the sequence alignment used.

Experimental data imposing topological constraints can be incorporated in this step. For example, the paramagnetic relaxation effect by the heme-iron on the nuclear magnetic resonance (NMR) spectrum of the substrate provided distance constraints between the iron and substrate protons for modeling CYP2D6/codeine complex *(14)*. Antonovic and coworkers designed photoaffinity probes that coordinated with the heme-iron on one side and labeled the nearby residue in the binding site on the other side, to identify amino acid residues within a certain distance (limited by the probe length) from the heme-iron *(64)*. Several other NMR studies *(65–68)* and photolabeling studies *(61,69,70)* have investigated the topological features in the active sites of various CYPs.

Assigning the coordinates to the conserved region is relatively straightforward; however, there are known "problem regions" in the CYP structure. The N-terminal membrane-anchor is absent in the bacterial CYPs (and removed from 2C5), however, this region is unlikely to participate in the interaction with the substrate/inhibitor so the structure is not so critical. The B′ region is very diverse in amino acid sequence as well as in length *(53)* among all isoenzymes. In bacterial CYPs, the F-G loop has high B-factors compared to the rest of the structure, indicating that this region is inherently flexible. Mammalian CYPs have an insertion in F-G loop, although not resolved in the 2C5 crystal. This extended F-G loop is thought to interact with the membrane and guide hydrophobic substrates into the binding site *(48)*. In modeling CYP2B6, the F-G loop was restored, based on the CYP102 structure, to complete the CYP2C5 structure *(28)* to be used as the template. For regions where no template atoms exist, adopting an extended conformation or searching in a fragment database for loops in other proteins, are the common approaches. To avoid insertions of such loops, unnecessary gaps must be eliminated in the sequence alignment step.

2.1.5. Refinement

The initial structure is then energy minimized. A molecular dynamics simulation is often performed in order to sample larger conformational space and to assess the stability of the resultant models. Several studies have suggested that the addition of water molecules into the binding site is necessary in order to preserve the structure of the active site *(11,45,62,71)*. The structure of the binding site could be distorted by false interactions among residues surrounding the binding pocket. Water molecules often stabilize the local regions by hydrogen bonding to the protein backbone. Water can be incorporated into the system by soaking the protein *(11,62,71)* and allowing the water molecules penetrate into the binding site in the course of molecular dynamics simulation. Although this approach allows the system to equilibrate, it is computationally demanding. Gorokhov and coworkers reported that four water molecules were detected in the interior of substrate-free CYP2A4 at the end of the 3 ns simulation in solution *(71)*. Alternatively, water molecules can be added into the binding site in a way that the local hydrogen bonding and steric interaction are optimized *(72)*.

2.1.6. Model Validation

The resultant model is subjected to validation, in purely structural and biological aspects. For stereochemical quality, PROCHECK *(73)*, PROVE *(74)*, and WhatIf *(75)* are among the widely used programs. Programs such as Errat

(76) or Verify3D *(77)* can examine the side chain environment of the models. This process determines if the structural properties of the computer-generated model are consistent with naturally occurring proteins, i.e., well-defined crystal structures.

In order to evaluate models in the biological context, known substrates may be docked into the modeled binding site. Interactions with the active site, such as number of hydrogen bonds, electrostatic interaction, and hydrophobic interaction, are compared with the observed substrate specificity and stereoselectivity. If the model is valid, its binding site should be able to accommodate the known substrates in the correct orientation, and the interaction energy with a range of substrates should correlate the binding affinities. The dockings can be guided by the crystal structures of CYP–substrate complexes *(45,46,54,78)* or by placing the reaction site [known or predicted *(79)*] in proximity to the catalytic heme-iron center. Most homology models, if not all, have been presented with the known substrate(s) docked into the active site to demonstrate that they can rationalize the experimental data. Although it is known that conformational changes often occur upon substrate binding *(45,80)*, it is usually not considered in the docking studies. This implies that the model is not necessarily disproved even if a known substrate does not fit into the binding site.

The effects of amino acid mutation on the substrate selectivity, preferences, and/or catalytic activity can be also used for testing the models. Mutants Ile477Ala, Ile480Ala, and Leu209Ala of CYP2B6 *(11)* and Leu362Ile and Leu362Ala of CYP2C9 *(26)* were predicted to impact the substrate binding by the homology models. These mutants were constructed and tested to confirm the validity of the models *(26,60)*. Valid models of the polymorphic CYPs, CYP2D6 and CYP2C19, are expected to rationalize the metabolic deficiencies caused by the certain alleles.

Finally, direct determinations of substrate orientation and distances between certain atoms by NMR or photolabeling experiments *(14,64)* provide invaluable information, and incorporating these measurements greatly improves the accuracy of the homology models.

2.2. Docking

In this section, we will examine docking methods as tools to probe the relation between structures and functions of the CYPs.

Alexlord and Brodie et al. were the first to distinguish the cytochrome P450 enzyme system in endoplasmic reticulum *(81,82)*. Subsequently, Garfinkel and Klingenberg identified CYP450 after realizing that the cytochrome P450–CO complex had a maximum absorption at 450 nm *(83,84)*. Since the early days of P450 discovery, several crystal structures of P450 have been solved *(54,80,86–91)*, but the first crystal structure dates back to 1985 (bacterial P450cam, CYP101) *(7,8)*.

Despite the availability of various spectroscopic techniques in determining CYP structures *(92–112)*, X-ray crystallography is considered to be the most reliable and realistic approach in depicting the 3D structure of any protein or enzyme system, and the CYP systems are no exception to this point of view. The X-ray structure can be thought of as a static snapshot of a very fluid system. That is, X-ray is our only way to provide the visual insight into capturing structures at the atomic level. The function of individual CYPs highlights the importance of their structures.; however, elucidating the structures for CYPs has been very challenging across the species, particularly for the mammalian enzyme. This difficulty in structural determination arises from the low solubility of the CYPs. CYP101-P450cam was the first structure to be determined, which led to solving several bacterial CYP structures. A major milestone was achieved with the crystallization of mammalian CYP2C5 *(80)*. In summary, solved crystal structures are publicly available for the bacterial (CYP101-P450cam, CYP102-P450BM3, CYP108-P450eryF), fungal (CYP55-P450nor), and rabbit (CYP2C5) isofoms *(85,80,86–88,91,113)*. Recently, Astex Technology determined the 3D crystal structure of two human CYPs, namely, CYP3A4 (October 2002) and CYP2C9 (December 2001) *(114)*.

Molecular recognition is the language of the cellular and the biochemical world *(115)*. The molecular recognition process typically involves binding of a ligand into a protein receptor. This event ultimately relies on the properties of the participants. In other words, "it takes two to Tango": the two partners define the interacting functional groups on the ligand and the receptors. The very specific interactions that define the recognition process can be viewed either as electronic or steric interactions *(116)*. Knowing the 3D structure of the target protein at the atomic level of detail is critical for structure-based drug design (SBDD). The SBDD approach provides a means for the design of a new molecule (*de novo* design, see the cross-methods portion of this review) or for the ability to search for bioactive compounds electronically (virtual screening). In order to utilize the available crystal structures for drug design, computational tools, namely docking, have been developed for generating the orientation of a drug (ligand) to its protein with a known 3D structure. The most fundamental docking algorithms treat molecules as rigid bodies and only explore the translational and rotational space of the molecules with respect to the binding domain of the receptor *(117)*. Simplifications are made by most docking programs in keeping the receptor molecule rigid and only allowing the conformational space of the ligand molecule to be realized *(115–122)*.

Therefore, the structures of CYPs along with all the existing homology models of the corresponding templates (please refer to the homology section in this chapter) provide the very basic information for examining CYPs from the docking point of view. Several heroic attempts have been made to use the structural information, by using docking techniques, to predict the binding of various molecules (inhibitors and substrates) in the CYPs active site *(32)*. Lewis et al. extracted a pharmacophore based on docking of a series of substrates to a homology model of CYP2A *(123)*. The specificity of various CYPs (1A2, 1A1, 2B6, 3A4) based on docking into the homology models constructed based on the bacterial structure of CYP102 *(124)* was also explored. Additional docking studies have been performed by Lewis et al. by using homology models of several CYP isoforms in conjugation with NMR paramagnetic shift measurements *(125)*. It is, however, the docking procedure described by Lewis et al. and others *(20,126–129)* that is very unclear and biased to a predetermined binding orientation of molecules of interest. Szklarz et al. used the combination of manual docking and MD methods to explore the homology model of human CYP1A1 *(18,32)*. Additionally, Szklarz and co-workers applied the same docking method to a homology construct of CYP3A4 and identified key residues in the active site that would not have been recognized without the docking investigation *(18)*. It was concluded that docking the substrate into the active site of the CYP1A1 model revealed several important residues that could be potential sites for further verification by site-directed mutagenesis. They further claimed that the binding constants of several substrates agreed with the experimental values *(18,130)*. Bathelt et al. used similar approach in determining the regioselectivity of CYP2B6 based on a limited number of residues at the binding pocket *(28)*. Docking a series of progesterone derivatives into the homology model of CYP2B1 has also illustrated the regioselectivity of CYP2B1 vs CYP2C5. Earlier docking studies using a CYP2B1 model provided explanations on regio- and stereospecificty of steroid hydroxylation *(11,60)*. Moreover, the docking of alkoxycoumarins into the active site of a CYP2B1 model validated the role of several residues studied by mutagenesis in substrate dealkylation *(131)*.

The mammalian crystal structure has proven to be very useful in docking studies. Spatzenegger and co-workers demonstrated that the differences in inhibitory functions between CYP2B4 and CYP2B5 are caused by both the inhibitor–residue contacts and residue–residue interactions *(132)*. In another situation, docking of 14 azole antifungal inhibitors indicated a similar binding mode toward CYP51, and the major interactions between the active site residues and the inhibitors were correctly identified *(133)*. Jones and his colleagues found the docking results of a terfenadine into the homology model of CYP2D6 (Modi et al.) substantiated the behavior of terfenadine as an inhibitor of CYP2D6 *(14,134)*.

De Voss et al. pioneered docking studies on bacterial CYP101 and its mutant. In this investigation of 16 potential substrates for CYP101, 15 (94%) compounds were predicted in accordance with the experimental data. The results are based on a modification to DOCK's *(135)* parameters to allow for

2.9 Å minimum contact distance: a minimum degree of freedom of motion is required for substrate positioning and function *(136,137)*. Zhang et al., however, used DOCK for determining potential ligands and substrates for the P450cam enzyme. In this study, the DOCK program was used to screen a library of 20,000 compounds from which initially 16 (and additional 10) candidates were selected. In order to have the highest predictivity for this set, it was recommended to use a minimum contact distance of 2.7 Å between the substrate and the active site atoms. Using this approach, it was possible to distinguish substrates from non-substrates *(136)*. CYPs 1A2, 2D6, and 3A4 were explored through rigid and flexible docking by DOCK, and special insight was provided for substrate specificity of each isoform *(25)*. Kollman's group also used DOCK in metabolic studies involving CYP3A4 *(138)*. They investigated the regiospecificites of sirolimus and everolimus using docking in combination with molecular dynamics (MD) and quantum mechanics (QM) calculations, and the qualitative results were in agreement to the experiments *(138)*.

Since the early days of the structure-based approaches to CYP modeling, a combination of pharmacophore and 3D structures have been implemented by using docking models *(17,139)*. Wang and Halpert *(33)* identified the complementarily of the pharmacophore, constructed from a set of CYP2B6 substrates, to the homology model of CYP2B6 based on the docking results. Thus, the lack of structural information was well complemented by the presence of the pharmacophore model. A similar docking investigation was performed on the homology models of the CYP2Cs, and the outcome indicated an agreement between the docking and the pharmacophore model in rationalizing the structure-based selectivity *(27)*. Anandatheerthavarada et al. performed docking to demonstrate that adrenodoxin and CYP P450 reductase (CPR) binds in a non-overlapping fashion to the same domain of P4540MT2 with different orientations, but CPR and bacterial flavodoxin compete for the same binding pocket *(140)*.

Other groups have used the docking approaches as a way of aligning molecules for creating 3D-QSAR models for specific CYPs *(26,141)*. For example, Afzelius et al. used GOLD *(142,143)* as a docking tool to select an appropriate alignment for a set of 29 of ligands bound to the 2C9 homology model (based on the 2C5 template) *(26)*. CYP2C8 has also been examined by GOLD *(144)*. The docking of amodiaquine into the active site of several CYP2C isoform models confirmed the experimental evidence of the specificity of 2C8 toward the metabolism of amodiaquine *(144)*. Docking approaches to 3D-QSAR could be a viable method to augment homology models *(144)*. Masimirebwa and colleagues used GOLD *(142,143)* to generate several conformations for further 3D-QSAR modeling using ALMOND *(145)* and GOLPE *(146)*. The resultant models expressed reasonable statistics ($q^2 = 0.58$ and $q^2 = 0.73$) *(126,147,148)*. See the QSAR section of this chapter for a more-detailed discussion.

Kirton reveals the Glu216 in CYP2D6 to be a major player in binding of basic substrates and Asp301 participates in positioning of the B'-C loop *(35)*. Park and Harris used AutoDock2.1's potential function along with the Larmarkian genetic algorithm available in AutoDock3.0 for docking a series of substrates *(120,149)*. They suggested that energy-based docking could be used as a screening tool for the initial determination of the site of metabolism in CYP2E1. When the initial docking orientations were refined with MD simulations, reasonable complexes in agreement with experiments were found *(149)*. Williams et al. were successful in verifying the contact residues around progesterone by docking progesterone into the active site of 2C5 using AutoDock *(6,59)*. As docking and homology techniques advance, the determination of specific residue functions in the active site will become more accurate. A very interesting study was performed by Keresu to initially validate FlexX and CScore for several available crystal structures of P450cam. The best combination of scores was reported to be docking with FlexX and scoring with the PMF/GOLD scoring functions. When this set up was exercised in a virtual screening experiment involving CYP3A4, the success rate in correctly classifying compounds was 344 out of 345 compounds *(150)*. However, Keresu's docking and scoring approach to CYPs is innovating in embracing structure-based virtual screening methods against CYPs.

Most docking efforts in the literature have been complementary to other methods with respect to understanding or rationalizing the behavior of certain substrates or inhibitors of cytochrome P450s (**Table 4**). Indeed, there have been several success stories and instances where a docking approach played an instrumental role in explaining the metabolic behavior of a certain CYP. It is, however, very premature to rely solely on docking techniques for understanding and predicting the interactions of unknown chemicals to any of the CYP isoforms. It is fair to mention that the limitations of docking technology, the shortcoming in structural information, and the errors associated with homology models make docking approaches to metabolism less reliable. As more mammalian, and specifically human, CYP structures become available, docking approaches will find their ways into the mainstream computational tactics for answering metabolism questions in the context of drug discovery.

3. Ligand-Based Design

3.1. Pharmacophore Models for CYPs

3.1.1. Introduction

Although little structural information is available for the CYP enzymes, the amount of experimental data on the substrates and inhibitors is growing rapidly. As a result, ligand-based analyses, quantitative structure-activity relationship

Table 4
A Collection of Docking Efforts Reported in the Literature

Docking method	Template X-ray	Human homology model	Group/year
AutoDock *(123)*	2C5 (3LVdH)	—	Williams et al. 2000 *(6)*
AutoDock3.0/MD	2C5 (3LVdH) and Bacterial P450	2E1	Park and Harris 2003 *(149)*
AutoDock	P450-BM3	Pharmacophore and 3D model of 1A2	Lozano and Lopez et al. 1997 and 2000 *(17,139, 148)*
DOCK3.0	CYP101 bacterial	L244 mutant	De Voss et al. 1995 and 1997 *(136,137)*
DOCK3.5	P450cam bacterial	—	Zhang et al. 1997, 1998 *(136,151)*
DOCK3.5	P450 terp, P450 eryF, P450 cam, P450 BM3	1A2, 2D6, 3A4	De Rienzo et al. 2000 *(25)*
DOCK4.01	P450 Bacterial	3A4 reported by Szklarz et al. *(32, 134)*	Kohn et al. 2001 *(138)*
FlexX/Cscore *(125,163)*	P450cam (1akd, 1phd, 1phe, 1phf, 1phg, 2cpp, 4cpp, 5cpp, 6cpp, 7cpp, 8cpp)	—	Keresu 2001 *(150)*
GOLD *(124)*	2C5	2C9	Afzelius et al. 2001 *(26)*
GOLD	2C5	2C8, 2C9, 2C18, 2C19	Ridderstrom et al. 2001 *(27)*
GOLD	2C5	2C9	Masimirebwa et al. 2002 *(147)*
GOLD	2C5 and P450 terp, P450 eryF, P450 cam, P450 BM3	2D6	Kirton et al. 2002 *(35)*
GOLD	2C5	2C8	Li et al. 2002 *(144)*
InsightII/docking	2C5	2B4, 2B5, 2B1	Spatzengger et al. 2000 *(132)*
InsightII/Affinity	2C5	2B6	Wang and Halpert 2001 *(33)*
InsightII/MD	2C5	2B1	Kumar et al. 2003 *(153)*
Manual docking /MD	2C5 (1dt6)	1A1	Szklarz et al. 2002 *(18,32)* and others *(20)*
Manual docking /MD	P450 Bacterial	3A4	Szklarz et al. 1997 *(18,32)*
Manual docking /MD	P450cam	2B1, 3A4	Szklarz et al. 1998 *(130)* and others *(19,154)*
Manual docking	P450cam	2B1	Szklarz et al. 1994, 1995 *(11,60,155)*

Table 4 *(continued)*

Docking method	Template X-ray	Human homology model	Group/year
Manual docking	P4502C17, BM3 and others *(148)*	P450MT2, Fln, CPR	Anandatheerthavarada et al. 2001 *(140)*
Manual docking /MD	2C5 and CYP BM3	2B6	Bathelt et al. 2002 *(28)*
Manual docking/MD	P450s (BM3, cam, terp, and eryF)	CYP51 (P45014DM)	Haitao et al. 2000 *(133)*
Manual docking	CYP102 bacterial	1A2, 1A1, 2B1, · 3A4	Lewis et al. 1995 *(124)*
Manual docking	P450cam	2B1	Kobayashi et al. 1998 *(131)*
Manual docking	P450terp, P450cam, P450BM3 *(140)*	2D6	Jones et al. 1998 *(134)*
Manual docking	102	2A6 human	Lewis et al. 1999 *(123)*
Manual docking /NMR	102(1fag)	1A2, 2A6, 2B6, 2C9, 2D6, 2E1, 3A4	Lewis et al. 1999 *(125)*

(QSAR), and pharmacophore modeling have been widely used to find structural features capable of explaining various interactions with CYPs, e.g., binding, inhibition, and CYP selectivity. In general terms, pharmacophore models represent the three-dimensional arrangement of the functional groups and/or features of the ligand that are recognized by the receptor. Pharmacophores can be constructed without knowledge of the binding site, assuming that the ligands share a common mechanism for the biological activity (i.e., binding to the same site in the same mode). The pharmacophore approach has been applied to CYP inducers as well as substrates/inhibitors. This section summarizes the pharmacophore models currently available for the major human drug-metabolizing enzymes, CYP1A2, 2A6, 2B6, 2C9, 2C19, 2D6, and 3A.

3.1.2. CYP1A2

The substrates for CYP1A family were characterized as lipophilic planar poly- or heteroaromatic molecules possessing a large area-to-depth ratio *(156,157)*. A theoretical model was proposed by studying the caffeine N-demethylation by CYP1A2 and inhibition of this metabolic reaction by other xanthine derivatives *(158)*. The minima of molecular electrostatic potential (MEP) distribution formed a triangular pattern in the xanthine plane, and the site of metabolism was located at a distance of approx 3 Å from the MEP minimum. This result suggested that three hydrogen bond donor sites exist within the active site of CYP1A2. The first pharmacophore model was generated by a study of inhibitory potency of caffeine N-demethylation for a series of quinolone antibacterial agents *(159)*. The keto group, the carboxylate group, and the core nitrogen at position 1 were suggested to be important for binding to the active site of CYP1A2. For all competitive inhibitors, the MEP distribution over these regions was very similar to that of caffeine. A QSAR analysis of the inhibition of the caffeine N-demethylation for flavonoids led to the conclusion that the volume to surface area ratio was the most significant factor *(160)*, consistent with the previously defined planar characteristics. This study also reported a negative correlation between the number of free hydroxyl groups and the decrease of inhibitory potency by glycosylation of the free hydroxyls. Docking of 13 CYP1A2 substrates, both specific and nonspecific, into a homology model characterized the substrates as generally neutral with a molecular volume less than 200 Å^3, and a total interaction energy greater than −40 kcal/mol *(25)*.

3.1.3. CYP2A6

CYP2A6 is responsible for the majority of coumarin 7-hydroxylase and nicotine C-oxidase activity in hepatic tissue. Substrate selectivity of 2A6 and 2A5 (mouse enzyme) was studied using 23 lactone-containing compounds *(161)*. The properties near the lactone moiety and the size of the substitution in the 7-position of coumarin were shown to be important for inhibition of coumarin 7-hydroxylation catalyzed by CYP2A6 and 2A5. CYP2A5 can accommodate larger substitution on the coumarin ring system than CYP2A6. A homology model of CYP2A6 was generated based on the CYP102 crystal structure and 12 structurally diverse substrates were docked into the modeled active site *(123)*. The overlay of the docked substrates suggested the following features as the CYP2A6 selectivity template: (1) hydrogen bond acceptors located at around 6.8 and 5.0 Å from the preferred site of metabolism (potential donor residue: Thr212, Gln104 and Asn295), (2) aromatic ring of which its center located at about 4 Å from the oxidation site; and (3) the two hydrogen bond acceptor sites 2.5 Å apart from each other. These features characterize the inhibitors pilocarpine and 8-methoxypsoralen as well.

3.1.4. CYP2B6

CYP2B6 is known to metabolize several clinically important drugs, such as benzphetamine, cinnarizine, bupropion, verapamil and lidocaine. It is unclear, however, if CYP2B6 is the primary enzyme to metabolize those drugs. Lewis and coworkers presented a substrate template by superimposing 12 substrates that were docked into the binding site of the homology model of CYP2B6 *(162)*. Visual inspections of the overlaid ligands led to these general characteristics of CYP2B6 substrate: (1) medium-sized non-planar molecules with some displaying V-shaped geometries; (2) relatively hydrophobic character and usually possessing an aromatic ring; (3) hydrogen bond acceptor group close to the site of metabolism; and (4) a basic nitrogen atom close to the site of metabolism in some cases.

A 3D pharmacophore model was developed using Catalyst (Accelrys, San Diego, CA) for 21 substrates *(163)*. It comprised three hydrophobes and one hydrogen bond acceptor region. The three hydrophobic regions are located at 5.3, 3.1, and 4.6 Å from the hydrogen bond acceptor, and have intermediate angles of 72.8° and 67.6°. Along with the Catalyst model, a PLS analysis of MS-WHIM descriptors, global descriptors of molecular surface properties, was reported. In this model, size, positive electrostatic potential, hydrogen bonding acceptor capacity, and hydrophobicity were the important factors, consistent with the Catalyst model. Both approaches yielded statistically valid models.

A homology model of CYP2B6 based on the CYP2C5 crystal structure was combined with the pharmacophore approach in a recent study *(33)*. Pharmacophore models were re-derived using Catalyst for the same set of compounds used in the earlier study *(163)*. The substrates were overlaid by their reaction sites in this study. The resultant eight hypotheses were clustered into two groups corresponding to the structurally distinct compounds of the two lowest K_m, bezyloxyresorufin and 7-ethoxy-4-trifluoromethyl-coumarin (7-EFC). As Catalyst attempts to map all functions in a hypothesis to one of the two most active molecules, it generated two kinds of pharmacophores primary based on bezyloxyresorufin (1.3 μM) and 7-EFC (1.7 μM). Both models consisted of two hydrophobes and one hydrogen bond acceptor. Benzyloxyresorufin and 7-EFC were then docked into the binding site and the pharmacophores were found to complement the active site. Their locations slightly differed within the binding site indicating that two binding modes might exist. No hydrogen bonding from the docked substrate to the protein could be formed, suggesting a possible water bridging.

3.1.5. CYP2C9

This is the most highly expressed member of the CYP2C subfamily in hepatic tissues. It is a polymorphic enzyme, and is involved in the metabolism of a number of anti-inflammatory drugs.

By comparing activities of 10 tienilic acid derivatives, it was concluded that the presence of a negative charge on the substrate at physiological pH is very important not only for the catalytic activity but also for recognition of the enzyme *(164)*. This is supported by the fact that many of the CYP2C9 substrates are indeed negatively charged at pH 7.4 (pK_a below 7). Although there are neutral compounds that bind to the enzyme quite tightly, the anions generally bind even tighter *(165,166)*. A pharmacophore model was developed for three tienilic acid analogs and additional substrates. The crystal structures, when available, or energy-minimized structures of the 12 substrates were overlaid by their hydroxylation sites. Two rigid compounds, phenytoin and (S)-warfarin were used as the templates. This substrate superposition was supported by an NMR study measuring distances between the heme-iron and the substrate protons *(66)*. The model featured (1) anionic heteroatom (A⁻) at a distance of approx 4 Å from a hypothetical cationic site (C⁺) of the protein, (2) distance between the hydroxylation site (Hy) and the anionic site (A⁻) is 7.8 ± 1.6 Å, and (3) angle of 82 ± 15° between A⁻Hy and A⁻C⁺ *(164)*. This pharmacophore model was able to include a strong inhibitor of CYP2C9, sulfaphenazole *(167)*. The anionic site (A⁻) of this molecule was the SO_2N^- group, and the aniline nitrogen interacts with heme-iron resulting a strong binding. The *N*-phenyl group of sulfaphenazole was well located in the hydrophobic region of their previous model *(164)*. Therefore, the hydrophobic feature was added to the model.

Instead of the cation–anion interaction, hydrogen bonding was used to develop a pharmacophore model of CYP2C9 *(168)*. Eight substrates and an inhibitor, sulfaphenazole, were overlaid by their hydroxylation sites using phenytoin as the template. The resultant pharmacophore consisted of the hydroxylation site (Hy), hydrogen bond donor heteroatom (D) located at a distance of 6.7 ± 1.0 Å, and the angle between Hy-D and the hydrogen bond of 133 ± 21°, implying a larger binding site.

Jones and coworkers studied the structure–activity relationship of CYP2C9 using 27 coumarin ring–containing compounds with inhibitory potency of (S)-warfarin 7-hydroxylation *(169)*. A hypothetical active site was constructed based on the crystal structure of CYP101 and the alignment of the coumarin compounds. The predicted protein–ligand interaction included two electrostatic interactions arising from anionic sites of the substrate, a steric interaction involving I helix, and an aromatic binding (π-stacking). An analysis of the combined pharmacophore-homology model for CYP2C9 identified Phe110 and Phe114 as potential π-stacking site. Introducing mutations of Phe110Leu, Phe110Tyr, Val113Leu, and Phe114Leu, they proved that Val113 and Phe114 were indeed in the hydrophobic interaction site *(170)*. The pharmacophore was further refined with additional 14 compounds *(171)*. From the resultant combined model, Arg105 was predicted to be the anionic interaction site and the carboxyl oxygen at the C-2 position of coumarin was likely to interact with Asp293. A mutation study indicated, however, that Arg105 was not important for the enzyme activity *(172)*. Instead, mutations of Arg97Ala and Arg108Ala showed significantly lower activity with diclofenac compared to the wild-type enzyme.

3D pharmacophore models for competitive inhibitors of CYP2C9 were built using Catalyst *(173)*. Three different metabolic reactions, diclofenac 4′-hydroxylation, (S)-warfarin 7-hydroxylation, and tolbutamide 4-hydroxylation, were considered. The general characteristics of the three models were similar with distances between a hydrogen bond acceptor and a second hydrogen bond acceptor/donor being 3.4–5.7 Å and the hydrophobic feature was positioned 3–5.8 Å from the hydrogen bond acceptor. The models were consistent with the previous study *(171)*.

A homology model of CYP2C9 based on the crystal structure of CYP2C5 was used to derive the structure–activity relationship for 21 structurally diverse, competitive inhibitors *(26)*. The compounds were docked into the binding site in order to generate initial conformers to be analyzed. The docked protein–ligand complexes identified a number of residues within the substrate recognition site (SRS) 1, 2, 4, 5, and 6 *(50)* including Val113 and Phe114, the sites previously proposed by others *(170,171)*. Two of the predicted interaction sites, Leu102 and Leu362, were confirmed by mutation studies *(27,172)*. The active site of the CYP2C9 homology model was also used to represent the envelope of the substrate/inhibitor. Such "inverse pharmacophore" generated with the GRID interaction field was able to accommodate diclofenac docked into the active site *(27)*. Another study described the use of alignment independent molecular descriptors from GRIND *(174)* for a pharmacophore model generation *(175)*. The GRIND descriptors represent important GRID-interactions as a function of the distance instead of the actual positions. The resultant model is not as visually interpretable as the standard pharmacophore models, but it comprises the spatial arrangement of the potential interaction regions.

Another combined model was developed for 16 substrates *(176)*. In this study, the pharmacophore model and the CYP2C5-based homology model were developed independently. Sixteen substrates were overlaid based on the oxidation site, hydrogen bond donor/acceptor, and hydrophobic/aromatic group, using 58C80 as the template. The pharmacophore (overlaid substrates) was able to fit into the active site of the homology model without steric clash, implying a large degree of complementarity. The combined model indicated that two amino acid residues, Arg108 and Phe476, were important for substrate binding. The acidic or hydrogen bond accepting group was shown to be interacts with Arg108, consistent with the mutation study *(172)*. The aromatic moieties within the substrates were placed to form a π-stacking interaction with Phe476. Although some large compounds could interact with Phe114, the model showed that Phe114 was partially shielded by the side chain of Arg108; therefore, the authors suggested that role of Phe114 was to stabilize the other critical interaction rather than directly interacting with the substrate.

3.1.6. CYP2C19

This isoenzyme is well known by the (S)-mephenytoin 4′-hydroxylase polymorphism. CYP2C19 shares 97% of amino acids with CYP2C9. In the active site region, only three conservative changes of amino acids are present. Comparison between the homology models of CYP2C9 and CYP2C19 indicated that the selectivity arises from the substrate access channel rather than interactions in the binding site. The proposed access channel between the F-G loop and B′ helix was negatively charged in CYP19, but not in CYP2C9. Therefore, negatively charged molecules would be repelled and cannot reach the active site *(176)*.

3.1.7. CYP2D6

CYP2D6 is the most-studied polymorphic enzyme due to its significant clinical relevance. It metabolizes a number of cardiovascular drugs, beta-adrenergic blocking agents, tricyclic antidepressants, and others. The first attempt to characterize the CYP2D6 (debrisoquine 4-hydroxylase) substrates identified the distance between the basic nitrogen and the site of oxidation to be approx 5 Å for 11 substrates *(177)*. Furthermore, all substrates had a hydrophobic domain near the oxidation site and a carboxylate group on the protein was suggested to interact with the basic nitrogen atom of the substrate. Meyer and coworkers studied substrates that were known to be affected by the CYP2D6 polymorphism. The common features for the substrates were lipophilic domain and basic nitrogen, same as previously reported *(177)*. The distance between the basic nitrogen and the reaction site was 7 Å for dextromethorphan O-demethylation and bufuralol 1′ hydroxylation and overlaid structures highlighted that the aromatic rings were nearly co-planar. In addition, the same distance (7 Å) was observed for a number of other substrates but this model could not explain the debrisoquine 4-hydroxylation *(178)*.

A pharmacophore model was generated by manually superposing the metabolic sites of 13 known substrates using debrisoquine as the template *(179)*. The heme group was included based on the crystal structure of CYP101/camphor complex. The distance between the basic nitrogen atom and the hypothetical anion location lies within 2.5 – 4.5 Å. The intramolecular distance between the metabolic sites and the basic nitrogen had a large range of 4.5–8 Å, thus questioning the previous studies suggesting 5 Å or 7 Å.

Koymans et al. argued that this 2 Å difference could be explained by the interaction to one or other oxygen atom of the same carboxylate group (the distance between the two oxygen atoms in a carboxylate is about 2.2 Å) *(180)*. The structural features found for 16 substrates and 23 metabolic reactions were in good agreement with the previous models. All substrates exhibit a coplanar conformation near the oxidation site and have negative molecular electrostatic potentials in a part of this planar domain, induced by a π-system, an oxygen atom, or a nitrogen atom, approx 3 Å away from the oxidation site. This model was able to correctly predict 13 out of 14 oxidative metabolic routes for 4 compounds, and 2 out of 3 metabolites for GBR12909 *(181)*. To complement the substrate model, homology modeling based on CYP101, 102, and 108 was carried out *(13)*. Asp301 was identified as the residue forming an ionic hydrogen bond with the basic nitrogen, and this was supported by the site-directed mutagenesis experiments *(182)*. The heme group and I helix containing Asp301 were incorporated into the substrate model and the steric restrictions were included *(183)*. The model was further extended by an addition of four larger substrates *(184)*. This model was used to develop a CYP2D6 selective fluorescent probe (change fluorescence-λ upon transformation), 7-methoxy-4-(aminomethyl)coumarin *(185)*.

A combined protein and pharmacophore model was developed for 40 substrates *(186)*. Although the pharmacophore and the homology models were derived independently, the pharmacophore was docked into the active site without major steric clash, showing a high degree of complementarity. The site of oxidation was positioned 3–3.5 Å above the heme iron, and the planar region of the pharmacophore was roughly perpendicular to the plane of the heme. Of 40 substrates, 3 compounds were classified as "5 Å substrate," and 6 compounds were classified as "10 Å substrate." Considering that the majority was classified into "7 Å substrate," a water-bridging with the "5 Å substrate" was suggested instead of interactions with the one of two carboxylate oxygens of Asp301 side chain *(180)*. Molecular orbital calculations in conjunction with the distance constraints (5, 7, or 10 Å) were used to determine the site of oxidation if the experimental data were unavailable or ambiguous. Minimization of each substrate in the presence of protein showed that the "10 Å substrate" possibly interacted with Glu216, as suggested previously *(187)*, and that Phe481 was the key residue for the π-π stacking interaction. The importance of Phe481 was later confirmed by a mutagenesis experiment *(188)*. This model was extended to include CYP2D6 mediated N-dealkylation reactions *(189)*. A pharmacophore was constructed for 14 compounds known to undergo N-dealkylation by overlaying the substrates using MPTP as the template. Although the basic nitrogen and Asp301 (or Glu216) were the most important sites of interaction for the hydroxylation/O-dealkylation pharmacophore, hydrophobic interaction with Phe481 (Leu121 and Leu213 were also suggested in the model) was the major interaction for the N-dealkylation pharmacophore with the protein. Accordingly, the orientations of these two pharmacophores in the binding site were slightly different. The combined model was able to correctly predict six out of eight observed metabolites.

Several pharmacophore models were developed for the CYP2D6 inhibitors. The first model was presented based on 31 competitive inhibitors of bufuralol 1′-hydroxylation *(190)*. The initial pharmacophore was constructed with six strong $(K_i < 7 \ \mu M)$ inhibitors using ajmalicin as the template, and the model was refined with additional compounds. Features observed in the model were very similar to that of substrate pharmacophores: tertiary nitrogen atom that is protonated at physiological pH and flat hydrophobic region that is almost perpendicular to the N-H axis and maximally extends up to a distance of 7.5 Å from the nitrogen atom. Compounds with high inhibitory potency showed additional functional groups with negative molecular electrostatic potential and hydrogen bond acceptor properties at distances of 4.8–5.5 Å and 6.6–7.5 Å, respectively from the nitrogen atom. The same set of compounds $(n = 31)$ was used to generate a pharmacophore model by Catalyst and compared with a model based on a different set of compounds *(191)*. Whereas all compounds were competitive inhibitors of CYP2D6 catalyzed bufuralol 1′-hydroxylation, the second set of compounds was structurally more diverse than the first set, which contained related structures *(190)*. The first compound set resulted in a pharmacophore with five features—three hydrophobes, one hydrogen donor, and one hydrogen bond acceptor—and the pharmacophore for the second set included four common structural features—two hydrophobes, one hydrogen bond acceptor, and one hydrogen bond donor. Validation of these models showed that the pharmacophore model for structurally related compounds was statistically more significant, suggesting that there existed multiple binding modes for the diverse structures.

While the basic nitrogen is the "signature" of the CYP2D6 substrate/inhibitor, there are several compounds that are missing the basic nitrogen, still bind to this enzyme very tightly. For instance, spirosulfonamide is a CYP2D6 substrate with high-affinity $(K_m = 7 \ \mu M)$ and is lacking the basic nitrogen atom *(192)*. Mutation of ASP301 to neutral amino acids did not affect the binding affinity of this compound, but did affect the metabolic turnover to the same extent as for the classic substrates with the basic nitrogen, bufuralol. This indicates that the role of Asp301 is complex rather than electrostatic interaction with a positively charged atom in the ligands.

3.1.8. CYP3A4

Substrates of CYP3A4 cover a wide range of lipophilic drugs that are characterized by different size and shape. Homology models have suggested that the active site of CYP3A4 is large *(18,25)*. This is consistent with the structural diversity of the substrates. It has been proposed that there are multiple binding subpockets in the active site *(193)*, and a number of studies have provided evidences that CYP3A4 accommodates two or more substrates in the active site simultaneously *(193–196)*. Furthermore, the inhibition potency is thought to be substrate-dependent *(197–199)*. This complexity of how this enzyme interacts with the ligands makes construction of predictive models challenging.

Thirty-eight substrates with various biotransformation pathways were mapped into a pharmacophore with four features: two hydrogen bond acceptors, one hydrogen bond donor, and one hydrophobic region *(200)*. The distance between the two hydrogen bond acceptors was 7.7 Å, while the hydrophobe and hydrogen bond donor were 6.6 Å and 6.4 Å, respectively, from one of the hydrogen bond acceptors. Within the training set, carbamazepine, nifedipine, and testosterone are known to activate their own metabolism (autoactivator), and a pharmacophore for these three substrates was determined to comprise three hydrophobes and one hydrogen bond acceptor.

Pharmacophore models of CYP3A4 inhibitors for three different metabolic reactions were generated *(201)*. The first model for 14 competitive inhibitors of midazolam 1′-hydroxylation contained three hydrophobes at distance of 5.2, 7.0, and 8.8 Å from a hydrogen bond acceptor. The second model was generated with 32 inhibitors of cyclosporin A hydroxylation and that resulted in five features: two hydrogen bond acceptors 5.2 Å apart and three hydrophobes at distances of 4.2–7.1 Å from one of the hydrogen bond acceptors. The third model for 22 quinine 3-hydroxylation inhibitors had four features—one hydrophobe at distances of 8.1–16.3 Å from the two farthest of three hydrogen bond acceptors. A recent study reported pharmacophore models of 7-benzyloxy-4-trifluoromethyl-coumarine (BFC) O-dealkylation inhibitor for CYP3A4, 3A5 and 3A7 *(202)*. Fourteen compounds (inhibition mechanism unknown) were used to generate the models. All three models contain one hydrogen bond acceptor and a cluster of three hydrophobes. While the models of CYP3A5 and 3A7 were nearly identical, the CYP3A4 pharmacophore was characterized by the large distance (14.3 Å) between the furthest hydrophobic region (aromatic ring) and the hydrogen bond acceptor. The current CYP3A4 pharmacophore models indicate that hydrogen bond acceptor is an essential feature for substrate/inhibitor, in a good agreement with a homology model of the active site *(203)*.

4. QSAR Approaches for Metabolism Prediction: the P450 Isozyme

QSAR approaches have proven to be useful in the drug discovery process in cases where little or no structural information of the protein or enzyme is available. In the case of metabolism, QSAR is an attempt to find a consistent relationship between inhibition or induction data and a series of descriptors accounting for structural differences among the molecules in the dataset. Presently, these relationships are generally discovered through the application of statistical techniques, including but not limited to multiple linear regression (MLR), partial least squares (PLS), hierarchical clustering, neural networks (NN), and *k* nearest neighbor (*k*NN).

QSAR methods can be divided into several categories dependent on the nature of descriptors chosen. In classical one-dimensional (1D) and two-dimensional (2D) QSAR analyses, scalar, indicator, or topological variables are examples of descriptors used to explain differences in the dependent variables. 3D-QSAR involves the usage of descriptors dependent on the configuration, conformation, and shape of the molecules under consideration. These descriptors can range from volume or surface descriptors to HOMO (highest occupied molecular orbital) and LUMO (lowest unoccupied molecular orbital) energy values obtained from quantum mechanics (QM) calculations.

Another class of 3D descriptors is molecular interaction field (MIF) descriptors, with its well-known example of Comparative Molecular Field Analysis *(204,205)* (CoMFA). In CoMFA, the steric and electrostatic fields are calculated for each molecule by interaction with a probe atom at a series of grid points surrounding the aligned molecules in 3D space. These interaction energy fields are correlated with the property of interest. The 3D nature of the CoMFA technique provides a convenient tool for visualization of the significant features of the resulting models.

GRID *(206)* is another example of a 3D MIF-based program that is used to determine energetically favorable binding sites on molecules of known structure by calculating the energies of interactions between a chemical group ("the probe") and the target molecule. GOLPE *(146)* is typical of the type of program that can used for variable selection and statistical analysis of the molecular field interactions calculated by GRID. Almond *(145)* is a similar MIF technique except that it uses the alignment-independent descriptors, GRIND (GRid INdependent Descriptors). Almond's PCA and PLS algorithms are used to establish a relationship between the dependent variable and the descriptors before visualizing these interactions.

In this part of the chapter, QSAR models developed to predict or interpret the metabolism of the CYP enzyme will be explored. The following sections are structured according to individual CYP isoforms and the various types of descriptors and algorithms used to develop the models.

4.1. CYP1A2

CYP1A2 is known to play a significant role in the metabolism of aromatic amines, estradiol, and other drugs. Furthermore, it is known that CYP1A2 is induced by cigarette smoke and charcoal-broiled meat.

In 1993, Fuhr et al. *(159)* correlated electrostatic and volume descriptors for a series of quinolone antibacterials with their percentage of inhibition effect of caffeine 3-demethylation in CYP1A2. The descriptors were derived with the SYBYL *(207)* and ALCHEMY II *(208)* software packages. It was shown that

Table 5
QSAR Expressions for CYP1A2

	QSAR equation	r^{2a}	s^b	$r^2_{\text{test set}}{}^c$	F^d	n^e
1	Inhibition = 196 + 1.56 MINI7 + 27.9 CORE2 – 189 CMAX7 + 0.41 VOL1 *(218,238)*					44
2	$-\log IC_{50}$ = 52.0 - 31.5 V/S – 3.43 10^{-3} Phi + 6.12 σ + 2.4 10^{-4} dV + 0.52 dL + 0.63 μ + 6.57 C4′ – 2.42 C3 + 1.03 C5 *(218,221,238)*	0.602				16
3	$-\log IC_{50}$ = 2.289 σ – 2.295 E_{HOMO} – 2.580 Cp_3 + 2.761 Cp_3′ –15.795 *(224)*	0.867	0.346	0.626		14
4	NN1^f: $-\log IC_{50}$ = f (σ, E_{HOMO}, Cp_3, Cp_3′) *(224)*	0.946	0.219	0.671		14
5	NN2: $-\log IC_{50}$ = f (Steric, C_3, Cp_3 and Cp_4′) *(224)*	0.984	0.121	0.800		14
6	ΔG_{bind} = 0.3 μ – 0.90 l/w + 2.11 ΔE – 0.50 N_{HB} – 22.41 *(225)*	0.941	0.420		22.30	11
7	log induction = 0.23 log P – 0.40 l/w – CR + 2.67 *(229)*	0.980	0.209		98.60	12
8	$pEC_{50}{}^{PCBss}$ = 0.33 a/d^2 – 3.22 E_{HOMO} + 0.84 length – 36.44 *(229)*	0.903	0.308		31.50	14

^{a}Coefficient of determination for a given training set; ^{b}standard error; ^{c}coefficient of determination for a given test set; ^{d}F-value; ^{e}number of observations; and ^{f}neural network.

Eq. 1: MINI7 is the electrostatic minimum generated by the substituent at position 7 (kcal/mol), CORE2 describes position-8 of the core (value was 0 for naphthyridines and for quinolines with H at this position, and was 1 in the presence of F substituent), CMAX7 reflects the maximum charge of the substituent at position 7 (kcal/mol), and VOL1 indicates the volume of the substituent at position-1 (in Å).

Eq. 2: V/S is the volume to surface ratio; Phi, the torsion angle between the C2 atom and the B ring; σ, the Hammett coefficient of the B ring; dV, volume difference between substrate and flavonoid; dL, length of the C3 side chain; (μ, dipole moment; and C3, C5, and C4′ the electron density occurring at these atoms.

Eq. 3,4,5: σ, the Hammett coefficient of the B ring; HOMO, the highest occupied molecular orbital energy; Cp_3 and Cp_3′, the HOMO π coefficients of C_3 and C_3′.

Eq. 6: ΔG_{bind}, free energy of binding; μ, molecular dipole moment; l/w, ratio of molecular length to width; ΔE, $E_L - E_H$, difference between the energy of the lowest unoccupied to the highest occupied molecular orbital; N_{HB}, number of active site hydrogen bonds formed between substrate and human CYP1A2.

Eq. 7: log P, logarithm of the octanol/water partition coefficient; l/w, ratio of molecular length to width; CR, COMPACT radius where CR=sqrt $[\Delta E - 7)^2 + (a/d^2 - 15)^2]$.

Eq. 8: pEC50, Ah receptor binding affinity in EC_{50}; a/d^2, ratio of molecular area to depth-square; E_{HOMO}, energy of highest occupied molecular orbital in the ligand molecule.

the electrostatic features of the caffeine derivative and the antibacterials were similar for the core nitrogen regions (**Eq. 1, Table 5**).

Lee et al. *(160)* investigated flavonoids, another molecular class of inhibitors for CYP1A2, in 1998. INSIGHT II *(209)* and MOPAC *(210)* were used to sketch the molecules and to calculate their electrostatic and shape descriptors. As observed in **Eq. 2**, **Table 5**, the volume to surface area ratio (V/S) had the greatest effect on the inhibitory activity. Hence, small molecules with a small V/S ratio have high inhibitory activity.

Another QSAR study utilizing 14 flavonoid derivatives in the training set and 5 flavonoid derivatives in the test set was performed by Moon et al. *(211)* using both multiple linear regression analysis and neural networks. Both statistical methods identified that the Hammett constant σ, the HOMO energy, the non-overlap steric volume, the partial charge of C_3 carbon atom, and the HOMO π-coefficient of C_3, C_3', and C_4' carbon atoms of flavonoids play an important role in inhibitory activity (**Eqs. 3–5**, **Table 5**).

Equation 6 in **Table 5** summarizes a QSAR study reported by Lewis et al. *(212)*, where the free energy of binding (ΔG_{bind} determined by K_m values) correlates closely with a combination of four shape and electrostatic descriptors. Recently, Lewis et al. *(213)* examined six series of compounds (polyaromatic hydrocarbons, nitrobenzofurans, food mutagens, benzanthracence, chrysenes, aminobiphenyl derivatives), which exhibit indirect mutagenic activity. These compounds need to be metabolized to reactive intermediates to become carcinogenic, which is frequently done by the CYP1A1. Molecular orbital calculations were performed via the MOPAC using the AM1 Hamiltonian method *(214)*. The results revealed that mutagenic activity could be correlated to the frontier orbital energies in the form of E_{HOMO}, E_{LUMO}, or the energy gap ΔE (= $E_{LUMO} - E_{HOMO}$) between the HOMO and LUMO energy *(214)*. It is shown in a study of 11 aminobiphenyls that the degree of correlation can be improved by including shape descriptors and hydrophobicity (in form of a HPLC determined lipophilicity parameter). The correlation coefficient *(r)* varied between 0.81 and 0.97 with a standard error (s) of 0.21–1.05. Moreover, it has been revealed that in some cases (e.g., PAHs, chrysenes, and benzanthracence) the frontier orbital electron density on key atoms can be used to generate a predictive model *(213)*. These results might be valuable for the prediction of the site of metabolism.

The Ah (aryl hydrocarbon) receptor, which is known to regulate enzymes of the CYP1 family, plays an important role in determining toxicity. Hence, several attempts have been made to model the relationship between the receptor binding and structure of xenobiotic chemicals. In 1996, Mekenyan et al. *(215)* showed interest in halogenated aromatic hydrocarbons and their effect for AhR binding affinity. For 30 polychlorinated biphenyls (PCBs), 38 polychlorinated dibenzofurans (PCDFs), and 26 polychlorinated dibenzo-p-dioxins (PCDDs) frontier orbital energies were calculated using the PM3 Hamilton. Using E_{HOMO} and E_{LUMO}, charge transfer and a physicochemical parameter such as log P, the authors were able to fit –log (1/IC$_{50}$) values. The regression coefficient (r^2) ranges between 0.721 and 0.899. The predictive power of these models, assessed as a crossvalidated r^2, or q^2, ranged between 0.722 and 0.841. Lewis et al. *(216)* published in 2002 several QSAR models generated via linear stepwise multiple regression analysis. **Equations 7** and **8** in **Table 5** show the structure–activity relationships for nuclear receptor ligands active against the Ah (aryl hydrocarbon) receptor.

In 1992, Waller and McKinney *(217)* published the results of a CoMFA study on a series of 78 polyhalogenated aromatic compounds with respect to their ability to bind to cytosolic Ah receptor. Bravi and Wikel *(218)* later utilized this same dataset and a combination of size descriptors, the positive molecular electrostatic potential, and hydrogen bonding acceptor properties calculated using the MS-WHIM (Molecular Surface—Weighted Holistic Invariant Molecular) *(219)* methodology to develop a predictive model ($q^2 = 0.723$). The most surprising fact was that the hydrogen bonding acceptor property was found as a favorable descriptor, which would mean hydrogen binding acceptor capacity might decrease pEC_{50}.

A 3D-QSAR study by Lozano et al. investigated the metabolism of heterocyclic amines by human cytochrome P450 1A2 *(148,220)*. In this study, COMBINE *(221–223)* and GRID/GOLPE were used to compare interaction fields of the ligand–protein complex with only the ligand structure. The best correlation for the ligand–enzyme interaction energies was obtained for 12 heterocyclic amines using two latent variables. The resultant model was revealed to be statistically robust $r^2 = 0.90$ and internally consistent $q^2 = 0.74$. For the GRID/GOLPE analysis, molecular interaction fields were calculated for each ligand using a phenolic OH probe. The best relationship was obtained after smart region definition *(224)* using two latent variables. Smart region definition is an algorithm developed by Pastor et al. that groupes energy descriptors into regions, where the variables contain the some chemical and statistical information. This leads to the generation of more stable and easier to interpet models. A model with excellent predictability of $q^2 = 0.79$ was achieved. The author showed that active compounds have the possibility to create hydrogen bonds with Thr223 and possess hydrophobic or bulky groups in the vicinity of the catalytic center.

4.2. CYP2A6/CYP2A5

With the solution of a new mammalian microsomal P450 crystal structure *(6)*, Lewis et al. *(226)* took the opportunity to evaluate the structure binding affinity (ΔG_{bind}) relationship of six substrates of CYP2A6, based on K_m published by Rendic et al. *(227)*. It was found that the binding affinity correlated to a combination of log P and the number of active site hydrogen bonds ($r = 0.97$). These findings proved the importance of the substrate's lipophilicity and hydro-

Table 6
QSAR Expressions for CYP2A5

QSAR equation	r^{2a}	s^b	F^c	n^d
1 $\Delta G_{bind} = -0.77\ N_{HB} - 0.78 \log P - 4.45$ *(239)*	0.94	0.343	21.20	6
2 $pK_i = 7.31 \log P - 7.26 \log M_r - 5.17 \log D_{7.4} +$ $0.80\ HB_A - 24.12$ *(241)*	0.94	0.415	12.36	8

[a]Coefficient of determination for a given training set; [b]standard error; [c]F-value; [d]number of observations.

Eq. 1: ΔG_{bind}, free energy of binding; N_{HB}, number of active site hydrogen bonds formed between substrate and human CYP2A6; $\log P$, logarithm of the octanol/water partition coefficient.

Eq. 2: pK_i, inhibition constant; M_r, relative molecular mass; $\log D_{7.4}$, logarithm of the distribution coefficient at pH 7.4; HB_A, number of hydrogen bond acceptors.

gen binding capability. The author mentioned that the major contribution to the overall binding energy is caused by hydrogen bonds. The importance of hydrogen bonding characteristic as influencing factor for inhibition of CYP2A6 has also been pointed out by Lewis *(225,228)* (**Eqs. 1** and **2** in **Table 6**).

The MS-WHIM methodology has been applied to study the binding affinity of 16 coumarin type inhibitors of CYP2A5. Bravi and Wikel *(218)* obtained a model using 48 descriptor with a cross-validated r^2 of 0.706. The most important features identified by the MS-WHIM property selectors are the size, a positive molecular electrostatic potential together with hydrogen bonding acceptor features of the ligands.

Poso et al. *(161)* performed a study to compare the inhibition of coumarin 7-hydroxylation of 28 lactone derivatives in mammalian CYP2A5 and human CYP2A6, since these enzymes are to 82% similar in their amino acid sequence. Moreover, the researcher analyzed the structure activities relationship using CoMFA and GOLPE/GRID. After a semi-empirical treatment within MOPAC the classical CoMFA interaction fields as well as the interaction energies using phenolic hydroxyl probe in GRID were determined. The 3D QSAR models produced with both methods were statistically indifferent (all models have internal and external q^2 values over 0.7). Using contour maps it was shown that the size of the substituent in the position 7 is an important feature for pIC_{50}. In addition, the CYP2A6 map revealed an unfavorable negative charge near the lactone moiety.

4.3. CYP2B1/CYP2B6

In general, the CYP2B subfamily is involved in the detoxication of exogenous substrates such as phenobarbital, which is also the recognized chemical

Table 7
QSAR Expressions for CYP2B6

	QSAR equation	r^{2a}	s^b	F^c	n^d
1	$\log k_D = -0.036V - 18.201\ Q_H + 5.677$ *(242,243)*	0.960	0.150	103.00	10
2	$\Delta G_{bind} = -0.231V - 792.95\ Q_L + 3.640$ *(242,243)*	0.980	0.837	133.80	10
3	$pK_i = 0.934 \log P - 0.193 \log P^2 + 0.88$ *(241)*	0.978	0.216	114.53	8
4	$\log k_{inact} = -0.003\ MW + 21.594\ QC - 0.813$ *(245)*	0.698	0.175	13.843	15
5	$\Delta G_{bind} = -3.99\ N_{HB} -5.41\ HB_D -1.92\ HB_A$ $- 4.19$ *(238)*	0.941	0.550	27.00	10

^{a}Coefficient of determination for a given training set; ^{b}standard error; ^{c}*F*-value; ^{d}number of observations.

Eq. 1: $\log k_D$, dissociation constant; V, solvent-accessible surface molecular volume (Å³); Q_H, greatest population in highest occupied molecular orbital for methyl group hydrogen atoms.

Eq. 2: ΔG_{bind}, free energy of binding; Q_L, greatest population in lowest unoccupied molecular orbital for methyl group hydrogen atoms.

Eq. 3: pK_i, inhibition constant; $\log P$, logarithm of the octanol/water partition coefficient

Eq. 4: $\log k_{inact}$, rate constant of inactivation; MW, molecular weight; QC, charge of the first carbon atom of the alkyl chain C5.

Eq. 5: ΔG_{bind}, free energy of binding; N_{HB}, number of active site hydrogen bonds formed between substrate and human CYP2B6; HB_D, number of hydrogen bond donor.

inducer of this isoform. Mostly, substrates of the CYP2B subfamily consist of two aromatic ring systems and a central tetrahedral carbon atom, which adopts "V" shape. Furthermore, it is known that CYP2B substrates usually posses high lipophilicity.

Lewis et al. *(124,229)* presented one of the first QSAR studies in 1995. This research investigated possible quantitative structure–activity relationships within a series of 10 pair-substituted toluene derivatives processing different binding affinity with CYP2B4, the rabbit ortholog of this subfamily. The dissoasiation constant ($\log k_D$) and binding affinity could be well correlated with molecular volume, but the correlations could be significantly improved by adding electronic structural parameter (**Eqs. 1** and **2** in **Table 7**).

Ekins et al. *(163)* used the rat ortholog 2B6 to generate a pharmacophore model and compared these findings with a partial least squares (PLS) model using MS-WHIM descriptors. The model was constructed using 16 B-lymphoblastoids and yielded a good cross-validated r^2 of 0.607. The analysis included molecular surface properties (size) together with positive elec-

Table 8
QSAR Expressions for CYP2C9

QSAR equation	r^{2a}	s^b	F^c	n^d
1 ΔG_{bind} = 8.62 log $D_{7.4}$ – 8.02 log P – 6.26 pK_a + 0.57 HB$_D$ + 42.74 *(238)*	0.980	0.230	29.50	8

[a]Coefficient of determination for a given training set; [b]standard error; [c]*F*-value; [d]number of observations.

Eq. 1: ΔG_{bind}, free energy of binding; log $D_{7.4}$, logarithm of the distribution coefficient at pH 7.4; pK_a, negative logarithm of the dissociation constant; HB$_D$, number of hydrogen bond donors.

trostatic potential, hydrogen bonding acceptor capacity, and hydrophobicity. Four out of five structurally diverse substrates for CYP2B6 could be predicted with residuals lower than one log unit. Nanbo A. and Nanbo T. *(230)* investigated the mechanism of N-demethylation of N,N-demethylaniline catalyzed by P450 by evaluating the relationship of the enzyme CYP2B1 activity with electronic properties. This study suggests that one electron is being transferred from the nitrogen to P450 resulting a cationic α-amino radical, which undergoes hydroxylation and N-demethylation.

A series of eight aliphatic amines was studied as inhibitors of CYP2B1 *(228)*. A linear combination of frontier orbital energies resulted in a correlation coefficient *(r)* = 0.98, while a quadratic expression of log *P* yielded an *r* = 0.989 (**Eq. 3** in **Table 8**). Based on the latter equation, it was determined that the optimal log *P* for the CYP2B1 substrates was 2.42, which related to an optimal length of 10 or 11 carbon atoms of the alkyl chain in these molecules. These results were supported by a QSAR and CoMFA study performed by Lesigiarska et al. *(231)*. Lesigiarska et al. *(231)* used 15 xanthates, which were geometry optimized using MOPAC and the PM3 Hamilton *(232)*. Several semiempirical parameters together with various shape descriptors were used to explain variations in the CYP2B1 inhibitory activity (**Eq. 4, Table 7**). The compounds were divided into two groups dependent on the lengths of methylene chain. The inactivation potency of the group with the shorter chain correlated with the charge of the first carbon atom of the chain. Hence, this atom might represent a potential target for metabolic attack. In the second group, the group with longer side chains, a decrease in the activation potency was observed with an increase in the side chain lengths.

An additional study performed by Lewis et al. *(225)* revealed the major contribution of hydrogen bonded interactions, as evident in **Eq. 5, Table 7**. For 10 substrates the combination of hydrogen bond donor and acceptors together with the number of active site hydrogen binds resulted in a good correlation coefficient *(r)* of 0.97.

Xanthates have been shown to be potent inhibitors for human CYP2B6. In a QSAR analysis performed by Lesigiarska ct al. *(231)* fifteen xanthates were tested to better understand the mechanism of interaction with the enzyme. The compounds were energy minimized using MOPAC and the PM3 Hamiltonian. After aligning the molecules using the dithiocarbonate group as a frame of reference, CoMFA fields were calculated using a sp^3 carbon as the probe atom. A PLS analysis with 14 of 15 compounds produced a $q^2 > 0.7$ with three or four latent variables. As mentioned above, the authors divided that dataset into two groups dependent on the length of methylene groups. It was shown that there is hardly any relationship visible in the group with less methylene groups. In the second group consisting of nine compounds, a q^2 of 0.72 was calculated with four components for the electrostatic CoMFA fields and two components for steric fields only. These fields revealed a dependency of the alkyl chain length and the charge of the first carbon atom with the biological activity, which is in accordance to the 3D QSAR findings.

4.4. CYP2C9/CYP2C5/3

CYP2C9 was identified as one of the most important P450s involved in human drug metabolism *(176)*. It is involved in the metabolism of many commonly used drugs such as taxol, warfarin, and omeparazole.

Ekins et al. *(173)* computed MS-WHIM descriptors for 29 compounds to obtain a 3D QSAR set. Computing multiple conformers of the inhibitors resulted in the generation of a 4D QSAR model. For each conformer, weighted MS-WHIM descriptors were calculated, which resulted in a maximum of 504 descriptors. It was not possible to create a valuable predictive 3D model for the inhibition of (S) warfin 7-hydroxylation. Nevertheless, the 4D QSAR model generated a q^2 of 0.64 using five components. The significant descriptors were the negative electrostatic potential, hydrogen bond acceptor and donor properties, and hydrophobicity.

In Lewis et al.'s *(225)* QSAR study, eight CYP2C9 substrates where examined. In this case, it appeared as if the acid dissociation constant pK_a, the compounds' lipophilicity, and the number of hydrogen bond donor atoms are important features (**Eq. 1, Table 8**). These suggestions are supported by a good correlation with the binding affinity.

Afzelius et al. *(26)* reported a study that describes the generation of a three-dimensional QSAR model for 25 competitive CYP2C9 inhibitors in the training set and 8 inhibitors in the test set. The GRID interaction fields using the DRY and OH probe were used as descriptors. The resulting predictive model

$(r^2 = 0.947, q^2 = 0.730)$ was able to predict the external dataset within 0.5 log unit of the experimental value.

A new method of determining the site of metabolism of CYP2C9 substrates has been introduced by Zamora et al. *(233)*. In this approach, the ligands as well as the protein active pocket were characterized with GRID descriptors using the probe atoms N, Dry, and O. The descriptors of the protein and the ligand were binned in a distance-space-dependent way (e.g., for the ligand, the distance between the different hydrogen atoms and classified atoms were calculated; for the protein; the interaction pattern has been translated into distances from the reactive center of the enzyme). The distance bin occurring from the protein was compared with the fingerprint bin of the ligand using Carbó's similarity index, after which each hydrogen atom got ranked. As the authors point out, in more than 90% of CYP2C9 catalyzed oxidative reactions, the hydrogen atom ranked at the first, second, or third position were experimentally reported as site of oxidation.

The first CoMFA QSAR study for CYP2C9, performed by Jones et al. *(169)*, used an active analog of 9 (S)-11 (R)-cyclocoumarol as a template to align 27 semiempirical geometry optimized compounds. A partial least square analysis revealed a prediction capability with cross-validated r^2 (q^2) of 0.70. Moreover, that model suggested a π-π stacking region together with two cationic interaction sites as important features. Rao et al. *(171)* used a diverse test set of 14 coumarin derivatives along with the same alignment rule found in the pharmacophore study of Jones et al. *(169)* to refine the CoMFA study. It was interesting to note that the test set consisted primarily of sulfonamide derivatives. Yet, the researchers were able to predict 13 of 14 compounds within 1 log residual.

Afzelius et al. *(175)* computed alignment independent GRIND descriptors in ALMOND for a dataset of 21 inhibitors and 21 non-inhibitors. A discriminate model was generated by assigning zeros to the non-inhibitors and ones to the inhibitors. The model ($r^2 = 0.74$, $q^2 = 0.64$) was tested with 14 competitive and 25 non-inhibitors, which were not utilized to generate to model; 74% of these compounds were correctly classified and 13% were in a border region. In a second model ($r^2 = 0.77$, $q^2 = 0.60$), the K_i values for 21 competitive inhibitors were used as the continuous dependent variable together with GRIND descriptors generated using Dry, O, and N1 probe as independent variables. This model was capable of predicting 11 of 12 test compounds within a 0.5 log error margin of K_i.

4.5. CYP2D6

Although CYP2D6 represents only 1.5% of the human P450, it participates in the metabolism of over 30% of clinically prescribed drugs. Moreover, CYP2D6 is absent in 5–9% of the Caucasian populations. This deficiency in drug oxidation is known as debrisoquine/sparteine polymorphism, which affects the metabolism of numerous drugs. Hence, interest in this subenzyme started fairly early. It was in 1985, that Wolff manually aligned substrates containing a basic nitrogen at 5 Å from the center of oxidation *(177)*.

Ekins et al. *(191)* used a previously published dataset by Snyder et al. *(190)* and their own laboratory results to generate a pharmacophore model and 3D/4D QSAR models with MS-WHIM descriptors derived from inhibition data of 1′-hydroxybufuralol. Inhibition data generated in the Eli Lilly laboratory resulted in a 3D predictive model with a high degree of internal consistency ($q^2 = 0.54$) using a combination of three molecular properties: negative potential, hydrogen bond donor, and hydrophobicity. A 4D (multiple conformers) model did not improve the predictability of the model, which suggests that the range of single conformations sufficiently described the conformational space. The same trend was reproduced for a dataset by Strobl et al. *(190)* using 28 of 31 inhibitors. The 3D and 4D QSAR models produced similar q^2 values (>0.5). It is worthwhile mentioning that the QSAR model produced from merged data from Snyder and the Eli Lilly research laboratories show no sign of prediction capability using a more realistically "five random groups repeated up to 100 times (5RG × 100)" cross-validation approach, whereas Strobl's dataset still results in a $q_{5RG \times 100}$ of 0.48. Snyder et al. *(234)* used a dataset containing of 52 compounds collected from the literature to enhance the understanding in CYP2D6 substrates requirements. A genetic algorithm was applied to find the best model between log K_m and MS-WHIM descriptors (**Eq. 1, Table 9**). The obtained model has a r^2 of 0.69 and a q^2 of 0.58 using all 52 compounds.

Lewis et al. *(228)* used a dataset of 11 inhibitors to produce a QSAR model. The best model ($r = 0.979$; **Eq. 2, Table 9**) was found using a combination of relative molecular mass, lipophilicity, number of hydrogen bond acceptors, and number of basic nitrogens. However, a model with only two descriptors (pK_i and log $D_{7.4}$) was found with $r = 0.97$. The author argues that for protonated nitrogens found in the dataset the log $D_{7.4}$ descriptors from the simpler regression model is the ionization-corrected lipophilicity at pH 7.4 (log P in **Eq. 2, Table 9**), which is an important feature supported by site-directed mutagenesis. Another study of CYP2D6 substrates (**Eq. 3, Table 9**) performed by Lewis et al. *(225)* explained the binding affinity with the relative mass of substrate together with number of hydrogen bonds and π-π stacking interactions.

4.6. CYP2E1

CYP2E1's substrates are small molecular weight aromatic hydrocarbons or their methyl derivatives, as the enzyme's active site is relative small and restricted. In a recently published study from Lewis et al. *(235)* eight alkyl benzenes, which undergo oxidative metabolism via human CYP2E1, were used to

Table 9
QSAR Expressions for CYP2D6

	QSAR equation	r^{2a}	s^b	F^c	n^d
1	$\log K_m = -9.72 + 3.15$ JWMWDW4 $+ 1.23$ JWMWKW2 $+ 5.19$ JWMWH3W2 $+ 7.25$ JWMWH2W1 $- 1.37$ JWMWP2W5 *(252)*	0.690			52
2	$pK_i = 0.014$ M$_r$ $- 0.477 \log P - 0.567$ HB$_A$ $- 1.794$ $N_B - 3.557$ *(241)*	0.958	0.048	35.10	11
3	$\Delta G_{bind} = 492.03 \log$ M$_r$ $- 0.88$ M$_r$ $- 5.08$ N$_{HB} - 3.76$ $N_{\pi\text{-}\pi} - 947.68$ *(238)*	0.884	0.37	9.60	10

[a]Coefficient of determination for a given training set; [b]standard error; [c]F-value; [d]number of observations.

Eq. 1: JWMWDW4, hydrogen bond acceptor capacity total density; JWMWKW2, positive molecular electrostatic potential total shape; JWMWH3W2, positive molecular electrostatic potential emptiness 3rd direction; JWMWH2W1, unitary weight emptiness 3rd direction; JWMWP2W5, hydrogen bond donor capacity proportion 2nd direction.

Eq. 2: K_i, inhibition constant; M$_r$, relative molecular mass; log P, logarithm of the octanol/water partition coefficient; HB$_A$, number of hydrogen bond acceptors; N_B, number of basic nitrogens.

Eq. 3: ΔG_{bind}, free energy of binding; M$_r$, relative molecular mass; N_{HB}, number of active site hydrogen bonds formed between substrate and human CYP2D6; $N_{\pi\text{-}\pi}$, number of π-π stacking interactions formed between substrate and enzyme active sites.

perform a QSAR study. As seen in **Eq. 1, Table 10**, the rate constant V_{max} shows a quadratic dependence to the difference in E_{LUMO} and E_{HOMO}. These results are consistent with a previous study *(30)*, where it was found that π-π stacking interactions between aromatic rings are important for the binding of substrates.

Lewis et al. *(225)* also used 10 CYP2E1 substrates to generate a QSAR model with a combination of the total number of hydrogen bond acceptor and donor, the number of active site π-π stacking interactions, and the relative molecular mass (**Eq. 2, Table 10**). It was also shown that only three descriptors (hydrogen bond acceptor and donor, π-π stacking interactions, and the log of the relative molecular mass) could satisfactorily explain the binding affinity. A early publication from Lewis et al. *(236)* on a series of 20 nitriles of varying rates revealed a correlation between molecular polarizibility and excitation energy.

Waller et al. *(237)* performed a CoMFA study to analyze the metabolic rates of CYP2E1 in rodents as intrinsic clearance of a 12 chlorinated volatile organic compounds (VOCs). After superimposition, the steric and electrostatic field interaction energies, the HINT (*h*ydropathic *int*eractions) energy *(238)*, and molecular orbital field were calculated in addition to clogP. The "best" model

Table 10
QSAR Expressions for CYP2E1

	QSAR equation	r^{2a}	s^b	F^c	n^d
1	$\log V_{\max} = 44.301\ \Delta E - 2.369\ \Delta E^2 - 203.75$ *(253)*	0.910	0.099	40.40	7
2	$\Delta G_{\mathrm{bind}} = 0.56\ HB - 2.18\ N_{\pi\text{-}\pi} - 3.37\ \log M_r$ $- 0.36\ N_{\mathrm{HB}} + 1.86$ *(238)*	0.980	0.2287	73.10	10

^{a}Coefficient of determination for a given training set; ^{b}standard error; ^{c}*F*-value; ^{d}number of observations.

Eq. 1: $\log V_{\max}$, rate constant for CYP2E mediated metabolism; ΔE, $E_{\mathrm{LUMO}} - E_{\mathrm{HOMO}}$.

Eq. 2: ΔG_{bind}, free energy of binding; HB, total number of hydrogen bond acceptors and donors; M_r, relative molecular mass; N_{HB}, number of active site hydrogen bonds formed between substrate and human CYP2E1.

using only one field at the time was generated with the energies of the HOMO as descriptors, lead to a q^2 of -0.186 and r^2 of 0.178. The most internally consistent model was generated from a combination of steric, electrostatic, LUMO and HINT fields, resulting in a q^2 of 0.527 and r^2 of 0.953. Based on the contribution of these fields to the model, the author was able to suggest a model for the metabolic process; for example, the electrostatic fields contribute with 44% to the overall model, which can be related to the recognition process between substrate and enzyme, based on long-range interactions.

4.7. CYP3A4

The CYP3 family constitutes the major portion (40–60%) of the human hepatic cytochrome P450. CYP3A4 occurs in the mammalian liver as well as mammalian small intestines, and is known to metabolize nearly 50% of all market drugs. It is therefore not surprising that much research has been performed on CYP3A4. Lewis et al. *(203,239)* and Ekins et al. *(200,201,240)* have investigated the metabolism of CYP3A4 since 1996. Here, we intend to review only most recent investigations.

Singh et al. *(79)* published in 2003 a novel approach to predict the interaction sites ("hot spots") in a molecule metabolized by CYP3A4. Once identified, these "hot spots" on the molecules can be modified to avoid metabolism. The assumption of this study is that the CYP3A4 susceptibility is largely dependent on the electronic environment surrounding the hydrogens in any molecules. Hence, the hydrogen abstraction energy was calculated using the MOPAC with the AM1 Hamiltonian for 50 CYP3A4 substrates. Moreover, the research group designed a novel "fingerprint" (and using a special PLS called trend vector) to capture the hydrogen's topological environment in a molecule. Using PLS, a correlation was identified between the fingerprint and the hydrogen abstraction energy. The model displayed reasonable statistical results of $r^2 = 0.98$ with a standard error $s = 2.06$ kcal/mol. The model revealed that only hydrogen atoms with hydrogen abstraction energies smaller than 27 kcal/mol in combination with an exposed surface area greater than 8 Å are susceptible to CYP3A4 mediated metabolism. These findings identified 78% of the experimentally known major metabolic sites.

Wang and coworkers *(33)* presented their research efforts at the 221st American Chemical Society National Meeting 2001; 31 dillapiol derivatives were used to generate a QSAR model. The analyses indicated a parabolic correlation between the inhibitory effect and the log P of dillapoils.

The dependence of induction of CYP3A, as determined by the percentage increase in ethylmorphine N-demethylase activity, was studied by Lewis et al. *(241)* by performing a QSAR study on 14 steroids (**Eq. 1, Table 11**). It was shown that the best model ($r = 0.89$) includes a combination of the compounds lipophilicity in the form of log P, the area/depth^2 feature and ΔE, which is the difference between the HOMO and LUMO energics. An additional study (**Fq. 2, Table 11**) of Lewis et al. *(238)* performed on 10 CYP3A4 substrates strengthen the importance of the HOMO and LUMO energies in combination with the number of active site hydrogen bond and π-π stacking interactions. The author underlined Koopman's theorem *(116)* by pointing out that the frontier orbital energies could be associated with electron donor/acceptor properties of the substrate molecules. The relatively low correlation coefficient can be explained by the fact that the dataset used had a large range of K_D values (1.8–348 μM).

Ekins et al. *(201)* used the MS-WHIM descriptors to construct 3D and 4D QSAR models for the log($1/K_i$) of 14 competitive inhibitors of CYP3A. The 3D QSAR of the CYP3A4-mediated midazolam 1′-hydroxylation was shown to be predictive yielding a leave-one-out (LOO) q^2 value of 0.32. Although the 4D QSAR methodology includes conformational changes, it did not provide for a significant improvement over the 3D QSAR (LOO q^2 0.44). Two other datasets *(242,243)* were used to create 3D and 4D QSAR models. In both datasets, it was not possible to build predictive 3D QSAR models; however, 4D QSAR models were constructed (LOO $q^2 = 0.41$–0.56).

Molnar *(244)* has investigated a novel and innovative method to study CYP3A4 inhibition. It is argued that CYP3A4 has highly structurally diverse inhibitors; hence, the probability that these inhibitors will bind in different binding modes is great. Because 3D-QSAR methods assume the same or similar binding mode, 2D descriptors and neural networks were proposed as better alternives; 145 inhibitors and 145 non-inhibitors were classified using a YES/NO scheme. The 2D Unity fingerprints were chosen as descriptor set.

Table 11
QSAR Expressions for CYP3A4

	QSAR equation	r^{2a}	s^b	F^c	n^d
1	Log A = 0.25 a/d^2 – 0.50 ΔE + 0.08 log P + 8.27 (*263*)	0.792	0.196	12.30	14
2	ΔG_{bind} = 1.92 E_L – 2.99 E_H – 0.52 N_{HB} + 3.55 $N_{\pi-\pi}$ – 35.10 (*238*)	0.922	0.360	13.00	10
3	Induction = 0.85 HB_A + 0.68 HBD – 0.051 M_r + 32.87 log M_r – 66.59 (*269*)	0.922	0.556	13.40	9
4	Induction = 10.64 l/w – 0.88 μ – 0.016 M_r – 5.01 E_L – 4.58 (*269*)	0.960	0.470	17.50	8
5	Induction = 1.01 N_{HB} – 0.336 μ – 0.321 E_L + 1.056 (*269*)	0.960	0.367	44.50	10
6	Induction = 1.09 N_{HB} – 0.615 a/d^2 – 2.147 l/w + 1.235 (*269*)	0.960	0.315	61.20	10

[a]Coefficient of determination for a given training set; [b]standard error; [c]*F*-value; [d]number of observations.

Eq. 1: log A, logarithm of the percentage increase in ethylmorphine N-demethylase activity; a/d^2, ratio of molecular area to depth-square; ΔE, E_L – E_H, difference between the energy of the lowest unoccupied to the highest occupied molecular orbital; log P, logarithm of the octanol/water partition coefficient.

Eq. 2: ΔG_{bind}, free energy of binding; E_L, energy of the lowest unoccupied molecular orbital; E_H, energy of the highest occupied molecular orbital; N_{HB}, number of active site hydrogen bonds formed between substrate and CYP3A4; $N_{\pi-\pi}$, number of π-π stacking interactions formed between substrate and enzymes active site.

Eq. 3: Induction: fold induction of CYP3A4 in the presence of hGR; HB_A, number of hydrogen bond acceptors; HB_D, number of hydrogen bond donor; M_r, relative molecular mass.

Eq. 4: Induction: fold induction of CYP3A4 in the presence of hGR; l/w, ratio of molecular length to width; M_r, relative molecular mass; E_L, energy of the lowest unoccupied molecular orbital.

Eq. 5: Induction: fold induction of CYP3A4 in the presence of hGR; N_{HB}, number of active site hydrogen bonds formed between substrate and CYP3A4; μ, molecular dipole moment; E_L, energy of the lowest unoccupied molecular orbital.

Eq. 6: Induction: fold induction of CYP3A4 in the presence of hGR; N_{HB}, number of active site hydrogen bonds formed between substrate and CYP3A4; a/d^2, ratio of molecular area to depth.

A feedforward neural network consisting of 31 hidden and one output neuron was generated; 97% inhibitors and 95% non-inhibitors of the training set were predicted correctly; 36 inhibitors and 36 non-inhibitors of a test set, which have not been used to generate the model, were predicted with 91.7% accuracy for inhibitors and 88.9% for non-inhibitor.

Schneider et al. (*245*) used 333 one and two-dimensional descriptors to create a virtual screening filter for CYP 3A4 inhibition. After the application of a space-filling subset selection algorithm, a total of 311 compounds were classified in as either low ($IC_{50} < 1$ µM) or high ($IC_{50} > 50$ µM) inhibitors. The 10 most relevant descriptors for the final PLS analyses are total number of hetero and aromatic atoms, total number of aromatic atoms, total number of aromatic bonds, total number of aromatic rings, total number of carbon atoms, molecular refractivity, total number of bonds, graphic mass index, atomic connectivity index rank 3 and rank 1. The Matthews correlation coefficient was used in contrast to the commonly used cross-validated r^2. The final PLS analysis was capable of reclassifying 95% of the compounds correctly; 90% of the compounds in a semi-independent test set were predicted in agreement with the experimental data.

Lewis et al. *(246)* studied 10 CYP3A4 inducers, where induction is mediated via human glucorticoid receptor (hGR). A good correlation ($r = 0.98$, **Eq. 3–6, Table 11**) between the induction and a combination of structural parameters including: relative molecular mass, dipole moment, LUMO energy, and rectangularity can be achieved. Lewis proposed that the dipole moment and LUMO energy are indicating a potential for hydrogen bonding between ligand and receptors, whereas the molecular mass can be related to desolvation *(216)*.

Wang *(247)* and coworker's 3D QSAR model for 31 dillapiol revealed that the activity was correlated with the steric bulk of the substitutes in position 5 and 6 and with the electron density of the groups at position 6. Unfortunately, no more information about that work has been found.

4.8. Other CYPs and relevant articles

Work on CYP51 has been done by Ji et al. *(247)*, Talele et al. *(248)*, and Lewis et al. *(228,250)*. P450 aromatase has been explored via QSAR by Baston et al. *(251–253)* and others *(126,252–256)*.

Some of the earliest QSAR studies on CYPs were performed by Basak *(257)*, Murray *(258)*, and Marshall *(205)*. Gao et al. *(259)* explored the influence of electronic parameters of CYP substrates in 1996. The findings of Basak that electronic terms would cancel out have been proven wrong by many research papers published in the following decades. Tyrakowska et al. *(260)* indicated via QSARs based on calculated molecular orbital descriptors that the k_{cat} (maximum velocity converted per nmol of P450 per min) for CYP catalyzed C4-hydroxylation rates of aniline derivatives of different species (rats, rabbit, mice, and human) are closely related to the highest occupied molecular orbital energy (E_{HOMO}), $r \geq 0.97$. Several reviews published by Lewis et al. *(212,216,228,261–265)* and Ekins *(240)* should also be mentioned.

5. Databases, Software Systems, Useful Web Pages, and Services

The burst in biologic and information technology in conjunction with the combinatorial chemistry advances is making many targets become available for the pharmaceutical industry at a rapid pace. Therefore, it is necessary to use our collective knowledge, contained in corporate and commercial databases, to screen the incoming avalanches of compounds to find the next blockbuster medicines faster, cheaper, and cleaner.

In pharmaceutical companies, the available ADME/T data in general and metabolism information in particular are focused around lead compounds. It is realized that most projects are lacking sufficient relative ADME/T data in terms of quality, quantity, and the useful range of data for modeling *(266)*. Moreover, it is very difficult to acquire data for inactive compounds with regard to the ADME/T endpoints. Additionally, our functional metabolism information is limited only to several chemical scaffolds (chemotypes). As a result, the challenge of finding "good" datasets has become the "holy grail" in ADME/T modeling. Clearly, more comprehensive datasets of known drugs and related series are required to provide the foundation of predictive models.

The biotechnology revolution has made an undeniable impression on the field of metabolism. For example, it is common, to seek *in vitro* metabolic data based on human CYPs. Currently, Cerep, Cyprotex, Novascreen, and many others *(267–271)* are providing larger and larger metabolism datasets, computational tools, and models, often in conjunction with other biological endpoints. However, the qualities of these datasets are yet to be established.

Having access to metabolism data in the early discovery stage is invaluable. For example, hepatic metabolism data could be used to characterize the pharmacokinetic behavior of a perspective lead. Several studies have reported how metabolism databases and software systems have been used at various settings *(272)*. In this section, we will provide an overview of recent databases, software systems, websites, tools, and services that could be potential starting points for metabolism modeling at various stages in drug discovery process *(271,273)*.

5.1. Databases and Software Systems

5.1.1. ArQule

ArQule provides professional services and products including metabolism models for CYP 3A4, 2D6, and 2C9. The metabolism models are based on combined empirical/quantum chemical approaches and are aimed at predicting the site of metabolism, enzyme–substrate binding affinities (2D6 and 2C9), and relative rates of metabolism at discrete sites within a molecule *(274)*.

5.1.2. Cerep

Cerep evaluates hits, leads, and new compounds from the metabolic point of view using liver microsomes and recombinant cytochrome P450s *(275)*. The results of these metabolic screening studies offer insight to the rate of metabolic pathways, in vivo pharmacokinetic properties, and drug–drug interactions.

Table 12
A Summary of Tests Available from Cerep

Enzyme *(275)*	Assay
CYP1A2 inhibition	Metabolic stability (liver S9, monkey, *Cynomolgus*)
CYP2B6 inhibition	Metabolic stability (liver S9, dog, beagle)
CYP2C9 inhibition	Metabolic stability (liver S9, rat, Sprague-Dawley)
CYP2C19 inhibition	Metabolic stability (liver S9, mouse, CD1)
CYP2D6 inhibition	Metabolic stability (CYP2D6)
CYP2E1 inhibition	Metabolic stability (CYP3A4)
CYP3A4 inhibition (BFC substrate)	Plasma stability (human)
CYP3A4 inhibition (BzRes substrate)	Half-life determination (liver micros., human)
CYP3A4 inhibition (Testosterone substrate)	Half-life determination (liver S9, human)
CYP3A5 inhibition	Apparent V_{max}/K_m (CYP2D6)
Time-dependent inhibition CYP3A4 (half-life)	Apparent V_{max}/K_m (CYP3A4)
Metabolic stability (liver micros. human)	Metabolite detection (liver micros, human)
Metabolic stability (liver micros. monkey, Cynomolgus)	Metabolite characterization (liver micros., human)
Metabolic stability (liver micros. dog, Beagle)	Glutathione conjugate detection
Metabolic stability (liver micros. rat, Sprague-Dawley)	Glutathione conjugate characterization
Metabolic stability (liver micros. mouse, CD1)	Glucuronide conjugate detection
Metabolic stability (liver S9, human)	Glucuronide conjugate characterization

Cerep also provides modeling tools and models for in silico prediction of new compounds. In vitro metabolism data are described in **Table 12**.

5.1.3. Cloe Screen

Cyprotex, using Cloe Screen™, evaluates pharmacokinetic properties in vitro and establishes a broad portfolio of in vitro assays that allows researchers to investigate the metabolism parameters for drug discovery and development. This company supplies the following data and assays *(276)*: microsomal stability, hepatocyte metabolic stability, cytochrome P450 inhibition (3A4, 2D6, 1A2, 2C9 and 2C19), cytochrome P450 identification, and cytochrome P450 induction.

5.1.4. COMPACT

COMPACT, Computer-Optimized Molecular Parametric Analysis of Chemical Toxicity, allows researchers to examine, using both electrostatic and steric parameters, the ability of xenobiotics to form complexes with CYP1A2, CYP2A6, CYP2B6, CYP2C8, CYP2C9, CYP2C19, CYP2D6, CYP2E1, CYP3A4, and CYP4A11. However, it should be realized that the system has limitations in detecting toxic agents that are participating in enzymatic oxidation *(4,277–279)*. COMPACT provides the ability to collectively employ diverse *in silico* techniques for a rapid screening of novel compounds. In addition, COMPACT involves the use of molecular modeling and related techniques for the evaluation of human drug metabolism *(4,277–279)*.

5.1.5. Cytochrome P450 Database (CPD)

Many references have been made to the Cytochrome P450 Database (CPD), which is maintained by the institute for Biomedical Chemistry and Center for Molecular Design in Russia *(280–283)*. This institute has complied amino acid sequences, gene structures and chromosomal location, substrate specificity, impression of P450 nomenclature, structure and function of the P450 superfamily, information on P450-catalyzed reactions, and inducibility of the superfamily of cytochromes P450. CPD comes with its own software (available on compact disk and online). However, accessing this site online is extremely slow, and its usage is very impractical.

5.1.6. Drug Interaction Database

The database contains information taken from approx 4000 research papers related to in vivo and in vitro drug interaction in humans. The database is searchable using a number of queries and is updated on a monthly basis *(284)*.

5.1.7. GenTest

This database, collected from hundreds of human cytochrome P450 reactions, is a collection of information on human cytochrome P450 metabolism *(285)*. For each substance in the database, information can be found regarding therapeutic category, human cytochrome P450 or P450 family with which the chemical interacts, chemical reaction which occurs, classification of the interacting chemical/drug substance with a human P450 as well as literature citations for this information. The Human P450 metabolism database is extracted from the published data from original papers, reviews, or abstracts at scientific conferences. The database is updated regularly. In addition, GenTest provides commercial kits and services for high throughput P450 inhibition in screening, human, dog, and rat cytochromes P450 systems *(227,245)*.

5.1.8. Human Drug Metabolism Database

IUPAC is constructing a human drug metabolism database model on the internet *(286)*. This effort is based on the premise that very few published datasets are available for modeling *(287,288)*, and even fewer sources outside the major pharmaceuticals are providing metabolism databases for various use by modeling groups. A version of this dataset is expected to be available in 2003, and it ultimately will serve as a standard for how new molecules are metabolized in humans.

5.1.9. iDEA

Lion Biosciences is the supplier of the iDEA™ Metabolism software package as well as other ADME/T services *(289)*. The iDEA software simulates metabolism and predicts a compound's metabolic behavior in humans. The Metabolism Module consists of a data expert module to perform data fitting and analysis of collected in vitro data and the physiological metabolism model. The physiological metabolism model is constructed from proprietary database of 64 clinically tested compounds. Additionally, the metabolism module automatically calculates the Michaelis-Menten constants K_m and V_{max} for the kinetic analysis of metabolism turnover *(289)*.

5.1.10. Integrity Database

Prous Science provides a database for drug discovery and development encompassing all the areas in drug discovery, including metabolism. Integrity enables researchers to combine chemistry and genomics data with pharmaco-dynamics and pharmacokinetics databases. All the data are cumulated through available public records, literature, conferences, and patents. This database is a very useful system to acquire public information *(290)*.

5.1.11. META/METAPC

The META system *(291–293)* is an expert system, based on well-established sources, for predicting the sites of potential enzymatic attack and the metabolites formed by metabolic transformations. The program uses dictionaries of biotransformation operators, which are created by experts to represent known metabolic paths. Currently, META can be combined with one of the following dictionaries: mammalian metabolism, aerobic biodegradation, anaerobic biodegradation, and metabolic transformation reactions *(291)*.

The program is capable of predicting the metabolites that could be generated from a novel xenobiotic. A genetic algorithm has been used to build and prioritize the biotransformation dictionaries. Moreover, quantum chemical parameters and structural descriptors were implemented in predicting the regioselectivity of ring oxidation in polynuclear aromatic hydrocarbons and the site of oxidation *(292,294–296)*.

5.1.12. MetaCyc

The MetaCyc database is the result of a collaborative effort between SRI International (see the website and useful links on this document), the Carnegie Institution, and Stanford University in creating a comprehensive database collected from literature and cyber sources. The MetaCyc database contains metabolic pathways (with citations), reactions, enzymes, and substrates. This database does not offer genomic data, but it does supply its own software and visualization tools *(297)*.

6.1.13. EcoCyc

Encyclopedia of *Escherichia coli* Genes and Metabolism is a bioinformatics database combining the biochemical and genomic information of *E. coli* allowing a better understanding of *E. coli* at the system level. It is linked to other biological databases and contains structures, genomics, and bibliographic data of *E. coli*. EcoCyc allows for visualizing of genes on chromosomes, a biochemical reaction, or pathway. EcoCyc also allows for computational investigations of the metabolism, design, evaluation, and simulation of metabolic pathways *(298)*.

5.1.14. MDL® Metabolite Database

MDL Metabolite is a metabolism information system that provides a database, registration system, and graphical interface *(299,300)*. The database (in vivo and in vitro studies including name, EC number, and isoenzyme) uses information from multiple sources to construct structural metabolic database entries for all parent compounds *(299)*. The system provides the user with the capability to create, edit, and register metabolic reactions. The available data spans the last 100 years of research extracted mainly from *Biotransformations of Drugs* (1977–1983), *Pharmacokinetics* (1986–1990), original metabolism literature, new drug applications (1990–present), and Proceedings from International Society for the Study of Xenobiotics (ISSX) meetings. It contains 8,590 parent compounds, 53,373 transformations, and 34,537 molecules. The Metabolite Database is updated semiannually *(301)*.

5.1.15. MetabolExpert

MetabolExpert *(302–304)* is composed of databases (including animal metabolism, plant metabolism, photodegradation chemistry, and soil degradation chemistry), a knowledge-base system, and prediction tools. The biotransformation database is based on known biotransformations and common metabolic pathways. The transformation knowledge-base system consists of literature-driven rules *(305,306)*. MetabolExpert uses matching basic biotransformations to the compound's structure for predicting the possible metabolites. Additionally, it includes models with validations and quantitative predictions *(307)*.

5.1.16. Metabolism Database

This Accelrys provided database is based on the journals of the Royal Society of Chemistry (RSC) *(308)*. It primarily contains information on the metabolic fate of chemicals (including pharmaceuticals, agrochemicals, food additives, and environmental and industrial chemicals) in vertebrates, invertebrates, and plants. New entries can be added, and the database may be searched graphically. This database can be combined with various computational tools from Accelrys for target-specific analysis and modeling. Metabolic pathways are organized alphanumerically, and future releases are scheduled to include a comprehensive survey of the metabolism literature *(308,309)*.

5.1.17. METEOR

METEOR uses a knowledge-based approach of structure–metabolism rules (biotransformations) to predict the metabolic fate of a query structure *(310)*. The system, developed and marketed by LHASA Limited, evolved out of the DEREK program. DEREK is a knowledge-based system that contains alerts capturing structural toxicity and relies on the available mechanisms of toxicity and metabolism. The rules in DEREK cover various toxicological endpoints (carcinogenicity, mutagenicity, skin sensitization, teratogenicity, irritation, and respiratory sensitization) for toxicity prediction *(311–313)*.

METEOR's biotransformation rules are generic reaction descriptors, and the versatile structural representation used in the system allows each atom or bond to have specific physicochemical properties. This approach provides more details than simple hard-coded functional group descriptors *(313)*, but this flexibility also can give rise to an avalanche of data. METEOR manages the amount of data by predicting which metabolites are to be formed rather than all the possible outcomes *(310,312,314,315)*. At high certainty levels, when chosen, only the more likely biotransformations are requested. At lower likelihood levels, the more common metabolites are also selected for examination. Currently, METEOR knowledge-based biotransformations are exclusively for mammalian biotransformations (phase I and phase II) *(314,315)*.

5.1.18. NOVASCREEN

NOVASCREEN provides a screening assay platform, pharmcoinformatics databases, and data mining tools and algorithms to create a map of the molecular recognition patterns and functional activity relationships between drug targets and drug-like chemical compounds. The following CYP data are commercially available: CYP1A2, CYP2A6, CYP2C9*1 (Arg 144), CYP2C19, CYP2D6 and CYP3A *(316)*.

5.2. Useful Links

5.2.1. The ICGEB (International Center for Engineering and Biotechnology)

This link (http://www.icgeb.org/~p450srv/) is a website with various links to several research laboratories, many research papers, proposals, databases, and proceedings. In addition, it contains a list of sequences of the CYP superfamily and its homologs from different enzyme systems *(273,317)*.

5.2.2. David R. Nelson's Webpage

This webpage (http://drnelson.utmem.edu/CytochromeP450.html) includes several links to talks, papers, presentations, and other useful information on P450. Moreover, this site has a very strong emphasis on structure- and sequence-related aspects of the CYP super family *(318,319)*. Other sites, such as KEGG (Kyoto Encyclopedia of Genes and Genomes is a bioinformatics resource for understanding higher-order functional meanings and utilities of the cell or the organism from its genome information), also have links to the Nelson's website (http://www.genome.ad.jp/kegg/kegg.html; http://www.genome.ad.jp/kegg/metabolism.html).

5.2.3. The International Society of Xenobiotics

The International Society of Xenobiotics is providing useful information on the P450 systems through many links to P450 research groups, the Nomenclature Committee (http://www.imm.ki.se/CYPalleles/) and drug interactions tables *(319)*.

5.3. Useful Services

5.3.1. PanVera Corps.

PanVera offers CYP450 Screening Kits, which allow for performing miniaturized CYP HTS. Vivid(r) CYP450 Screening Kits are designed to quantify the inhibition of the predominant human CYP isozymes (CYP3A4, CYP3A5, CYP2B6, CYP2D6, CYP2C9, CYP2C19, CYP1A2, and 2E1) involved in hepatic drug metabolism *(320)*.

5.3.2. SRI International

SRI evaluates drug metabolism and drug interactions, using human and animal (rat, dog, and monkey) tissue models based on human hepatocytes. It also extends services for the metabolite profiling of drug candidates using hepatocytes, liver and small intestine microsomes, and S9 microsomes containing a single enzyme. The analysis is conducted by various spectroscopic and analytical techniques. Moreover, it provides predictions on drug interactions due to inhibition or induction of drug metabolizing enzymes and metabolite formation by enzymes (phase I and II). Additionally, information on pharmacogenetic effects on human drug metabolism could be made available *(321)*.

5.3.3. XenoTech, LLC

XenoTech offers a selection of services for drug metabolism-related research including liver and pulmonary microsomes and S9, cryopreserved hepatocytes from human and six other relevant species, antibodies directed against CYP enzymes, recombinant CYPs, and bDNA probe sets *(322)*.

5.3.4. Human Biologics International

Human Biologics International offers various in vitro data, screens (Hepato-Screen™), kits, and analysis software (HepatoSoft™) for CYP inhibition, reactions, and stability *(323)*.

5.3.5. MDS, Inc.

MDS offers studies and designs (stability/profile screens, enzyme inhibition, drug–drug interactions, CYP450 identification, enzyme induction) to provide diverse in vitro metabolism screenings *(324)*. For example, in determining which CYP enzymes are involved in the metabolism of a drug candidate, the variation in human rate of metabolite formation with the variation in CYP activity in human microsomal samples from a panel of 10–15 donors are examined. The metabolism of the drug candidate is determined by various analytical methods in the panel of human liver microsomal samples and then it compared to known marker activities for individual CYP enzymes *(324)*.

5.3.6. CytroChroma, Inc.

Cytochroma has developed an approach for identifying cytochrome P450s (human, fungi, parasite, bacteria) through the use of molecular biology tools and the information about cytochrome P450 structure *(325)*. Cytochroma uses a bioinformatics approach to take advantage of the wealth of gene sequence information in public databases to identify new members of the cytochrome P450 family. Cytochroma claims to have identified 6 proprietary human cytochrome P450s *(325)*.

5.3.7. Metabolic Solutions, Inc.

The erythromycin breath test, provided by Metabolic Solutions, is a rapid and a quantitative measure of in vivo CYP3A4 activity. The test is for designed to be used as an investigational tool for assessing CYP3A4 activity during pharmacological research *(326–328)*.

5.3.8. TNO Pharma

TNO Pharma has developed a panel of 10 3T3-fibroblast–derived cell lines that express individual human CYP450 enzymes. At present, three are co-expressing human oxidoreductase. These cell lines can be used for metabolism and inhibition studies, cytotoxicity studies, and small-scale metabolite production *(329)*.

5.3.9. Ricerca, LLC.

Ricerca offers in vivo and in vitro ADMET services. Specifically, it provides in vitro assays for CYP inhibition, metabolism, ADME, pharmacokinetic, and metabolism profiling *(330)*.

5.3.10. Affymetrix, Inc.

This is the provider of GeneChip® cytochrome P450 assay for detection of 18 polymorphisms present in two human CYP genes (2D6 and 2C19 genes). In addition, Affymetrix offers specialty classification and subclassification systems, which operates based on the CYP450 database collected from 574 protein sequences *(281,282,331,332)*, for gene families such as the cytochrome P450 *(332)*.

5.3.11. Pharmagene, plc.

Pharmagene offers various services on metabolism predictors, drug–drug interactions, toxicity, Cytochrome P450 (CYP450), hepatocytes, MetMatrix™, and drug metabolism *(333)*.

6. Cross-Methods

Several research techniques are commonly used in the field of QSAR (quantitative structure–activity relationship). Nevertheless, this research area is constantly on the search to develop better, faster, or different methods. In this section, we intend to point out some ongoing research efforts that are exploring unique pathways with the same goal of better understanding the metabolism process of CYPs.

Classification trees are used to predict membership of cases or objects in the classes of a categorical dependent variable from their measurements on one or more predictor variables. Lewis et al. *(334)* used the concept of classification trees to design a decision tree for human P450 substrates. The intention was to predict which CYP isozyme will interact with which substrates, based on physicochemical parameters. The resulting classifiers are the volume, the charge, and the area/depth^2 shape descriptor of the substrate. Based on the volume descriptor, one is able to distinguish between CYP2E1 (low volume), CYP3A (high volume), and the other subenzymes. These medium volume subenzymes can be partitioned based on the pK_a; where acid compounds tend to interact with CYP2C9 and basic molecules with CYP2D6. The remaining isozymes are finally split up based on the shape descriptor (area/depth^2), where a low value indicates interaction with CYP2B6, medium values specify interactions with CYP2A6, and finally a high area/depth^2 value identifies interaction with CYP1A2. Another decision tree published in *Drug Discovery Today* by Lewis et al. *(361)* introduced an additional branch of the previously published decision tree, so that based on the COMPACT ratio (CR), a descriptor dependent on ΔE and the area/depth^2 of the substrate, one is able to distinguish between CYP 1 substrates (CR<12) and CYP2/CYP3 substrates, if the compact ratio is greater than 12.

Keseru and Molnar et al. *(336)* introduced a *novel metabolic fingerprint*, METAPRINT, for the assessment of metabolic similarity and diversity in combinatorial chemical libraries. Metaprint contains information of the metabolic routes and metabolites, predicted by MetabolExpert as well as *clog*P and molecular weight information for each metabolite and parent compound. This approach could be advantageous for the design of cassettes for dosing pharmacokinetic experiments. Another method to predict the metabolic route was developed by Singh et al. *(79)* for CYP 3A4 substrates. Here, a *trend vector*, describing the hydrogen's topological environment in a molecule, was successfully related to the hydrogen abstraction energy. Snyder et al. have applied a *genetic algorithm* as a method to select variables in a study of 50 CYP 2D6 substrates. *Neural networks*, an alternative statistical method, were used to explore the dependency of CYP1A2 flavonoids IC$_{50}$ values *(211)* as well as CYP 3A4 inhibition data *(244)* and structural descriptors. Gasteiger et al. *(337)* presented self-organizing neural network models to investigate the selectivity of CYP 2D6 against CYP3A4, 2D9, and 2C19 at the 225th ACS National Meeting. Gironés et al. *(254)* used alignment-depended molecular quantum similarities as descriptors of a partial least square model to exhibit the influences in binding affinity of aromatase of 50 steroids ($r^2 = 0.839$, $q^2 = 0.734$). *Weighted path numbers* as a set of descriptors have been used to study the inhibitory effects of 19 aliphatic alcohols on microsomal P450 p-hydroxylation of anilines *(338)*, where a path is a sequence of adjacent edges that do not pass through the same vertex more than once. The best statistical model could be achieved using path lengths of 4 ($r = 0.975$, $r_{cv} = 0.943$). Finally, *de novo design* strategies have been investigated by Ji et al. *(248)* for CYP51 and Halpert et al. *(339)*.

7. Future Perspective

An overview of the current understanding of the structures and functions for members of the CYP family has been presented in this chapter. There has been great interest in expanding our view of the structures and functions of members of this family of enzymes due to the key role these enzymes play in phase I metabolism of pharmaceutical compounds. It is has been demonstrated that a greater understanding of these proteins at the structural level can facilitate the development of predictive models for metabolism. By incorporating these models into the early drug discovery stages, it may prove possible to weed out those compounds that may demonstrate metabolic liabilities in preclinical and clinical trials.

In fact, the ability to accurately estimate and/or predict ADME-related properties has prompted some to suggest a new paradigm for drug discovery. As discovery technologies such as combinatorial chemistry and high throughput screening become the norm, it has been suggested that screening collections be censored of compounds with the potential to possess adverse ADME properties. As an example, the rise in the popularity of using the Lipinski "rule of five" *(340)* in identifying *a priori* those compounds that may possess poor solubility profiles is highly indicative of the industry-wide desire to "attrit" compounds in a fail fast, fail early manner.

While the application of models for CYP-substrate interactions, as presented herein, may be used to provide further support to eliminate compounds, real or virtual, from consideration prior to synthesis and/or activity assessment, it has been suggested that models of this type may be of greater utility in a drug discovery paradigm in which biological activity and ADME related properties are simultaneously optimized in an interactive and iterative fashion *(341)*. Although Lipinski-type filtering is commonplace in the pharmaceutical industry, the latter approach is beginning to emerge as ADME models become available. In addition, a review of the biotechnology and small pharmaceutical company sector will reveal numerous companies that incorporate this latter paradigm into their corporate mission statements.

8. Summary

The cost to bring a new drug to market has risen from $318 million to $802 million from 1991 to 2000, respectively. Clinical costs represent the majority of this spend ($467 million vs $335 million in 2000). In addition, the increase in clinical costs over this same time period ($104 million in 1991 vs $467 million in 2000) far exceeded that of the increase in preclinical costs ($214 million in 1991 vs $335 million in 2000) *(2)*. In order to maintain profitability and growth, given the current economic and regulatory and healthcare realities discussed in the introduction, the average-sized pharmaceutical company must release one average-sized new product every two years for each percentage of market share that it holds. As an example, it is calculated that the new company formed by the merger of Pfizer and Pharmacia will require four to five new product launches per year to sustain itself *(342)*. In order to meet this demand in productivity while minimizing the total cost required to bring a new drug to market, it is becoming increasingly important for the discovery units of pharmaceutical organizations to deliver high-quality compounds for preclinical and clinical assessments. The virtual screening of compounds using models (macromolecular, pharmacophore, or structure–activity relationship) based on structural information about or physicochemical requirements for substrates of the various CYP isoforms implicated in the metabolism of pharmaceuticals has the potential to accelerate the discovery effort and reduce the overall drug development costs by promoting higher quality candidate compounds for clinical assessment.

References

1. Grabowski, H. and Vernon, J. (1996) Longer patents for increased generic compeition in the US: the Waxman-Hatch act after one decade. *Pharmacoeconomics* **10,** 110–123.
2. DiMasi, J. A., Hansen, R. W., and Grabowski, H. G. (2003) The price of innovation: new estimates on drug development costs. *J. Health Econ.* **22,** 151–185.
3. Cheng, A., Diller, D. J., Dixon, S. L., Egan, W. J., Lauri, G., and Merz, K. M. (2002) Computation of the physio-chemical properties and data mining of large molecular collections. *J. Comput. Chem.* **23,** 172–183.
4. Lewis, D. F. V. (2001) COMPACT: A structural approach to the modelling of cytochromes P450 and their interactions with xenobiotics. *J. Chem. Technol. Biotechnol.* **76,** 237–244.
5. Danielson, P. B. (2002) The cytochrome P450 superfamily: biochemistry, evolution and drug metabolism in humans. *Curr. Drug. M.* **3,** 561–597.
6. Williams, P. A., Cosme, J., Sridhar, V., Johnson, E. F., and McRee, D. E. (2000) Mammalian microsomal cytochrome P450 monooxygenase: structural adaptations for membrane binding and functional diversity. *Mol. Cell* **5,** 121–31.
7. Poulos, T. L., Finzel, B. C., Gunsalus, I.C., Wagner, G. C., and Kraut, J. (1985) The 2.6 Å crystal structure of pseudomonas pudita cytochrome P-450. *J. Biol. Chem.* **260,** 16,122–16,130.
8. Poulos, T. L., Finzel, B. C., and Howard, A. J. (1986) Crystal structure of substrate-free *Pseudomonas putida* cytochrome P-450. *Biochemistry* **25,** 5314–5322.
9. Ferenczy, G. G. and Morris, G. M. (1989) The active site of cytochrome P-450 nifedipine oxidase: a model-building study. *J. Mol. Graph.* **7,** 206–11.
10. Koymans, L. M., Vermeulen, N. P., Baarslag, A., and Donne-Op den Kelder, G. M. (1993) A preliminary 3D model for cytochrome P450 2D6 constructed by homology model building. *J. Comput. Aid. Molec. Design* **7,** 281–9.

11. Szklarz, G. D., Ornstein, R. L., and Halpert, J. R. (1994) Application of 3-dimensional homology modeling of cytochrome P450 2B1 for interpretation of site-directed mutagenesis results. *J. Biomol. Struct. Dyn.* **12**, 061–078.

12. Lewis, D. F. and Lake, B. G. (1995) Molecular modelling of members of the P4502A subfamily: application to studies of enzyme specificity. *Xenobiotica* **25**, 585–98.

13. de Groot, M. J., Vermeulen, N. P., Kramer, J. D., van Acker, F. A., and Donne-Op den Kelder, G. M. (1996) A three-dimensional protein model for human cytochrome P450 2D6 based on the crystal structures of P450 101, P450 102, and P450 108. *Chem. Res. Toxicol.* **9**, 1079–91.

14. Modi, S., Paine, M. J., Sutcliffe, M. J., Lian, L. Y., Primrose, W. U., Wolf, C. R., and Roberts, G. C. (1996) A model for human cytochrome P450 2D6 based on homology modeling and NMR studies of substrate binding. *Biochemistry* **35**, 4540–50.

15. Tan, Y., White, S. P., Paranawithana, S. R., and Yang, C. S. (1997) A hypothetical model for the active site of human cytochrome P4502E1. *Xenobiotica* **27**, 287–99.

16. Chang, Y. T., Stiffelman, O. B., Vakser, I. A., Loew, G. H., Bridges, A., and Waskell, L. (1997) Construction of a 3D model of cytochrome P450 2B4. *Protein Eng.* **10**, 119–129.

17. Lozano, J. J., Lopez-de-Brinas, E., Centeno, N. B., Guigo, R., and Sanz, F. (1997) Three-dimensional modelling of human cytochrome P450 1A2 and its interaction with caffeine and MeIQ. *J. Comput. Aid. Mol. Design* **11**, 395–408.

18. Szklarz, G. D. and Halpert, J. R. (1997) Molecular modeling of cytochrome P450 3A4. *J. Comput. Aid. Molec. Design* **11**, 265–72.

19. Dai, R., Pincus, M. R., and Friedman, F. K. (1998) Molecular modeling of cytochrome P450 2B1: mode of membrane insertion and substrate specificity. *J. Protein Chem.* **17**, 120–129.

20. Dai, R., Zhai, S., Wei, X., Pincus, M. R., Vestal, R. E., and Friedman, F. K. (1998) Inhibition of human cytochrome P450 1A2 by flavones: a molecular modeling study. *J. Protein Chem.* **17**, 643–50.

21. Lewis, D. F. V. (1999) Homology modelling of human cytochromes P450 involved in xenobiotic metabolism and rationalization of substrate selectivity. *Exp. Toxicol. Pathol.* **51**, 369–374.

22. Lewis, D. F. and Lake, B. G. (1999) Molecular modelling of CYP4A subfamily members based on sequence homology with CYP102. *Xenobiotica* **29**, 763–81.

23. Payne, V. A., Chang, Y. T., and Loew, G. H. (1999) Homology modeling and substrate binding study of human CYP2C9 enzyme. *Proteins: Struct., Funct., Genet.* **37**, 176–190.

24. Payne, V. A., Chang, Y. T., and Loew, G. H. (1999) Homology modeling and substrate binding study of human CYP2C18 and CYP2C19 enzymes. *Proteins: Struct., Funct., Genet.* **37**, 204–217.

25. De Rienzo, F., Fanelli, F., Menziani, M. C., and De Benedetti, P. G. (2000) Theoretical investigation of substrate specificity for cytochromes P450 IA2, P450 IID6 and P450 IIIA4. *J. Comput. Aid. Molec. Design* **14**, 93–116.

26. Afzelius, L., Zamora, I., Ridderstrom, M., Andersson, T. B., Karlen, A., and Masimirembwa, C. M. (2001) Competitive CYP2C9 inhibitors: enzyme inhibition studies, protein homology modeling, and three-dimensional quantitative structure-activity relationship analysis. *Mol. Pharmacol.* **59,** 909–919.

27. Ridderstrom, M., Zamora, I., Fjellstrom, O., and Andersson, T. B. (2001) Analysis of selective regions in the active sites of human cytochromes P450, 2C8, 2C9, 2C18, and 2C19 homology models using GRID/CPCA. *J. Med. Chem.* **44,** 4072–4081.

28. Bathelt, C., Schmid, R. D., and Pleiss, J. (2002) Regioselectivity of CYP2B6: homology modeling, molecular dynamics simulation, docking. *J. Mol. Model.* **8,** 327–35.

29. Bapiro, T. E., Hasler, J. A., Ridderstrom, M., and Masimirembwa, C. M. (2002) The molecular and enzyme kinetic basis for the diminished activity of the cytochrome P450 2D6.17 (CYP2D6.17) variant: potential implications for CYP2D6 phenotyping studies and the clinical use of CYP2D6 substrate drugs in some African populations. *Biochem. Pharmacol.* **64,** 1387–1398.

30. Lewis, D. F. (2002) Homology modelling of human CYP2 family enzymes based on the CYP2C5 crystal structure. *Xenobiotica* **32,** 305–323.

31. Sechenykh, A. A., Dubanov, A. V., Skvortsov, V. S., et al. (2002) Computer model of 3D structure of cytochrome P450 2B4. *Vopr. Med. Khim.* **48,** 526–538.

32. Szklarz, G. D. and Paulsen, M. D. (2002) Molecular modeling of cytochrome P450 1A1: enzyme-substrate interactions and substrate binding affinities. *J. Biomol. Struct. Dyn.* **20,** 155–162.

33. Wang, Q. and Halpert, J. R. (2002) Combined three-dimensional quantitative structure-activity relationship analysis of cytochrome P450 2B6 substrates and protein homology modeling. *Drug Metab. Dispos.* **30,** 86–95.

34. Kirton, S. B., Baxter, C. A., and Sutcliffe, M. J. (2002) Comparative modelling of cytochromes P450. *Adv. Drug Deliv. Rev.* **54,** 385–406.

35. Kirton, S. B., Kemp, C. A., Tomkinson, N. P., St -Gallay, S., and Sutcliffe, M. J. (2002) Impact of incorporating the 2C5 crystal structure into comparative models of cytochrome P450 2D6. *Proteins* **49,** 216–231.

36. Venhorst, J., ter Laak, A. M., Commandeur, J. N., Funae, Y., Hiroi, T., and Vermeulen, N. P. (2003) Homology modeling of rat and human cytochrome P450 2D (CYP2D) isoforms and computational rationalization of experimental ligand-binding specificities. *J. Med. Chem.* **46,** 74–86.

37. Lewis, D. F. V., Lake, B. G., Bird, M. G., Loizou, G. D., Dickins, M., and Goldfarb, P. S. (2003) Homology modelling of human CYP2E1 based on the CYP2C5 crystal structure: Investigation of enzyme-substrate and enzyme-inhibitor interactions. *Toxicol. in Vitro* **17,** 93–105.

38. Lewis, D. F., Lake, B. G., Dickins, M., and Goldfarb, P. S. (2003) Homology modelling of CYP2A6 based on the CYP2C5 crystallographic template: enzyme-substrate interactions and QSARs for binding affinity and inhibition. *Toxicol. in Vitro* **17,** 179–90.

39. Lewis, D. F. (2003) Essential requirements for substrate binding affinity and selectivity toward human CYP2 family enzymes. *Arch. Biochem. Biophys.* **409,** 32–44.

40. Pearson, W. R. (1990) Rapid and sensitive sequence comparison with FASTP and FASTA. *Methods Enzymol.* **183,** 63–98.

41. Altschul, S. F., Madden, T. L., Schaffer, A. A., et al. (1997) Gapped BLAST and PSI-BLAST: a new generation of protein database search programs. *Nucleic Acids Res.* **25,** 3389–3402.

42. Berman, H. M., Westbrook, J., Feng, Z., et al. (2000) The Protein Data Bank. *Nucleic Acids Res.* **28,** 235–242.

43. Thompson, J. D., Higgins, D. G., and Gibson, T. J. (1994) CLUSTAL W: improving the sensitivity of progressive multiple sequence alignment through sequence weighting, position-specific gap penalties and weight matrix choice. *Nucleic Acids Res.* **22,** 4673–4680.

44. Martin, A. C., MacArthur, M. W., and Thornton, J. M. (1997) Assessment of comparative modeling in CASP2. *Proteins* **Suppl. 1,** 14–28.

45. Haines, D. C., Tomchick, D. R., Machius, M., and Peterson, J. A. (2001) Pivotal role of water in the mechanism of P450BM-3. *Biochemistry* **40,** 13,456–13,465.

46. Cupp-Vickery, J. R., Garcia, C., Hofacre, A., and McGee-Estrada, K. (2001) Ketoconazole-induced conformational changes in the active site of cytochrome P450eryF. *J. Mol. Biol.* **311,** 101–110.

47. Mizuguchi, K., Deane, C. M., Blundell, T. L., and Overington, J. P. (1998) HOMSTRAD: a database of protein structure alignments for homologous families. *Protein Sci.* **7,** 2469–2471.

48. Peterson, J. A. and Graham, S. E. (1998) A close family resemblance: the importance of structure in understanding cytochromes P450. *Structure* **6,** 1079–1085.

49. Heinemann, F. S. and Ozols, J. (1983) The complete amino acid sequence of rabbit phenobarbital-induced liver microsomal cytochrome P-450. *J. Biol. Chem.* **258,** 4195–4201.

50. Gotoh, O. (1992) Substrate recognition sites in cytochrome P450 family 2 (CYP2) proteins inferred from comparative analyses of amino acid and coding nucleotide sequences. *J. Biol. Chem.* **267,** 83–90.

51. Nelson, D. R. and Strobel, H. W. (1988) On the membrane topology of vertebrate cytochrome P-450 proteins. *J. Biol. Chem.* **263,** 6038–6050.

52. Nelson, D. R. and Strobel, H. W. (1989) Secondary structure prediction of 52 membrane–bound cytochromes P450 shows a strong structural similarity to P450cam. *Biochemistry* **28,** 656–660.

53. Hasemann, C. A., Kurumbail, R. G., Boddupalli, S. S., Peterson, J. A., and Deisenhofer, J. (1995) Structure and function of cytochromes P450: a comparative analysis of three crystal structures. *Structure* **3,** 41–62.

54. Poulos, T. L., Finzel, B. C., and Howard, A. J. (1987) High-resolution crystal structure of cytochrome P450cam. *J. Mol. Biol.* **195,** 687–700.

55. Alwyn Jones, T. and Kleywegt, G. J. (1999) CASP3 comparative modeling evaluation. *Proteins* **Suppl. 3,** 30–46.

56. Holm, L. and Sander, C. (1996) The FSSP database: fold classification based on structure-structure alignment of proteins. *Nucleic Acids Res.* **24,** 206–209.

57. Jones, D. T. (1999) Protein secondary structure prediction based on position-specific scoring matrices. *J. Mol. Biol.* **292,** 195–202.
58. Rost, B., Sander, C., and Schneider, R. (1994) PHD—an automatic mail server for protein secondary structure prediction. *Comput. Appl. Biosci.* **10,** 53–60.
59. Domanski, T. L. and Halpert, J. R. (2001) Analysis of mammalian cytochrome P450 structure and function by site-directed mutagenesis. *Curr. Drug. M.* **2,** 117–137.
60. Szklarz, G. D., He, Y. A., and Halpert, J. R. (1995) Site-directed mutagenesis as a tool for molecular modeling of cytochrome P450 2B1. *Biochemistry* **34,** 14,312–14,322.
61. Gartner, C. A. (2003) Photoaffinity ligands in the study of cytochrome p450 active site structure. *Curr. Med. Chem.* **10,** 671–689.
62. Chang, Y. T. and Loew, G. H. (1999) Homology modeling and substrate binding study of human CYP4A11 enzyme. *Proteins* **34,** 403–415.
63. Sali, A. and Blundell, T. L. (1993) Comparative protein modelling by satisfaction of spatial restraints. *J. Mol. Biol.* **234,** 779–815.
64. Antonovic, L., Hodek, P., Smrcek, S., Novak, P., Sulc, M., and Strobel, H. W. (1999) Heterobifunctional photoaffinity probes for cytochrome P450 2B. *Arch. Biochem. Biophys.* **370,** 208–215.
65. Lee, H., Ortiz de Montellano, P. R., and McDermott, A. E. (1999) Deuterium magic angle spinning studies of substrates bound to cytochrome P450. *Biochemistry* **38,** 10,808–10,813.
66. Poli-Scaife, S., Attias, R., Dansette, P. M., and Mansuy, D. (1997) The substrate binding site of human liver cytochrome P450 2C9: an NMR study. *Biochemistry* **36,** 12,672–12,682.
67. Modi, S., Gilham, D. E., Sutcliffe, M. J., et al. (1997) 1-Methyl-4-phenyl-1,2,3,6-tetrahydropyridine as a substrate of cytochrome P450 2D6: allosteric effects of NADPH-cytochrome P450 reductase. *Biochemistry* **36,** 4461–4470.
68. Koerts, J., Rietjens, I. M., Boersma, M. G., and Vervoort, J. (1995) 1H NMR T1 relaxation rate study on substrate orientation of fluoromethylanilines in the active sites of microsomal and purified cytochromes P450 1A1 and 2B1. *FEBS Lett.* **368,** 279–284.
69. Ohnishi, T., Miura, S., and Ichikawa, Y. (1993) Photoaffinity labeling of cytochrome P-450(11beta) with methyltrienolone as a probe for the substrate binding region. *BBA-Protein Struc. Mol. Enzym.* **1161,** 257–264.
70. Yun, C. H., Hammons, G. J., Jones, G., et al. (1992) Modification of cytochrome P450 1A2 enzymes by the mechanism-based inactivator 2-ethynylnaphthalene and the photoaffinity label 4-azidobiphenyl. *Biochemistry* **31,** 10,556–10,563.
71. Gorokhov, A., Negishi, M., Johnson, E. F., et al. (2003) Explicit water near the catalytic I helix Thr in the predicted solution structure of CYP2A4. *Biophys. J.* **84,** 57–68.
72. Zhao, D., Gilfoyle, D. J., Smith, A. T., and Loew, G. H. (1996) Refinement of 3D models of horseradish peroxidase isoenzyme C: predictions of 2D NMR assignments and substrate binding sites. *Proteins* **26,** 204–216.

73. Laskowski, R. A., Moss, D. S., and Thornton, J. M. (1993) Main-chain bond lengths and bond angles in protein structures. *J. Mol. Biol.* **231,** 1049–1067.

74. Pontius, J., Richelle, J., and Wodak, S. J. (1996) Deviations from standard atomic volumes as a quality measure for protein crystal structures. *J. Mol. Biol.* **264,** 121–136.

75. Rodriguez, R., Chinea, G., Lopez, N., Pons, T., and Vriend, G. (1998) Homology modeling, model and software evaluation: three related resources. *Bioinformatics* **14,** 523–528.

76. Colovos, C. and Yeates, T. O. (1993) Verification of protein structures: patterns of nonbonded atomic interactions. *Protein Sci.* **2,** 1511–1519.

77. Luthy, R., Bowie, J. U., and Eisenberg, D. (1992) Assessment of protein models with three-dimensional profiles. *Nature* **356,** 83–85.

78. Podust, L. M., Poulos, T. L., and Waterman, M. R. (2001) Crystal structure of cytochrome P450 14alpha-sterol demethylase (CYP51) from Mycobacterium tuberculosis in complex with azole inhibitors. *Proc. Natl. Acad. Sci. USA* **98,** 3068–3073.

79. Singh, S. B., Shen, L. Q., Walker, M. J., and Sheridan, R. P. (2003) A model for predicting likely sites of CYP3A4-mediated metabolism on drug-like molecules. *J. Med. Chem.* **46,** 1330–1336.

80. Ravichandran, K. G., Boddupalli, S. S., Hasermann, C. A., Peterson, J. A., and Deisenhofer, J. (1993) Crystal structure of hemoprotein domain of P450BM-3, a prototype for microsomal P450's. *Science* **261,** 731–736.

81. Brodie, B., Axelrod, J., Cooper, J. R., et al. (1955) Detoxication of drugs and other foreign compounds by liver microsomes. *Science* **121,** 603–604.

82. Axelrod, J. (1955) The enzymatic demethylation of ephidrine. *J. Pharmacol. Exp. Ther.* **114,** 430–438.

83. Garfinkel, D. (1958) Studies on pig liver microsomes. I. enzymic and pigment composition of different microsomal fractions. *Arch. Biochem. Biophys.* **77,** 493–509.

84. Klingenberg, M. (1958) Pigments of rat liver microsomes. *Arch. Biochem. Biophys.* **75,** 376–386.

85. Hasemann, C. A., Ravichandran, K. G., Peterson, J.A., and Deisenhofer, J. (1994) Crystal structure and refinement of cytochrome at 2.3 Å resolution. *J. Mol. Biol.* **236,** 1169–1185.

86. Raag, R. and Poulos, T. L. (1989) Crystal structure of the carbon-monoxide-substrate-cytochrome. *Biochemistry* **28,** 7586–7592.

87. Poulos, T. L. and Howard, A. J. (1987) Crystal structure of metyrapone- and phenylimidazole-inhibited complexes of cytochrome. *Biochemistry* **26,** 8165.

88. Raag, R. and Poulos, T. L. (1991) Crystal structures of cytochrome complexed with camphane, thiocamphor and adamantane: factors controlling P450 substrate hydroxylation. *Biochemistry* **30,** 2674–2684.

89. Raag, R., Li,H., Jones, B. C., and Poulos,T. L. (1993) Inhibitor-induced conformational change in cytochrome. *Biochemistry* **32,** 4571–4578.

90. Raag, R. and Poulos, T. L. (1989) The structural basis for substrate-induced changes in redox potential and spin equilibrium in cytochrome. *Biochemistry* **28,** 917–922.

91. Raag, R., Swanson, B. A., Poulos, T.L., and Ortiz de Montellano, P. R. (1990) Formation, crystal structure and rearrangement of a cytochrome P- iron-phenyl complex. *Biochemistry* **29**, 8119–8126.

92. Lewis, D. V. F. (1996) *Cytochrome P450: structure, function and mechanism.* Taylor and Francis, London.

93. Raucy, J. L. and Allen, S. W. (2001) Recent advances in P450 research. *Pharmacogenomics J.* **1**, 178–186.

94. Lewis, D. V. F. (1986) Physical methods in the study of the active site geometry of cytochrome P450. *Drug Metab. Rev.* **17**, 1–66.

95. Hawkes, B. K. and Dawson, J. H. (1992) Oxygen activation by mono-oxygenase. Active site structure and mechanisms of action. *Frontiers in Biotransformation* **7**, 216–278.

96. Hildebrandt, P. (1992) Resonance Raman spectroscopy of cytochrome P450. *Frontiers in Biotransformation* **7**, 166–215.

97. Schenkman, J. B., Sligar, S. G., and Cinti, D. L. (1981) Substrate interaction with cytochrome P450. *Pharmacol. Ther.* **12**, 43–71.

98. Coon, M. J. and White, R. J. (1980) Cytochrome P450: a versatile catalyst in mono-oxygenation reactions. In *Metal ion activation of dioxygen.* Wiley, New York.

99. Hanson, L. K., Eaton, W. A., Sligar, S. G., Gunsalus, I.C., Gouterman, M., and Connell, C. R. (1976) Origin of the anomalous Soret Spectra carboxy cytochrome P450. *J. Am. Chem. Soc.* **98**, 2672–2674.

100. Hanson, L. K., Sligar, S. G., and Gunsalus, I. C. (1977) Electronic structure of P450. *Croat. Chem. Acta* **49**, 237–250.

101. Gibson, G. G. and Tamburini, P. P. (1984) Cytochrome P450 spin state: inorganic biochemistry of heme iron ligation and functional significance. *Xenobiotica* **14**, 27–47.

102. Gibson, G. G. and Skett, P. (1994) *Introduction of drug metabolism.* Chapman and Hall, London.

103. Dawson, J. H. and Sono, M. (1987) Cytochrome P450 chloroperoxidase: thiolate-ligand heme enzymes. Spectroscopic determination of their active site structure and mechanistic implication of thiolate ligation. *Chem. Rev.* **87**, 1255–1276.

104. Dawson, J. H., Andersson, L. A., and Song, M. (1982) Spectroscopic investigations of ferric cytochrome P-450-CAM ligand complexes. *J. Biol. Chem.* **257**, 3606–3617.

105. Dawson, J. H., et al. (1986) Oxygenated cytochrome P450cam and chloroperoxidase: direct evidence for sulfur donor ligation trans todioxygen and structural characterization using EXAFS spectroscopy. *J. Am. Chem. Soc.* **108**, 8114–8116.

106. Champion, P. M., et al. (1982) Resonance Raman detection of an Fe-S bond in cytochrome P45cam. *J. Am. Chem. Soc.* **104**, 5469–5473.

107. Munro, A. W., et al. (1992) Investigating the function of cytochrome P450 BM-3: a role for the phylogenetically conserved tryptophane residue. *Biochem. Soc. Trans.* **21**, 66.

108. Munro, A. W., et al. (1994) Resonance Raman spectroscopic studies on intact cytohrome P450–BM3. *Biochem. Soc. Trans.* **22**, 54.

109. Egawa, T., et al. (1991) Observation of the O-O stretching Raman band for cytochrome P450cam under catalytic conditions. *J. Biol. Chem.* **266,** 10,246–10,248.

110. Jung, C., et al. (1992) Substrate analouge induced changes of the CO-stretching mode in cytochrome P450cam -carbon monoxide complex. *Biochemistry* **31,** 12,855–12,862.

111. Nagai, M., et al. (1991) Unusual CO bonding geometry in abnormal subunits of hemoglobin M Boston hemoglobin M Saskatoon. *Biochemistry* **30,** 6495–6503.

112. Sharrock, M., et al. (1976) Cytochrome P45cam and its complexes. Mossbauer parameters of the heme iron. *Biochim. Biophys. Acta* **420,** 8–26.

113. (2003) www.rcsb.org/pdb.

114. AstexTechnology (2003) http://www.astex-technology.com/servlet/astex.

115. Wermuth, C. G. (1999) *The practice of medicinal chemistry.* Academic Press, San Diego, CA.

116. Leach, R. A. (1996) *Molecular modelling and applications.* Addison Wesely Longman Limited, Singapore.

117. Kuntz, D. I., et al. (1982) Geometric approach to macromolecule-ligand interactions. *J. Mol. Biol.* **161,** 262.

118. Li, R., Chen, X., Gong, B., et al. (1996) Structure-based design of parasitic protease inhibitors. *Bioorg. Med. Chem.* **4,** 1421–1427.

119. Kuntz, D. I. (1992) Structure-based strategies for drug design and discovery. *Science* **257,** 1078–1082.

120. Morris, G. M., et al. (1998) Automated docking using a Lamarckian genetic algorithm and an empirical binding free energy function. *J. Comput. Chem.* **19,** 1638–1662.

121. Jones, G., Willett, P., and Glen, R. C. (1995) A genetic algorithm for flexible molecular overlay and pharmacophore elucidation. *J. Comput. Aid. Molec. Design* **9,** 532–549.

122. Rarey, M., Kramer, B., Lengauer, T., and Klebe, G. (1996) A fast flexible docking method using an incremental construction algorithm. *J. Mol. Biol.* **261,** 470–489.

123. Lewis, D. F. V., Dickins, M., Lake, B. G., Eddershaw, P. J., Tarbit, M. H., and Goldfarb, P. S. (1999) Molecular modelling of the human cytochrome P450 isoform CYP2A6 and investigations of CYP2A substrate selectivity. *Toxicology* **133,** 1–33.

124. Lewis, D. F., Lake, B. G., and Parke, D. V. (1995) Molecular orbital-generated QSARs in a homologous series of alkoxyresorufins and studies of their interactive docking with P450s. *Xenobiotica* **25,** 1355–1369.

125. Lewis, D. F. V., Wiseman, A., and Tarbit, M. H. (1999) Molecular modeling of lanosterol 14-alpha-demethylase (CYP51) from Saccharomyces cerevisiae via homology with CYP102, a unique bacterial cytochrome P450 isoform: quantitative structure-activity relationships (QSARs) within two related series of antifungal azole derivatives. *J. Enz. Inhib.* **14,** 175–192.

126. Cavalli, A., Greco, G., Novellino, E., and Recanatini, M. (2000) Linking CoMFA and protein homology models of enzyme-inhibitor interactions: an application to non-steroidal aromatase inhibitors. *Bioorg. Med. Chem.* **8,** 2771–2780.

127. Cavalli, A. and Recanatini, M. (2002) Looking for selectivity among cytochrome P450s inhibitors. *J. Med. Chem.* **45**, 251–254.

128. Lewis, D. F. and Moereels, H. (1992) The sequence homologies of cytochromes P-450 and active-site geometries. *J. Comput. Aid. Molec. Design* **6**, 235–252.

129. Ahmed, S. (1999) Modelling the active site of the P-450 family of enzymes involved in steroidogenesis-Potentially a novel approach to the initial (computer based) screening of compounds against the P-450 family of enzymes. *J. Pharm. Pharmacol.* **51**, 254.

130. Szklarz, G. D. and Halpert, J. R. (1998) Molecular basis of P450 inhibition and activation: implications for drug development and drug therapy. *Drug Metab. Dispos.* **26**, 1179–1184.

131. Kobayashi, Y., Fang, X., Szklarz, G. D., and Halpert, J. R. (1998) Probing the active site of cytochrome P450 2B1: metabolism of 7- alkoxycoumarins by the wild type and five site-directed mutants. *Biochemistry* **37**, 6679–6688.

132. Spatzenegger, M., Wang, Q., He, Y. Q., Wester, M. R., Johnson, E. F., and Halpert, J. R. (2001) Amino acid residues critical for differential inhibition of CYP2B4, CYP2B5, and CYP2B1 by phenylimidazoles. *Mol. Pharmacol.* **59**, 475–484.

133. Ji, H., Zhang, W., Zhou, Y., et al. (2000) A three-dimensional model of lanosterol 14alpha-demethylase of Candida albicans and its interaction with azole antifungals. *J. Med. Chem.* **43**, 2493–2505.

134. Jones, B. C., Hyland, R., Ackland, M., Tyman, C. A., and Smith, D. A. (1998) Interaction of terfenadine and its primary metabolites with cytochrome P450 2D6. *Drug Metab. Dispos.* **26**, 875–882.

135. DesJarlais, R. L., Sheridan, R. P., Dixon, J. S., Kuntz, I. D., and Venkataraghavan, R. (1986) Docking flexible ligands to macromolecular receptors by molecular shape. *J. Med. Chem.* **29**, 2149–2153.

136. De Voss, J., Zhang, Z., Sibbesen, O., and de Montellano, O. (1997) Substrate docking algorithms and prediction of the substrate specificity of cytochrome P450-cam and its L244 mutant. *J. Am. Chem. Soc.* **119**, 5489.

137. De Voss, J. and Ortiz de Montellano, R. (1995) Computer-assisted, structure-based prediction of substrate for cytochrome P450cam. *J. Am. Chem. Soc.* **117**, 4185–4186.

138. Kuhn, B., Jacobsen, W., Christians, U., Benet, L. Z., and Kollman, P. A. (2001) Metabolism of sirolimus and its derivative everolimus by cytochrome P450 3A4: Insights from docking, molecular dynamics, and quantum chemical calculations. *J. Med. Chem.* **44**, 2027–2034.

139. Lopez de Brinas, E., et al. (2000) European symposium on QSAR: molecular modeling and prediction of bioactivity, Copenhagen, Denmark.

140. Anandatheerthavarada, H. K., Amuthan, G., Biswas, G., et al. (2001) Evolutionarily divergent electron donor proteins interact with P450MT2 through the same helical domain but different contact points. *EMBO J.* **20**, 2394–2403.

141. Jalaie, M. and Erickson, J. A. (2000) Approaches to molecular alignments for CoMFA. *J. Comput. Aid. Molec. Design* **14**, 181–197.

142. Jones, G., Willett, P., Glen, R. C., A. Leach, R., and Taylor, R. (1995) Molecular recognition of receptor sites using a genetic algorithm with a description of desolvation. *J. Mol. Biol.* **246,** 43–53.

143. Jones, G., Willett, P., Glen, R. C., A. Leach, R., and Taylor, R. (1997) Development and validation of a genetic algorithm for flexible docking. *J. Mol. Biol.* **267,** 727–748.

144. Li, X. Q., Bjorkman, A., Andersson, T. B., Ridderstrom, M., and Masimirembwa, C. M. (2002) Amodiaquine clearance and its metabolism to N-desethylamodiaquine is mediated by CYP2C8: A new high affinity and turnover enzyme-specific probe substrate. *J. Pharmacol. Exp. Ther.* **300,** 399–407.

145. ALMOND. Multivariate Infometric Analysis S.r.l., Perugia.

146. Baroni, M., Costantino, G., Cruciani, G., Riganelli, D., Valigi, R., and Clementi, S. (1993) Generating optimal linear PLS estimations (GOLPE): an advanced chemometric tool for handling 3D-QSAR problems. *Quant. Struct.-Act. Relat.* **12,** 9–20.

147. Masimirembwa, C. M., Ridderstrom, M., Zamora, I., and Andersson, T. B. (2002) Combining pharmacophore and protein modeling to predict CYP450 inhibitors and substrates. *Methods Enzymol.* **357,** 133–144.

148. Lozano, J. J., Pastor, M., Cruciani, G., et al. (2000) 3D-QSAR methods on the basis of ligand-receptor complexes. Application of COMBINE and GRID/ GOLPE methodologies to a series of CYP1A2 ligands. *J. Comput. Aid. Molec. Design* **14,** 341–353.

149. Park, J. and Harris, D. (2003) Construction and assessment of models of CYP2E1: predictions of metabolism from docking, molecular dynamics, and density functional calculations. *J. Med. Chem.* **46,** 1645–1660.

150. Keseru, G. M. (2001) A virtual high throughput screen for high affinity cytochrome P450cam substrates. Implications for in silico prediction of drug metabolism. *J. Comput. Aid. Molec. Design* **15,** 649–657.

151. Zhang, Z., Sibbesen, O., and Johnson. R. A. (1998) The substrate specificity of cytocrome P450cam. *Bioorg. Med. Chem.* **6,** 1501–1508.

152. Clark, R. D., Strizhev, A., Leonard, J. M., Blake, J. F., and Matthew, J. B. (2002) Consensus scoring for ligand/protein interactions. *J. Mol. Graph.* **20,** 281–295.

153. Kumar, S., Scott, E. E., Liu, Hong, and Halpert, J. (2003) A rational approach to re-engineer cytochrome P450 2B1 regioselectivity based on the crystal structure of cytochrome P450 2C5. **278,** 17,178–17,184.

154. Szklarz, G. D. and Halpert, J. R. (1997) Use of homology modeling in conjunction with site-directed mutagenesis for analysis of structure-function relationships of mammalian cytochromes P450. *Life Sci.* **61,** 2507–2520.

155. He, K., He, Y. A., Szklarz, G. D., Halpert, J. R., and Correia, M. A. (1996) Secobarbital-mediated inactivation of cytochrome P450 2B1 and its active site mutants. Partitioning between heme and protein alkylation and epoxidation. *J. Biol. Chem.* **271,** 25,864–25,872.

156. Lewis, D. F., Ioannides, C., and Parke, D. V. (1986) Molecular dimensions of the substrate binding site of cytochrome P-448. *Biochem. Pharmacol.* **35,** 2179–2185.

157. Ioannides, C. and Parke, D. V. (1987) The cytochromes P-448—a unique family of enzymes involved in chemical toxicity and carcinogenesis. *Biochem. Pharmacol.* **36,** 4197–4207.

158. Sanz, F., Lopez-de-Brinas, E., Rodriguez, J., and Manaut, F. (1994) Theoretical study on the metabolism of caffeine by cytochrome p-450 1A2 and its inhibition. *Quant. Struct.-Act. Relat.* **13,** 281–284.

159. Fuhr, U., Strobl, G., Manaut, F., Anders, E. M., Soergel, F., and Lopez de Brinas, E. (1993) Quinolone antibacterial agents: relationship between structure and in vitro inhibition of the human cytochrome P450 isoform CYP1A2. *Mol. Pharmacol.* **43,** 191–199.

160. Lee, H., Yeom, H., Kim, Y. G., et al. (1998) Structure-related inhibition of human hepatic caffeine N3-demethylation by naturally occurring flavonoids. *Biochem. Pharmacol.* **55,** 1369–1375.

161. Poso, A., Gynther, J., and Juvonen, R. (2001) A comparative molecular field analysis of cytochrome P450 2A5 and 2A6 inhibitors. *J. Comput. Aid. Molec. Design* **15,** 195–202.

162. Lewis, D. F., Lake, B. G., Dickins, M., Eddershaw, P. J., Tarbit, M. H., and Goldfarb, P. S. (1999) Molecular modelling of CYP2B6, the human CYP2B isoform, by homology with the substrate-bound CYP102 crystal structure: evaluation of CYP2B6 substrate characteristics, the cytochrome b5 binding site and comparisons with CYP2B1 and CYP2B4. *Xenobiotica* **29,** 361–393.

163. Ekins, S., Bravi, G., Ring, B. J., et al. (1999) Three-dimensional quantitative structure activity relationship analyses of substrates for CYP2B6. *J. Pharmacol. Exp. Ther.* **288,** 21–29.

164. Mancy, A., Broto, P., Dijols, S., Dansette, P. M., and Mansuy, D. (1995) The substrate binding site of human liver cytochrome P450 2C9: an approach using designed tienilic acid derivatives and molecular modeling. *Biochemistry* **34,** 10,365–10,375.

165. Miners, J. O. and Birkett, D. J. (1998) Cytochrome P4502C9: an enzyme of major importance in human drug metabolism. *Br. J. Clin. Pharmacol.* **45,** 525–538.

166. He, M., Korzekwa, K. R., Jones, J. P., Rettie, A. E., and Trager, W. F. (1999) Structural forms of phenprocoumon and warfarin that are metabolized at the active site of CYP2C9. *Arch. Biochem. Biophys.* **372,** 16–28.

167. Mancy, A., Dijols, S., Poli, S., Guengerich, P., and Mansuy, D. (1996) Interaction of sulfaphenazole derivatives with human liver cytochromes P450 2C: molecular origin of the specific inhibitory effects of sulfaphenazole on CYP 2C9 and consequences for the substrate binding site topology of CYP 2C9. *Biochemistry* **35,** 16,205–16,212.

168. Jones, B. C., Hawksworth, G., Horne, V. A., et al. (1996) Putative active site template model for cytochrome P4502C9 (tolbutamide hydroxylase). *Drug Metab. Dispos.* **24,** 260–266.

169. Jones, J. P., He, M., Trager, W. F., and Rettie, A. E. (1996) Three-dimensional quantitative structure-activity relationship for inhibitors of cytochrome P4502C9. *Drug Metab. Dispos.* **24,** 1–6.

170. Haining, R. L., Jones, J. P., Henne, K. R., et al. (1999) Enzymatic determinants of the substrate specificity of CYP2C9: role of B′-C loop residues in providing the pi-stacking anchor site for warfarin binding. *Biochemistry* **38**, 3285–3292.

171. Rao, S., Aoyama, R., Schrag, M., Trager, W. F., Rettie, A., and Jones, J. P. (2000) A refined 3-dimensional QSAR of cytochrome P450 2C9: computational predictions of drug interactions. *J. Med. Chem.* **43**, 2789–2796.

172. Ridderstrom, M., Masimirembwa, C., Trump-Kallmeyer, S., Ahlefelt, M., Otter, C., and Andersson, T. B. (2000) Arginines 97 and 108 in CYP2C9 are important determinants of the catalytic function. *Biochem. Biophys. Res. Commun.* **270**, 983–987.

173. Ekins, S., Bravi, G., Binkley, S., et al. (2000) Three- and four-dimensional-quantitative structure activity relationship (3D/4D-QSAR) analyses of CYP2C9 inhibitors. *Drug Metab. Dispos.* **28**, 994–1002.

174. Pastor, M., Cruciani, G., McLay, I., Pickett, S., and Clementi, S. (2000) GRid-INdependent descriptors (GRIND): a novel class of alignment-independent three-dimensional molecular descriptors. *J. Med. Chem.* **43**, 3233–3243.

175. Afzelius, L., Masimirembwa, C. M., Karlen, A., Anderson, T. B., and Zamora, I. (2002) Discriminant and quantitative PLS analysis of competitive CYP2C9 inhibitors versus non-inhibitors using alignment independent GRIND descriptors. *J. Comput. Aid. Molec. Design* **16**, 443–458.

176. De Groot, M. J., Alex, A. A., and Jones, B. C. (2002) Development of a combined protein and pharmacophore model for cytochrome P450 2C9. *J. Med. Chem.* **45**, 1983–1993.

177. Wolff, T., Distlerath, L. M., Worthington, M. T., et al. (1985) Substrate specificity of human liver cytochrome P-450 debrisoquine 4-hydroxylase probed using immunochemical inhibition and chemical modeling. *Cancer Res.* **45**, 2116–2122.

178. Meyer, U. A., Gut, J., Kronbach, T., Skoda, C., Meier, U. T., Catin, T., and Dayer, P. (1986) The molecular mechanisms of two common polymorphisms of drug oxidation—evidence for functional changes in cytochrome P-450 isozymes catalysing bufuralol and mephenytoin oxidation. *Xenobiotica* **16**, 449–464.

179. Islam, S. A., Wolf, C. R., Lennard, M. S., and Sternberg, M. J. (1991) A three-dimensional molecular template for substrates of human cytochrome P450 involved in debrisoquine 4-hydroxylation. *Carcinogenesis* **12**, 2211–2219.

180. Koymans, L., Vermeulen, N. P., van Acker, S. A., et al. (1992) A predictive model for substrates of cytochrome P450-debrisoquine (2D6). *Chem. Res. Toxicol.* **5**, 211–219.

181. de Groot, M. J., Bijloo, G. J., Hansen, K. T., and Vermeulen, N. P. (1995) Computer prediction and experimental validation of cytochrome P4502D6-dependent oxidation of GBR 12909. *Drug Metab. Dispos.* **23**, 667–669.

182. Ellis, S. W., Hayhurst, G. P., Smith, G., et al. (1995) Evidence that aspartic acid 301 is a critical substrate-contact residue in the active site of cytochrome P450 2D6. *J. Biol. Chem.* **270**, 29,055–29,058.

183. de Groot, M. J., Bijloo, G. J., Martens, B. J., van Acker, F. A., and Vermeulen, N. P. (1997) A refined substrate model for human cytochrome P450 2D6. *Chem. Res. Toxicol.* **10**, 41–48.

184. de Groot, M. J., Bijloo, G. J., van Acker, F. A., Fonseca Guerra, C., Snijders, J. G., and Vermeulen, N. P. (1997) Extension of a predictive substrate model for human cytochrome P4502D6. *Xenobiotica* **27,** 357–368.

185. Onderwater, R. C., Venhorst, J., Commandeur, J. N., and Vermeulen, N. P. (1999) Design, synthesis, and characterization of 7-methoxy-4-(aminomethyl)coumarin as a novel and selective cytochrome P450 2D6 substrate suitable for high-throughput screening. *Chem. Res. Toxicol.* **12,** 555–559.

186. de Groot, M. J., Ackland, M. J., Horne, V. A., Alex, A. A., and Jones, B. C. (1999) Novel approach to predicting P450-mediated drug metabolism: development of a combined protein and pharmacophore model for CYP2D6. *J. Med. Chem.* **42,** 1515–1524.

187. Lewis, D. F., Eddershaw, P. J., Goldfarb, P. S., and Tarbit, M. H. (1997) Molecular modelling of cytochrome P4502D6 (CYP2D6) based on an alignment with CYP102: structural studies on specific CYP2D6 substrate metabolism. *Xenobiotica* **27,** 319–339.

188. Hayhurst, G. P., Harlow, J., Chowdry, J., et al. (2001) Influence of phenylalanine-481 substitutions on the catalytic activity of cytochrome P450 2D6. *Biochem. J.* **355,** 373–379.

189. de Groot, M. J., Ackland, M. J., Horne, V. A., Alex, A. A., and Jones, B. C. (1999) A novel approach to predicting P450 mediated drug metabolism CYP2D6 catalyzed N-dealkylation reactions and qualitative metabolite predictions using a combined protein and pharmacophore model for CYP2D6. *J. Med. Chem.* **42,** 4062–4070.

190. Strobl, G. R., Von Kruedener, S., Stockigt, J., Guengerich, F. P., and Wolff, T. (1993) Development of a pharmacophore for inhibition of human liver cytochrome P-450 2D6: molecular modeling and inhibition studies. *J. Med. Chem.* **36,** 1136–1145.

191. Ekins, S., Bravi, G., Binkley, S., et al. (1999) Three and four dimensional-quantitative structure activity relationship (3D/4D-QSAR) analyses of CYP2D6 inhibitors. *Pharmacogenetics* **9,** 477–489.

192. Guengerich, F. P., Miller, G. P., Hanna, I. H., et al. (2002) Diversity in the oxidation of substrates by cytochrome P450 2D6: Lack of an obligatory role of aspartate 301-substrate electrostatic bonding. *Biochemistry* **41,** 11,025–11,034.

193. Domanski, T. L., He, Y. A., Khan, K. K., Roussel, F., Wang, Q., and Halpert, J. R. (2001) Phenylalanine and tryptophan scanning mutagenesis of CYP3A4 substrate recognition site residues and effect on substrate oxidation and cooperativity. *Biochemistry* **40,** 10,150–10,160.

194. Korzekwa, K. R., Krishnamachary, N., Shou, M., et al. (1998) Evaluation of atypical cytochrome P450 kinetics with two-substrate models: evidence that multiple substrates can simultaneously bind to cytochrome P450 active sites. *Biochemistry* **37,** 4137–4147.

195. Shou, M., Grogan, J., Mancewicz, J. A., et al. (1994) Activation of CYP3A4: Evidence for the simultaneous binding of two substrates in a cytochrome P450 active site. *Biochemistry* **33,** 6450–6455.

196. Hosea, N. A., Miller, G. P., and Guengerich, F. P. (2000) Elucidation of distinct ligand binding sites for cytochrome P450 3A4. *Biochemistry* **39,** 5929–5939.

197. Wang, R. W., Newton, D. J., Liu, N., Atkins, W. M., and Lu, A. Y. (2000) Human cytochrome P-450 3A4: in vitro drug-drug interaction patterns are substrate-dependent. *Drug Metab. Dispos.* **28,** 360–366.

198. Stresser, D. M., Blanchard, A. P., Turner, S. D., et al. (2000) Substrate-dependent modulation of CYP3A4 catalytic activity: analysis of 27 test compounds with four fluorometric substrates. *Drug Metab. Dispos.* **28,** 1440–1448.

199. Kenworthy, K. E., Bloomer, J. C., Clarke, S. E., and Houston, J. B. (1999) CYP3A4 drug interactions: correlation of 10 in vitro probe substrates. *Br. J. Clin. Pharmacol.* **48,** 716–727.

200. Ekins, S., Bravi, G., Wikel, J. H., and Wrighton, S. A. (1999) Three-dimensional-quantitative structure activity relationship analysis of cytochrome P-450 3A4 substrates. *J. Pharmacol. Exp. Ther.* **291,** 424–433.

201. Ekins, S., Bravi, G., Binkley, S., et al. (1999) Three- and four-dimensional quantitative structure activity relationship analyses of cytochrome P-450 3A4 inhibitors. *J. Pharmacol. Exp. Ther.* **290,** 429–438.

202. Ekins, S., Stresser, D. M., and Andrew Williams, J. (2003) In vitro and pharmacophore insights into CYP3A enzymes. *Trends Pharmacol. Sci.* **24,** 161–166.

203. Lewis, D. F., Eddershaw, P. J., Goldfarb, P. S., and Tarbit, M. H. (1996) Molecular modelling of CYP3A4 from an alignment with CYP102: identification of key interactions between putative active site residues and CYP3A-specific chemicals. *Xenobiotica* **26,** 1067–1086.

204. Cramer, I. I. I. R. D., Patterson, D. E., and Bunce, J. D. (1988) Comparative molecular field analysis (CoMFA). 1. Effect of shape on binding of steroids to carrier proteins.

205. Marshall, G. R. and Cramer, R. D., 3rd. (1988) Three-dimensional structure-activity relationships. *Trends Pharmacol. Sci.* **9,** 285–289.

206. Pastor, M., Cruciani, G., and Watson, K. (1997) A strategy for the incorporation of water molecules present in a ligand binding site into a 3D QSAR analysis. *J. Med. Chem.* **40,** 4089–4102.

207. Tripos Associates, I. SYBYL. St. Louis, MO.

208. Tripos Associates, I. Alchemy II. St. Louis, MO.

209. Accelrys, InsightII, San Diego, CA.

210. MOPAC, Creative Arts Building 181, Indiana University, Bloomington, IN 47405.

211. Moon, T., Chi, M. H., Kim, D.-H., Yoon, C. N., and Choi, Y.-S. (2000) Quantitative structure-activity relationships (QSAR) study of flavonoid derivatives for inhibition of cytochrome P450 1A2. *Quant. Struct.-Act. Relat.* **19,** 257–263.

212. Lewis, D. F. V., Modi, S., and Dickins, M. (2002) Structure-activity relationship for human. *Drug Metab. Rev.* **34,** 69–82.

213. Lewis, D. F., Ioannides, C., and Parke, D. V. (2003) A quantitative structure-activity relationship (QSAR) study of mutagenicity in several series of organic

chemicals likely to be activated by cytochrome P450 enzymes. *Teratog. Carcinog. Mutagen* **23 Suppl. 1,** 187–193.

214. Dewar, M. J. S., Zoebisch, E. G., Healy, E. F., and Stewart, J. J. P. (1985) AM1: a new general purpose quantum mechanical molecular model. *J. Am. Chem. Soc.* **107,** 3902–3909.

215. Mekenyan, O. G., Veith, G. D., Call, D. J., and Ankley, G. T. (1996) A QSAR evaluation of Ah receptor binding of halogenated aromatic xenobiotics. *Environ. Health Perspect.* **104,** 1302–1310.

216. Lewis, D. F., Jacobs, M. N., Dickins, M., and Lake, B. G. (2002) Quantitative structure–activity relationships for inducers of cytochromes P450 and nuclear receptor ligands involved in P450 regulation within the CYP1, CYP2, CYP3 and CYP4 families. *Toxicology* **176,** 51–57.

217. Waller, C. L. and McKinney, J. D. (1992) Comparative molecular field analysis of polyhalogenated dibenzo-p-dioxins, dibenzofurans, and biphenyls. *J. Med. Chem.* **35,** 3660–3666.

218. Bravi, G. and Wikel, J. H. (2000) Application of Ms-WHIM descriptors 1. Introduction of new molecular surface properties and 2. prediction of binding affinity data. *Quant. Struct.-Act. Relat.* **19,** 29–38.

219. Bravi, G., Gancia, E., Mascagni, P., Pegna, M., Todeschini, R., and Azaliani, A. (1997) MS-WHIM, new 3D theoretical descriptors derived from molecular surface properties: a comparative 3D QSAR study in a series of steroids. *J. Comput. Aid. Molec. Design* **11,** 79–92.

220. Lozâno, J. J., Pastor, M., Gago, F., Cruciani, G., Centeno, N. B., and Sanz, F. (1998)

221. Ortiz, A. R., Pisabarro, M. T., Gago, F., and Wade, R. C. (1995) Prediction of drug binding affinities by comparative binding energy analysis. *J. Med. Chem.* **38,** 2681–2691.

222. Ortiz, A. R., Pastor, M., Palomer, A., Cruciani, G., Gago, F., and Wade, R. C. (1997) Reliability of comparative molecular field analysis models: effects of data scaling and variable selection using a set of human synovial fluid phospholipase A2 inhibitors. *J. Med. Chem.* **40,** 1136–1148.

223. Perez, C., Pastor, M., Ortiz, A. R., and Gago, F. (1998) Comparative binding energy analysis of HIV-1 protease inhibitors: incorporation of solvent effects and validation as a powerful tool in receptor-based drug design. *J. Med. Chem.* **41,** 836–852.

224. Pastor, M., Cruciani, G., and Clementi, S. (1997) Smart region definition: a new way to improve the predictive ability and interpretability of three-dimensional quantitative structure-activity relationships. *J. Med. Chem.* **40,** 1455–1464.

225. Lewis, D. F., Modi, S., and Dickins, M. (2002) Structure-activity relationship for human cytochrome P450 substrates and inhibitors. *Drug Metab. Rev.* **34,** 69–82.

226. Lewis, D. F. and Lake, B. G. (2002) Species differences in coumarin metabolism: a molecular modelling evaluation of CYP2A interactions. *Xenobiotica* **32,** 547–561.

227. Rendic, S. and Di Carlo, F. J. (1997) Human cytochrome P450 enzymes: a status report summarizing their reactions, substrates, inducers, and inhibitors. *Drug Metab. Rev.* **29**, 413–580.

228. Lewis, D. F. V. and Dickins, M. (2001) Quantitative structure-activity relationships (QSARs) within series of inhibitors for mammalian cytochromes P450 (CYPs). *J. Enz. Inhib.* **16**, 321–330.

229. Lewis, D. F., Ioannides, C., and Parke, D. V. (1995) A quantitative structure-activity relationship study on a series of 10 para-substituted toluenes binding to cytochrome P4502B4 (CYP2B4), and their hydroxylation rates. *Biochem. Pharmacol.* **50**, 619–625.

230. Nanbo, A. and Nanbo, T. (2002) Mechanistic study on N-demethylation catalyzed with P450 by quantitative structure activity relationship using electronic properties of 4-substituted N,N-dimethylaniline. *Quant. Struct.-Act. Relat.* **21**, 613–616.

231. Lesigiarska, I., Pajeva, I., and Yanev, S. (2002) Quantitative structure-activity relationship (QSAR) and three-dimensional QSAR analysis of a series of xanthates as inhibitors and inactivators of cytochrome P450 2B1. *Xenobiotica* **32**, 1063–1077.

232. Stewart, J. J. P. (1989) Optimization of parameters for semiemprirical parameters. 1. Method. *J. Comput. Chem.* **10**, 209–220.

233. Zamora, I., Afzelius, L., and Cruciani, G. (2003) Predicting drug metabolism: a site of metabolism prediction tool applied to the cytochrome P450 2C9. *J. Med. Chem.* **46**, 2313–2324.

234. Snyder, R., Sangar, R., Wang, J. B., and Ekins, S. (2002) Three-dimensional quantitative structure activity relationship for CYP2D6 substrates. *Quant. Struct.-Act. Relat.* **21**, 357–368.

235. Lewis, D. F., Sams, C., and Loizou, G. D. (2003) A quantitative structure-activity relationship analysis on a series of alkyl benzenes metabolized by human cytochrome P450 2E1. *J. Biochem. Mol. Toxicol.* **17**, 47–52.

236. Lewis, D. F., Ioannides, C., and Parke, D. V. (1994) Interaction of a series of nitriles with the alcohol-inducible isoform of P450: computer analysis of structure-activity relationships. *Xenobiotica* **24**, 401–408.

237. Waller, C. L., Evans, M. V., and McKinney, J. D. (1996) Modeling the cytochrome P450-mediated metabolism of chlorinated volatile organic compounds. *Drug Metab. Dispos.* **24**, 203–210.

238. Kellogg, G. E., Semus, S. F., and Abraham, D. J. (1991) HINT: a new method of empirical hydrophobic field calculation for CoMFA. *J. Comput. Aid. Molec. Design* **5**, 545–552.

239. Lewis, D. F. and Lake, B. G. (1998) Molecular modelling and quantitative structure-activity relationship studies on the interaction of omeprazole with cytochrome P450 isozymes. *Toxicology* **125**, 31–44.

240. Ekins, S., De Groot, M. J., and Jones, J. P. (2001) Pharmacophore and three-dimensional quantitative structure. *Drug Metab. Dispos.* **29**, 936–944.

241. Lewis, D. F., Ioannides, C., Parke, D. V., and Schulte-Hermann, R. (2000) Quantitative structure-activity relationships in a series of endogenous and synthetic

steroids exhibiting induction of CYP3A activity and hepatomegaly associated with increased DNA synthesis. *J. Steroid Biochem. Mol. Biol.* **74,** 179–185.

242. Pichard, L., Domergue, J., Fourtanier, G., Koch, P., Schran, H. F., and Maurel, P. (1996) Metabolism of the new immunosuppressor cyclosporin G by human liver cytochromes P450. *Biochem. Pharmacol.* **51,** 591–598.

243. Zhao, X. J. and Ishizaki, T. (1997) Metabolic interactions of selected antimalarial and non-antimalarial drugs with the major pathway (3-hydroxylation) of quinine in human liver microsomes. *Br. J. Clin. Pharmacol.* **44,** 505–511.

244. Molnar, L. and Keseru, G. M. (2002) A neural network based virtual screening of cytochrome P450 3A4 inhibitors. *Bioorg. Med. Chem. Lett.* **12,** 419–421.

245. Zuegge, J., Fechner, U., Roche, O., Parrot, N. J., Engkvist, O., and Schneider, G. (2002) A fast virtual screening filter for cytochrome P 450 3A4 inhibition liability of compound libraries. *Quant. Struct.-Act. Relat.* **21,** 249–256.

246. Lewis, D. F. V., Ogg, M. S., Goldfarb, P. S., and Gibson, G. G. (2002) Molecular modelling of the human glucocorticoid receptor (hGR) ligand-binding domain (LBD) by homology with the human estrogen receptor a (hERa) LBD: Quantitative structure-activity relationships within a series of CYP3A4 inducers where induction is mediated via hGR involvement. *J. Steroid Biochem. Mol. Biol.* **82,** 195–199.

247. Wang, K., Budzinski, J. W., Foster, B. C., Durst, T., Arnason, J. T., and Compadre, C. M. (2001) Molecular modeling and 3D- QSAR analysis of the inhibition of cytochrome P450 3A4 (CYP3A4) by dillapiol and its derivatives. *Abstr. Pap. Am. Chem. Soc.* **269,** 0065–7727.

248. Ji, H., Zhang, W., Zhang, M., et al. (2003) Structure-based de novo design, synthesis, and biological evaluation of non-azole inhibitors specific for lanosterol 14alpha-demethylase of fungi. *J. Med. Chem.* **46,** 474–485.

249. Talele, T. T. and Kulkarni, V. M. (1999) Three-dimensional quantitative structure-activity relationship (QSAR) and receptor mapping of cytochrome P-450(14 alpha DM) inhibiting azole antifungal agents. *J. Chem. Inf. Comput. Sci.* **39,** 204–210.

250. Lewis, D. F., Wiseman, A., and Tarbit, M. H. (1999) Molecular modelling of lanosterol 14 alpha-demethylase (CYP51) from *Saccharomyces cerevisiae* via homology with CYP102, a unique bacterial cytochrome P450 isoform: quantitative structure-activity relationships (QSARs) within two related series of antifungal azole derivatives. *J. Enz. Inhib.* **14,** 175–192.

251. Baston, E., Klein, C. D., Grimminger, W., Hebecker, N., and Hartmann, R. W. (2001) Synthesis, evaluation and QSAR studies of highly potent aromatase inhibitors of the piperidinedione type. *Anticancer Drug Des.* **16,** 37–47.

252. Oprea, T. I. and Garcia, A. E. (1996) Three-dimensional quantitative structure-activity relationships of steroid aromatase inhibitors. *J. Comput. Aid. Molec. Design* **10,** 186–200.

253. Recanatini, M. and Cavalli, A. (1998) Comparative molecular field analysis of non-steroidal aromatase inhibitors: an extended model for two different structural classes. *Bioorg. Med. Chem.* **6,** 377–388.

254. Gironés, X. and Carbo-Dorca, R. (2002) Molecular quantum similarity-based QSARs for binding affinities of several steroid sets. *J. Chem. Inf. Comput. Sci.* **42**, 1185–1193.

255. Recanatini, M., Bisi, A., Cavalli, A., et al. (2001) A new class of nonsteroidal aromatase inhibitors: design and synthesis of chromone and xanthone derivatives and inhibition of the P450 enzymes aromatase and 17 alpha-hydroxylase/C17,20-lyase. *J. Med. Chem.* **44**, 672–680.

256. You, L., Sar, M., Bartolucci, E., Ploch, S., and Whitt, M. (2001) Induction of hepatic aromatase by p,p'-DDE in adult male rats. *Mol. Cell. Endocrinol.* **178**, 207–214.

257. Basak, S. C. (1988) Binding of Barbiturates to Cytochrome P450: A QSAR study using log P and topological indices. *Med. Sci. Res.* **16**, 281–282.

258. Murray, M., Marcus, C. B., and Wilkinson, C. F. (1985) Quantitative structure-acvitity relationships in the displacement of the dihydrosafrole metabolite-cytochrome P-450 complex. *Quant. Struct.-Act. Relat.* **4**, 18–22.

259. Gao, H. and Hansch, C. (1996) QSAR of P450 oxidation: on the value of comparing kcat and km with kcat/km. *Drug Metab. Rev.* **28**, 513–526.

260. Tyrakowska, B., Cnubben, N. H., Soffers, A. E., Wobbes, T., and Rietjens, I. M. (1996) Comparative MO-QSAR studies in various species including man. *Chem.-Biol. Interact.* **100**, 187–201.

261. Bird, M. G., Lewis, D. F., Whitman, F. T., Lewis, R. J., Przygoda, R. T., and Witz, G. (2001) Application of process chemistry and SAR modelling to the evaluation of health findings of lower olefins. *Chem. Biol. Interact.* **135–136**, 571–584.

262. Lewis, D. F. (2000) Structural characteristics of human P450s involved in drug metabolism: QSARs and lipophilicity profiles. *Toxicology* **144**, 197–203.

263. Lewis, D. F. (2002) Molecular modeling of human cytochrome P450-substrate interactions. *Drug Metab. Rev.* **34**, 55–67.

264. Lewis, D. F. and Dickins, M. (2002) Factors influencing rates and clearance in P450-mediated reactions: QSARs for substrates of the xenobiotic-metabolizing hepatic microsomal P450s. *Toxicology* **170**, 45–53.

265. Lewis, D. F., Modi, S., and Dickins, M. (2001) Quantitative structure-activity relationships (QSARs) within substrates of human cytochromes P450 involved in drug metabolism. *Drug Metab. Drug Interact.* **18**, 221–242.

266. Ekins, S., Waller, C. L., Swaan, P. W., Cruciani, G., Wrighton, S. A., and Wikel, J. H. (2000) Progress in predicting human ADME parameters in silico. *J. Pharm. Tox. Methods* **44**, 251–271.

267. (2003) Genomatica http://www.genomatica.com/.

268. Incyte. (2003) DrugMatrix: http://www.incyte.com/control/researchproducts/insilico/drugmatrix.

269. (2003) GastroPlus Simmulation Plus Inc. http://www.simulations-plus.com/products/module_metabolism.html.

270. (2003) Oxford BioMedica plc. http://www.oxfordbiomedica.co.uk.

271. van de Waterbeemd, H. and Gifford, E. (2003) ADMET in silico modelling: towards prediction paradise? *Nature* **2**, 192–204.

272. Erhardt, P. W. (1999) *Drug metabolism: databases and high throughput testing during drug design and development.* Blackwell Science Inc., Oxford, UK.

273. van de Waterbeemd, H. and De Groot, M. (2002) Can the internet help to meet the challenges in ADME and e-ADME? *SAR QSAR Environ. Res.* **13,** 391–401.

274. ArQule. (2003) http://www.arqule.com/insilico/admet1.html.

275. Cerep. (2003) http://www.cerep.fr/Cerep/Utilisateur/index.asp.

276. Cyprotex. (2003) Cloe Screen™ www.Cyprotex.com.

277. Lewis, D. F., Ioannides, C., and Parke, D. V. (1998) An improved and updated version of the compact procedure for the evaluation of P450-mediated activation. *Drug Metab. Rev.* **30,** 709–737.

278. Lewis, D. F., Ioannides, C., and Parke, D. V. (1998) Further evaluation of COMPACT, the molecular orbital approach for the prospective safety evaluation of chemicals. *Mutat. Res.* **412,** 41–54.

279. Lewis, D. F., Iannides, C., and Parke, D. V. (1995) A retrospective evaluation of COMPACT predictions of the outcome of NTP rodent carcinogenicity testing. *Environ. Health Perspect.* **103,** 176–184.

280. Archakov, A. (2003) http://cpd.ibmh.msk.su.

281. Archakov, A. I. and Bachmanova, G. I. (1995) Cytochrome P450 database for prediction of drugs' fate in living systems. *In Vitro Toxicology* **8,** 49–54.

282. Archakov, A. I. and Bachmanova, G. I. (1995) The usage of cytochrome P450 database (CPD) for prediction of the drugs' fate in living systems. *Alt. Meth. Tox. Life Sci.* **11,** 205–212.

283. Archakov, A., et al. (2001) Inventory of the cytochrome P450 superfamily. *J. Mol. Model.* **7,** 140–142.

284. Washington, U. O. (2003) Drug Interaction Database: http://depts.washington.edu/didbase/index.shtml.

285. GenTest. (2003) GenTest: http://www.gentest.com/human_p450_database/index.html.

286. Erhardt, P. W., IUPAC. (2003) Human Drug Metabolism Database: http://www.iupac.org/projects/2000/2000-010-1-700.html.

287. Highuch, T. V. S. (1975) *Pro-drugs as novel drug delivery systems.* American Chemical Society, Washington, D.C.

288. Smith, J. N. (1968) The comparative metabolism of xenobiotics. *Adv. Comp. Physiol. Biochem.* **3,** 173–232.

289. LionBioscience. (2003) iDEA™: http://www.lionbioscience.com/solutions/products/idea/modules.

290. Science, P. (2003) Porus Science, Integrity database: http://www.prous.com.

291. Multicase. (2003) http://www.multicase.com/products/prod05.htm.

292. Klopman, G., Dimayuga, M., and Talafous, J. (1994) A program for the evaluation of metabolic transformation of chemicals. *J. Chem. Inf. Comput. Sci.* **34,** 1320–1325.

293. Talafous, J., Sayre, L. M., Mieyal, J. J., and Klopman, G. (1994) META 2. A dictionary model of mammalian xenobiotic metabolism. *J. Chem. Inf. Comput. Sci.* **34,** 1326–1333.

294. Klopman, G., Tu, M. H., and Talafous, J. (1997) META 3. A genetic algorithm for metabolic transform priorities optimization. *J. Chem. Inf. Comput. Sci.* **37,** 329–334.
295. Klopman, G., Tu, M. H., and Fan, B. T. (1999) META 4. Prediction of the metabolism of polycyclic aromatic hydrocarbons. *Theor. Chem. Acc.* **102,** 33–38.
296. Klopman, G. and Tu, M. (1999) META. *A program for the prediction of the products of mammal metabolism of xenobiotics.* Blackwell Science, Oxford, UK.
297. MetaCyc. (2003) http://biocyc.org/metacyc.
298. EcoCyc. (2003) http://biocyc.org/ecocyc.
299. Snyder, R., et al. (1999) *Metabolite.* Blackwell Science, Oxford, UK.
300. SciVision/MDL. (2003) SciVision, Metabolite: http://www.scivision.com/products/products.html.
301. MDL Headquarters, M. I. S., Inc., 14600 Catalina Street, San Leandro, CA 94577, USA. (2003) http://mdl.com/products/products.html.
302. Darvas, F. (1988) Predicting metabolic pathways by logic programming. *J. Mol. Graph.* **6,** 80–86.
303. Compudrug. (2003) http://www.compudrug.com.
304. Darvas, F. (1987) *QSAR in environmental toxicology*, Kaiser, K. (ed.), pp. 71–81.
305. Testa, B. and Jenner, P. (1976) *Drug metabolism: chemical and biochemical aspects.* New York.
306. Pfeifer, S. and Borchert, H. (1963) *Biotransformation von Arzneimitteln.* Berlin.
307. Darvas, F., et al. (1999) *Drug Metabolism*, Erhardt, P. W. (ed.), Blackwell Science, Oxford, UK, pp. 237–270.
308. Hawkins, D. (1989) A survey of the biotransformation of drugs and chemicals. *R. Soc. Chem.* 1–8.
309. Hayward, J. (1999) *Synopsis.* Blackwell Science, Oxford, UK.
310. METEOR. (2003) http://www.chem.leeds.ac.uk/luk/meteor/index.html. http://www.chem.leeds.ac.uk/.
311. Greene, N. (1999) In *Drug metabolism*, Erhardt, P. W. (ed.), Blackwell Science, Oxford, UK, pp. 289–296.
312. Greene, N., Judson, P., Langowski, J., and Marchant, C. A. (1999) Knowledge-based expert systems for toxicity and metabolism prediction: DEREK, StAR, and METEOR. *SAR QSAR Environ. Res.* **10,** 299–313.
313. Langowski, J. and Long, A. (2002) Computer systems for the prediction of xenobiotic metabolism. *Adv. Drug. Deliv. Rev.* **54,** 407–415.
314. Tonnelier, C. A. G., Fox, J., Judson, P. N., Krause, P. J., Pappas, N., and Patel, M. (1997) Representation of chemical structures in knowledge-based systems: the StAR system. *J. Chem. Inf. Comput. Sci.* **37,** 117–123.
315. Judson, P. N., Fox, J., and Krause, P. J. (1996) Using new reasoning technology in chemical information systems. *J. Chem. Inf. Comput. Sci.* **36,** 621–624.
316. NOVASCREEN. (2003) www.NOVASCREEN.com.
317. Fabian, P. and Degtyarenko, K. N. (1997) The directory of P450-containing systems in 1996. *Nucleic Acids Res.* **25,** 274–277.
318. David, R. N. s. W. (2003) David, R. Nelson's webpage: http://drnelson.utmem.edu/CytochromeP450.html.

319. Flockart, D. (2003) The International Scociety of Xenobiotics: http://issx.org/p450pg.htm, http://medicine.iupui.edu/flockhart.

320. PanVera. (2003) PanVera Corps.: http://www.PanVera.com.

321. SRI. (2003) SRI International: http://www.sri.com.

322. XenoTech. (2003) XenoTech, LLC: http://www.xenotechllc.com/.

323. (2003) Human Biologics International: http://www.humanbiologics.com.

324. (2003) MDS Panlabs Inc.: http://www.mdsps.com.

325. (2003) CytoChroma, Inc.: http://www.cytochroma.com.

326. (2003) Metabolic Solutions, Inc.: http://www.metsol.com.

327. Harris, R. Z., Tsunoda, S. M., Mroczkowski, P., Wong, H., and Benet, L. Z. (1996) The effects of menopause and hormone replacement therapies on prednisolone and erythromycin pharmacokinetics. *Clin. Pharmacol. Ther.* **59,** 429–435.

328. Tateishi, T., Graham, S. G., Krivoruk, Y., and Wood, A. J. J. (1995) Omeprazole does not affect measured CYP3A4 activity using the erythromycin breath test. *Br. J. Clin. Pharmacol.* **40,** 411–412.

329. (2003) TNO Pharma: http://www.pharma.tno.nl.

330. (2003) Ricerca, LLC: http://www.ricerca.com/.

331. Nelson, D. R. (2002) Mining databases for cytochrome P450 genes. *Methods Enzymol.* **357,** 3–15.

332. (2003) Affymetrix, Inc.: http://www.affymetrix.com/index.affx.

333. (2003) Pharmagene, plc.: http://www.pharmagene.com.

334. Lewis, D. F. V. (2000) On the recognition of mammalian microsomal cytochrome P450 substrates and their characteristics: Towards the prediction of human p450 substrate specificity and metabolism. *Biochem. Pharmacol.* **60,** 293–306.

335. Lewis, D. F. and Dickins, M. (2002) Substrate SARs in human P450s. *Drug Discov. Today* **7,** 918–925.

336. Keseru, G. and Molnar, L. (2002) METAPRINT: a metabolic fingerprint. Application to cassette design for high-throughput ADME screening. *J. Chem. Inf. Comput. Sci.* 437–444.

337. Gasteiger, J. (2003) In "225th ACS National Meeting."

338. Amic, D., Lucic, B., Nikolic, S., and Trinajstic, N. (2001) Predicting inhibition of microsomal p-hydroxylation of aniline by aliphatic alcohols: a QSAR approach based on the weighted path numbers. *Croat. Chem. Acta* **74,** 237–250.

339. Halpert, J. R. (1995) Structural basis of selective cytochrome P450 inhibition. *Annu. Rev. Pharmacol. Toxicol.* **35,** 29–53.

340. Lipinski, C. A. (2000) Drug-like properties and the causes of poor solubility and poor permeability. *J. Pharm. Tox. Methods* **44,** 235–249.

341. Oprea, T. I. (2002) Virtual screening in lead discovery: a viewpoint. *Molecules* **7,** 51–62.

342. Ansell, J. (2003) Quantifying new product need: productivity target considered at company level. *Pharmaceutical Industry Dynamics*, 1–15.

Index

A

Absorption, distribution,
    metabolism, excretion
    (ADME), 216, 394–396, 489
    databases and software systems,
        489–495
Atomic properties
    binary, 264–265
    general, 265–267

B

Bioisosterism, 428
Biological promiscuity, 116–117

C

Chemical graphs, 6–10
    hydrogen-suppressed, 7–8
    maximum common substructure,
        7–9
Chemical space representations, 35–
    40
    binning, 282
    dimensionality, 36–37
    dimension reduction, 37–40,
        281–282
Chemometrics, 171–172
Chirality, 144, 428–429
Chromosomes, 287
Classical sets, 4, 43–44
Clustering, 279–280, 303–304
Compound classification, 285–287,
    296, 311–312

Cytochrome P450 isozymes, 450–451
    docking models, 459–463
    homology models, 450–459
    pharmacophore models, 463–473
    quantitative structure-activity
        relationship models, 473–488

D

Database access, 67–72
Data shaving, 94–97
Descriptors
    3D-log$P$, 219–223, 256
    3D pharmacophore, 358–360
    BCUTs, 18–19, 282–283, 365–367
        receptor relevance, 367–368
    constitutional, 302, 327
    correlation, 267–268, 295
    descriptor medians, 293
    electron density derived, 401,
        411–412
    encoding, 268–271
    general, 302–303, 339–341
    grid cell occupancy, 164
    VSA, 265–267
Distance metrics (*see* Feature
    vectors)
Diversity (*see also* Molecular
    similarity), 51, 58
    design, 308–310
    selection, 295–296
Docking, 370–371, 439, 459–463
Drug-like features, 340–341, 355, 450